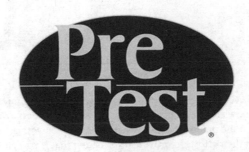

Emergency Medicine

PreTest® Self-Assessment and Review

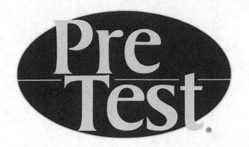

Emergency Medicine

PreTest® Self-Assessment and Review

Fifth Edition

Adam J. Rosh, MD, MS, FACEP
Attending Physician
Department of Emergency Medicine
Southern Ohio Medical Center
Portsmouth, Ohio

Ciara J. Barclay-Buchanan, MD, FACEP
Associate Vice Chair of Operations
Associate Professor (CHS)
BerbeeWalsh Department of Emergency Medicine
University of Wisconsin School of Medicine and Public Health
Madison, Wisconsin

New York   Chicago   San Francisco   Athens   London   Madrid   Mexico City
Milan   New Delhi   Singapore   Sydney   Toronto

1 2 3 4 5 6 7 8 9 LCR 26 25 24 23 22 21

ISBN 978-1-260-46894-6
MHID 1-260-46894-1

This book was set in Minion Pro by KnowledgeWorks Global Ltd.
The editors were Bob Boehringer and Peter J. Boyle.
The production supervisor was Richard Ruzycka.
Project management was provided by Garima Poddar, KnowledgeWorks Global Ltd.

This book is printed on acid-free paper.

Cataloging-in-publication data for this book is on file at the Library of Congress.

McGraw Hill Education books are available at special quantity discounts to use as premiums and sales promotions or for use in corporate training programs. To contact a representative, please visit the Contact Us pages at www.mhprofessional.com.

Contributors

Nicole A. Bonk, MD
Assistant Professor (CHS)
Department of Family Medicine and
 Community Health
University of Wisconsin School of Medicine
 and Public Health
Madison, Wisconsin
Gastrointestinal Bleeding

Shannon M. Burke, MD
Resident, Class of 2021
BerbeeWalsh Department of Emergency
 Medicine
University of Wisconsin School of Medicine
 and Public Health
Madison, Wisconsin
Fever

Lauren J. Curato, DO, FACEP
Assistant Professor
Department of Emergency Medicine
Columbia University Vagelos College of
 Physicians and Surgeons
New York-Presbyterian Hospital
New York, New York
Chest Pain and Cardiac Dysrhythmias

Bram A. Dolcourt, MD
Associate Residency Program Director
Sinai-Grace Hospital, Detroit Medical
 Center
Assistant Professor
Department of Emergency Medicine
Medical Toxicology
Wayne State University
Detroit, Michigan
Poisoning and Overdose

Joshua Gauger, MD, MBA
Assistant Medical Director
Assistant Professor (CHS)
BerbeeWalsh Department of Emergency
 Medicine
University of Wisconsin School of Medicine
 and Public Health
Madison, Wisconsin
Trauma, Shock, and Resuscitation

Jonah Gunalda, MD
Assistant Professor
Clerkship Director
Department of Emergency Medicine
University of Mississippi Medical Center
Jackson, Mississippi
Abdominal and Pelvic Pain
Altered Mental Status
Headache, Weakness, and Dizziness
Professionalism, Ethics, and Communication

Megan E. Gussick, MD
Assistant Professor
Assistant Medical Director, Division of
 Prehospital Medicine
BerbeeWalsh Department of Emergency
 Medicine
University of Wisconsin School of Medicine
 and Public Health
Madison, Wisconsin
Wound Care

Corlin Jewell, MD
Education Fellow
BerbeeWalsh Department of Emergency
  Medicine
University of Wisconsin School of Medicine
  and Public Health
Madison, Wisconsin
Environmental Exposures

Aaron Kraut, MD
Residency Program Director
Assistant Professor (CHS)
BerbeeWalsh Department of Emergency
  Medicine
University of Wisconsin School of Medicine
  and Public Health
Madison, Wisconsin
Fever

Nicholas A. Kuehnel, MD
Medical Director, Pediatric Emergency
  Medicine
Assistant Professor (CHS)
BerbeeWalsh Department of Emergency
  Medicine
University of Wisconsin School of Medicine
  and Public Health
Madison, Wisconsin
Pediatrics

Michael Mancera, MD, FAEMS
Associate EMS Medical Director
Assistant Professor (CHS)
BerbeeWalsh Department of Emergency
  Medicine
University of Wisconsin School of Medicine
  and Public Health
Madison, Wisconsin
Prehospital, Disaster, and Administration

Benjamin R. Parva, MD
Resident, Class of 2022
Department of Emergency Medicine
University of Mississippi Medical Center
Jackson, Mississippi
Altered Mental Status

Kaitlin Ray, MD
Assistant Residency Program Director
Assistant Professor (CHS)
BerbeeWalsh Department of Emergency
  Medicine
University of Wisconsin School of Medicine
  and Public Health
Madison, Wisconsin
Musculoskeletal Injuries

Dana Resop, MD
Assistant Director of Clinical Ultrasound
Assistant Professor
BerbeeWalsh Department of Emergency
  Medicine
University of Wisconsin School of Medicine
  and Public Health
Madison, Wisconsin
Vaginal Bleeding
Ultrasound in Emergency Medicine

Adam J. Rosh, MD, MS, FACEP
Attending Physician
Department of Emergency Medicine
Southern Ohio Medical Center
Portsmouth, Ohio

Daniel Rutz, MD
Assistant Professor (CHS)
BerbeeWalsh Department of Emergency
  Medicine
University of Wisconsin School of Medicine
  and Public Health
Madison, Wisconsin
Eye Pain and Visual Change
Endocrine Emergencies
Psychosocial Disorders
Emerging Infectious Diseases

Jessica Schmidt, MD, MPH
Assistant Ultrasound Director,
  Medical Student Education
Director of Global Health
Assistant Professor (CHS)
BerbeeWalsh Department of Emergency
  Medicine
University of Wisconsin School of Medicine
  and Public Health
Madison, Wisconsin
Ultrasound in Emergency Medicine

Lauren M. Titone, MD
Assistant Professor
Department of Emergency Medicine
Columbia University Irving Medical Center
Vagelos College of Physicians and Surgeons
New York, New York
Shortness of Breath

Contents

Gastrointestinal Bleeding

Musculoskeletal Injuries

Headache, Weakness, and Dizziness

Pediatrics

Vaginal Bleeding

Ultrasound in Emergency Medicine

Environmental Exposures

Eye Pain and Visual Change

Introduction

Emergency Medicine: PreTest® Self-Assessment and Review, Fifth Edition, is intended to provide medical students, as well as house officers and physicians, with a convenient tool for assessing and improving their knowledge of emergency medicine. The 570 questions in this book are similar in format and complexity to those included in step 2 of the United States Medical Licensing Examination (USMLE). They may also be a useful study tool for step 3, the National Board of Medical Examiners (NBME) Emergency Medicine and other clerkship examinations.

Each question in this book has a corresponding answer and a short discussion of various issues raised by the question and its answer. For multiple-choice questions, the **one best** response to each question should be selected. A listing of subject-based recommended readings follows each chapter.

To simulate the time constraints imposed by the qualifying examinations for which this book is intended as a practice guide, the student or physician should allot approximately 1 minute for each question. After answering all questions in a chapter, as much time as necessary should be spent reviewing the explanations for each question at the end of the chapter. Attention should be given to all explanations, even if the examinee answered the question correctly. Those seeking more information on a subject should refer to the recommended reading lists or to other standard texts in emergency medicine.

Acknowledgments

A hearty thanks goes out to my family for their love and support, Danielle, Ruby, Rhys, and especially my parents, Karl and Marcia; the dedicated medical professionals of the emergency departments at New York University/ Bellevue Hospital, and Wayne State University/Detroit Receiving Hospital; Catherine Johnson for giving me this opportunity, and my patients, who put their trust in me, and teach me something new each day.

Adam J. Rosh

I am forever grateful for the incredible women who shaped my path in academic medicine: Drs. Gloria Kuhn, Melissa Barton, Michelle Lall, and Azita Hamedani; the many talented emergency medicine residents and medical students of both Wayne State University/Sinai-Grace Hospital and University of Wisconsin for allowing me to be a part of your education; Adam Rosh and McGraw Hill for this amazing opportunity; and most of all, my family for loving and supporting me along the way: especially my husband, Steve, our boys CJ and Owen, my mom, and my dad.

Ciara J. Barclay-Buchanan

Chest Pain and Cardiac Dysrhythmias

Lauren J. Curato, DO, FACEP

Questions

The following scenario applies to questions 1-3.

A 38-year-old woman presents to the emergency department (ED) with chest pain and mild shortness of breath that began the night before. She was able to sleep without difficulty, but awoke in the morning with persistent pain that worsens with a deep breath. Upon walking up a flight of stairs, she became very short of breath, prompting her ED visit. On physical exam, she was noted to be tachycardic and have left calf pain. She has no past medical history (PMH), but has smoked half pack per day for 15 years and is on an oral contraceptive.

1. What is the most common electrocardiogram (ECG) finding for this patient's diagnosis?
a. $S_1Q_3T_3$ pattern
b. Atrial fibrillation (AF)
c. Right-axis deviation
d. Right bundle-branch block (RBBB)
e. Sinus tachycardia

2. Which of the following tests is best to confirm the suspected diagnosis?
a. Brain natriuretic peptide (BNP)
b. Cardiac troponin
c. Chest X-ray (CXR)
d. Computed tomography angiography (CTA) chest
e. D-dimer

3. Which of the following is an indication for the administration of thrombolytics for this diagnosis?

a. Bilateral proximal clot
b. Hypotension
c. Persistent tachycardia
d. Right atrial dilation
e. Elevated BNP

4. A 70-year-old man with a long history of hypertension presents to the ED complaining of intermittent palpitations for 1 week. He denies chest pain, shortness of breath, nausea, and vomiting. He recalls feeling similar episodes of palpitations a few months ago but they resolved spontaneously. His blood pressure (BP) is 130/75 mm Hg, heart rate (HR) is 140 beats/minute, respiratory rate (RR) is 16 breaths/minute, and oxygen saturation is 99% on room air. An ECG is seen in the figure. Which of the following is the most appropriate next step in management?

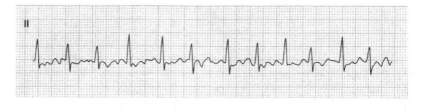

a. Sedate the patient for immediate synchronized cardioversion with 100 J
b. Prepare patient for emergent cardiac catheterization
c. Administer oral warfarin
d. Administer intravenous (IV) amiodarone
e. Administer IV diltiazem

The following scenario applies to questions 5 and 6.

A 54-year-old woman presents to the ED because of increased weakness. Her daughter states the patient has been increasingly tired, occasionally confused, and has not been eating her usual diet for the past 3 days. The patient has a history of end-stage renal disease (ESRD) requiring dialysis for the past 5 years. On examination, the patient is alert and oriented to person only. The remainder of her examination is normal. An initial 12-lead ECG is performed as seen in the figure.

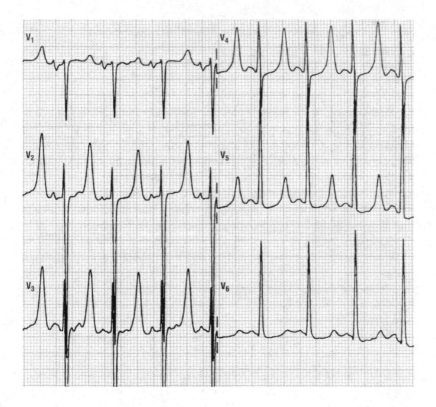

5. Which of the following electrolyte abnormalities best explains these findings?

a. Hypokalemia
b. Hyperkalemia
c. Hypocalcemia
d. Hypercalcemia
e. Hyponatremia

6. Which of the following medications is most important to administer first?

a. Albuterol
b. Calcium gluconate
c. Dextrose
d. Insulin
e. Kayexalate

7. A 29-year-old tall, thin man presents to the ED for shortness of breath for 2 days. In the ED, he is in no acute distress. His BP is 115/70 mm Hg, HR is 81 beats/minute, RR is 16 breaths/minute, and oxygen saturation is 98% on room air. Cardiac, lung, and abdominal examinations are normal. An ECG reveals sinus rhythm at a rate of 79 beats/minute. A chest radiograph shows a small right-sided (<10% of the hemithorax) pneumothorax. A repeat CXR 6 hours later reveals a decreased pneumothorax. Which of the following is the most appropriate next step in management?

a. Discharge the patient with follow-up in 24 hours
b. Perform needle decompression in the second intercostal space, midclavicular line
c. Insert a 20 F chest tube into right hemithorax
d. Observe for another 6 hours
e. Admit for pleurodesis

8. A 42-year-old man is brought to the ED by emergency medical services (EMS). He has a history of alcohol use with multiple presentations for intoxication. Today, the patient complains of acute onset, persistent chest pain associated with dysphagia, and pain upon flexing his neck. His BP is 115/70 mm Hg, HR is 101 beats/minute, RR is 18 breaths/minute, and oxygen saturation is 97% on room air. As you listen to his heart, you hear a crunching sound. His abdomen is soft with mild epigastric tenderness. The ECG is sinus tachycardia without ST-T–wave abnormalities. On chest radiograph, you note lateral displacement of the left mediastinal pleura. What is the most likely diagnosis?

a. Aspiration pneumonia
b. Acute pancreatitis
c. Pericarditis
d. Esophageal perforation
e. Aortic dissection

9. A 65-year-old man with a history of hypertension presents to the ED with sudden-onset tearing chest pain that radiates to his jaw. His BP is 205/110 mm Hg, HR is 90 beats/minute, RR is 20 breaths/minute, and oxygen saturation is 97% on room air. He appears apprehensive. On cardiac examination, you hear a diastolic murmur at the right sternal border. A CXR reveals a widened mediastinum. You call for a stat bedside transesophageal echocardiogram (TEE) which confirms your suspected diagnosis. Which of the following medications should be administered first in the treatment of this patient?

a. Amiodarone
b. Esmolol
c. Nicardipine
d. Nifedipine
e. Nitroprusside

10. A 32-year-old woman presents to the ED with a fever of 101°F over the last 3 days associated with generalized fatigue, myalgias, and mild shortness of breath that worsens with exertion. On cardiac exam, you detect a murmur. Her abdomen is soft and nontender with an enlarged spleen. Skin examination demonstrates track marks to the antecubital fossa. Chest radiograph reveals multiple patchy infiltrates in both lung fields. Laboratory results reveal white blood cells (WBCs) 14,000/μL with 91% neutrophils, hematocrit 33%, and platelets 250/μL. An ECG reveals sinus rhythm with first-degree heart block. Which of the following is the most appropriate next step in management?

a. Diagnose community-acquired pneumonia and discharge with oral antibiotics and outpatient follow-up
b. Order liver function tests and a Monospot and advise her to refrain from vigorous activities until cleared
c. Treat with IV antibiotics and admit to the hospital for community-acquired pneumonia
d. Obtain four sets of blood cultures, order an echocardiogram, start IV antibiotics, and admit to the hospital for suspected endocarditis
e. Place the patient on isolation and order three sets of sputum cultures for AFB, consult infectious disease, and admit to the hospital for suspected tuberculosis

The following scenario applies to questions 11-13.

A 61-year-old woman was walking to the grocery store when she started feeling chest pressure in the center of her chest. She became diaphoretic and felt short of breath. On arrival to the ED by EMS, her BP is 130/70 mm Hg, HR is 76 beats/minute, and oxygen saturation is 98% on room air. An ECG is performed as seen in the figure.

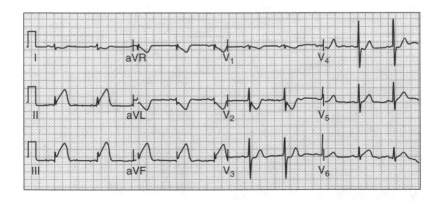

11. Which of the following best describes the location of this patient's myocardial infarction (MI)?

a. Anteroseptal
b. Anterior
c. Lateral
d. Inferior
e. Posterior

12. Which of the following therapeutic agents has been shown to independently reduce mortality in the setting of acute MI?

a. Nitroglycerin
b. Aspirin
c. Unfractionated heparin
d. Lidocaine
e. Diltiazem

13. This patient's ECG demonstrates an ST-segment elevation myocardial infarction (STEMI). You activate the STEMI team in anticipation of the patient going to the cardiac catheterization laboratory for percutaneous coronary intervention (PCI). Which of the following time intervals is gold standard for "door to balloon" time in acute STEMI?

a. 45 minutes
b. 60 minutes
c. 75 minutes
d. 90 minutes
e. 120 minutes

14. A 21-year-old woman presents to the ED complaining of light-headedness. Her symptoms appeared 45 minutes ago. She has no other symptoms and is not on any medications. She has a medical history of mitral valve prolapse. Her BP is 105/55 mm Hg and HR is 170 beats/minute. Physical examination is unremarkable. After administering the appropriate medication, her HR slows down and her symptoms resolve. You repeat a 12-lead ECG that shows a rate of 89 beats/minute with a regular rhythm. The PR interval measures 100 milliseconds and there is a slurred upstroke of the QRS complex. Based on this information, which of the following is the most likely diagnosis?

a. Ventricular tachycardia
b. Atrial flutter with 3:1 block
c. AF
d. Lown-Ganong-Levine (LGL) syndrome
e. Wolff-Parkinson-White (WPW) syndrome

15. A 65-year-old man presents complaining of chest pain. He was out to a restaurant having a steak and drinking wine when he suddenly felt a piece of steak "get stuck" in his chest. He coughed and then vomited, but it did not resolve the sensation. He attempted to drink water, but spit it back up. In the ED, he complains of dysphagia and is occasionally retching. On examination, his BP is 130/80 mm Hg, HR is 75 beats/minute, RR is 16 breaths/minute, and oxygen saturation is 99% on room air. He appears in no respiratory distress. CXR is negative for air under the diaphragm. Which of the following is the most appropriate next step in management?

a. Administer 1 mg glucagon intravenously while arranging for endoscopy
b. Administer a meat tenderizer, such as papain, to soften the food bolus
c. Administer 10 mL syrup of ipecac to induce vomiting and dislodge the food bolus
d. Perform the Heimlich maneuver until the food dislodges
e. Call surgery consult to prepare for laparotomy

16. A 59-year-old man presents to the ED with left-sided chest pain and shortness of breath that began 2 hours prior to arrival. He states the pain is pressure-like and radiates down his left arm. He is diaphoretic. His BP is 160/80 mm Hg, HR is 86 beats/minute, and RR is 15 breaths/minute. ECG reveals 2-mm ST-segment elevation in leads I, aVL, and V_3 to V_6. Which of the following is an *absolute* contraindication to receiving thrombolytic therapy?

a. Systolic blood pressure (SBP) greater than 180 mm Hg
b. Patient takes aspirin daily
c. Total hip replacement 3 months ago
d. Peptic ulcer disease
e. Previous hemorrhagic stroke

17. A 67-year-old woman is brought to the ED by paramedics complaining of dyspnea, fatigue, and palpitations. Her BP is 80/50 mm Hg, HR is 139 beats/minute, and RR is 20 breaths/minute. Her skin is cool and she is diaphoretic. Her lung examination reveals bilateral crackles and she is beginning to have chest pain. Her ECG shows a narrow complex irregular rhythm with a rate in the 140's. Which of the following is the most appropriate immediate treatment for this patient?

a. Diltiazem
b. Metoprolol
c. Digoxin
d. Coumadin
e. Synchronized cardioversion

The following scenario applies to questions 18 and 19.

A 61-year-old woman with a history of congestive heart failure (CHF) is at a family picnic when she starts complaining of shortness of breath. Her daughter brings her to the ED where she is found to have mild tachypnea, an oxygen saturation of 85% on room air, and rales halfway up both of her lung fields. Her BP is 185/90 mm Hg and pulse rate is 101 beats/minute. On examination, her jugular venous pressure (JVP) is 6 cm above the sternal angle. There is lower extremity pitting edema.

18. Which of the following is the most appropriate first-line medication to lower cardiac preload?

a. Metoprolol
b. Morphine sulfate
c. Nitroprusside
d. Nitroglycerin
e. Oxygen

19. You have successfully lowered this patient's preload; however, her respiratory status worsens. She develops increased work of breathing, accessory muscle usage, and is diaphoretic. Which of the following is the most appropriate next action?

a. Noninvasive positive pressure ventilation
b. Rapid sequence endotracheal intubation
c. High-flow nasal cannula
d. Ketamine infusion
e. Morphine sulfate

20. A 27-year-old otherwise healthy man presents to the ED with a laceration on his thumb that he sustained while cutting a bagel. You irrigate and repair the wound and are about to discharge the patient when he asks you if he can receive an ECG. It is not busy in the ED so you perform the ECG, as seen in the figure. Which of the following is the most appropriate next step in management?

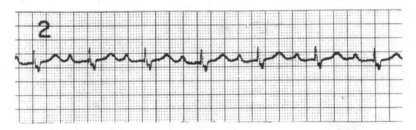

(Reproduced, with permission, from Tintinalli J, Kelen G, Stapczynski J. Emergency Medicine: A Comprehensive Study Guide. New York, NY: McGraw Hill, 2004:193.)

a. Admit the patient for placement of a pacemaker
b. Admit the patient for a 24-hour observation period
c. Administer aspirin and send cardiac biomarkers
d. Repeat the ECG because of incorrect lead placement
e. Discharge the patient home

The following scenario applies to questions 21 and 22.

A 61-year-old woman with a history of diabetes and hypertension is brought to the ED by her daughter. The patient started feeling short of breath approximately 12 hours ago and then noticed a tingling sensation in the middle of her chest and became diaphoretic. An ECG reveals ST depression in leads II, III, and aVF. You believe that the patient had a non–ST-elevation MI (NSTEMI).

21. Which of the following cardiac markers begins to rise within 3 to 6 hours of chest pain onset, peaks at 12 to 24 hours, and returns to baseline in 7 to 10 days?

a. Myoglobin
b. Creatine kinase (CK)
c. Creatine kinase-MB (CK-MB)
d. Troponin I
e. Lactic dehydrogenase (LDH)

22. If the patient in this scenario is found to have an MI, which of the following is considered a core measure in management?

a. Administration of anticoagulants
b. Aspirin on arrival
c. β-Blocker administration in the ED
d. Performance of baseline CXR
e. Serial ECGs

23. A 27-year-old man complains of chest palpitations and light-headedness for the past hour. He has no past medical history and is not taking any medications. He drinks beer occasionally on the weekend and does not smoke cigarettes. His BP is 110/65 mm Hg, HR is 180 beats/minute, and oxygen saturation is 99% on room air. An ECG reveals a regular rhythm, rate of 180 beats/minute, and QRS complex of 90 milliseconds. There are no discernable P waves. Which of the following is the most appropriate medication to treat this dysrhythmia?

a. Digoxin
b. Lidocaine
c. Amiodarone
d. Adenosine
e. Bretylium

The following scenario applies to questions 24 and 25.

A 70-year-old man presents to the ED with paramedics. The patient collapsed in the street and bystanders performed cardiopulmonary resuscitation (CPR). Paramedics found the patient to be in ventricular fibrillation. They performed CPR and defibrillation according to ACLS protocols after which they obtained return of spontaneous circulation and proceeded to intubate the patient. Initial ED vital signs are BP 85/45 mm Hg, HR 105 beats/minute, and oxygen saturation 94%. An ECG is shown in the figure.

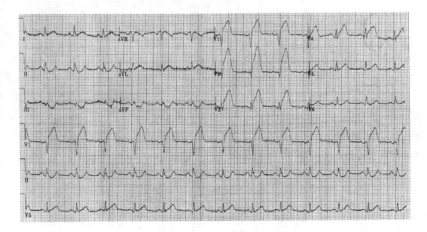

24. Which coronary artery is most likely occluded?

a. Acute marginal branch
b. Left anterior descending artery
c. Right coronary artery (RCA)
d. Posterior descending artery
e. There is no arterial occlusion; this is hyperkalemia

25. Which of the following is the most appropriate definitive treatment?

a. IV heparin infusion
b. Electrical cardioversion
c. IV calcium gluconate
d. Thrombolytic therapy
e. Percutaneous angioplasty

26. A 55-year-old man presents to the ED at 2:00 AM with left-sided chest pain that radiates down his left arm. He takes a β-blocker for hypertension, a proton-pump inhibitor for gastroesophageal reflux disease, and a statin for high cholesterol. He also took sildenafil the previous night for erectile dysfunction. His BP is 130/70 mm Hg and HR is 77 beats/minute. The patient's chest pain has been constant since starting after exertion and you are concerned for unstable angina. Which of the following medications is contraindicated in this patient?

a. Aspirin
b. Unfractionated heparin
c. Nitroglycerin
d. Metoprolol
e. Morphine sulfate

27. A 71-year-old man is playing cards with some friends when he starts to feel a pain in the left side of his chest. The fingers in his left hand become numb and he feels short of breath. His wife calls the ambulance and he is brought to the hospital. In the ED, an ECG is performed. Which of the following best describes the order of ECG changes seen in an MI?

a. Hyperacute T wave, ST-segment elevation, Q wave
b. Q wave, ST-segment elevation, hyperacute T wave
c. Hyperacute T wave, Q wave, ST-segment elevation
d. ST-segment elevation, Q wave, hyperacute T wave
e. ST-segment elevation, hyperacute T wave, Q wave

The following scenario applies to questions 28 and 29.

A 22-year-old college student went to the health clinic complaining of a fever over the last 5 days, fatigue, myalgias, and a bout of vomiting and diarrhea. The clinic doctor diagnosed him with acute gastroenteritis and told him to drink more fluids. Three days later, the student presents to the ED complaining of constant substernal chest pain. He also feels short of breath. His BP is 120/75 mm Hg, HR is 122 beats/minute, RR is 18 breaths/minute, temperature is 100.9°F, and oxygen saturation is 96% on room air. An ECG is performed revealing sinus tachycardia. A chest radiograph is unremarkable. Laboratory tests are normal except for slightly elevated WBC.

28. Which test will help make the diagnosis in this patient?

a. Erythrocyte sedimentation rate (ESR)
b. Procalcitonin
c. C-reactive protein (CRP)
d. Troponin
e. LDH

29. Which of the following is the most common cause of this patient's condition?

a. *Streptococcus viridans*
b. Influenza A
c. Coxsackie B virus
d. Atherosclerotic disease
e. Cocaine abuse

30. A 23-year-old elementary school teacher is brought to the ED after collapsing in her classroom. She remembers feeling light-headed and dizzy and the next thing she remembers is being in an ambulance. There was no seizure activity. She has no medical problems and does not take any medications. Her father died of a "heart problem" at 32 years of age. She does not smoke or use drugs. BP is 120/70 mm Hg, pulse rate is 71 beats/minute, RR is 14 breaths/minute, and oxygen saturation is 100% on room air. Her physical examination and laboratory results are all normal. A rhythm strip is seen in the figure. Which of the following is the most likely diagnosis?

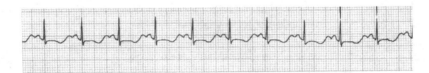

a. WPW syndrome
b. Long QT syndrome (LQTS)
c. LGL syndrome
d. Complete heart block
e. Atrial flutter

31. A 55-year-old man presents to the ED with chest pain and shortness of breath. His BP is 76/40 mm Hg, HR is 89 beats/minute, RR is 28 breaths/minute, and oxygen saturation is 90% on room air. Physical examination reveals crackles midway up both lung fields and a new holosystolic murmur that is loudest at the apex and radiates to the left axilla. ECG reveals ST elevations in the inferior leads. Chest radiograph shows pulmonary edema with a normal-sized cardiac silhouette. Which of the following is the most likely cause of the cardiac murmur?

a. Critical aortic stenosis
b. Papillary muscle rupture
c. Pericardial effusion
d. CHF
e. Aortic dissection

32. An 82-year-old woman is brought to the ED by her daughter for worsening fatigue, dizziness, and light-headedness. The patient denies chest pain or shortness of breath. She has not started any new medications. Her BP is 140/70 mm Hg, HR is 37 beats/minute, and RR is 15 breaths/minute. An IV is started and blood is drawn. An ECG is seen in the figure. Which of the following is the most appropriate next step in management?

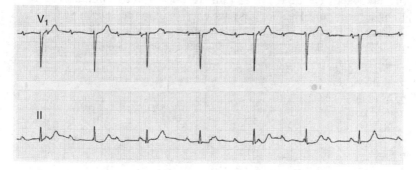

(Reproduced, with permission, from Fuster V, et al. Hurst's The Heart. New York, NY: McGraw Hill, 2004: 904.)

a. Bed rest for the next 48 hours and follow-up with her primary-care physician
b. Administer aspirin, order cardiac enzymes, and admit to the cardiac care unit (CCU)
c. Place a magnet on her chest to turn off her pacemaker
d. Admit for cardiac monitoring and echocardiogram
e. Place on a cardiac monitor, place external pacing pads on the patient, and admit to the CCU

33. A 19-year-old man is brought to the ED by EMS for an episode of syncope that occurred during a basketball game. A friend states that the patient dropped to the ground shortly after scoring a basket on a fast break. On examination, you note a prominent systolic ejection murmur along the left sternal border and at the apex. An ECG reveals left ventricular (LV) hypertrophy, left atrial enlargement, and septal Q waves. You suspect the diagnosis and ask the patient to perform the Valsalva maneuver while you auscultate his heart. Which of the following is most likely to occur to the intensity of the murmur with this maneuver?

a. Decrease
b. Increase
c. Remain unchanged
d. Disappear
e. The intensity stays the same, but the heart skips a beat

34. A 55-year-old man with hypertension and a one-pack-per-day smoking history presents to the ED complaining of three episodes of severe heavy chest pain this morning that radiated to his left shoulder. In the past, he experienced chest discomfort after walking 20 minutes that resolved with rest. The episodes of chest pain this morning occurred while he was reading the newspaper. His BP is 155/80 mm Hg, HR is 76 beats/minute, and RR is 15 breaths/minute. He does not have chest pain in the ED. An ECG reveals sinus rhythm with a rate of 72 beats/minute. Initial troponin I is negative. Which of the following best describes this patient's diagnosis?

a. Variant angina
b. Stable angina
c. Unstable angina
d. NSTEMI
e. STEMI

The following scenario applies to questions 35 and 36.

A 58-year-old man is brought to the ED for an episode of syncope at dinner. His wife found him suddenly slumping in the chair and losing consciousness for a minute. The patient recalls having some chest discomfort and shortness of breath prior to the episode. His rhythm strip, obtained by EMS, is shown in the following figure.

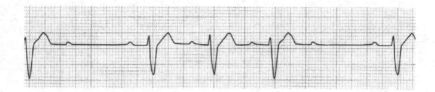

35. Which of the following best describes these findings?
a. Mobitz type I
b. Mobitz type II
c. First-degree atrioventricular (AV) block
d. Atrial flutter with premature ventricular contractions (PVCs)
e. Sinus bradycardia

36. As you are examining the patient described in the previous question, he starts to complain of chest discomfort and shortness of breath and has another syncopal episode. His ECG is shown in the figure. Which of the following is the most appropriate next step in management?

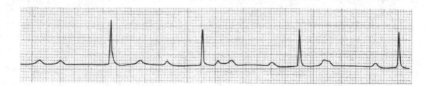

a. Call cardiology consult
b. Cardiovert the patient
c. Administer metoprolol
d. Administer amiodarone
e. Apply transcutaneous pacemaker

The following scenario applies to questions 37 and 38.

A 31-year-old kindergarten teacher presents to the ED complaining substernal chest pain that is sharp in nature. The pain is worse when she is lying down on the stretcher and improves when she sits up. She smokes cigarettes occasionally and was told she has borderline diabetes. She denies any recent surgery or travel. Her BP is 145/85 mm Hg, HR is 99 beats/minute, RR is 18 breaths/minute, and temperature is 100.6°F. Examination of her chest reveals clear lungs and a cardiac friction rub. Her abdomen is soft and nontender to palpation. Her legs are not swollen. Chest radiography and echocardiography are unremarkable. Her ECG is shown in the figure.

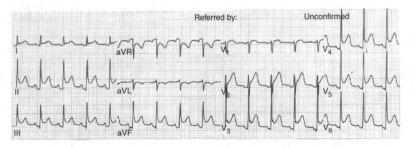

(Reproduced, with permission, from Fuster V, et al. Hurst's The Heart. New York, NY: McGraw Hill, 2004: 304.)

37. Which of the following is the most appropriate next step in management?

a. Order heparin and obtain a CTA to evaluate for a pulmonary embolism (PE)
b. Prescribe ibuprofen and discharge the patient home
c. Administer aspirin, heparin, clopidogrel, and admit for acute coronary syndrome (ACS)
d. Administer thrombolytics, if the pain persists
e. Prescribe oral antibiotics and discharge the patient home

38. The same patient returns to the ED 1-week later reporting shortness of breath and worsening chest pain. She cannot catch her breath and becomes light-headed with minimal activity. Her vitals include BP 80/42 mm Hg, HR 124 beats/minute, and RR 24 breaths/minute. She is afebrile. On physical examination, you note distended neck veins, distant muffled heart sounds, and cool extremities. Her ECG demonstrates sinus tachycardia with low voltage throughout all leads. What is the most likely diagnosis?

a. Acute myocarditis
b. Tension pneumothorax
c. Cardiac tamponade
d. Dressler's syndrome
e. Pleural effusion

39. You are evaluating a 70-year-old man for an ankle sprain. While in the ED, his automatic implantable cardioverter-defibrillator (AICD) begins firing. When he is placed on the cardiac monitor, you note that he is in a sinus rhythm with a rate of 80 beats/minute. You also obtain a quick point of care metabolic panel and blood gas, both of which are normal. The AICD continues to fire while the patient is resting on the stretcher and in sinus rhythm. Which of the following is the most appropriate next step in management?

a. Send the patient back to the radiology suite for another radiograph to desensitize his AICD
b. Administer pain medication and wait until the device representative arrives at the hospital to turn off the AICD
c. Admit the patient to the telemetry unit to monitor his rhythm and find the cause of his AICD discharge
d. Place a magnet over the AICD generator to inactivate it
e. Make a small incision over his chest wall and remove the AICD generator and leads

Chest Pain and Cardiac Dysrhythmias

Answers

1. The answer is e. The patient most likely has a **PE** originating from a thrombus in her left calf. The diagnosis of PE is usually made with a CTA or less commonly a ventilation-perfusion scan performed in nuclear medicine. The most common ECG abnormalities in the setting of PE are **sinus tachycardia and nonspecific ST-T–wave abnormalities.** Other ECG abnormalities may be present and suggestive of PE, but the absence of ECG abnormalities has no significant predictive value. Moreover, 25% of patients with proven PE have ECGs that are unchanged from their baseline state.

With a large PE, the right heart becomes strained. Classic ECG findings of right heart strain and acute cor pulmonale are tall, peaked P waves in lead II (P pulmonale), right-axis deviation **(c)**, incomplete or complete right bundle-branch block **(d)**, a $S_1Q_3T_3$ pattern **(a)**, or AF **(b)**. The finding of $S_1Q_3T_3$ pattern is nonspecific and insensitive in the absence of clinical suspicion for PE. Unfortunately, only 20% of patients with proven PE have any of these classic ECG abnormalities.

2. The answer is d. CTA is more than 90% sensitive and specific for diagnosing PE. While all the other answer choices are important in the work up of a patient with shortness of breath and chest pain, they will not definitively diagnose PE. The blood tests, BNP **(a)** and cardiac troponin **(b),** are important markers that can help to risk stratify patients with known PE as these can be released when there is right ventricular (RV) strain. Patients without RV Strain can be treated with anticoagulants alone while patients with evidence of RV strain need to be assessed for thrombolytic therapy. The main purpose of a CXR **(c)** in the work up of this patient is to rule out alternative causes of chest pain and dyspnea. The most common finding on CXRs in patients with PE is a normal CXR. The D-dimer **(e)** is a blood test that measures the presence of the breakdown of fibrin in an intravascular thrombus. Its concentration varies with clot burden. The D-dimer is helpful to rule out thrombosis when it is negative in patients with low pre-test probability; however, a positive D-dimer is nonspecific (specificity 50-60%) thus further imaging is required.

3. The answer is b. The use of **fibrinolytic therapy** in PE is reserved mostly for patients with **massive PE and hemodynamic collapse.** Massive PE is defined as a proximal embolus with **sustained hypotension** (SBP < 90 mm Hg for 15 minutes or a 40 mm Hg drop from baseline) or hypotension requiring inotropic support or any RV strain. Other causes of hypotension must be excluded. Additionally, patients who lose pulses or suffer from persistent profound bradycardia also fall into this category.

The use of systemic fibrinolytic therapy in submassive PE is less clear. Based on the MOPPET (Moderate Pulmonary Embolism Treated With Thrombolysis) trial in 2013 (1), it appears that the use of fibrinolytics in this population leads to a reduction in the development of long-term pulmonary hypertension. Catheter-directed thrombolytics (if available) may be safer and equally effective. The definition of submassive PE includes those scenarios where there is no persistent hypotension of requirement of inotropic support, but there is evidence of either RV strain [RV dilation on echocardiogram or CT, RV dysfunction on echocardiogram, elevated BNP, electrocardiogram (EKG) changes such as new RBBB or anteroseptal T-wave inversions or ST elevations or depressions] or myocardial necrosis. The presence of bilateral proximal clot **(a)** reflects significant clot burden, but does not guide therapy beyond traditional anticoagulation. Persistent tachycardia **(c)** is common in patients with pulmonary emboli given the additional work required of the myocardium with increased pulmonary afterload. RV dilation **(d)** is a surrogate marker for right heart strain when it is identified on echocardiography. This also implies some degree of RV dysfunction supporting the definition of a submassive PE. Elevation of BNP **(e)** is seen as a result of myocardial stretch. It is frequently identified in patients with pulmonary emboli and may be associated with worse prognosis. Evidence of myocardial necrosis required for the definition of submassive PE is reflected by a positive troponin.

4. The answer is e. AF is a rhythm disturbance of the atria that results in irregular and chaotic ventricular conduction. This irregular electrical activity can lead to reduced cardiac output from a loss of coordinated atrial contractions and a rapid ventricular rate, both of which may limit diastolic filling and stroke volume of the ventricles. AF may be chronic or paroxysmal (sudden onset lasting minutes to days). On the ECG, fibrillatory waves are accompanied by an irregular QRS pattern. The main ED treatment for stable AF is **rate control.** This can be accomplished by many agents, but the agent most commonly used is **diltiazem,** a calcium channel blocker (CCB) with excellent AV nodal blocking effects.

If a patient is unstable, he should be immediately cardioverted (a). However, this patient is stable and asymptomatic; therefore, the goal in the ED is rate control. Catheterization (b) would be correct if the patient exhibited ST-segment elevations on the ECG. If the patient is in AF for more than 48 hours, he needs to be anticoagulated (c) prior to cardioversion because of the risk of atrial thrombus. In general, a patient with stable AF undergoes an echocardiogram to evaluate for thrombus. If there is a thrombus present, patients are placed on warfarin for 2 to 3 weeks and cardioversion takes place when their international normalized ratio (INR) is therapeutic. If no clot is seen on echocardiogram, heparin is administered and cardioversion can take place immediately. Long-term anticoagulation is usually completed with warfarin or the new anticoagulant agents. Amiodarone (d) is an antidysrhythmic agent that sometimes achieves rate control in AF; however, it is not a first-line agent and in the ED the primary goal is rate control, not rhythm control.

5. The answer is b. Patients with ESRD, who require dialysis, are prone to electrolyte disturbances. This patient's clinical picture is consistent with **hyperkalemia** (normal potassium is 3.5-5 mmol/L). The ECG can provide valuable clues to the presence of hyperkalemia. As potassium levels rise, **peaked T waves** are the first characteristic manifestation. Further rises are associated with progressive ECG changes, including **loss of P waves and widening of the QRS complex.** Eventually, the QRS widens further and assumes a **sine-wave pattern,** followed by ventricular fibrillation or asystole. ECG findings of hyperkalemia are very specific, but a screening ECG is not sensitive enough to rule out hyperkalemia.

ECG manifestations of hypokalemia (a) include flattening of T waves, ST-segment depression, and U waves. Hypocalcemia (c) manifests as QT prolongation, whereas hypercalcemia (d) manifests as shortening of the QT interval. There are no classic ECG findings with hyponatremia (e).

6. The answer is b. Elevated potassium is cardiotoxic by a few methods that lead to membrane excitability. It increases the resting membrane potential of the myocyte, causes slow depolarization and decreased length of time of depolarization. When potassium levels are very high, the depolarization threshold increases leading to decreased cardiac function. There are three ways to treat hyperkalemia: antagonize the membrane action of potassium, drive extracellular potassium into cells, and remove potassium from the body. All of the answer choices are treatments used in hyperkalemia but it is important to start with **calcium gluconate (b)** in this patient with ECG abnormalities of hyperkalemia. **Calcium works rapidly to stabilize the cardiac membrane** by increasing depolarization threshold and increasing cardiac conduction speed (thereby narrowing the QRS complex). It does not actually decrease potassium levels, thus other treatments are required. Calcium gluconate is more frequently used than calcium chloride, which ideally is given via central access to prevent local tissue necrosis. Albuterol **(a)** and insulin **(d)** both work by shifting potassium intracellularly by stimulating the Na-K-ATPase pump. Dextrose **(c)** does not affect potassium levels but works to counteract the hypoglycemia that can result from administration of Insulin. Oral kayexalate **(e)** is a cation exchange resin that works to remove potassium from the body through the stool but it takes hours to work and is thus not effective in the acute management of hyperkalemia. In this patient who has ESRD, hemodialysis will be the definitive treatment to reduce her potassium level.

7. The answer is a. The patient has a **primary spontaneous pneumothorax (PTX)**, which occurs in individuals without clinically apparent lung disease. In contrast, secondary spontaneous pneumothorax occurs in individuals with underlying lung disease, especially chronic obstructive pulmonary disease (COPD). For otherwise healthy, young patients with a small primary spontaneous PTX (<20% of the hemithorax), observation alone may be appropriate. The intrinsic reabsorption rate is approximately 1% to 2% a day and accelerated with the administration of 100% oxygen. Many physicians treat with oxygen; **observe these patients for 4 to 6 hours** and then **repeat the CXR**. If the repeat CXR shows no increase in the size of the PTX, the patient can be **discharged with follow-up in 24 hours**. If outpatient follow-up cannot be appropriately arranged, the patient can return to ED in 24 hours for reevaluation or they can be admitted to the hospital for observation. Air travel and underwater diving (changes in atmospheric pressure) must be avoided until the PTX completely resolves.

Needle decompression **(b)** is a temporizing maneuver for patients with suspected tension PTX. Tube thoracostomy **(c)** is used in secondary spontaneous PTX, traumatic PTX, and PTX greater than 20% of the hemithorax. In some scenarios, a pigtail catheter may be used in place of a full tube thoracostomy. Unless there is a change in his status, the patient does not need to be observed for another 6 hours **(d)**. A pleurodesis **(e)** is an operative intervention to prevent recurrence of PTX. It is performed on patients with underlying lung disease or recurrent pneumothorax.

8. The answer is d. **Esophageal perforation** (Boerhaave syndrome) is a potentially life-threatening condition that can result from any Valsalva-like maneuver, which rapidly increases esophageal pressure (including childbirth, vomiting or retching, coughing, and heavy lifting). The most common cause of esophageal perforation is iatrogenic, such as a complication from upper endoscopy. The classic physical examination finding is **mediastinal or cervical emphysema**. This is noted by feeling air under the skin on palpation of the chest wall or by a **crunching** sound heard on auscultation, also known as **Hamman sign**. Radiographic signs of pneumomediastinum can be subtle. Lateral displacement of the mediastinal pleura by mediastinal air creates a linear density paralleling the mediastinal contour. On the lateral projection, mediastinal air can be seen in the retrocardiac space.

Aspiration pneumonia (**a**) is an inflammation of lung parenchyma precipitated by foreign material entering the tracheobronchial tree. Alcoholics are prone to aspiration pneumonia because of ethanol's sedating effect and subsequent decrease of the normal protective airway reflexes. Chest radiograph findings are often delayed with atelectasis typically being the first finding. The right lower lung is the most common site of infiltrate because of the right mainstem bronchus' more vertical angle and larger size compared to the left. Alcoholics have a high incidence of pancreatitis (**b**), which can present with epigastric tenderness and vomiting; however, mediastinal air is not present on radiography. The physical examination hallmark of acute pericarditis (**c**) is the friction rub. The rub may be caused by friction between inflamed or scarred visceral and parietal pericardium or may result from friction between the parietal pericardium and adjacent pleura. Additionally, this patient's ECG did not exhibit the ST elevations and PR depressions typically seen in pericarditis. Aortic dissection (**e**) usually occurs in patients with chronic hypertension or connective tissue disorders. While CXR in aortic dissection is not specific, a widened mediastinum is classically taught. They should not have Hamman sign.

9. The answer is b. The patient's clinical picture of chronic hypertension, acute-onset tearing chest pain, diastolic murmur of aortic insufficiency, and CXR with a widened mediastinum is consistent with an **aortic dissection.** The goal is to decrease the blood pressure and the HR to decrease the shearing forces on the vessel wall that could worsen the dissection. The goal SBP is 100 to 120 mm Hg and HR less than 60 beats/minute. **Esmolol** is a titratable and short-acting β-blocker. It should be **given first** as it decreases the blood pressure and shearing forces and reduces the reflex tachycardia that occurs with vasodilatory agents.

Amiodarone (a) is an antidysrhythmic agent used to treat ventricular arrhythmias which this patient does not have. Nicardipine (c) and nifedipine (d) are both CCB that cause vasodilation and decreased peripheral resistance. Nicardipine can be used as a second-line agent in place of nitrates or when β-blockers are not well tolerated (it seems to have little effect on HR). Nifedipine is only available in oral form which is not acceptable in this acute situation, and it can increase HR. Nitroprusside (e) is a vasodilator that relaxes vascular smooth muscle to reduce afterload and preload by producing NO. This may be added as an agent to further control blood pressure after the β-blocker has already been initiated.

10. The answer is d. The incidence of **endocarditis in an intravenous drug user (IVDU)** is estimated to be 40 times that of the general population. Unlike the general population, endocarditis in IVDUs is typically **right sided** with the majority of cases involving the **tricuspid valve**. Patients with IVDU-related endocarditis usually have no evidence of prior valve damage. The most common organism in IVDU-related endocarditis is *Staphylococcus aureus*. Patients may present with fever, cardiac murmur, cough, pleuritic chest pain, and hemoptysis. Right-sided murmurs, which vary with respiration, are typically pathologic, and more specific for the diagnosis. In patients with right-sided endocarditis and septic pulmonary emboli, pulmonary complaints, infiltrates on chest radiographs, and moderate hypoxia have been described in greater than 33% of patients. Without a good history and physical examination, these symptoms and signs may mislead the physician to identify the lung as the primary source of infection (a and c). **Blood cultures** will be positive in more than 98% of IVDU-related endocarditis patients if **three to five sets** are obtained. Diagnosis generally requires microbial isolation from a blood culture or demonstration of typical lesions on echocardiography. TEE is the most sensitive imaging modality for demonstrating vegetations and tricuspid valve involvement in IVDU-related endocarditis. Initial antibiotic treatment should be directed against *S. aureus* and *Streptococcus* species.

Mononucleosis (b) presents with fever, sore throat, and lymphadenopathy. Patients may also have an enlarged spleen putting them at high risk for traumatic injury. However, mononucleosis does not cause a heart murmur or patchy infiltrates on chest radiograph. Liver function tests (LFTs) are abnormal in more than 90% of patients with infectious mononucleosis. Tuberculosis (e) generally does not present with chest pain or cardiac murmur; the most common symptom is cough and it is usually hemoptysis that causes concern to prompt ED visit.

11. The answer is d. The standard 12-lead ECG identifies patients having an acute STEMI upon presentation in the ED. It is important to identify the anatomic location of an acute MI to estimate the amount of endangered myocardium. The RCA supplies the AV node and inferior wall of the left ventricle in 90% of patients. **Inferior wall MIs** are characterized by **ST elevation in at least two of the inferior leads (II, III and, aVF)**. Reciprocal ST changes (ie, ST depression) in the anterior precordial leads (V_1-V_4) in the setting of an inferior wall acute MI. The RCA also provides perfusion to the right ventricle and it is important to identify RV involvement with a right-sided ECG. If there is RV involvement, patients are preload dependent and therapy that decreases preload (eg, nitroglycerin and morphine) should be avoided. In general, the more elevated the ST segments and the more ST segments that are elevated, the more extensive the injury.

The anteroseptal wall **(a)** of the heart is supplied by the left anterior descending coronary artery (LAD). An acute MI is identified by ST elevation in leads V_1, V_2, and V_3. The LAD also supplies the anterior wall **(b)** of the heart and LAD infarction exhibits ST elevations in leads V_2, V_3, and V_4. The lateral wall **(c)** of the heart is supplied by the left circumflex coronary artery and an infarct exhibits ST elevations in leads I, aVL, V_5, and V_6. A posterior MI **(e)** refers to the posterior wall of the left ventricle. It occurs in 15% to 20% of all MIs and usually in conjunction with inferior or lateral infarction. In a posterior MI, deep ST depressions are seen in V_1, V_2, and V_3, or ST elevations on a posterior ECG. The following figure summarizes the distribution.

I	aVR	V_1	V_4
Lateral		Septal	Anterior
II	aVL	V_2	V_5
Inferior	High Lateral	Septal	Lateral
III	aVF	V_3	V_6
Inferior	Inferior	Anterior	Lateral

12. The answer is b. **Aspirin** is an antiplatelet agent that should be administered early to all patients suspected of having an ACS, unless there is a contraindication. The ISIS-2 (Second International Study of Infarct Survival trial (2)) provides the strongest evidence that aspirin **independently reduces the mortality (by 23%)** of patients with acute MI.

Nitroglycerin (a) provides benefit to patients with ACS by reducing preload and dilating coronary arteries. However, there is no mortality benefit with its use and is contraindicated in inferior wall MI. Unfractionated heparin (c) acts indirectly to inhibit thrombin, preventing the conversion of fibrinogen to fibrin and thus inhibiting clot propagation. ASA and heparin are synergistic in their effects in preventing death. Routine use of lidocaine (d) as prophylaxis for ventricular arrhythmias in patients who have experienced an acute MI has been shown to increase mortality rates. Use of CCBs like diltiazem (e) in the acute setting has come into question, with some trials showing increased adverse effects.

13. The answer is d. When a patient is diagnosed with an STEMI, the standard of care for therapy is immediate reperfusion with PCI. The Joint Commission evaluates the **time from arrival (door) to reperfusion (balloon)**. Hospitals accredited as STEMI centers are held to this standard. Based on clinical trials evaluating outcomes in MI, the time window for door to balloon is **90 minutes.**

All other answer choices (a, b, c, and e) are incorrect.

14. The answer is e. **WPW syndrome** is caused by an **accessory electrical pathway (ie, bundle of Kent)** between the atria and ventricles. The primary significance of WPW syndrome is that it predisposes the individual to the development of reentry tachycardias. The classic ECG findings include a **short PR interval (<120 milliseconds), widened QRS interval (>100 milliseconds)**, and a **delta wave** (slurred upstroke at the beginning of the QRS). When conduction occurs, anterograde down the AV node and then retrograde up the accessory pathway (orthodromic), the ECG will appear normal. When the impulse occurs, anterograde down the accessory pathway and retrograde up the AV node (antidromic), the QRS complex will be wide. In the presence of antidromic conduction (conduction first through the bypass tract), the normal slowing effect of the AV node is lost and rapid ventricular response rates (>200 beats/minute) can occur. The most dangerous circumstance is in AF where impulses occur at a rate greater than 300 beats/minute. This can quickly lead to ventricular fibrillation. **Procainamide** is the drug most commonly associated with the acute treatment of WPW, and nodal agents like β-blockers and CCBs are avoided because they will promote conduction solely through the accessory pathway increasing the risk of rhythm deterioration.

Ventricular tachycardia (a) may be difficult to distinguish from WPW. In a young patient with classic ECG findings, however, WPW is more likely. Nonetheless, it is prudent to avoid AV nodal blocking agents in any wide-complex tachycardia. Atrial flutter (b) will have flutter waves that take on a sawtooth pattern. AF (c) is an irregular rhythm. LGL syndrome (d) is classified as a preexcitation syndrome (similar to WPW) in which a bypass tract is present. LGL is characterized by an individual who is prone to tachydysrhythmias and has a PR interval less than 120 milliseconds. Unlike WPW, the QRS complex is normal (no delta wave).

15. The answer is a. The patient most likely has a **partial or complete obstruction of his lower esophagus** secondary to the steak he consumed. This most commonly occurs near the **gastroesophageal junction**. Administration of **glucagon may** cause enough **relaxation of the esophageal smooth muscle** in the lower esophageal sphincter to allow passage of the bolus. The dose is 1-2 mg slow intravenous pyelogram (IVP) over 2 minutes. Potential side effects include nausea and vomiting. The success rate of glucagon is generally considered to be poor and may be no better than placebo. Some authors suggest it is likely worth a try while awaiting gastroenterology consultation for endoscopy (EGD) which is the recommended definitive management.

Meat tenderizer (b), once used for this situation, is now contraindicated secondary to the possibility of perforation as a result of its proteolytic effect on an inflamed esophageal mucosa. Syrup of ipecac (c) was used in situations of toxic ingestions to induce vomiting, but is no longer recommended. Also, vomiting should be avoided in our patient to avoid risk of esophageal perforation and aspiration. The Heimlich maneuver (d) can be a lifesaving procedure but is not necessary in this patient who is not in respiratory distress. Respiratory compromise may occur when a foreign body lodges in the oropharynx, proximal esophagus, or is large enough that it impinges on the trachea. Laparotomy (e) is not indicated for esophageal foreign bodies.

16. The answer is e. Thrombolytic therapy can be administered to patients having an acute STEMI that is **within 12 hours** from symptom onset. Contraindications to fibrinolytic therapy are those that increase the risk of hemorrhage. The most catastrophic complication is intracranial hemorrhage.

Absolute contraindications include the following:

- History of any intracranial hemorrhage
- Known intracranial neoplasm or cerebral vascular malformation
- Ischemic stroke within 3 months
- Active internal bleeding (excluding menses)
- Suspected aortic dissection or pericarditis
- Significant closed-head or facial trauma within 3 months

Systolic BP greater than 180 mm Hg is a relative contraindication (**a**). However, if thrombolytics are going to be administered and the patient's SBP is greater than 180 mm Hg systolic and or more than 110 mm Hg diastolic, antihypertensive medication can be administered to lower the SBP to below 180 mm Hg. Anticoagulation is a relative contraindication (**b**). Many patients who suffer from a STEMI are on aspirin and other antiplatelet and anticoagulant therapies. Major surgery less than 3 weeks prior to administration of thrombolytics is a relative contraindication (**c**). Active peptic ulcer disease is a relative contraindication (**d**).

17. The answer is e. This patient is hypotensive, exhibiting signs and symptoms of acute heart failure (eg, dyspnea, fatigue, respiratory crackles, and chest pain), and is in AF (irregular, narrow complex rhythm) with rapid ventricular response (HR 140's). Any patient with **unstable vital signs** with a tachydysrhythmia should receive a dose of sedation and undergo **synchronized cardioversion** starting at 100 J.

Diltiazem (**a**) is used as a rate-control agent for patients in AF. If the patient was not hypotensive or exhibiting signs of heart failure, diltiazem could be used to slow the ventricular response. Metoprolol (**b**) is sometimes used to control ventricular rate in AF; however, it is contraindicated in patients with acute heart failure due to its significant effect on inotropy. Digoxin (**c**) is another option to control the ventricular response in AF; however, its relatively slow onset (ie, hours) precludes it from use in the acute setting. Coumadin (**d**) is an anticoagulant that is administered to a select group of patients in AF. Anticoagulation reduces the risk of embolic stroke and other embolic events by two-thirds. The decision to anticoagulate is based upon weighing the benefit of reduction of embolic events with the risk of bleeding. The American Heart Association (AHA) and the

European Society of Cardiology (ESC) recommend using the CHA2DS2-VAS2 score (congestive heart failure, hypertension, age ≥75 years, diabetes mellitus, prior stroke or TIA or thromboembolism, vascular disease, age 65 to 74 years, sex category).

18. The answer is d. This patient has **decompensated CHF with pulmonary edema. Nitroglycerin** is the most effective and most rapid means of **reducing preload** in a patient with CHF. Nitrates decrease myocardial preload and, to a lesser extent, afterload. Nitrates increase venous capacitance, including venous pooling, which decreases preload and myocardial oxygen demand. It is most beneficial when the patient who presents with acute CHF is also hypertensive. It can be administered via the sublingual, intravenous, or transdermal route.

Metoprolol **(a)**, a β-blocker, is contraindicated in acute decompensated heart failure. Morphine sulfate **(b)** reduces pulmonary congestion through a central sympatholytic effect that causes peripheral vasodilation. This decreases central venous return and reduces preload. However, morphine sulfate is a respiratory depressant and may lead to hypoventilation and is most commonly avoided now in cases of acute heart failure. Nitroprusside **(c)** is a mixed venous and arteriolar dilator thereby reducing both pre- and afterload. It can be used in patients with acute pulmonary edema (APE) but is less commonly used because of challenges with administration (sensitivity to light and toxicity). This patient is hypoxic with an oxygen saturation of 85% and requires supplemental oxygen **(e)**. In the acute setting, this patient should be placed on a nonrebreather with 100% oxygen flowing through the mask; however, oxygen administration via this method does not decrease preload.

19. The answer is a. This patient has a worsening respiratory status in the setting of APE. With the increased RR and work of breathing, the patient is at risk of developing respiratory failure and needs assistance. This patient is a perfect candidate for the use of **noninvasive positive pressure ventilation**, either in the form of continuous positive airway pressure **(CPAP) or bilevel positive airway pressure (BiPAP).** CPAP provides a constant flow of positive pressure to the patient delivered through a tight-fitting face mask. BiPAP provides a baseline level of positive pressure at all times and an increase in pressure when the patient takes a breath. Noninvasive ventilation supports the patient by decreasing the patient's work of breathing, providing supplemental O_2, pushing edema out of the alveoli, and allowing the alveoli to remain open during exhalation. The use of noninvasive ventilation in this population of patients with APE decreases rates of intubation and mortality. BiPAP and CPAP are equally efficacious for CHF patients. Patients must be awake and able to participate in the respiratory effort and not at risk for emesis and aspiration in order for it to be successful.

Rapid sequence endotracheal intubation (**b**) is indicated for patients with APE who are too somnolent or even potentially too agitated to take part in noninvasive positive pressure ventilation. High-flow nasal cannula (**c**) is becoming increasingly popular in the ED as a supplemental oxygen source delivered at very high rates through nasal cannula. It may provide a small amount of positive pressure but not nearly the amount of CPAP or BiPAP. It is frequently used in patients with significant hypoxia who are unable to tolerate noninvasive ventilation and have "do not intubate" orders. A ketamine infusion (**d**) is sometimes used with limited evidence for patients who are agitated and may benefit from noninvasive ventilation. As a dissociative sedative, it allows patients to maintain their respiratory drive and muscle tone while at the same time providing enough sedation for compliance with noninvasive therapy. It is also used in delayed sequence intubation where noninvasive ventilation is used as bridging therapy for preoxygenation in preparation for intubation. Morphine sulfate (**e**) was frequently used in the past for patients with APE. However, given its effect of respiratory depression, it should be avoided in this population.

20. The answer is e. The patient's ECG shows a sinus rhythm at a rate of 70 beats/minute with a **first-degree heart block.** *First-degree heart block* is defined as prolonged conduction of atrial impulses without the loss of any impulse. On an ECG, this translates to a **PR interval more than 200 milliseconds** with a narrow QRS complex (<120 milliseconds). First-degree heart block is most often a **normal variant** without clinical significance, occurring in 1% to 2% of healthy young adults. This variant requires no specific treatment.

A pacemaker (**a**) is considered in patients with a second-degree type II AV block or third-degree complete heart block. An observation period is not required (**b**), as the prolonged PR interval is a normal variant in this individual. Aspirin and cardiac biomarkers are sent for patients thought to have ACS (**c**). There is no evidence that the ECG leads are placed incorrectly (**d**).

21. The answer is d. Serum cardiac markers are used to confirm or exclude myocardial cell death and are considered the gold standard for the diagnosis of MI. While there are many markers currently used, the most sensitive and specific markers are **troponin I** and **T.** A rise in these levels, as seen in the figure, is diagnostic for an acute MI. Troponin levels **rise within 3 to 6 hours of chest pain onset, peak at 12 to 24 hours,** and **remain elevated for 7 to 10 days.**

Myoglobin (**a**) is found in both skeletal and cardiac muscles and released into the bloodstream when there is muscle cell death. It tends to rise within 1 to 2 hours of injury, peaks at 4 to 6 hours, and returns to baseline in 24 hours. CK (**b**) is an enzyme found in skeletal and cardiac muscles. Following acute MI, increases in serum CK are detectable within 3 to 8 hours with a peak at 12 to 24 hours after injury and normalize within 3 to 4 days. CK-MB (**c**) is an isoenzyme found in cardiac muscle and released into the bloodstream upon cell death. It rises 4 to 6 hours after acute MI, peaks at 12 to 36 hours, and returns to normal within 3 to 4 days. LDH (**e**) is an enzyme found in muscle and rises 12 hours after acute MI, peaks at 24 to 48 hours, and returns to normal at 10 to 14 days.

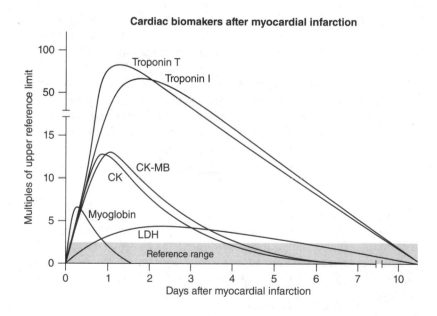

Cardiac biomakers after myocardial infarction

22. The answer is b. Federal regulatory agencies have established **core measures** related to multiple diagnoses. These include pneumonia, acute MI, sepsis, and CHF. Care provided in the ED is monitored carefully for compliance with these measures. These measures are evaluated for any patient with a discharge diagnosis of an acute MI. For the purposes of the ED, the core measure that applies is the **administration of aspirin on arrival**. This means that all patients with an MI must receive an aspirin in the ED.

The administration of anticoagulants (**a**) is considered the standard of care but not a core measure that is monitored by The Joint Commission. β-Blocker administration in the ED (**c**) is no longer considered the standard of care. Previously, β-blockers were administered acutely for acute MI; however, when administered acutely, it was associated with increased rates of heart failure, particularly if given intravenously. However, β-blockers are part of the overall regimen for an acute MI and must be prescribed at the time of discharge (a core measure). The performance of a baseline CXR (**d**) does not play a significant role acutely in the management of MI. We frequently evaluate for other causes of chest pain or shortness of breath with the CXR. It is also sometimes useful in the assessment of the mediastinum when considering aortic dissection as the cause of a patient's pain. Serial ECGs (**e**) are helpful to monitor the evolution of an acute MI. There is no standard for how many and how often an ECG should be performed.

23. The answer is d. *Narrow-complex tachycardias* are defined as rhythms with a QRS complex duration less than 100 milliseconds and a ventricular rate greater than 100 beats/minute. Although virtually all narrow-complex tachydysrhythmias originate from a focus above the ventricles, the term **supraventricular tachycardia (SVT)** is conventionally used to denote those rhythms aside from sinus tachycardia, atrial tachycardia, AF, and atrial flutter [eg, atrioventricular nodal reentry tachycardia (AVNRT) and atrioventricular reentry tachycardia (AVRT)]. **Adenosine**, an ultrashort-acting AV nodal blocking agent, is typically used to treat SVTs. Because it is so fast acting, it must be delivered through a large vein (eg, the antecubital fossa) with a rapid IV fluid bolus. The initial dose is 6 mg IVP, if this does not work, the dose can be increased to 12 mg IVP and repeated. In addition to adenosine, **maneuvers that increase vagal tone** have been shown to slow conduction through the AV node. Some of these maneuvers include carotid sinus massage, Valsalva maneuver, and facial immersion in cold water.

Digoxin (**a**) is an antidysrhythmic and ionotropic but it has a slow onset that may take several hours or more to work as its maximal effect is at 2 to 6 hours. If SVT is refractory to adenosine, diltiazem, esmolol or metoprolol are options. Lidocaine (b) and amiodarone (c) are effective in treating narrow-complex tachycardias, but they are agents generally used to treat wide-complex or ventricular tachycardias. Bretylium (e) is no longer available in the United States as it has a poor safety profile.

24.   The answer is b. This ECG depicts an **acute anteroseptal wall MI with ST elevations in leads V_1 to V_4.** The anterior wall of the heart including the septum is represented by leads V_1 to V_4 on ECG and the heart muscle is supplied by the **left anterior descending artery**. It is not surprising that this patient presented after a VFib arrest. Patients presenting with anterior wall MI do worse than those with inferior wall MI due to the damage to the left ventricle with higher incidence of heart failure and mortality.

The acute marginal artery (a) is a branch of the RCA and it supplies the right ventricle. The RCA (c) supplies the inferior wall if the heart represented by leads II, III, aVF. The circumflex artery (d) supplies the lateral wall and can be represented by leads I and aVL on ECG. This ECG is not consistent with hyperkalemia (e). Be careful not to confuse the tall hyperacute T-waves of ischemia that lead to ST segment elevation with peaked T-waves of hyperkalemia.

25.   The answer is e. The preferred treatment for STEMI is **primary PCI**. It has shown to improve long-term mortality over thrombolytic therapy (d). The patient is also hypotensive secondary to **cardiogenic shock.** As a stabilizing measure, the patient may require an intra-aortic balloon pump. This is a mechanical device that is used to decrease myocardial oxygen demand while at the same time increasing cardiac output. By increasing cardiac output, it also increases coronary blood flow and therefore myocardial oxygen delivery. It is inserted through the femoral artery. Heparin (a) is an antithrombin agent and should be administered early in patients with ACS, acute MI, and dynamic EKG changes, but is not definitive treatment.

The patient does not have a dysrhythmia and therefore should not be cardioverted (b). Calcium gluconate (c) is the agent of choice for individuals with ECG signs of hyperkalemia. It does not have a role in the management of acute MI.

26.   The answer is c. Sildenafil is a selective cyclic guanosine monophosphate (GMP) inhibitor that results in smooth-muscle relaxation and vasodilation by the release of nitric oxide. It is used in men for erectile dysfunction and also sometimes pulmonary hypertension. It is **contraindicated to administer nitroglycerin** to individuals who have taken sildenafil in the previous 24 hours. The combination of nitroglycerin and sildenafil can lead to **hypotension and death**. If nitrates are co-administered with sildenafil, the patient should be closely monitored for hypotension. Fluid resuscitation and pressor agents may be needed to restore BP.

Aspirin (**a**) is contraindicated in individuals with an allergy or active bleeding. Heparin (**b**) is contraindicated in individuals with heparin-induced thrombocytopenia, and those who are actively bleeding. Metoprolol is contraindicated in hypotensive individuals (**d**). Morphine sulfate (**e**) is contraindicated in patients with respiratory depression. All of the other answer choices are medications that can be used to treat unstable angina.

27. The answer is a. The earliest ECG finding of an acute myocardial infarction (AMI) is the **hyperacute T wave**, which may appear minutes after the interruption of blood flow. The hyperacute T wave, which is short-lived, evolves to progressive **elevation of ST segments**. In general, **Q waves** represent established myocardial necrosis and usually develop within 8 to 12 hours after a STEMI, though they may be noted as early as 1 to 2 hours after the onset of complete coronary occlusion.

All other answer choices (**b, c, d, and e**) are ordered incorrectly.

28. The answer is d. The patient has **myocarditis**. **Flu-like complaints**, such as fatigue, myalgias, nausea, vomiting, diarrhea, and fever, are usually the earliest symptoms and signs of myocarditis. **Tachycardia is common and can be disproportionate to the patient's temperature (ie, HR faster than what is expected)**. This may be the only clue that something more serious than a simple viral illness exists. Approximately 12% of patients also complain of chest pain. Given the inflammation of the myocardial muscle, typically **cardiac enzymes are elevated** in these patients.

The ESR (**a**) is a nonspecific marker of inflammation. This test is elevated when someone is acutely infected, but also in a host of inflammatory conditions like the autoimmune diseases. Procalcitonin (**b**) is used as a serum marker for occult infection. It has gained popularity in its use as a screening test for sepsis of a bacterial nature. Like ESR, CRP (**c**) is another nonspecific marker of inflammation. It will elevate in many conditions and will not help the physician to narrow the diagnosis to a specific organ system. LDH (**e**) is not a useful test in this case. LDH is often used in the evaluation of patients for possible *Pneumocystis jiroveci*. It is also helpful in identifying patients with hemolysis. Prior to the development of better troponin and CK assays, LDH was used as a "cardiac enzyme" but due to its lack of specificity for myocardium, it is no longer used.

29. The answer is c. The **Enteroviruses**, especially the **coxsackie B virus**, predominate as causative agents of viral myocarditis in the United States. Coxsackie B virus usually causes infection during the summer months. Some other causes of myocarditis include adenovirus, parvovirus B19, influenza, human immunodeficiency virus (HIV), *Mycoplasma, Trypanosoma cruzi,* and steroid abuse.

S. viridans **(a)** is a common cause of acute bacterial endocarditis, an infection of a cardiac valve. The influenza virus **(b)** rarely causes myocarditis. It is more commonly associated with myalgias, cough, diarrhea, and headache. The young and old populations are at the greatest risk for pulmonary complications. Myocarditis can masquerade as an acute MI because patients with either may have severe chest pain, ECG changes, elevated cardiac enzymes, and heart failure. Patients with myocarditis are usually young and have few risk factors for CAD **(d)**. Cocaine **(e)** use can cause chest pain, tachycardia, and even an MI. It does not lead to flu-like symptoms.

30. The answer is b. LQTS is a **congenital disorder** characterized by a prolongation of the QT interval on ECG and a propensity to ventricular tachydysrhythmias, which may lead to syncope, cardiac arrest, or sudden death in otherwise healthy individuals. The QT interval on the ECG, measured from the beginning of the start of the Q-wave to the end of the T wave, represents the duration of ventricular depolarization (activation) and repolarization (recovery) of the ventricular myocardium. In general, **HR corrected QT intervals (QTc) values above 440 ms in men and 460 ms in women are considered abnormal**. The QT interval shortens at faster HRs and lengthens with slower HRs. There is increased risk of torsades de pointes with QTc intervals of more than 500 ms. LQTS has been recognized as the **Romano-Ward syndrome** (ie, familial occurrence with autosomal dominant inheritance, QT prolongation, and ventricular tachydysrhythmias) or the **Jervell and Lange-Nielsen syndrome** (ie, familial occurrence with autosomal recessive inheritance, congenital deafness, QT prolongation, and ventricular arrhythmias). Patients with LQTS are usually diagnosed after a cardiac event (ie, syncope, cardiac arrest) has already occurred. In some situations, LQTS is diagnosed after sudden death in family members. Some individuals are diagnosed with LQTS based on an ECG showing QT prolongation.

β-Blockers are drugs of choice for patients with LQTS. The protective effect of β-blockers is related to their adrenergic blockade diminishing the risk of cardiac arrhythmias. Implantation of **cardioverter-defibrillators** appears to be the most effective therapy for high-risk patients.

WPW syndrome **(a)** is characterized by a shortened PR interval (<120 milliseconds), a slurred upstroke of the QRS complex (delta wave), and a wide QRS complex (>100 milliseconds) as seen on the resting ECG. It is caused by an accessory pathway (bundle of Kent) that predisposes individuals to tachydysrhythmias. LGL syndrome **(c)** is classified as a pre-excitation syndrome in which an accessory (James tract) is present. LGL is characterized by an individual who is prone to tachydysrhythmias and has a short PR interval less than 120 milliseconds, but a normal QRS complex and no delta wave. Complete heart block **(d)** is characterized by the absent conduction of all atrial impulses resulting in complete electrical and mechanical AV dissociation. Both the atria and ventricles depolarize regularly but in no relation to each other. Atrial flutter **(e)** is distinguished by broad sawtooth flutter waves that are regular depolarizations prior to a QRS. Atrial depolarization occurs at a rate of 250 to 350 beats/min with QRS complexes at a fraction of the rate (commonly 150 beats/min).

31. The answer is b. The patient's presentation is consistent with **acute mitral valve regurgitation** because of a **ruptured papillary muscle** in the setting of an AMI. Ruptured papillary muscle is an early complication of AMI and this presentation of acute deterioration with a new, harsh systolic murmur should prompt immediate cardiac surgery consultation. This patient is in cardiogenic shock and should be treated with vasopressor and inotropic support. An intra-aortic balloon pump is a bridge to the definitive surgical treatments of valve repair or replacement that can be used. CXR characteristically reveals pulmonary edema with a normal heart size. The characteristic murmur of mitral regurgitation is a **holosystolic murmur that is loudest at the apex**.

Critical aortic stenosis **(a)** produces a loud systolic murmur that is best heard at the second right intercostal space and radiates to the carotids. The classic finding of a pericardial effusion **(c)** is decreased breath sounds. With a large-sized effusion or one that rapidly accumulates, patients may develop pericardial tamponade which will cause distended neck veins and hypotension. CHF **(d)** does not cause a murmur but rather an extra heart sound (S_3). Aortic dissection **(e)** is associated with a murmur of aortic insufficiency if the dissection involves the aortic valve.

32. The answer is e. The patient's ECG reveals **third-degree (or complete) heart block.** It is a disorder of the cardiac conduction system, where there is no conduction through the AV node and electrical dissociation of the atria and ventricles. This may occur secondary to MI, drug intoxication, infection, or infiltrative diseases. On the ECG, **complete heart block is represented by QRS complexes being conducted at their own regular rate independent of the P waves which are also conducting at their own regular rate.** Individuals with second-degree type II or third-degree complete heart block are considered unstable. **External pacing pads** should be placed on them, followed by a transvenous pacer if their BP is unstable. They may require a permanent pacemaker for irreversible complete heart block.

Clearly, this patient has an unstable rhythm and should not be discharged home (**a**). The patient should receive aspirin and have cardiac biomarkers obtained; however, the ABCs must be followed and the patient's rhythm is currently unstable (**b**). Placement of the magnet over the pacemaker turns off the sensing function of the pacemaker and temporarily converts the pacemaker from the demand mode to a fixed-rate mode (**c**). This assesses whether the pacing function is intact and the pacing stimulus can capture the myocardium. There is no evidence in this patient's medical history that she has a pacemaker. Cardiac monitoring and echocardiogram (**d**) are generally used to continuously monitor a patient's rhythm and cardiac function. This patient will likely undergo rhythm- and function-assessment as an inpatient.

33. The answer is b. The patient has **hypertrophic cardiomyopathy (HCM)**, which is characterized by LV hypertrophy without associated ventricular dilation. The hypertrophy is usually asymmetric, involving the septum to a greater extent than the free wall. Patients are at increased risk of **dysrhythmias and sudden death**. Syncope is usually exertion-related and is caused by a dysrhythmia or a sudden decrease in cardiac output. The murmur associated with HCM is a prominent **systolic ejection murmur** heard along the left sternal boarder and at the apex with radiation to the axilla. The murmur is a result of LV outflow obstruction and mitral regurgitation. It is **increased** with maneuvers that decrease LV end-diastolic volume, such as the Valsalva maneuver, sudden standing, and exercise. The most common cardiovascular cause of sudden death in the athlete is HCM. A patient with suspected HCM should avoid physical exertion until cardiology follow-up and further testing has been completed. If the patient has pre-syncope, syncope, angina, or dysrhythmia (such as this patient), he or she should be admitted to the hospital for an echocardiogram and cardiology consultation.

The Valsalva maneuver will decrease the duration of all other murmurs except mitral valve prolapse and HCM (a). All other choices (c, d, and e) are incorrect as described in the explanation earlier.

34. The answer is c. The patient exhibits **unstable angina**, which is defined as new-onset angina, angina occurring at rest lasting longer than 20 minutes, or angina deviating from a patient's normal pattern. Unstable angina is considered the harbinger of an acute MI and, therefore, should be evaluated and treated aggressively. Patients may be pain free and have negative cardiac biomarkers with unstable angina. In general, unstable angina is treated with oxygen, aspirin, clopidogrel, low-molecular-weight or unfractionated heparin, and further risk stratification in the hospital.

Variant or prinzmetal angina (a) is caused by coronary artery vasospasm at rest with minimal coronary artery disease. It is sometimes relieved by exercise or nitroglycerin. It is generally treated with CCBs. Patients with prinzmetal angina may have ST elevations on their ECG that are indistinguishable from an acute MI. Stable angina (b) is described as transient episodic chest discomfort resulting from MI. The discomfort is typically predictable and reproducible, with the frequency of attacks constant over time. The discomfort is thought to be caused by fixed, stenotic atherosclerotic plaques that narrow a blood vessel lumen and reduce coronary blood flow. NSTEMI (d) and STEMI (e) result from myocardial necrosis with release of cardiac biomarkers (eg, troponin) into the bloodstream.

35. The answer is b. The rhythm strip shows **second-degree AV block type II or Mobitz type II.** Mobitz II presents with a prolonged PR interval (PR >0.2 second) and random dropped beats (ie, P wave without QRS complex). The PR intervals are always the same duration. The block is below the level of the AV node, generally the His-Purkinje system. This heart block reflects serious cardiac pathology and may be seen with an anterior wall MI, which is the case with this patient.

Mobitz type I (a) (also called Wenckebach phenomenon) shows progressive prolongation of PR interval with each beat until AV conduction is lost causing a dropped beat. First-degree AV block (c) presents with prolonged PR interval (PR >0.2 second) without loss of AV conduction. This block is asymptomatic. Atrial flutter (d) is a tachydysrhythmia with rapid atrial beat and variable conduction through the AV node. It has a characteristic "sawtooth" appearance of atrial flutter waves. Sinus brady-cardia (e) is similar to sinus rhythm except that the rate is less than 60 and generally greater than 45 beats/minute. There are several etiologies of sinus bradycardia; some are normal (ie, young person, well-trained athlete) and some pathologic (ie, β-blocker overdose, cardiac ischemia).

36. The answer is e. The rhythm strip findings are consistent with **third-degree AV block**, also called *complete heart block*. It is characterized by absent conduction through the AV node, resulting in the dissociation of atrial and ventricular rhythms. The ECG shows independent P waves and QRS complexes. Mobitz type II often progresses to third-degree heart block, as seen in this case. The immediate step in managing complete heart block is applying a **transcutaneous pacemaker** for ventricular pacing as a tem-porizing measure in the unstable or hypotensive patient. Pacer pads should always be applied to the patient even when stable, in case the need arises for emergent pacing. If the transcutaneous pacemaker cannot achieve capture, or does not improve hemodynamics, an emergent **transvenous pacemaker** placement is needed. In cases of irreversible complete heart block, patients need **implantable ventricular pacemakers** for definitive management. In addition, the underlying cause of the block needs to be addressed.

Consulting cardiology (a) is a good choice as they will implant a perma-nent pacemaker and manage any underlying cardiac disease. However, the patient must first be stabilized. Cardioversion (b) is used to treat unstable patients with reentrant arrhythmias, such as AF. It is not helpful in a setting of conduction abnormality, such as heart block. Metoprolol (c), a β-blocker, is contraindicated in complete heart block. This agent prolongs AV nodal conduction. Amiodarone (d) is an antidysrhythmic used in patients with wide-complex tachycardias or AF.

37. The answer is b. The classic presentation of **pericarditis** includes **chest pain, a pericardial friction rub, and ECG abnormalities.** A prodrome of fever and myalgias may occur. Pericarditis chest pain is usually subster-nal and varies with respiration. It is typically **relieved by sitting forward and worsened by lying down.** The physical examination hallmark of acute pericarditis is the **pericardial friction rub.** The earliest ECG changes are seen in the first few hours to days of illness and include **diffuse ST-segment elevation** seen in leads I, II, III, aVL, aVF, and V_2 to V_6. Most patients with acute pericarditis will have concurrent **PR-segment depression.** The mainstay of treatment includes supportive care with **anti-inflammatory**

medications [(ie, nonsteroidal anti-inflammatory drugs (NSAIDs)]. Corticosteroids have been shown to increase the risk of recurrence and therefore should only be used when NSAIDs are contraindicated.

PE (**a**) can present with substernal chest pain that is sharp in nature and worse with inspiration. However, the patient does not exhibit any risk factors for a PE. It is very important to be able to differentiate an acute MI from acute pericarditis because thrombolytic therapy is contraindicated in pericarditis as it may precipitate hemorrhagic tamponade (**d**). Unlike the ECG in an acute MI, the ST elevations in early pericarditis are concaved upward rather than convex upward (**c**). Subsequent tracings do not evolve through a typical MI pattern and Q waves do not appear. Antibiotics (**e**) are not routinely used to treat pericarditis.

38. The answer is c. This patient is presenting with signs and symptoms of **pericardial tamponade** from a **pericardial effusion** caused by her pericarditis. Prior to discharging a patient with suspected pericarditis, an echocardiogram should be performed to rule out a pericardial effusion. A pericardial effusion is an abnormal accumulation of fluid in the pericardial space and is a known complication of pericarditis. Tamponade results when the fluid in the pericardium causes compression of the myocardium resulting in decreased blood flow into the heart, thereby causing decreased stroke volume and decreased cardiac output. This patient is presenting with symptoms of classic **Beck's Triad: hypotension, distended neck veins, and muffled heart sounds.** Echocardiogram or ED point-of-care cardiac ultrasound can easily make this diagnosis. **Pericardiocentesis** is indicated for this unstable patient.

Acute myocarditis (**a**) is when the virus attacks the heart muscle itself and should be considered in young patients with history of viral illness and fulminant heart failure as myocarditis can lead to dilated cardiomyopathy that causes CHF and hypotension; it does not cause pericardial effusion. Tension pneumothorax (**b**) can occur after a traumatic or spontaneous pneumothorax but is more common after traumatic. While patients can have distended neck veins and hypotension, they also have absent lung sounds over the affected side and tracheal deviation. This is treated emergently with needle thoracostomy followed by chest tube placement. Dressler Syndrome (**d**), also known as postcardiac injury syndrome, is a type of pericarditis thought to be immune mediated that occurs in the late course after myocarditis and can also occur after percutaneous cardiac procedures. Signs and symptoms include fever, chest pain, and a pericardial friction rub. It can also lead to pericardial effusions and tamponade. A pleural effusion (e) is when fluid accumulates in the pleural space between the visceral and parietal pleura of the lung. It is generally viewed as a manifestation of underlying disease with CHF, pneumonia, malignancy, and PEs being responsible for most cases.

39. The answer is d. AICDs are placed in patients at high risk for fatal dysrhythmias (eg, ventricular tachycardia and fibrillation). In these patients, AICDs decrease the risk of sudden death from approximately 40% per year to less than 2% per year. Occasionally, it may become necessary to temporarily deactivate an AICD, as in the case of inappropriate shock in the setting of a stable rhythm (such as seen with the patient in question). The patient in this scenario is receiving a shock while he is in sinus rhythm. Some potential causes of inappropriate shock delivery include false sensing of SVTs, muscular activity (eg, shivering), sensing T waves as QRS complexes, nonsustained tachydysrhythmias, and AICD failure. AICDs are generally **inactivated by placing a magnet over the AICD generator.** Although there is some variability depending on the generation of the AICD, most EDs have a special donut magnet that is reserved for this function. If the patient subsequently experiences a dysrhythmia in the setting of having his or her defibrillator turned off, the physician should use the bedside defibrillator to treat the patient. It is important to note that if a patient with an AICD is in cardiac arrest and it discharges, this poses no threat to the rescuer administering chest compressions. Additionally, if a patient with an AICD is in cardiac arrest and the AICD is not delivering appropriate shocks, standard defibrillator pads or paddles can be used as long as they are 10 cm from the implanted device.

Sending the patient back to the radiology suite (a) will not temporarily turn off the AICD. However, radiographs are important in detecting AICD lead fractures. Most patients carry a manufacturer card and it is often possible to contact the AICD company. However, it is not appropriate to wait for a representative (b) to arrive at the hospital to deactivate the AICD. The patient will require interrogation of his AICD to confirm that he was not having runs of a shockable rhythm. Either a cardiologist or company representative has the ability to do this. However, it is ill advised to let the AICD inappropriately deliver shocks to the patient while you administer pain medication (c). The AICD should not be removed (e) from the chest wall in the ED. If this procedure is required (eg, the device was a source of infection), it should be performed by a cardiothoracic surgeon in the operating room.

Recommended Readings

Amsterdam EA, Wenger NK, Brindis RG, et al. 2014 AHA/ACC guideline for the management of patients with non–ST-elevation acute coronary syndromes: executive summary: a report of the American College of Cardiology/American Heart Association Task Force on Practice Guidelines. *Circulation*. 2014;130:2354-2394.

Baigent C, Collins R, Appleby P, et al. ISIS-2: 10 year survival among patients with suspected myocardial infarction in randomized comparison of intravenous streptokinase, oral aspirin, both, or neither. The ISIS-2 (Second International Study of Survival) Collaborative Group. *BMJ*. 1998;316(7141):1337-1343.

Brown JE. Chapter 23. Chest pain. In: Marx JA, Hockberger RS, Walls RM, et al, eds. *Rosen's Emergency Medicine: Concepts and Clinical Practice*. 9th ed. Philadelphia, PA: Saunders, 2018.

Fuster V, Harrington RA, Narula J, Eapen ZJ. *Hurst's The Heart*. 14th ed. New York, NY: McGraw-Hill, 2017: 904.

LeWinter MM. Clinical practice. Acute pericarditis. *N Engl J Med*. 2014;371:2410-2416.

Meyer G. Effective diagnosis and treatment of pulmonary embolism: improving patient outcomes. *Arch Cardiovasc Dis*. 2014;107:406-414.

Sharifi M, Bay C, Skrocki L, et al. Moderate pulmonary embolism treated with thrombolysis (from the "MOPETT" Trial). *Am J Cardiol*. 2013;111(2):273-277.

Thompson JJ, Brady WJ. Chapter 68. Acute coronary syndrome. In: Marx JA, Hockberger RS, Walls RM, et al, eds. *Rosen's Emergency Medicine: Concepts and Clinical Practice*. 9th ed. Philadelphia, PA: Saunders, 2018.

Tintinalli J, Kelen G, Stapczynski J. *Emergency Medicine: A Comprehensive Study Guide*. 9th ed. New York, NY: McGraw-Hill, 2019: 193.

Wolf SJ, Shih RD, Smith MD, et al. Clinical policy: Critical issues in the evaluation and management of adult patients in the emergency department with asymptomatic elevated blood pressure. *Ann Emerg Med*. 2013;62:52-68.

Shortness of Breath

Lauren M. Titone, MD

Questions

The following scenario applies to questions 40 and 41.

A 55-year-old woman with a past medical history of hypertension presents to the emergency department (ED) because her tongue and lips feel swollen. During the history, she tells you she recently started a new blood pressure (BP) medication. Her only other medication is a baby aspirin. Her vitals at triage are BP 130/70 mm Hg, heart rate (HR) 85 beats/minute, respiratory rate (RR) 16 breaths/minute, temperature 98.7°F, and oxygen saturation 99% on room air. On physical examination, you detect mild lip and tongue swelling. Over the next hour, you notice that not only are her tongue and lips getting more swollen, but that her face is also starting to swell.

40. Which is the most likely causative agent?

a. Metoprolol
b. Furosemide
c. Aspirin
d. Lisinopril
e. Diltiazem

41. Which of the following is true regarding this condition?

a. Steroids will help minimize the swelling
b. The mechanism of action is through inhibition of prostaglandin production
c. It can occur at any point when taking the causative medication
d. The uvula is spared when significant oral swelling is present
e. Urticaria is a common skin finding

42. A 45-year-old woman presents to the ED immediately after landing at the airport from a transatlantic flight. She states that a few moments after landing, she felt short of breath with pain in her chest during deep inspiration. She takes oral contraceptive pills and levothyroxine. She is a social drinker and smokes cigarettes occasionally. Her BP is 130/75 mm Hg, HR is 105 beats/minute, RR is 20 breaths/minute, temperature is 98.9°F, and oxygen saturation is 97% on room air. You send her for a venous duplex ultrasound of her legs, which is positive for a deep vein thrombosis (DVT). What are the most appropriate initial steps in management for this patient?

a. Place the patient on a cardiac monitor and administer unfractionated heparin if no contraindications to anticoagulation exist
b. Place the patient on a cardiac monitor and order a chest computed tomography (CT) scan to confirm a pulmonary embolism (PE)
c. Place the patient on a cardiac monitor and administer aspirin
d. Instruct the patient to walk around the ED so that she remains mobile and does not exacerbate thrombus formation
e. Place the patient on a cardiac monitor and administer warfarin if no contraindications to anticoagulation exist

The following scenario applies to questions 43 and 44.

A tall, thin 18-year-old man presents to the ED with acute onset of dyspnea while at rest. The patient reports sitting at his desk when he felt a sharp pain on the right side of his chest that worsened with inspiration. His past medical history is significant for peptic ulcer disease. He reports taking a 2-hour plane trip a month ago. His initial vitals include a BP of 120/60 mm Hg, HR of 100 beats/minute, RR of 16 breaths/minute, and an oxygen saturation of 97% on room air. On physical examination, you note decreased breath sounds on the right side.

43. Which of the following tests should be performed next?

a. Echocardiogram
b. D-dimer
c. Ventilation perfusion scan (V/Q scan)
d. Upright abdominal radiograph
e. Chest radiograph

44. If a bedside ultrasound was performed, which of the following might you expect to find on scanning of the right thorax?

a. B-lines
b. A-lines
c. Lung point
d. Hepatization
e. Sinusoid sign

45. A 30-year-old woman with no significant past medical history presents to the ED complaining of chest pain, shortness of breath, and coughing up blood-streaked sputum. The patient states that she traveled to Moscow a month ago. Upon returning to the United States, the patient developed a persistent cough associated with dyspnea. She was seen by her primary care physician who diagnosed her with bronchitis and prescribed an inhaler. However, over the following weeks, the patient's symptoms worsened and she developed pleuritic chest pain. In the ED, she lets you know that she smokes half a pack per day. Her vitals include BP of 105/65 mm Hg, HR of 124 beats/minute, RR of 22 breaths/minute, temperature of 99°F, and an oxygen saturation of 94% on room air. Physical examination is non-contributory. Her electrocardiogram (ECG) reveals sinus tachycardia with large R waves in V_1 to V_3 and inverted T waves. Given this patient's history and presentation, what is the most likely etiology of her symptoms?

a. *Mycoplasma pneumoniae* pneumonia
b. Q fever pneumonia
c. *Pneumocystis jirovecii* pneumonia (PJP)
d. PE
e. Acute respiratory distress syndrome (ARDS)

46. A 24-year-old woman is brought to the ED after being found on a nearby street, hunched over, and in mild respiratory distress. Upon arrival, she is tachypneic at 28 breaths/minute with an oxygen saturation of 97% on a nonrebreather face mask. On physical examination, the patient appears to be in mild distress with supraclavicular retractions. Scattered wheezing is heard throughout bilateral lung fields. Which of the following medications should be administered first?

a. Corticosteroids
b. Magnesium sulfate
c. Epinephrine
d. Anticholinergic nebulizer treatment
e. β_2-agonist nebulizer treatment

47. A 65-year-old woman with human immunodeficiency virus (HIV) arrives to the ED in respiratory distress. A chest radiograph shows bilateral multifocal pneumonia. Despite maximum medical management, the patient decompensates and requires emergent intubation. An endotracheal tube (ETT) is placed, the balloon is inflated, the tube is attached to a bag-valve-mask (BVM), and several breaths are given. Upon auscultation, you note absent breath sounds over the left lung fields and asymmetric chest rise. Her vitals show an oxygen saturation of 98% on 100% fraction of inspired oxygen (Fio_2), BP of 123/74 mm Hg, HR of 88 beats/minute, and temperature of 101°F. Which of the following is the most appropriate initial step in management?

a. Remove the ETT and re-intubate
b. Perform a needle decompression of the left hemithorax
c. Retract the ETT 2 cm
d. Obtain a stat portable chest X-ray
e. Administer inhaled bronchodilators

48. You are evaluating a patient with shortness of breath and you appreciate decreased breath sounds at the left-lung base. You suspect the patient has a small pleural effusion. Which of the following X-ray views of the chest is most likely to detect this small pleural effusion?

a. Supine
b. Lateral decubitus with the right side down
c. Lateral decubitus with the left side down
d. Lateral
e. Posterior-anterior (PA)

The following scenario applies to questions 49 and 50.

A 32-year-old firefighter presents to the ED in acute respiratory distress. He was taken to the ED shortly after extinguishing a large fire in a warehouse. His initial vitals include a BP of 120/55 mm Hg, HR of 90 beats/minute, RR of 18 breaths/minute, and oxygen saturation of 98% on 2 L nasal cannula (NC). An ECG shows a first-degree heart block. On physical examination, there are diffuse rhonchi bilaterally. The patient is covered in soot and the hairs in his nares are singed.

49. Which of the following is most likely responsible for this patient's respiratory distress?

a. Reactive airway disease
b. Foreign-body aspiration
c. Decompression sickness
d. Thermal burns
e. Pneumothorax

50. You perform nasopharyngoscopy on this patient and notice that there appears to be soot throughout the upper airway. The patient remains in respiratory distress. Which of the following is the most appropriate next action?

a. Continuous albuterol nebulizers
b. Humidified oxygen and observation
c. Corticosteroids
d. Rapid sequence endotracheal intubation
e. Transfer to a hyperbaric chamber

The following scenario applies to questions 51 and 52.

51. A 76-year-old man presents to the ED in acute respiratory distress, gasping for breath while on oxygen via a nonrebreather face mask. Paramedics state he was found on a bench outside of his apartment in respiratory distress. Initial vitals include a BP of 170/90 mm Hg, HR of 90 beats/minute, RR of 33 breaths/minute, and oxygen saturation of 90%. On physical examination, the patient is coughing up pink, frothy sputum, has rales two-thirds of the way up both lung fields, and pitting edema of his lower extremities. A chest radiograph reveals bilateral perihilar infiltrates, an enlarged cardiac silhouette, and a small right-sided pleural effusion. After obtaining IV access and placing the patient on a monitor, which of the following medical interventions is most appropriate?

a. Morphine sulfate
b. Nitroglycerin only
c. Nitroglycerin and a loop diuretic
d. Aspirin
e. Antibiotics

52. Which of the following laboratory abnormalities is most likely based on his disease process?

a. Elevated D-dimer
b. Leukocytosis
c. Elevated troponin
d. Anemia
e. Elevated B-type natriuretic peptide (BNP)

The following scenario applies to questions 53 and 54.

A 67-year-old man is brought to the ED in respiratory distress. His initial vitals include a BP of 145/88 mm Hg, HR of 112 beats/minute, RR of 18 breaths/minute, and oxygen saturation of 92% on room air. He is also febrile at 102°F. After obtaining IV access, placing the patient on a cardiac monitor, and administering oxygen via NC, a chest radiograph is performed and shows patchy alveolar infiltrates with consolidation in the lower lobes. On review of systems, the patient tells you that he had five to six watery bowel movements a day for the last 2 days with a few bouts of emesis.

53. Which of the following infectious etiologies is most likely responsible for this patient's presentation?
a. *Streptococcus pneumoniae*
b. *Haemophilus influenzae*
c. *M. pneumoniae*
d. *Chlamydophila pneumoniae*
e. *Legionella pneumophila*

54. Which of the following laboratory abnormalities would you expect secondary to the causative organism?
a. Hyponatremia
b. Hyperkalemia
c. Hypocalcemia
d. Elevated blood urea nitrogen (BUN)
e. Thrombocytopenia

The following scenario applies to questions 55 and 56.

A 32-year-old woman presents to the ED with a 1-month history of general malaise, mild cough, and subjective fevers. She is HIV positive and 6 months ago her CD4 count was 220. She is not on antiretroviral therapy or any other medications. Initial vitals include a BP of 130/60 mm Hg, HR of 88 beats/minute, RR of 12 breaths/minute, and oxygen saturation of 91% on room air. Her chest radiograph shows bilateral diffuse interstitial infiltrates as shown in the illustration. Subsequent laboratory tests are unremarkable except for leukopenia and an elevated lactate dehydrogenase (LDH) level.

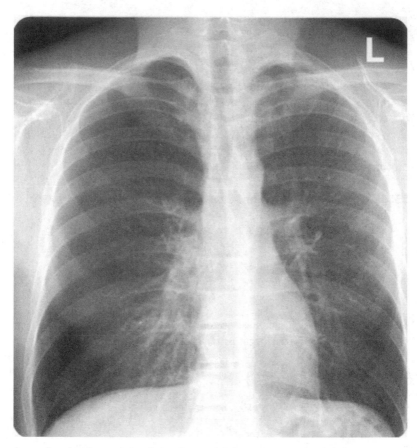

(Reproduced with permission from Adam J. Rosh, MD, and Rosh Review.)

55. Which of the following is the most likely organism responsible for her clinical presentation?

a. *Coccidioides immitis*
b. *Mycobacterium tuberculosis*
c. *Pneumocystis jirovecii*
d. *M. pneumoniae*
e. *H. influenzae*

56. Which of the following is an indication for corticosteroid administration in this patient?

a. LDH above 450 U/L
b. Oxygen saturation of 94%
c. History of asthma
d. RR above 20 breaths/minute
e. Partial pressure of oxygen (PaO_2) less than 70 mm Hg

57. A 27-year-old woman presents to the ED complaining of an intensely pruritic rash all over her body, abdominal cramping, and chest tightness. She states that 1 hour ago she was at dinner and accidentally ate soup containing seafood. She has a known anaphylactic allergy to shrimp. Her BP is 115/75 mm Hg, HR is 95 beats/minute, RR is 20 breaths/minute, temperature is 98.9°F, and oxygen saturation is 97% on room air. She appears anxious and her skin is flushed with scattered urticarial lesions. Auscultation of her lungs reveals scattered wheezes with decreased air entry. Which of the following is the most appropriate next step in management?

a. Administer oxygen via nonrebreather, place a large-bore IV, begin IV fluids, and administer methylprednisolone intravenously
b. Administer oxygen via nonrebreather, place a large-bore IV, begin IV fluids, and administer methylprednisolone and diphenhydramine intravenously
c. Administer oxygen via nonrebreather, place a large-bore IV, begin IV fluids, administer methylprednisolone and diphenhydramine intravenously, and give intramuscular epinephrine
d. Administer oxygen via nonrebreather, place a large-bore IV, begin IV fluids, and start nebulized albuterol
e. Administer oxygen via nonrebreather, place a large-bore IV, begin IV fluids, and start nebulized racemic epinephrine

58. A 42-year-old man presents to the ED via ambulance after activating emergency medical services (EMS) for dyspnea. He is currently on NC oxygen and received one nebulized treatment of a β_2-agonist by the paramedics. His initial vitals include a RR of 16 breaths/minute with an oxygen saturation of 96% on 2 L via NC. The patient appears to be in mild distress with some intercostal retractions. Upon chest auscultation, there are minimal wheezes and decreased air movement over bilateral lower lung fields. The patient's symptoms completely resolve after two more nebulizer treatments. Which of the following medications, in addition to a rescue β_2-agonist inhaler, should be prescribed for outpatient use?

a. Magnesium sulfate
b. Epinephrine autoinjector
c. Corticosteroids
d. Cetirizine
e. Ipratropium

59. A 43-year-old man is brought to the ED after being found intoxicated on the street. He is currently arousable and expresses a request to be left alone. Initial vitals include BP of 125/80 mm Hg, HR of 92 beats/minute, RR of 14 breaths/minute, and oxygen saturation of 93% on room air. His rectal temperature is 101.2°F. A chest radiograph shows infiltrates involving the right-lower lobe. Given this clinical presentation, what initial antibiotic coverage is most appropriate for this patient?

a. Gram-negative coverage only
b. Gram-positive coverage only
c. Broad-spectrum with anaerobic coverage
d. *P. jirovecii* coverage
e. Antifungal therapy

The following scenario applies to questions 60 and 61.

A 32-year-old man is brought into the ED by EMS with fever, shortness of breath, and stridor. The patient was treated the previous day in the ED for a viral syndrome and discharged home. His BP is 90/50 mm Hg, HR is 110 beats/minute, RR is 28 breaths/minute, and temperature is 101.2°F. A chest radiograph reveals a widened mediastinum. The patient is endotracheally intubated, given a 2 L bolus of normal saline, and started on antibiotics. His BP improves to 110/70 mm Hg and he is transferred to the intensive care unit (ICU). The patient's friend accompanied him to the hospital and discloses that the patient is a drum maker and frequently works with animal hides.

60. What is the most likely organism that is responsible for this patient's presentation?

a. *S. pneumoniae*
b. *Corynebacterium diphtheriae*
c. *Coxiella burnetii*
d. *H. influenzae*
e. *Bacillus anthracis*

61. Which of the following antibiotics is the treatment of choice for this condition?

a. Ceftriaxone
b. Ciprofloxacin
c. Azithromycin
d. Clindamycin
e. Cefazolin

62. A 62-year-old man presents to the ED with gradual dyspnea over the last few months, in addition to a 20-lb unintentional weight loss. He reports that he is a daily smoker and has not seen a physician in years. On physical examination, he is not in respiratory distress. There are decreased breath sounds on the right as compared to the left. A chest radiograph indicates blunting of the right costophrenic angle with a fluid line and a spiculated nodule in the right-upper lung. A thoracentesis is performed. Which of the following most likely characterizes his pleural effusion?

a. Transudative effusion
b. Exudative effusion
c. Transudative and exudative effusion
d. Fluid-to-blood LDH ratio less than 0.6
e. Fluid-to-blood protein ratio less than 0.5

63. A 57-year-old woman with a history of end-stage renal disease on hemodialysis presents with a fever and shortness of breath. On examination, she is noted to have rales in the right-mid lung. Her indwelling tunneled catheter through which she receives dialysis is neither erythematous nor tender. Her chest X-ray confirms right-middle lobe pneumonia. Which of the following is the most appropriate antibiotic choice?

a. Moxifloxacin
b. Ceftriaxone and azithromycin
c. Azithromycin
d. Vancomycin, cefepime, and azithromycin
e. Ampicillin/sulbactam and ciprofloxacin

64. Which of the following statements is true regarding pertussis infection?

a. Infection is more severe in adults than children
b. The organism is typically identified on routine sputum culture
c. Treatment is with a macrolide antibiotic
d. Antibiotics do not alter the course of illness
e. The first phase of illness involves paroxysms of cough

The following scenario applies to questions 65 and 66.

A 68-year-old man is brought in by EMS after being found sleeping underneath a nearby bridge. The patient frequently sleeps in shelters or outdoors. He complains of a cough that is productive of blood-streaked sputum which has been present for 2 months. Patient also endorses weight loss, night sweats, and general malaise over the same period of time. He does not know of any active medical problems; however, he has not sought medical treatment for many years. On exam, the patient appears cachectic, but in no acute distress. His BP is 115/63 mm Hg, HR is 82 beats/minute, RR 22 breaths/minute, temperature oxygen saturation is 93% on room air, and his temperature is 99.7°F. A chest X-ray is performed and demonstrates bilateral cavitary lesions located in the upper lobes.

65. Which of the following is true regarding this patient's diagnosis?

a. The initial infection usually causes severe symptoms
b. Active disease is diagnosed via an intradermal injection of purified protein derivative (PPD)
c. The disease is typically treated with a 5-day course of antibiotics
d. Nursing home residents are considered a low-risk population
e. The most common site of extra-pulmonary disease is the lymphatic system

66. Which of the following isolation precautions should be used when treating this patient?

a. Airborne
b. Contact
c. Droplet
d. Droplet and contact
e. Standard

67. A 57-year-old woman presents to the ED complaining of progressively worsening shortness of breath and abdominal distention over the last two weeks. She suffers from alcohol use disorder and consumes on average one pint of liquor per day for the last 10 years. On exam, the patient has yellow tinged sclera, a distended and nontender abdomen, and palmar erythema. She also has dullness to percussion and decreased tactile fremitus over the right-lower lung fields correlating with a pleural effusion noted on chest radiograph. What is the most likely physiologic cause of her pleural effusion?

a. Increased intravascular hydrostatic pressure
b. Decreased intravascular osmotic pressure
c. Increased intravascular osmotic pressure
d. Decreased intravascular hydrostatic pressure
e. Increased vascular permeability

68. A 45-year-old man presents to the ED in respiratory failure. His RR is 35 breaths/minute and his oxygen saturation is 88% on a nonrebreather face mask. The patient is endotracheally intubated and placed on a ventilator with 100% Fio_2. An arterial blood gas (ABG) is obtained 1 hour later and shows a Pao_2 of 80 mm Hg. A chest radiograph shows diffuse bilateral opacities. Based on the information provided, what is the most appropriate initial tidal volume setting in milliliters per kilogram (mL/kg)?

a. 4 mL/kg of ideal body weight (IBW)
b. 6 mL/kg of IBW
c. 6 mL/kg of actual body weight
d. 10 mL/kg of IBW
e. 10 mL/kg of actual body weight

Shortness of Breath

Answers

40. The answer is d. The patient has **angioedema**, a rare, but significant side effect of **angiotensin-converting enzyme inhibitors (ACE-I), such as lisinopril**. This type of angioedema is usually limited to the **lips, tongue, and face** and is frequently asymmetric. In severe cases, the tongue, uvula, and pharyngeal or laryngeal structures can be involved. Diagnosis is often aided by the use of nasopharyngoscopy to directly visualize these posterior structures. In cases of severe tongue, uvular, or vocal cord edema, the patient may develop **airway compromise** and emergent intubation or surgical cricothyrotomy is indicated. The medication should be immediately discontinued. Angioedema can also be caused by a type I hypersensitivity reaction or a hereditary C1 esterase deficiency.

None of the other medications listed cause angioedema (**a, b, c, and e**).

41. The answer is c. One of the curious things about ACE-I–induced angioedema is that it **can occur at any point in the course of a person taking this medication**. This is unlike a true type I hypersensitivity reaction which occurs immediately after exposure to the allergen.

The typical treatments for allergic reactions used in emergency practice are not effective against ACE-I angioedema; therefore, steroids (**a**) will not help minimize the swelling. These agents are often given in conjunction with antihistamines although they are not proven to have an effect. Most clinicians choose to give the agents in case the etiology is something other than ACE-I. The mechanism of action is related to the inhibition of bradykinin production caused by the ACE-I, not prostaglandins (**b**). Although in a mild case of angioedema, the swelling may only involve the lips and tongue, the uvula is not spared (**d**) in a severe case of angioedema. Urticaria (**e**) does not occur with ACE-I angioedema. Urticaria (or hives) are a manifestation of a type I hypersensitivity related to mast cell degranulation and histamine release which is often caused by allergen exposure and can lead to anaphylaxis.

42. The answer is a. The patient has a **confirmed venous thrombosis** and has symptoms consistent with a PE. The presence of a PE in this patient can be **presumed by a confirmed DVT with pulmonary symptoms**. All patients with concerns for PE need to be on **a monitor**. **Anticoagulation** is considered first-line therapy and should be administered promptly. Unfractionated heparin is frequently used in patients requiring hospitalization; however, low-molecular-weight (LMW) heparin or a direct oral anticoagulant (DOAC) can also be used given their rapid onset of action. Warfarin **(e)** should never be started without concomitant administration of heparin. After the international normalized ratio (INR) is at a therapeutic level (2-3 IU), heparin can be stopped and warfarin can be taken alone. Warfarin initially causes a temporary hypercoagulable state caused by warfarin's inhibition of the body's endogenous anticoagulants, proteins C and S.

A chest CT scan **(b)** is not urgently needed since a DVT is already confirmed by duplex ultrasound and should not delay administration of anticoagulation. Aspirin **(c)** is not effective in preventing propagation of a DVT. The patient requires an anticoagulant, not an antiplatelet agent. Although immobility **(d)** can lead to thrombus development and propagation, a patient with a diagnosed DVT requires urgent initiation of anticoagulation therapy as this is a more effective way to dissolve a previously formed clot.

43. The answer is e. A **spontaneous pneumothorax** typically presents with ipsilateral **pleuritic chest pain** and dyspnea while at rest. Physical findings tend to correlate with the degree of symptoms. Mild tachycardia, **decreased breath sounds** to auscultation, or **hyperresonance** to percussion are the most common findings. It typically occurs in **healthy young men of taller than average stature** without a precipitating factor. Mitral valve prolapse and Marfan syndrome are also associated with spontaneous pneumothorax. The most common condition associated with secondary spontaneous pneumothorax is chronic obstructive pulmonary disease (COPD). Although suggested by this patient's symptoms, the diagnosis of pneumothorax is generally made with a **chest radiograph**. The classic radiograph finding is the appearance of a thin, visceral, pleural line lying parallel to the chest wall, separated by a radiolucent band that is devoid of lung markings as shown in the figure below. The diagnosis can also be seen on point-of-care ultrasound by the absence of lung sliding. If clinical suspicion is high with a negative initial chest X-ray, inspiratory and expiratory films or a lateral decubitus film may be taken to evaluate for lung collapse.

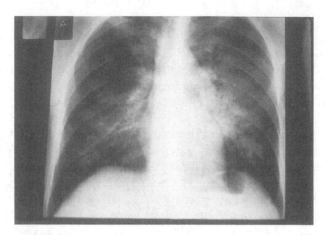

(Reproduced with permission from Knoop KJ, Stack LB, Storrow AB. Atlas of Emergency Medicine. New York, NY: McGraw Hill, 2002: 666.)

An echocardiogram (a) may be performed at a later time to evaluate for structural heart abnormalities but given the high likelihood of pneumothorax, a chest radiograph should be done first. A D-dimer (b) is a blood test used as a screening tool for pulmonary thromboembolism. A negative D-dimer can exclude the diagnosis of PE in patients with a low pretest probability. If the chest radiograph is unremarkable in this patient, sending a D-dimer may help in the workup of his dyspnea. A V/Q scan (c) also aides in the diagnosis of PE. CT angiography has emerged as a test with high sensitivity and specificity; therefore, V/Q scans are being used less frequently. They are generally reserved for institutions that do not have access to CT angiography or for individuals with a contraindication to CT angiography (eg, contrast dye allergy and renal insufficiency). An upright abdominal X-ray (d) may be helpful in the evaluation of the bowel for air fluid levels as seen in a bowel obstruction. If there is concern for a perforated viscous, the test of choice is an upright chest X-ray to identify air under the diaphragm.

44. The answer is c. The use of bedside point-of-care ultrasound in the ED has expanded to include thoracic imaging. It is helpful in evaluating the lung parenchyma for excess fluid and consolidation and also in the identification of a pneumothorax. For the evaluation of pneumothorax, the high-frequency probe is placed on the chest wall with the indicator marker toward the head. The intercostal space is identified in which you can see the layers of the chest wall (muscle, then pleural, and then the lung). In a normal lung, **lung sliding** is present and represents the movement of the visceral pleura again the parietal pleura. This can be directly visualized as a shimmering-like effect of the pleura that is accentuated with inspiration and expiration. Lung sliding will be absent in a pneumothorax as the visceral and parietal pleura are separated by air. The **lung point** is the most specific sign for pneumothorax on ultrasound and is the transition point between normal lung and pneumothorax.

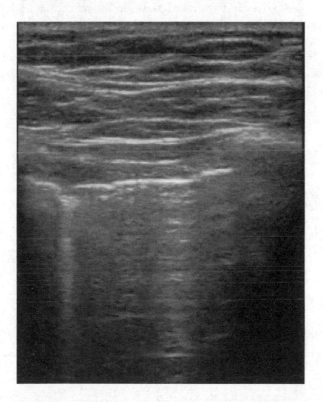

B-lines (**a**) are vertical lines spreading down into the lung parenchyma. They represent interstitial edema and are present in pulmonary edema. The more B-lines present the more edema within the lung. A-lines (**b**) are horizontal lines seen within the lung created by air artifact. They are present in a normal lung and may increase in cases of hyperinflation like asthma or COPD. Hepatization (**d**) is a process by which lung tissue consolidates and takes on the sonographic appearance of the liver. This typically occurs with pneumonia or atelectasis. The sinusoid sign (**e**) is obtained when a pleural effusion is present in the lung. When the ultrasound is placed in M-mode, the inspiratory movement of the lung toward the pleural line creates a sinusoid pattern.

45. The answer is d. In the history, there are details that lead you to suspect **PE**—obesity, recent travel, progressive dyspnea despite inhaler treatment, and blood-streaked sputum. Objectively, her ECG shows **right-heart strain** (large R waves and inverted T waves in the precordial leads V_1–V_3). This is caused by heart beating against the high resistance of the pulmonary vasculature causing back flow and resulting in right ventricular enlargement. There are several classic ECG findings in PE as shown in the figure. The lack of ECG changes, however, does not eliminate the possibility of a PE as up to 25% of patients with a PE have a normal ECG.

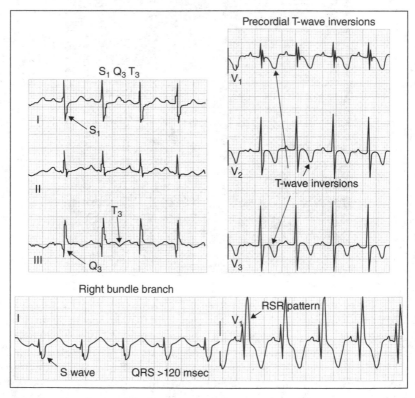

(Reproduced with permission from Adam J. Rosh, MD, and Rosh Review.)

This patient is tachycardic, tachypneic, and hypoxic; the cardinal signs of cardiovascular distress. **Dyspnea, pleuritic chest pain, or tachypnea** is present in 95% of patients with a PE. The classic triad of dyspnea, pleuritic chest pain, and hemoptysis is uncommon and present in less than 25% of patients.

M. pneumoniae (**a**) is the most common cause of atypical "walking" pneumonia. In addition to constitutional symptoms, patients may have conjunctivitis, pharyngitis, or bullous myringitis. The hallmark of the disease is the disparity between the patient's clinically benign appearance and the extensive radiographic findings. Q fever (**b**) is caused by *C. burnetii* and is typically spread by breathing in dust contaminated by animal feces, urine milk, or birth products. Infected individuals look ill, diaphoretic, and/or febrile. PCP (**c**) is seen almost exclusively in patients who are immunocompromised, such as those with acquired immunodeficiency syndrome (AIDS) or on chronic steroids or immunosuppressants. It is the most common opportunistic infection seen in HIV patients and is considered an AIDS defining illness. Patients typically present with dyspnea, nonproductive cough, and fever. Chest radiograph may be normal in up to 20% to 30% of patients. The classic chest radiograph of PCP demonstrates bilateral diffuse interstitial infiltrates in the perihilar region and extending laterally in a "bat-wing" pattern. The clinical hallmark of ARDS (**e**) is severe hypoxemia unresponsive to increased concentrations of inspired oxygen. Many different conditions can precipitate ARDS; however, gram-negative sepsis is the most common.

46. The answer is e. This patient is suffering from an **acute asthma exacerbation**. This is a reversible bronchospasm initiated by a variety of environmental factors that produce a narrowing and inflammation of the bronchial airways. The first-line treatment in order to open the airways is an **aerosolized β_2-agonist**, such as **albuterol sulfate**, which acts to decrease bronchospasm of the smooth muscle to improve linear air flow and oxygenation.

Corticosteroids (**a**) are an effective measure for decreasing the late inflammatory changes involved in asthma. Additionally, when administered in the first hour of arrival to the ED, corticosteroids decrease rates of admission and bounce back. Magnesium sulfate (**b**) works through smooth muscle relaxation and is initiated in cases of moderate to severe asthma where it has proven benefit in decreasing admission rates. Epinephrine (**c**) decreases bronchospasm through its bronchodilator effects but given its side-effect profile it should only be administered in patients deemed to be in severe respiratory distress. Anticholinergics (**d**) are effective in patients with COPD and are also administered in combination with a β_2-agonist to patients with an acute asthma exacerbation. However, they should never be given alone to treat asthma.

47. The answer is c. A common, but easily manageable complication of ETT placement is a **right mainstem bronchus intubation.** Due to the normal anatomy of the respiratory tree, if placed too deep, an ETT will preferentially enter the right mainstem bronchus. This will cause absent or diminished breath sounds on the left, asymmetric chest rise, and potentially hypoxia. Initial management is to retract the ETT tube several centimeters and auscultate bilaterally. If left undiagnosed, a right mainstem intubation can lead to barotrauma of the right lung and atelectasis of the left lung.

An esophageal intubation is possible, however, unlikely given that the patient has chest rise and a normal oxygen saturation. Re-intubating the patient (**a**) without an attempt at repositioning the tube could potentially be dangerous as it may require additional paralytics and sedation. The use of colorimetric end-tidal CO_2 detectors or quantitative waveform capnography is useful in determining esophageal versus tracheal intubation. Lack of breath sounds on the left can be due to a pneumothorax; however, this patient has no indication for an emergent needle decompression (**b**) which is reserved for a tension pneumothorax with hemodynamic instability. A tension pneumothorax typically causes mediastinal shift and decreased venous return leading to severe hypotension. This is possible after intubation and introduction of positive pressure to the pulmonary system; however, mainstem intubation is more common and should be ruled out first, especially when breath sounds are absent over the left. A portable chest X-ray (**d**) is necessary to confirm tube placement and can help diagnose a pneumothorax, however, is not the first appropriate step in this case. Bronchodilators (**e**) are often used in patients with COPD and asthma to help relax the smooth muscles of the airway.

48. The answer is c. Pleural effusions are most easily detected on a **lateral decubitus film with the affected side down**. In this scenario, this would be the patient's left side, not the right (**b**). Accumulations of 5 to 50 mL of fluid can be detected with this view.

Small effusions can be missed entirely on supine views (**a**) and are not generally apparent on PA views (**e**) and lateral views (**d**) until 200 mL or more of fluid is present. Point-of-care ultrasound is also a useful adjunct in the identification of pleural fluid.

49. The answer is d. The **singed nasal hairs** seen in this patient should give you a clue to the possibility of severe **thermal burns.** Although there is minimal external involvement, damage from the heat may extend deep into the pulmonary system through inspiration. This results in a severe inflammatory reaction causing **pneumonitis.** Early intubation is critical even when the patient does not appear to be in severe respiratory distress as the delayed effects of pneumonitis can be rapid in onset and fatal.

Although you should always consider a foreign-body aspiration **(b)** in the differential diagnosis of respiratory distress, it is not consistent with the history of this individual. Reactive airway disease **(a)** typically presents with wheezing and a pneumothorax **(e)** with decreased breath sounds. Decompression sickness **(c)** occurs when a scuba diver ascends too quickly and dissolved nitrogen bubbles reenter tissues and blood vessels.

50. The answer is d. This patient arrives in respiratory distress. In the setting of structural fires, there is always concern that the patient has deeper injuries not visualized externally. In this case, the patient has **singed nasal hairs** suggesting thermal burns deeper within the respiratory tract. Given his respiratory distress and evidence of airway burn, the appropriate next step is **prophylactic rapid sequence intubation.** In this case, nasopharyngoscopy is performed adding further evidence although his respiratory distress and singed nasal hairs are sufficient evidence for his need for intubation.

Continuous albuterol nebulizers **(a)** are helpful for patients with severe bronchospasm. This patient may have a component of bronchospasm from the smoke inhalation but his more pressing need is control of his airway before further soft tissue swelling takes place. Humidified oxygen and observation **(b)** are too conservative for this patient given his chance for quick decompensation. Corticosteroids **(c)** have no role in the treatment of inhalational injuries and are not indicated in this patient. A transfer to a hyperbaric chamber **(e)** may be indicated in cases of carbon monoxide poisoning which is always a concern in a structural fire. Carbon monoxide has a much higher affinity for hemoglobin than oxygen and when bound prevents oxygen delivery to tissues. Patients with signs of end-organ damage (ie, cardiac ischemia, syncope, and/or neurologic impairment) or high carbon monoxide levels may be transferred to a hyperbaric chamber.

51. The answer is c. Pulmonary edema can be divided into cardiogenic and noncardiogenic. Cardiogenic varieties are commonly seen in the ED and are usually a result of high intravascular hydrostatic pressures. It is seen in patients with myocardial ischemia (MI) or cardiac ischemia, cardiomyopathies, valvular heart disease, and hypertensive emergencies. **Nitroglycerin** acts to decrease the preload of the heart via venous dilation. Decreasing the preload decreases the amount of work the heart has to perform and allows it pump more effectively. A **loop diuretic** is used to induce diuresis and is also thought to act as a venous dilator. In conjunction with one another, these medications act to improve the overall functional capacity of the heart and decrease the amount of accumulating fluid in the lungs.

Morphine sulfate (**a**) is a potent opioid analgesic that also acts as a venous dilator. Its effects on preload and afterload are relatively minimal compared to nitroglycerin. It is also a respiratory depressant and should only be given in small quantities for patients with pulmonary edema, if at all. Aspirin (**d**) should be administered if there is suspicion of cardiac ischemia. If this patient had pneumonia, then antibiotics (**e**) should be given. However, the chest radiograph and clinical presentation are more consistent with acute pulmonary edema. If medical interventions are not stabilizing, preparation should be made for endotracheal intubation. Noninvasive bi level positive airway pressure devices may also be used as a temporalizing measure for oxygen delivery and to help redistribute pulmonary edema back into the intravascular space.

52. The answer is e. BNP can be used to aid in the diagnosis of the dyspneic patient. Congestive heart failure is characterized by a lack of adequate forward flow of blood due to impaired cardiac function. Poor forward flow leads to **increased end-diastolic volumes** in the left atria and ventricle. These increased volumes stretch the cardiac myocytes and increase tension on the chamber walls. In response to this stress, the heart releases BNP. Natriuretic peptides regulate the sympathetic nervous system to decrease afterload and increases natural diuresis by the kidney to decrease preload. Elevations in BNP can also be seen in pulmonary hypertension, PE, pneumonia, sepsis, and renal failure, so this test should be used in combination with history and physical exam findings. BNP can be falsely lowered by obesity and should be used with caution in patients with a high BMI.

A positive D-dimer (**a**) may be seen in PE, disseminated intravascular coagulopathy, or sepsis. A negative D-dimer can be useful in excluding a PE when there is a low pretest probability. Leukocytosis (**b**) may be present if the patient is suffering from an infectious, inflammatory, or malignant process. Troponin (**c**) is a biomarker released by cardiac myocytes during ischemia. This is seen during acute coronary syndrome or septic shock.

This patient is not experiencing chest pain and it is more likely they are suffering from fluid overload than acute cardiac ischemia. Anemia (d) is not frequently associated with congestive heart failure exacerbations.

53. The answer is e. *L. pneumophila* is an intracellular organism that lives in **aquatic** environment and is the causative agent of **Legionnaires' disease**. The organism may live in ordinary tap water and patients are infected by breathing in contaminated mist, frequently via air conditioning units. It is typically seen in the elderly and immunocompromised. Legionnaires' disease is more common in the summer, especially in August. Patients often experience a prodrome of 1 to 2 days of mild headache and myalgias followed by high fever, chills, and rigors. Cough is present in 90% of cases. Other **pulmonary manifestations** include dyspnea, pleuritic chest pain, and hemoptysis. **Gastrointestinal (GI) symptoms** include nausea, vomiting, diarrhea, and anorexia. **Neurologic symptoms** include headache, altered mental status, and rarely, focal symptoms. **Urine antigen testing** is highly specific and sensitive and, if available, very rapid in making the diagnosis.

S. *pneumoniae* (a) is the most common etiology of community-acquired pneumonia among adults. It is found in the nasopharynx of almost half of the population and may manifest itself as a lobar pneumonia. *H. influenzae* (b) is a common cause of pneumonia among patients with COPD, alcoholism, malnutrition, or malignancy. *M. pneumoniae* (c) is another common cause of community-acquired pneumonia in patients younger than the age of 40. It presents as a mild, nonproductive cough with low-grade temperature and the typical chest X-ray appearing much worse than expected with diffuse infiltrates. Bullous myringitis may also be an associated symptom. *C. pneumoniae* (d) is an intracellular parasite that is transmitted between humans by respiratory secretions or aerosols. It remains a relatively uncommon cause of pneumonia in the community.

54. The answer is a. *Legionella* pneumonia is different than other causes of pneumonia because it has characteristic laboratory findings. These include **hyponatremia** and **elevated liver function tests**. Clinically patients will also frequently have GI-related symptoms like vomiting and diarrhea when they have an active infection.

The other answer choices (b, c, d, and e) are not laboratory findings that are classically associated with this infection. Patients may have an elevated BUN secondary to dehydration if they have had decreased intake and GI losses with the infection, but it is not unique to *Legionella*.

55. The answer is c. PJP is a common opportunistic infection in the HIV/ AIDS population. It typically presents with mild subjective symptoms of cough and general malaise and is considered an AIDS defining illness along with diseases like cryptococcosis and histoplasmosis. Objectively, patients are **hypoxic** and have a chest radiograph with a bilateral interstitial process. Risk factors include a **CD4 count less than 200**. Serum LDH is also elevated in AIDS patients with PJP pneumonia and a negative test leads to a very low predictive value of active PJP. In fact, the greater the elevation in LDH, the worse the prognosis. Despite the classic PJP radiograph demonstrating bilateral diffuse interstitial infiltrates beginning in the perihilar region and extending into a "bat-wing" pattern, the chest radiograph may be normal in up to 30% of patients. In addition to Kaposi sarcoma involvement in the lungs, pulmonary infections, such as tuberculosis (TB), cytomegalovirus, and other fungal infections, should also be considered.

Coccidioidomycosis (**a**) is caused by the fungus *C. immitis*. The fungus is endemic in the southwestern United States. Confirmation of the diagnosis is made through direct observation of the fungus in smear or culture, or through the detection of serum antibodies. The chest radiograph generally reveals mediastinal or hilar adenopathy, pleural effusions, nodules, cavitations, or infiltrates. *M. tuberculosis* (**b**) is the causative organism of TB. Patients can present with chronic cough, hemoptysis, and constitutional symptoms. Because TB can present in a clinically similar fashion as PJP in immunocompromised individuals, it should also be ruled out in this patient. In classic reactivation TB, pulmonary lesions are located in the posterior segment of the right-upper lobe, apicoposterior segment of the left-upper lobe, and apical segments of the lower lobes. In the presence of HIV or other immunosuppressant disease, lesions are often atypical. Up to 20% of patients who are HIV positive with active TB disease have normal chest X-ray findings. *M. pneumoniae* (**d**) is a common cause of community-acquired pneumonia in patients younger than the age of 40. Radiographic findings are variable, but abnormalities are usually more striking than the findings on physical examination. *H. influenzae* (**e**) is common among patients with COPD, alcoholism, malnutrition, or malignancy.

56. The answer is e. The patient has PJP. This is one of the rare cases in infectious diseases where the administration of **steroids** is critical in some patients. As the organism is killed with the administration of antibiotics, a large inflammatory reaction is induced in the lung. This inflammatory reaction may actually lead to worsening respiratory distress and poorer outcomes.

Studies demonstrated that the administration of steroids to a subset of patients improved outcomes by limiting this inflammatory reaction. **Patients at risk** for this reaction, and therefore those who should receive steroids, include those with a **Pao$_2$ less than 70 mm Hg** or an **Alveolar-arterial (A-a) gradient of greater than 35 mm Hg**.

An elevated LDH is suggestive of PCP infection. A normal LDH value is a sensitive test for the exclusion of PJP. A value above 450 U/L **(a)** is not a cut off for steroid treatment. A higher LDH value does confer a worse prognosis for the infection, but does not help determine whether or not steroids are started. Oxygen saturation of 94% **(b)** suggests that a patient's Pao$_2$ may be below 70 mm Hg, but does not correlate perfectly. As it cannot be extrapolated from an oxygen saturation, an ABG is required to determine Pao$_2$ in these patients. A history of asthma **(c)** alone does not warrant steroid use; however, they should be administered if the patient has acute exacerbation of bronchospasm. RR above 20 breaths/minute **(d)** is one of the systemic inflammatory response syndrome (SIRS) criteria, but is not an indication for steroid administration.

57. The answer is c. The patient is having an **anaphylactic reaction** to the soup she ate which likely contained shrimp. Anaphylaxis refers to a severe systemic allergic reaction with variable features such as respiratory difficulty, cardiovascular collapse, pruritic skin rash, and abdominal cramping. Anaphylaxis is a hypersensitivity reaction caused by a **type I hypersensitivity IgE-mediated** reaction. Foods are the major cause in cases of anaphylaxis in which a source can be determined. Common foods that incite anaphylaxis include **nuts, shellfish,** and **eggs**. In the ED, attention is focused on reversing cardiovascular and respiratory disturbances. **Epinephrine** is the first drug of choice for patients with anaphylaxis and can often be lifesaving. The route of administration is chosen by the severity of the patient's presentation. In a patient with severe upper airway obstruction or worsening hypotension, IV epinephrine should be administered. Patients with relatively stable vital signs can receive intramuscular epinephrine. Many patients with known allergies carry epinephrine autoinjectors that they can self-administer in the outpatient setting. Antihistamines, both H$_1$ antagonists (**diphenhydramine**) and H$_2$ antagonists (famotidine), should be used in all cases. These drugs block the action of circulating histamines at target tissue receptors. Corticosteroids, such as **methylprednisolone,** have an onset of action approximately 4 to 6 hours after administration and are of limited value in the acute setting. Giving steroids early may, however, blunt the biphasic reaction of anaphylaxis and should be administered initially along with antihistamines.

Nebulized albuterol (d) is appropriate for treatment of anaphylaxis. Racemic epinephrine (e) is more commonly used for croup. They are both adjunctive therapies to assist with dilatation of the pulmonary tree but should never be given alone to treat anaphylaxis or prior to IM/IV epinephrine. Both diphenhydramine and methylprednisolone (**a and b**) should be given; however, the patient requires treatment with epinephrine first and foremost.

58. The answer is c. **Corticosteroids** have been shown to improve asthma symptoms in subsequent days after an exacerbation and prevent acute recurrences in patients who are deemed suitable to be discharged from the ED. An acceptable dosage is 40 to 60 mg prednisone daily for 3 to 10 days after the initial event. Inhaled steroids may also be an alternative to prevent relapses in more intractable cases and should be used daily with the guidance of the patient's primary care provider. Spacers are available to ensure adequate delivery of aerosolized medications deep into the alveoli.

Cetirizine (**d**) is an H_1 antagonist and is used primarily in the management of allergic rhinitis. Ipratropium (**e**) is an inhaled anticholinergic medication that is used in the management of COPD. Although it is usually administered in the acute care of asthma, it is not indicated for asthma maintenance. Adequate amounts of magnesium (**a**) should be obtained in the patient's diet. Epinephrine autoinjectors (**b**) are only indicated for those patients who suffer severe allergic reactions and are not routinely given to patients with asthma.

59. The answer is c. Aspiration of oropharyngeal or gastric contents into the lower airways may cause a pulmonary inflammatory response called pneumonitis. This inflammation can progress to **aspiration pneumonia**. Aspiration leading to pulmonary disease is often seen in those patients with **swallowing difficulties,** such as after a stroke, or a **relaxed lower esophageal sphincter** because of **alcohol use.** Given these factors, this patient is in a high-risk category for aspiration pneumonia. The small degree of angulation of the right mainstem bronchus makes the right lung at higher risk. Most particles easily travel down this route, ending up in the **right middle or lower lobe** of the lung. The patient's chest X-ray shows classic findings for aspiration pneumonia and **antibiotic coverage** should be **broad,** covering for both **gram-positive and gram-negative organisms including anaerobes,** which are commonly present in the GI tract.

Gram-negative organisms **(a)**, such as *H. influenzae, Pseudomonas aeruginosa, Klebsiella pneumoniae,* and *Escherichia coli,* are the most frequent causes of nosocomial pneumonia. Gram-positive organisms **(b)** such as *S. pneumoniae* and *Staphylococcus aureus* are most commonly associated with community-acquired pneumonia. *P. jirovecii* **(d)** is found in immunocompromised patients, such as those with AIDS or those receiving immunosuppressants secondary to organ transplantation. Patient with alcohol use disorder are also at risk for fungal pneumonia **(e)**; however, treatment should not be initiated unless there is high clinical suspicion.

60. The answer is e. Inhalation anthrax is a rare but life-threatening disease caused by inhalation of *B. anthracis* spores. Initially, the patient develops flu-like symptoms; however, within 24 to 48 hours, the clinical course may abruptly deteriorate to **septic shock, respiratory failure,** and **mediastinitis**. Chest X-ray may reveal a **widened mediastinum** due to hilar lymphadenopathy. Death usually results within 3 days and mortality rates exceed 90%. Anthrax is normally a disease of sheep, cattle, and horses. Working with **untreated animal hides** or **raw wool** increases the risk for anthrax exposure. There is no evidence for human-to-human transmission, but spores can be inhaled from a powdered form which was used in bioterrorism attacks in the early 2000s.

Though *S. pneumoniae* and *H. influenzae* **(a and d)** can cause respiratory failure, it is unlikely to occur in a healthy 32-year-old patient. Diphtheria **(b)** is a potentially life-threatening disease that is characterized by a gray-green pseudomembrane covering the tonsils and pharyngeal mucosa. *C. burnetii* **(c)** is the organism that causes Q fever. It is similar to *B. anthracis* in that sheep, cattle, and goats are the primary reservoirs. It can cause, hepatitis, headaches, and cardiac manifestation such as endocarditis and pericarditis. Deterioration due to Q fever is not as rapid as that seen in anthrax.

61. The answer is b. Ciprofloxacin is the treatment of choice for inhalational anthrax infection. Doxycycline is also considered first line and may cause fewer GI side effects than a fluoroquinolone. These treatments are preferred regardless of age despite the known side effects of fluoroquinolones and tetracyclines in the pediatric population. In combination with a vaccine, these antibiotics can also be used prophylactically in patients who may have had exposure. Traditionally anthrax infectious were treated with penicillin; however, there is some concern that weapons grade anthrax may be resistant so they are considered a less desirable agent until antibiotic sensitivity can be performed.

Cephalosporins (**a and e**) are not used due to resistance. The other antibiotics listed (**c, and d**) are also not effective against anthrax infection.

62. The answer is b. Given this patient's long-standing history of **tobacco** use and the presence of a nodule in the upper lung, it is likely that the pleural effusion is **exudative** as a result of an underlying **malignancy**. Other causes of exudative effusions include infection, connective tissue diseases, neoplasm, pulmonary emboli, uremia, pancreatitis, esophageal rupture— postsurgical, trauma, and drug induced. Pleural fluid analysis includes LDH, glucose, protein, amylase, cell count, Gram stain, culture, and cytology. Exudative effusions are defined by Light's criteria. The fluid must meet one of the following criteria to be considered exudative: fluid-to-blood LDH ratio greater than 0.6, a fluid-to-blood protein ratio greater than 0.5, or a pleural fluid LDH greater than two-thirds the serum LDH upper limit of normal.

A low fluid-to-blood protein or LDH ratio (**d and e**) is associated with a transudative effusion. Causes of transudative effusions (**a**) include CHF, hypoalbuminemia, cirrhosis, nephrotic syndrome, superior vena cava syndrome, and peritoneal dialysis. An effusion cannot be both exudative and transudative (**c**).

63. The answer is d. This patient has pneumonia. Although you are not given information about recent hospitalizations, the patient must be treated for **healthcare-associated pneumonia** because of the history of hemodialysis. Patients who are chronically on hemodialysis are at risk for healthcare-associated infections. The two infections that must be specifically covered are *P. aeruginosa* **and methicillin-resistant** *S. aureus* (**MRSA**). MRSA is a less common cause of pneumonia but the patient has an indwelling catheter which increases their risk and therefore necessitates coverage with an antibiotic such as vancomycin. Cefepime and piperacillin/tazobactam are often used to cover pseudomonas. It is important to remember that the patient must also receive coverage that is adequate for the usual pneumonia causing pathogens which is why azithromycin is still included as it provides coverage for atypical infections.

Moxifloxacin (**a**) is a broad-spectrum fluoroquinolone antibiotic that is frequently prescribed as a single agent for patients with community-acquired pneumonia. However, in this case, coverage with moxifloxacin alone is inadequate since it does not provide activity against *Pseudomonas* or MRSA. Ceftriaxone and azithromycin (**b**) are the alternative recommendation for coverage against community-acquired pneumonia, achieving good gram positive, gram negative, and atypical coverage. Azithromycin (**c**) alone is sometimes prescribed for outpatient therapy of community-acquired pneumonia. It does not provide adequate coverage for the spectrum of organisms which can infect a patient on long-term hemodialysis. Ampicillin/sulbactam and ciprofloxacin (**e**) provide very broad activity including likely some anaerobic coverage by the former. *Pseudomonas* coverage can be achieved with ciprofloxacin; however, ampicillin/sulbactam does not have activity against MRSA.

64. The answer is c. *Bordetella pertussis* is a gram-negative bacillus that causes a respiratory illness most commonly in the summer and fall months. Classically, the disease infects unvaccinated infants (<1-year-old). Over time, immunity conferred by the pediatric vaccine loses its effectiveness and as a result we have seen a resurgence of this infection, but overall incidence has decreased over the last 20 years. There are **three stages** of illness: (1) Catarrhal—characterized by sneezing, rhinorrhea, and coughing; (2) Paroxysmal—frequent coughing episodes followed by an inspiratory "whoop" and posttussive emesis; (3) Convalescent—chronic cough lasting several months. First-line treatment is with **macrolides**, preferably azithromycin, for 5 days. Trimethoprim/sulfamethoxazole for 14 days may also be used in the case of allergy.

Pertussis infections in the adult population (**a**) are less severe than that in infants and children and they can act as asymptomatic carriers. The organism is not easily identified on routine sputum culture (**b**) and definitive diagnosis usually requires polymerase chain reaction (PCR) via nasopharyngeal swabs or serologic detection of antibodies. Antibiotics (**d**) impact the course of illness but only when they are prescribed early. Treatment is most effective when started within the first week of symptoms. After 2 weeks of infection, the role of antibiotics is primarily to decrease transmission to others. Antitussives have not shown to be effective in reducing the cough symptoms. As mentioned earlier, the first phase of illness (**e**) is the catarrhal phase. The paroxysms of cough occur in phase 2.

65. The answer is e. This patient is suffering from active **reactivation TB** caused by the slow growing anaerobic rod *M. tuberculosis*. This bacterium settles in areas of high oxygen concentrations, so preferentially infects the lungs and more specifically the **apices**. More than one-third of the world's population is infected with the bacteria, and it is the second leading infectious cause of death worldwide. Risk factors include immigration from a high-risk area, HIV, residents and staff of prisons or shelters, alcoholics and IV drug users, and elderly and nursing home patients. When a patient is first infected, they enter the **primary TB** phase. This stage is usually **asymptomatic**, although some may experience symptoms of a common cold. Radiographic findings consistent with active primary TB are similar to those of lobar pneumonia with ipsilateral hilar adenopathy. Following the initial infection, the disease progresses to the **latent infection** phase. Here the bacteria lie dormant, many times for years, in granulomas called tubercles. Only 13% of those infected will go on to develop reactivation TB. Reactivation is most common in those with compromised immune systems. This phase is classically characterized by constitutional symptoms, cough, hemoptysis, pleuritic chest pain, and dyspnea as the infection spreads through the lungs. Findings on chest X-ray include cavitary or non-cavitary lesions in the upper lobes or superior segment of the lower lobes. Twenty percent of cases will have extrapulmonary manifestations and the most common site is the lymphatic system where it causes painless lymphadenopathy commonly referred to as **scrofula**.

After initial infection, most patients are asymptomatic and those with symptoms are usually very mild **(a)**. Twenty percent of patients with active TB have a negative test after injection of PPD making it an unreliable test **(b)**. PPD placement is best used for the diagnosis of latent TB. Active TB is often diagnosed via cultures and/or nucleic acid amplification (NAAT) tests of induced sputum. Due to the fact that *M. tuberculosis* is a very slow growing organism, treatment for TB includes a long course of antituberculous medications, often lasting 26 to 31 weeks **(c)**. Multiple drugs, including pyrazinamide, rifampin, isoniazid, and ethambutol are administered concurrently to overcome resistance. Nursing home residents **(d)** and the elderly are considered a high-risk population.

66. The answer is a. TB caused by *M. tuberculosis* is spread through **airborne particles** which are generated when an infected person speaks, coughs, sneezes, etc. These particles are small, measuring approximately 1 to 5 microns. Airborne precautions require standard precaution plus the use of an N95 or powered air-purifying respirator (PAPR). The patient should also be placed in a **negative pressure room**.

Contact precautions (**b**) are used to prevent transmission of multidrug-resistant organisms (MDRO) such as MRSA and vancomycin-resistant *enterococcus* (VRE). This involves standard precautions plus the use of a gown and gloves at all times when near the patient. Droplet precautions (**c**) are used for diseases that spread via such as influenza, mycoplasma, and *Neisseria meningitidis*. Droplets also spread via the air but the particles are larger than those spread via airborne transmission and thus do not require a respirator. These precautions include standard precautions plus the use of a face mask and eye protection. Droplet and contact precautions (**d**) would not be sufficient to protect providers from an airborne disease. Standard precautions (**e**) should be used during every patient encounter, regardless of their infectious status, and include proper hand hygiene and gloves when touching body fluids, nonintact skin, mucous membranes, and contaminated items.

67. The answer is b. This patient is showing signs of **portal hypertension** likely secondary to her long-term alcohol use. Alcoholism can lead to **alcoholic hepatitis.** Over time, this process replaces normal liver parenchyma with fibrotic tissue leading to **cirrhosis.** Signs of cirrhosis include abdominal distention due to buildup of **ascites,** electrolyte derangements, and **hepatic encephalopathy** from elevated ammonia levels. Decreased **albumin** production by the liver can also be seen with cirrhosis leading to decreased intravascular oncotic pressure. Albumin functions to keep fluid inside the vessels and therefore its absence causes fluid to leak out of the vessel and can lead to fluid collections such as abdominal ascites and **pleural effusions.** Effusions as well as upward displacement of the diaphragm from increased intra-abdominal pressure can cause dyspnea in patients with cirrhosis.

Increased intravascular hydrostatic pressure (**a**) is the cause of peripheral and pulmonary edema observed in patients with congestive heart failure. Decrease forward flow due to heart failure leads to a backup of fluid in the venous system. The increased fluid exerts hydrostatic pressure on the vessel walls and leaks out into the interstitium. Increased vascular permeability (**e**) is often seen in sepsis and inflammation and is the cause of distributive shock. As the integrity of the endothelial cells lining the vasculature decompensates, fluid leaks out causing a third-spacing effect as well as intravascular volume depletion. High intravascular oncotic pressure (**c**) would draw fluid into the vasculature from the interstitium. Decreased intravascular hydrostatic pressure (**d**) can be secondary to volume depletion from dehydration or hemorrhage and would not cause a pleural effusion.

68. The answer is b. This patient is suffering from **ARDS**. ARDS is a severe form of **acute lung injury** (ALI). It is characterized by hypoxemia that is resistant to oxygen therapy due to diffuse alveolar damage. ARDS can be caused by a variety of etiologies including pneumonia, smoke inhalation, aspiration, drowning, contusion/trauma, and septic shock. Chest radiographs can show a variety of findings; however, diffuse infiltrates consistent with alveolar edema are common. ARDS is characterized by a **Pao_2/Fio_2** ratio of less than 300 mm Hg. This patient's ratio is 80 mm Hg, placing him in the severe ARDS category. Due to the extensive nature of their lung injury, many patients suffering from ARDS require mechanical ventilation. While they can deliver high concentrations of oxygen, ventilators can also cause barotrauma to the alveoli and can worsen the disease process. A low tidal volume, lung-protective strategy is favored in order to minimize the volume of air forced into the lungs by the ventilator. Several recent trials have looked at the most effective ventilator strategies in ARDS and have found that the ideal starting tidal volume is **6 to 8 mL/kg of (predicted) IBW**. IBW is calculated using sex and height.

Actual body weight (**c and e**) may not accurately represent a patient's lung capacity and if used to calculate tidal volume can lead to significant lung injury. For example, two male patients who are 68 inches tall likely have the same lung capacity regardless of their measured body weight and therefore IBW is preferred. 4 mL/kg (**a**) and 10 mL/kg (**d**) are too low and high, respectively.

Recommended Readings

Braithwaite SA, Perina D. Chapter 22: Dyspnea. In: Walls RM, Hockberger RS, Gausche-Hill M, eds. *Rosen's Emergency Medicine: Concepts and Clinical Practice*. 9th ed. Philadelphia, PA: Elsevier, 2018.

Deakins KM. Year in review 2014: asthma. *Respir Care*. 2015;60:744-748.

Lewis C, Mathew C, Lewis C, Swartz J, et al. Acute Dyspnea. WikEM, The Global Emergency Medicine Wiki. September 14, 2019. Available at: https://wikem.org/wiki/Acute_dyspnea. Accessed May 22, 2020.

Lewis LN, Tozer J. Approach to Shortness of Breath. SAEM CDEM M4 Curriculum. 2019. Available at: https://www.saem.org/cdem/education/online-education/m4-curriculum/group-m4-approach-to/shortness-of-breath. Accessed May 22 2020.

Mosier JM, Hypes C, Joshi R, et al. Ventilator strategies and rescue therapies for management of acute respiratory failure in the emergency department. *Ann Emerg Med.* 2015;66(5):529-541.

Sovari AA, Kocheril AG, Baas AS. Cardiogenic Pulmonary Edema. Available at: http://emedicine.medscape.com/article/157452-overview. Accessed May 22, 2020.

Stapczynski JS. Chapter 62: Respiratory distress. In: Tintinalli JE, Ma O, Yealy DM, et al, eds. *Tintinalli's Emergency Medicine: A Comprehensive Study Guide.* 9th ed. New York, NY: McGraw-Hill, 2020.

Abdominal and Pelvic Pain

Jonah Gunalda, MD

Questions

69. An 81-year-old diabetic woman with a history of atrial fibrillation is transferred to your emergency department (ED) from the local nursing home with a note from the facility stating that she was complaining of abdominal pain and vomited once. Her vital signs in the ED are blood pressure (BP) 105/75 mm Hg, heart rate (HR) 95 beats/minute, respiratory rate (RR) 18 breaths/minute, and temperature 100.1°F. The patient appears very uncomfortable and has not stopped moaning in pain since arriving to the ED. You are surprised to find that her abdomen is soft and nontender on palpation. Which of the following diagnostic tests is most likely to reveal the cause of her symptoms?

a. Capsule endoscopy
b. Colonoscopy
c. Computed tomography (CT) angiography of the abdomen
d. Ultrasound
e. Abdominal radiograph

The following scenario applies to questions 70 and 71.

A 49-year-old man with a history of alcoholism presents to the ED with nausea, vomiting, and abdominal pain that began approximately 2 days ago. He usually drinks a six-pack of beer daily, but increased his drinking to two six packs daily over the last week because of increased stress at work. He notes decreased appetite over the last 3 days and states he has not had anything to eat in 2 days. His BP is 125/75 mm Hg, HR is 105 beats/minute, and RR is 20 breaths/minute. You note generalized abdominal tenderness on examination. Laboratory results reveal the following:

White blood cells (WBC) 9,000/μL

Hematocrit 48%

Platelets 210/μL

Aspartate transaminase
(AST) 85 U/L

Alanine transaminase
(ALT) 60 U/L

Alkaline phosphatase 75 U/L

Total bilirubin 0.5 mg/dL

Lipase 40 IU

Sodium 131 mEq/L

Potassium 3.5 mEq/L

Chloride 101 mEq/L

Bicarbonate 10 mEq/L

Blood urea nitrogen (BUN)
9 mg/dL

Creatinine 0.5 mg/dL

Glucose 190 mg/dL

Nitroprusside test weakly positive
for ketones

70. Which of the following is the mainstay of therapy for patients with this condition?

a. Normal saline (NS) infusion
b. Half normal saline (½NS) infusion
c. Glucose solution (D_5W) infusion
d. Solution containing both saline and glucose (D_5/NS or D_5 ½NS)
e. Insulin drip

71. The patient is admitted to the hospital for treatment. Several hours later, he becomes agitated, tremulous, and diaphoretic. He is tachycardic and hypertensive. He also reports auditory and visual hallucinations. What is the most likely cause of his symptoms?

a. Wernicke encephalopathy
b. Subdural hematoma
c. Alcohol withdrawal
d. Drug overdose
e. Underlying psychiatric illness

72. A 38-year-old woman presents to the ED with abdominal pain. She reports that over the past 2 days she gets pain in her right-upper quadrant (RUQ) shortly after eating. As you palpate her abdomen, you notice that she stops her inspiration for a brief moment due to increased pain. Her vitals include a BP of 130/75 mm Hg, HR of 95 beats/minute, RR of 16 breaths/minute, and temperature of 100.4°F. What is the initial diagnostic test of choice for this condition?

a. Plain film radiograph
b. CT scan
c. Magnetic resonance imaging (MRI)
d. Radioisotope cholescintigraphy [hepatobiliary iminodiacetic acid (HIDA) scan]
e. Ultrasonography

73. A 31-year-old man without significant past medical history presents to the ED complaining of severe pain in his left flank that radiates to his left testicle. It waxes and wanes in intensity. He also noticed some blood in his urine in the morning. He had an episode of similar pain last week that resolved spontaneously. His BP is 145/75 mm Hg, HR is 90 beats/minute, RR is 24 breaths/minute, and temperature is 98.9°F. As you examine the patient, he vomits and has trouble lying still in his stretcher. His abdomen is soft and nontender. Which of the following is the most appropriate next step in management?

a. Call surgery consult to evaluate the patient for appendicitis
b. Order an abdominal CT
c. Start intravenous (IV) fluids and administer an IV nonsteroidal anti-inflammatory drug (NSAID) and antiemetic
d. Perform an ultrasound to evaluate for an abdominal aortic aneurysm (AAA)
e. Perform an ultrasound to evaluate for testicular torsion

74. A 57-year-old woman presents to the ED with several hours of abdominal pain and vomiting. You examine her abdomen and note that it is distended and there is a small midline scar in the lower abdomen. Upon auscultation, you hear high-pitched "tinkling" bowel sounds. Palpation elicits pain in all four quadrants, but no rebound tenderness. She is guaiac negative. Which of the following is the most likely to be responsible for this patient's symptoms?

a. Travel to Mexico
b. Ethanol abuse
c. Previous hysterectomy
d. Previous hernia repair
e. Constipation

75. A 41-year-old homeless man walks into the ED complaining of abdominal pain, nausea, and vomiting. He tells you that he has been drinking beer continuously over the previous 18 hours. On examination, his vitals are BP 150/75 mm Hg, HR 104 beats/minute, RR 16 breaths/minute, temperature 99.1°F, and oxygen saturation 97% on room air. A finger stick glucose is 81 mg/dL. The patient is alert and oriented and his pupils are anicteric. You notice gynecomastia and spider angiomata. His abdomen is soft but tender in the RUQ. Laboratory tests reveal an AST of 212 U/L, ALT of 170 U/L, alkaline phosphatase of 98 U/L, total bilirubin of 1.9 mg/dL, international normalized ratio (INR) of 1.3, and WBC of 12,000/µL. Urinalysis shows 1+ protein. Chest X-ray is unremarkable. Which of the following is the most appropriate next step in management?

a. Place a nasogastric (NG) tube in the patient's stomach to remove any remaining ethanol
b. Order a HIDA scan to evaluate for acute cholecystitis
c. Administer hepatitis B immune globulin
d. Send viral hepatitis titers
e. Provide supportive care by correcting any fluid and electrolyte imbalances

76. A 48-year-old man with a past medical history of hepatitis C and cirrhosis presents to the ED complaining of abdominal pain and chills. His BP is 118/75 mm Hg, HR is 105 beats/minute, RR is 16 breaths/minute, temperature is 101.2°F, and oxygen saturation is 97% on room air. His abdomen is distended and diffusely tender. You perform a paracentesis and retrieve 1 liter of cloudy fluid. Laboratory analysis of the fluid shows a neutrophil count of 550 cells/mm^3. Which of the following is the most appropriate treatment?

a. Metronidazole
b. Vancomycin
c. Sulfamethoxazole/trimethoprim (SMX/TMP)
d. Neomycin and lactulose
e. Cefotaxime

The following scenario applies to questions 77 and 78.

A 24-year-old man woke up from sleep 1 hour ago with severe pain in his right testicle. He states that he is sexually active with multiple partners. On examination, the right scrotum is swollen, tender, and firm. You are unable to elicit a cremasteric reflex. His BP is 145/75 mm Hg, HR is 103 beats/minute, RR is 14 breaths/minute, temperature is 98.9°F, and oxygen saturation is 99% on room air.

77. Which of the following is the most appropriate next step in management?

a. Administer intramuscular (IM) ceftriaxone and oral azithromycin, then discharge home with urology follow-up
b. Swab his urethra for gonorrhea and *Chlamydia* culture and treat if positive
c. Send a urinalysis and treat for a urinary tract infection (UTI) if positive
d. Treat the patient for epididymitis and have him return if symptoms persist
e. Consult urology and order a STAT Doppler ultrasound of the testicle

78. Patients presenting with testicular torsion within what time period from symptom onset have the highest rate of testicular salvage?

a. 1 hour
b. 2 hours
c. 6 hours
d. 12 hours
e. 24 hours

79. A 28-year-old man presents to the ED complaining of constant, vague, diffuse abdominal pain. He reports decreased appetite and nausea since eating sushi last night. His BP is 125/75 mm Hg, HR is 96 beats/minute, RR is 16 breaths/minute, and temperature is 100.5°F. On examination, his abdomen is moderately tender in the right-lower quadrant (RLQ). Palpation of the left-lower quadrant (LLQ) elicits pain in the RLQ. Laboratory results reveal a WBC of 12,000/µL. Urinalysis shows 1+ leukocyte esterase. The patient is convinced that his symptoms are due to food poisoning from the sushi and is requesting an antacid. Which of the following is the most appropriate next step in management?

a. Order a plain radiograph to look for dilated bowel loops
b. Administer a proton-pump inhibitor (PPI) and observe for 1 hour
c. Send the patient for an abdominal ultrasound
d. Order an abdominal CT scan
e. Discharge the patient home with ciprofloxacin

80. A 23-year-old woman presents to the ED with LLQ pain that began suddenly and is associated with nausea and vomiting. This is the second time this month that she experienced pain in this location; however, this time it is more severe. Her BP is 120/75 mm Hg, HR is 109 beats/minute, RR is 18 breaths/minute, and temperature is 99.5°F. On examination, she appears extremely uncomfortable. Her abdomen is tender in the LLQ and she also has tenderness to palpation of the left adnexa on pelvic examination. Which of the following is the most appropriate initial diagnostic test for the patient?

a. CT scan of the abdomen/pelvis
b. MRI of the abdomen/pelvis
c. X-ray of the abdomen
d. Doppler ultrasound of the pelvis
e. Diagnostic laparoscopy

81. A 55-year-old man presents to the ED complaining of diffuse abdominal pain. He underwent a routine colonoscopy the previous day and reports that "everything was fine." The pain began upon waking up and is associated with nausea. He denies fever, vomiting, diarrhea, or rectal bleeding. His BP is 143/71 mm Hg, HR is 87 beats/minute, RR is 16 breaths/minute, temperature is 98.9°F, and oxygen saturation is 96% on room air. His abdomen is tense but only mildly tender. His chest radiograph is seen in the figure. Which of the following is the most likely diagnosis?

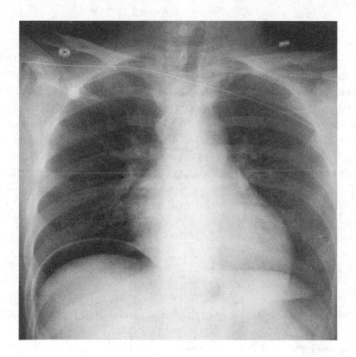

a. Ascending cholangitis
b. Acute pulmonary edema
c. Acute liver failure
d. Pancreatitis
e. Pneumoperitoneum

82. A 78-year-old woman is brought to the ED by emergency medical services (EMS) with vomiting and abdominal pain that began during the night. Her BP is 90/50 mm Hg, HR is 110 beats/minute, RR is 18 breaths/minute, and temperature is 101.2°F. She appears jaundiced. She winces when you palpate her RUQ. An ultrasound reveals dilation of the common bile duct and stones in the gallbladder. What is the most likely diagnosis?

a. Cholecystitis
b. Acute hepatitis
c. Cholangitis
d. Pancreatic cancer
e. Bowel obstruction

The following scenario applies for questions 83 and 84.

A 71-year-old obese man is brought to the ED complaining of constant left-mid abdominal pain with radiation into his back that began abruptly 1 hour ago. His past medical history is significant for hypertension, peripheral vascular disease, and kidney stones. He smokes a pack of cigarettes daily. His BP is 90/60 mm Hg, HR is 120 beats/minute, RR is 16 breaths/minute, and temperature is 98.9°F. Abdominal examination is unremarkable. An electrocardiogram (ECG) shows sinus tachycardia. An abdominal radiograph reveals normal loops of bowel and curvilinear calcification of the aortic wall.

83. Which of the following is the most likely diagnosis?

a. Biliary colic
b. Nephrolithiasis
c. Pancreatitis
d. Small bowel obstruction (SBO)
e. AAA

84. What is the best next step in the management of this patient?

a. Assess orthostatic vital signs after IV fluid bolus
b. Insert NG tube for gastric decompression
c. Consult vascular surgery and prepare for emergent transfusion
d. Obtain a right-sided ECG
e. Perform an emergent pericardiocentesis

85. A 51-year-old man presents to the ED complaining of epigastric pain that radiates to his back. He states that he drinks six packs of beer daily. His BP is 135/75 mm Hg, HR is 90 beats/minute, RR is 17 breaths/minute, and temperature is 100.1°F. Laboratory results reveal WBC 13,000/μL, hematocrit 48%, platelets 110/μL, amylase 1150 U/L, lipase 1450 IU, lactate dehydrogenase (LDH) 150 U/L, sodium 135 mEq/L, potassium 3.5 mEq/L, chloride 105 mEq/L, bicarbonate 23 mEq/L, BUN 15 mg/dL, creatinine 1.1 mg/dL, and glucose 125 mg/dL. Which of the following laboratory values are most specific for acute pancreatitis?

a. Elevated amylase
b. Hyperglycemia
c. Elevated lipase
d. Elevated LDH
e. Leukocytosis

86. A 40-year-old woman presents to the ED complaining of fever and 1 day of increasing pain in her RUQ. She denies nausea or vomiting or worsening of pain after eating. The patient returned from a trip to Mexico 6 months ago. About 2 weeks ago, she experienced intermittent diarrhea with blood-streaked mucus. Her BP is 130/80 mm Hg, HR is 107 beats/minute, RR is 17 breaths/minute, and temperature is 102°F. Physical examination reveals decreased breath sounds over the right lung base. Abdominal examination is notable for tenderness to palpation in RUQ. Murphy sign is negative. Her WBC is 20,500/µL. Chest radiograph reveals a small right pleural effusion. Which of the following is the most likely diagnosis?

a. Amebic abscess
b. Cholecystitis
c. Cryptosporidium
d. Enterobiasis
e. Pyogenic abscess
f. Begin fluid resuscitation, IV antibiotics, and observe the patient for 24 hours
g. Order an abdominal ultrasound, and administer antiemetics and analgesics

87. A 25-year-old woman presents to the ED with a 6-hour history of worsening lower abdominal pain, most severe in the RLQ. She also noticed some vaginal spotting in the morning. She also reports nausea, but no vomiting. Her last menstrual period was 2 months ago, but her cycles are always irregular. She is sexually active and has a history of pelvic inflammatory disease (PID). Her BP is 120/75 mm Hg, HR is 95 beats/minute, RR is 16 breaths/minute, and temperature is 99.2°F. Her abdomen is tender in the RLQ and pelvic examination reveals right adnexal tenderness. β-human chorionic gonadotropin (β-hCG) is positive. After establishing IV access, which of the following is the most appropriate next step in management?

a. Consult gynecology for emergent laparoscopy
b. Order an emergent CT scan of the abdomen
c. Perform a transvaginal ultrasound
d. Order a urinalysis
e. Swab her cervix and treat for *Neisseria gonorrhoeae* and *Chlamydia trachomatis*

88. A 68-year-old man presents to the ED by EMS from his nursing home for abdominal pain and abdominal distension. He appears chronically debilitated and uncomfortable. He is not obese, but his abdomen appears moderately distended. A digital rectal exam reveals no gross blood and an empty rectal vault. An abdominal radiograph is obtained and shown below. Which of the following is the most likely diagnosis?

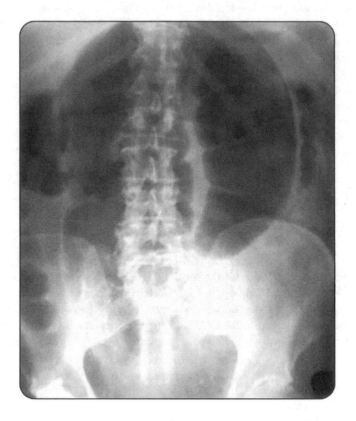

a. SBO
b. Sigmoid volvulus
c. Gastric outlet obstruction
d. Irritable bowel syndrome
e. Pneumoperitoneum

89. A 19-year-old woman presents to the ED with 1 hour of progressively worsening pain in her RLQ that began acutely. Shortly after the pain began, she felt nauseous and vomited twice. Her BP is 123/78 mm Hg, HR is 99 beats/minute, RR is 16 breaths/minute, and temperature is 99.1°F. The patient appears uncomfortable and is writhing in pain. Her abdomen is nondistended, diffusely tender with maximal tenderness in the RLQ. Pelvic examination is significant for right-sided adnexal tenderness. Laboratory results reveal WBC 10,000/μL, hematocrit 38%, and a negative urinalysis and β-hCG. Pelvic ultrasound reveals an enlarged right ovary with decreased flow. Which of the following is the most appropriate next step in management?

a. Admit to the gynecology service for observation
b. Administer IV antibiotics
c. Attempt manual detorsion
d. Order an abdominal CT
e. Consult gynecology for immediate laparoscopic surgery

90. An 18-year-old woman presents to the ED complaining of bilateral lower abdominal pain. She also describes the loss of appetite over the last 12 hours, but denies nausea and vomiting. Her BP is 124/77 mm Hg, HR is 110 beats/minute, RR is 16 breaths/minute, temperature is 102.1°F, and oxygen saturation is 100% on room air. Abdominal examination reveals lower abdominal tenderness bilaterally. Pelvic examination is notable for cervical motion tenderness and white cervical discharge. On laboratory evaluation, WBC is 20,500/μL and β-hCG is negative. Which of the following is the most appropriate next step in management?

a. Consult general surgery for appendectomy
b. Begin antibiotic therapy
c. Perform a culdocentesis
d. Consult gynecology for immediate laparoscopy
e. Order an abdominal plain film

91. A 73-year-old man comes to the ED with abdominal pain, nausea, and vomiting. His symptoms have progressively worsened over the past 2 to 3 days. The pain is diffuse and comes in waves. He denies fever or chills, but has a history of constipation. He reports no flatus for 24 hours. Physical examination is notable for diffuse tenderness and voluntary guarding. An abdominal radiograph is seen in the figure. Which of the following is the most likely diagnosis?

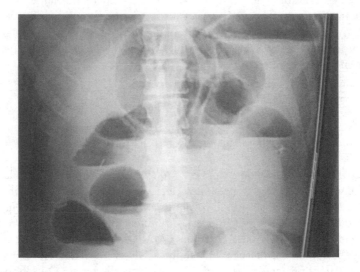

a. Constipation
b. SBO
c. Cholelithiasis
d. Large bowel obstruction
e. Inflammatory bowel disease

92. A 30-year-old man presents to the ED complaining of 2 days of worsening right flank pain that began abruptly. The pain radiates from his flank around to the abdomen and down toward the scrotum. He is in severe pain and actively vomiting. Vital signs are notable for an HR of 107 beats/minute and oral temperature of 101.2°F. A CT scan reveals a 9-mm obstructing stone of the left ureter with hydronephrosis. Urinalysis is positive for 2+ blood, 2+ leukocytes, 2+ nitrites, 40 to 50 WBC/hpf, and many bacteria. You administer pain medicine, antiemetics, and IV antibiotics. Which of the following is the most appropriate next step in management?

a. Consult urology and admit for possible surgical intervention
b. Observe in ED for 6 hours
c. Discharge with PO antibiotics and analgesics
d. Admit to medicine for IV antibiotics
e. Discharge with antibiotics, pain medicine, and instructions to drink large amounts of water and cranberry juice

93. You are working in the ED on a Sunday afternoon when four people present with acute-onset vomiting and crampy abdominal pain. They were all at the same picnic and ate most of the same foods. The vomiting began approximately 4 hours into the picnic. They deny having any diarrhea. You administer IV fluids and antiemetics and observe the patients. Over the next few hours, the vomiting stops, and their abdominal pain resolves. Which of the following is the most likely cause of their symptoms?

a. Scombroid
b. *Staphylococcus aureus*
c. *Clostridium perfringens*
d. *Campylobacter*
e. *Salmonella*

94. A 63-year-old man is brought to the ED by EMS complaining of severe abdominal pain that began suddenly 6 hours ago. His BP is 145/75 mm Hg and HR is 105 beats/minute and irregular. On examination, you note mild abdominal distention and diffuse abdominal tenderness without guarding. Stool is guaiac positive. Laboratory results reveal WBC 12,500/μL, hematocrit 48%, and lactate 4.2 U/L. ECG shows atrial fibrillation with a ventricular rate of 110 beats/minute. A CT scan is shown in the figure. Which of the following is the most likely diagnosis?

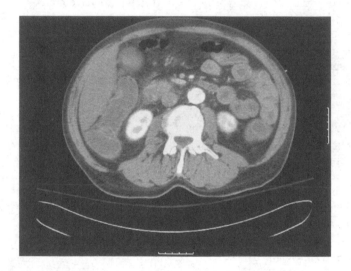

a. AAA
b. Mesenteric ischemia
c. Diverticulitis
d. SBO
e. Crohn's disease

95. A 24-year-old woman presents to the ED after being sexually assaulted. She is a college student with no past medical history. On physical examination, you observe vaginal trauma and scattered bruising and abrasions. Which of the following medications should be offered to the patient in this scenario?

a. Ceftriaxone, azithromycin, metronidazole, antiretroviral therapy, emergency contraception
b. Ceftriaxone, tetanus, metronidazole, antiretroviral therapy, emergency contraception

c. Ceftriaxone, azithromycin, tetanus, metronidazole, emergency contraception
d. Ceftriaxone, azithromycin, tetanus, antiretroviral therapy, emergency contraception
e. Ceftriaxone, azithromycin, tetanus, metronidazole, antiretroviral therapy, emergency contraception

96. A 21-year-old woman presents to the ED complaining of diarrhea, abdominal cramps, fever, anorexia, and weight loss for 3 days. Her BP is 127/75 mm Hg, HR is 91 beats/minute, and temperature is 100.8°F. Her abdomen is soft and nontender without rebound or guarding. WBC is 9200/µL, β-hCG is negative, and urinalysis is unremarkable. Stool is guaiac positive. She tells you that she has had similar symptoms four times over the past 2 months. Which of the following extraintestinal manifestations is associated with Crohn's disease but not ulcerative colitis?

a. Ankylosing spondylitis
b. Erythema nodosum
c. Nephrolithiasis
d. Thromboembolic disease
e. Uveitis

97. A 23-year-old woman presents to the ED complaining of pain with urination. She has no other complaints. Her symptoms started 3 weeks ago. During this time, she has been to the clinic twice, with negative urine cultures each time. Her condition has not improved with antibiotic therapy with sulfonamides or quinolones. Physical examination is normal. Which of the following organisms is most likely responsible for the patient's symptoms?

a. *S. aureus*
b. Herpes simplex virus
c. *Trichomonas vaginalis*
d. *Escherichia coli*
e. *C. trachomatis*

The following scenario applies to questions 98 and 99.

A 41-year-old alcoholic man with a history of cirrhosis and hepatitis C presents to the ED with bright red emesis. His temperature is 99.4°F, BP is 91/50 mm Hg, HR is 122 beats/minute, RR is 26 breaths/minute, and oxygen saturation is 95% on room air.

98. Which of the following conditions is the most common cause of upper gastrointestinal (GI) bleeding?

a. Esophageal varices
b. Gastritis
c. Mallory-Weiss tear
d. Gastric adenocarcinoma
e. Peptic ulcer disease

99. Which of the following should be added to this patient's medical therapy in the ED?

a. Octreotide
b. Ranitidine
c. Propranolol
d. Calcium carbonate
e. Azithromycin

100. NG tube placement is contraindicated in which of the following clinical scenarios?

a. A 3-month-old infant with poor weight gain and failure to thrive who has had rhinorrhea and cough for the past 3 days
b. A 78-year-old man with an SBO who is on warfarin for deep vein thrombosis (DVT)
c. A 19-year-old man with extensive facial trauma after an unhelmeted motorcycle accident
d. A 58-year-old man who is vomiting blood and takes ibuprofen daily for osteoarthritis
e. A 25-year-old female who is intubated and unresponsive following a polydrug overdose

101. A 35-year-old man with a history of human immunodeficiency virus (HIV) complains of severe throat pain. In addition, he reports that swallowing is extremely painful. He was previously on antiretroviral medications, but stopped them about 1 year ago. On physical examination, white material is noted on the tongue and palate that can be scraped off with a tongue blade. Which of the following medications should be started?

a. Acyclovir
b. Amoxicillin
c. Clotrimazole troches
d. Penicillin
e. Fluconazole

102. An obese 49-year-old woman with a history of hyperlipidemia and noninsulin-dependent diabetes mellitus presents to the ED with severe abdominal pain and nausea. Her temperature is 98.9°F, BP is 145/85 mm Hg, HR is 101 beats/minute, and RR is 22 breaths/minute. She has slight yellowing of the eyes. Her abdomen is tender in the RUQ, and she has mild scleral icterus. An RUQ ultrasound demonstrates a normal anterior gall-bladder wall thickness, no pericholecystic fluid, a negative sonographic Murphy's sign, and a common bile duct diameter of 1.0 cm. Which of the following is the most likely diagnosis?

a. Ascending cholangitis
b. Gallstone pancreatitis
c. Acalculous cholecystitis
d. Cholangiocarcinoma
e. Choledocholithiasis

103. A 41-year old woman presents to the ED 5 days after having an uncomplicated laparoscopic cholecystectomy. She began having abdominal pain yesterday and has had multiple episodes of nonbloody, nonbilious emesis today. She reports no bowel movement since her surgery and she is not passing flatus. She has mild diffuse abdominal tenderness without rebound or guarding. Her abdomen is not distended, and her bowel sounds are hypoactive. Which of the following metabolic abnormalities is associated with this patient's condition?

a. Hypernatremia
b. Hypocalcemia
c. Hyperphosphatemia
d. Hypokalemia
e. Hypermagnesemia

Abdominal and Pelvic Pain

Answers

69. The answer is c. This patient has **mesenteric ischemia** secondary to a **thromboembolism** from **atrial fibrillation.** The classic presentation of acute mesenteric ischemia is **sudden onset** of **poorly localized abdominal pain** in an individual with **underlying cardiac disease.** Arterial emboli are the most common cause of acute mesenteric ischemia, responsible for approximately 50% of cases. Most emboli are cardiac in origin, arising from mural thrombi or valvular lesions. Atrial fibrillation is an important risk factor for mesenteric ischemia owing to the propensity to form mural thrombi. Mesenteric ischemia can also occur as a result of thrombosis within mesenteric arteries, typically seen in patients with advanced atherosclerotic disease. Physical examination findings are notable for **"pain out of proportion to examination"** where a patient may be writhing from abdominal pain but have a soft, nontender abdomen. While mesenteric angiography remains the gold standard for diagnosis of acute mesenteric ischemia, **CT angiography has largely supplanted traditional angiography and is the initial test of choice for mesenteric ischemia.** Vascular surgery should be consulted emergently if mesenteric ischemia is suspected.

Capsule endoscopy **(a)**, colonoscopy **(b)**, and ultrasound **(d)** are not part of the initial management of mesenteric ischemia. Abdominal radiographs **(e)** may be abnormal, but are not sufficiently specific to diagnose mesenteric ischemia.

70. The answer is d. The patient's presentation is consistent with **alcoholic ketoacidosis (AKA).** This is an acute metabolic acidosis that occurs in chronic alcohol abusers with a **recent alcohol binge,** little or **no recent food intake,** and persistent vomiting. AKA is characterized by elevated serum ketone levels and an elevated anion gap ($\uparrow$ AG = Na $-$ [HCO$_3$ + Cl] > 12). A concomitant metabolic alkalosis is common, secondary to vomiting and volume depletion. AKA is the result of the following: (1) Starvation with glycogen depletion and counter-regulatory hormone production;

(2) A raised NADH/NAD+ ratio (related to the metabolism of ethanol); and (3) Volume depletion, resulting in ketogenesis. Typical signs and symptoms include nausea, vomiting, and abdominal pain. The fruity odor of ketones may be present on the patient's breath. Patients may also appear tremulous, and mental status may be impaired. In AKA, β-hydroxybutyrate is the predominant ketone produced, which is not detected well by the nitroprusside reaction (Acetest). Therefore, the degree of ketosis may be more severe than would be inferred from a nitroprusside reaction alone. The mainstay of treatment for AKA is hydration with glucose-containing fluids (**D₅NS or ½NS**). Thiamine should also be administered to prevent Wernicke encephalopathy.

Saline containing fluids alone (**a, b, and c**) do not correct AKA as quickly as fluids and carbohydrates combined. Insulin (**e**) is contraindicated in the treatment of AKA because it may cause life-threatening hypoglycemia in patients with depleted glycogen stores.

71. The answer is c. The patient has developed **alcohol withdrawal**. Symptoms of alcohol withdrawal usually **begin within 24 hours of cessation of alcohol** and subside after 2 to 3 days. Symptoms of alcohol withdrawal run a spectrum of severity ranging from mild symptoms (ie, anxiety and sleep disturbance) to more severe (ie, agitation, diaphoresis, tremor, nausea and vomiting, hallucinations, seizures, and autonomic instability). **Delirium tremens**, the most severe form of alcohol withdrawal, occurs in approximately 5% of patients with alcohol withdrawal. A hyperadrenergic state is characterized by agitation, disorientation, altered mental status, tremor, fever, tachycardia, delusions, and hallucinations. Hyperpyrexia, ketoacidosis, and circulatory collapse may ensue. The treatment for alcohol withdrawal includes close monitoring and liberal use of benzodiazepines. Patients with a history of alcohol withdrawal seizures and/or delirium tremens should be admitted to the hospital.

Wernicke encephalopathy (**a**) results from thiamine deficiency and is characterized by altered mental status, ataxia, and ophthalmoplegia. Acute alcohol withdrawal is more likely in this clinical scenario. Subdural hematoma (**b**) would be more likely in an individual with a history of trauma. The question stem does not suggest drug overdose (**d**). Psychiatric illness (**e**) can produce agitation and hallucinations, but the hyperadrenergic state is more characteristic of a toxic-metabolic process like alcohol withdrawal.

72. The answer is e. The patient's history and physical examination is consistent with **acute cholecystitis**. Because of the poor predictive value of the history, physical, and laboratory findings in cholecystitis, the most important initial imaging test is **RUQ ultrasound.** Ultrasound findings suggestive of acute cholecystitis include gallstones, gallbladder wall thickening and distention, and pericholecystic fluid.

CT scanning (**b**) may be useful when other intra-abdominal disorders are being considered. However, the sensitivity of a CT is less than that of ultrasound for acute cholecystitis. MRI (**c**) is not a first-line test for acute cholecystitis. HIDA scan (**d**) has a higher sensitivity and specificity than ultrasound, making it the most accurate study for cholecystitis; however, it is reserved for cases where ultrasound is negative or equivocal. Plain film radiographs (**a**) demonstrate stones in the gallbladder less than 25% of the time.

73. The answer is c. The patient's history of colicky flank pain that radiates to the groin and hematuria is consistent with a **ureteral stone.** Adequate **analgesia** is critical in treating a patient with a ureteral stone. IV **ketorolac** (an NSAID) is frequently administered as a first-line analgesic, but morphine or other opioids may be necessary for continued pain. In addition to analgesics, antiemetics are often administered for nausea and vomiting.

Appendicitis (**a**) is unlikely with a soft and nontender abdomen. An abdominal CT (**b**) will probably be necessary, but controlling the patient's pain is the first priority. An AAA (**d**) can present with flank pain; however, it is very rare in a 31 year old without significant past medical history. Testicular torsion (**e**) should always be considered in a patient with groin pain. In this case, a stone is more consistent with the history.

74. The answer is c. The patient presentation is suggestive of an **SBO.** Symptoms of an SBO include colicky abdominal pain, vomiting, abdominal distention, hyperactive bowel sounds, and decreased flatus. The most common cause of SBO is **postoperative adhesions,** responsible for more than 50% of cases. One of the more common procedures associate with SBO is a hysterectomy. Other common causes of SBO include hernia and neoplasm.

Hernias (**d**) are the second most common cause of obstruction. Traveling to Mexico (**a**) may lead to diarrhea and abdominal pain from infectious enteritis. Ethanol abuse (**b**) is associated with many causes of abdominal pain including gastritis and pancreatitis, but not obstruction. Constipation (**e**) does not usually produce vomiting.

75. The answer is e. The patient's clinical presentation is consistent with **alcoholic hepatitis,** which is a potentially severe form of alcohol-induced liver disease. The presentation can range from nausea and vomiting to fulminant hepatitis and liver failure. Laboratory tests may reveal moderate elevations of AST and ALT. In alcoholic hepatitis, the **AST is usually greater than ALT** (think "scotch" and "tonic" for AST > ALT). The patient may exhibit stigmata of chronic liver disease such as gynecomastia and spider angiomata. The management of alcoholic liver disease is **supportive, with fluid hydration and correction of electrolyte imbalances,** paying special attention to blood glucose (ethanol can suppress gluconeogenesis) and magnesium. Thiamine should also be administered to prevent Wernicke encephalopathy.

Suctioning the patient's stomach with a NG tube **(a)** is not indicated. A HIDA scan **(b)** is a diagnostic test for acute cholecystitis. Unless this is a known needle stick or mucosal exposure, hepatitis immune globulin **(c)** is not acutely indicated. Viral hepatitis titers **(d)** can be drawn if viral infection is suspected. However, this presentation is more suggestive of alcoholic hepatitis.

76. The answer is e. This patient with known liver disease has **spontaneous bacterial peritonitis (SBP)**. Diagnostic criteria for SBP include an ascitic fluid neutrophil count **greater than 250 cells/mm^3**. Pathogens associated with SBP include gram-negative rods like *E. coli* and *Klebsiella*, as well as *Streptococcus* sp, and *Streptococcus pneumoniae*. Therefore, the most appropriate antibiotic for treatment is a **third-generation cephalosporin** such as **cefotaxime.**

All other answer choices **(a, b, c, and d)** are inappropriate antibiotic choices.

77. The answer is e. This presentation of sudden onset severe testicular pain, a swollen tender testicle, and absent cremasteric reflex is very concerning for **testicular torsion**. Testicular torsion is a **urologic emergency** that occurs when the spermatic cord suspending the testicle twists, resulting in ischemia to the testicle. Urology should be consulted immediately and a STAT **Doppler ultrasound** ordered while awaiting urology evaluation. **Manual detorsion** can be attempted in most cases while arranging for definitive care in the operating room (OR). After appropriate analgesia, the testicle should be twisted laterally, like opening the pages of a book. The incidence has a bimodal peak, with most cases occurring during infancy and in puberty.

Administering ceftriaxone and azithromycin **(a)** and swabbing his urethra **(b)** is the management of urethritis. A urinalysis **(c)** should be carried out on most patients with scrotal pain, but in this case ruling out testicular torsion takes precedence. Although epididymitis **(d)** and torsion both present with testicular pain, epididymitis usually has more of a gradual onset, reaching a peak over hours to days, rather than sudden onset.

78. The answer is c. Prompt diagnosis and treatment of testicular torsion is paramount in saving the testicle. If the torsion is reduced **within 6 hours**, either with manual detorsion or via surgical intervention, there is a **90% chance of salvaging the testicle**. After 12 hours, the rate of salvage drops to 50% and after 24 hours, it drops to 10%.

All other answer choices (**a, b, d, and e**) are incorrect.

79. The answer is d. Appendicitis is the most common cause of the acute surgical abdomen. It can occur at any age, but is most frequently seen in adolescents and young adults. The classic presentation is the onset of dull **periumbilical pain, which eventually migrates to the RLQ**. Associated symptoms include anorexia, nausea, and vomiting. Low-grade fever may be present. **Rovsing's sign** refers to the elicitation of pain in the RLQ when the LLQ is palpated. Leukocytosis is often present, but a normal WBC count does not rule out appendicitis. Urinalysis may show pyuria if the inflamed appendix results in ureteral irritation. **Abdominal CT** is the test of choice in adults, with a reported sensitivity of up to 100% and specificity of 95%. CT findings of appendicitis include an enlarged appendix (> 6 mm), pericecal inflammation, and the presence of an appendicolith.

Dilated loops of bowel are suggestive of bowel obstruction (**a**). Many patients who ultimately are diagnosed with appendicitis initially believed they had food poisoning (**b**). However, the history and physical examination is concerning for appendicitis, so a CT should be ordered. Abdominal ultrasound is commonly used as an initial test in children and pregnant women with suspected appendicitis (**c**). Its sensitivity and specificity approach 90%, but may be inconclusive as a result of body habitus or with a retrocecal appendix. It would be inappropriate to discharge this patient home without first evaluating for appendicitis (**e**).

80. The answer is d. The patient's clinical picture is concerning for **ovarian torsion.** Ovarian torsion occurs when the **ovary twists on its stalk,** leading to obstruction of venous drainage, edema, and eventual ischemia. Most cases of ovarian torsion occur in the presence of an enlarged ovary, due to cyst, tumor, or abscess. Patients report severe pain that began abruptly. They may give a history of similar pain that resolved spontaneously. **Doppler ultrasound** is the diagnostic modality of choice for evaluating ovarian torsion, which demonstrates decreased or absent blood flow to the ovary. Ovarian torsion is a surgical emergency and gynecologist should be consulted for definitive surgical treatment.

Ultrasound is the test of choice, not a CT scan (**a**). MRI (**b**) and X-ray (**c**) have no role in the diagnosis of ovarian torsion. If the clinical suspicion is high and diagnostic tests are equivocal, laparoscopy (**e**) can be used to visualize the ovaries in vivo.

81. The answer is e. The patient has **pneumoperitoneum**. Complications of colonoscopy include hemorrhage, perforation with pneumoperitoneum, retroperitoneal abscess, pneumoscrotum, pneumothorax, volvulus, and infection. **Perforation of the colon** with **pneumoperitoneum** is usually evident immediately, but can take several hours to manifest. Perforation is usually secondary to intrinsic disease of the colon (ie, diverticulitis) or to vigorous manipulation during colonoscopy. Most patients require laparotomy. However, expectant management is appropriate in some patients with a late presentation (1-2 days later) who have no signs of peritonitis. The radiograph in the figure demonstrates **air under the diaphragm,** which is pathognomonic for pneumoperitoneum.

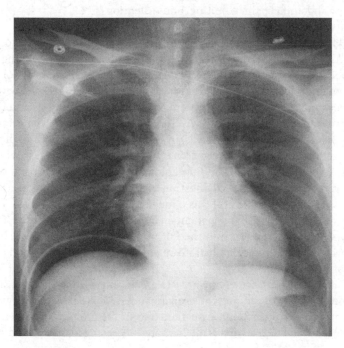

Ascending cholangitis (a) and pancreatitis (d) may occur as a complication from endoscopic retrograde cholangiopancreatography (ERCP). There is no evidence of pulmonary edema (b) in this radiograph. Liver failure with ascites (c) is not associated with pneumoperitoneum.

82. The answer is c. The patient's clinical picture is consistent with ascending **cholangitis,** a bacterial infection of the biliary tree caused by biliary tract obstruction. Obstruction may occur as a result of gallstones, stricture, or malignancy. The classic **"Charcot triad"** of ascending cholangitis is **RUQ pain, fever,** and **jaundice.** Cholangitis is a **surgical emergency** and patients can rapidly become septic. Ultrasound may demonstrate intrahepatic or ductal dilation. The presence of stones in the gallbladder suggests gallstones as the etiology of obstruction.

The patient has some features of cholecystitis (a), however, the presence of jaundice and dilated common and intrahepatic ducts is more suggestive of cholangitis. Acute hepatitis (b) does not have the same sonographic findings seen in cholangitis. Pancreatic cancer (d) can present with jaundice, but it is usually painless. Bowel obstruction (e) presents with intermittent crampy abdominal pain, vomiting, and distention.

83. The answer is e. The patient presents with multiple risk factors for an **AAA** including age older than 60, hypertension, cigarette smoking, and peripheral artery disease. Classically, AAA presents with severe abdominal pain, often sudden in onset, with radiation to the back. Flank or back pain may also be the presenting symptom. Physical examination may reveal a **pulsatile abdominal mass.** If the AAA is ruptured or leaking, vital signs are often unstable. A ruptured AAA is an emergent condition with high mortality, and patients require immediate management in the OR. Evidence of an AAA is seen on plain radiograph approximately 66% to 75% of the time, revealing curvilinear calcification of the aortic wall or a paravertebral soft tissue mass. However, CT has a much higher sensitivity for AAA, and is the test of choice in stable patients. Unstable patients with suspect ruptured AAA should be taken to the OR. A bedside ultrasound can also be performed, which may demonstrate an enlarged aorta and free fluid in the case of rupture.

Biliary colic (a) presents with RUQ pain after eating. Kidney stones (nephrolithiasis) (b) can present similarly to AAA. The classic kidney stone presentation is colicky flank pain radiating to the groin. The presence of hypotension and tachycardia is much more concerning for a ruptured AAA.

Pancreatitis (c) typically presents with mid-epigastric pain that radiates to the back and is associated with nausea and vomiting. Symptoms of SBO (d) include abdominal pain, distention, vomiting, and inability to pass flatus, and dilated bowel loops with air fluid levels on radiographs are characteristic.

84. The answer is c. A ruptured AAA causes imminent death unless emergently surgically repaired. Upon clinical suspicion or diagnosis based on imaging (eg, focused assessment with sonography in trauma examination, X-ray with displaced calcification), the emergency physician should **consult vascular surgery and prepare for emergent blood transfusion** until the patient is taken for operative intervention. Ideally, the patient will have adequate IV access with at least two large-bore (ie, 18-guage or larger) IVs for rapid fluid resuscitation. In the setting of a ruptured AAA, blood is the preferred fluid as the patient will rapidly become intravascularly depleted from hemoperitoneum.

Assessing orthostatic vital signs (a) is inappropriate in an already hypotensive patient. Inserting a NG tube (b) would be appropriate for management of an SBO. Obtaining a right-sided ECG (d) would be appropriate to evaluate for a possible right-sided myocardial infarction (MI). Obtaining an ECG will only delay definitive management. A pericardiocentesis (e) is indicated for the management of acute pericardial tamponade from rapid development of a pericardial effusion.

85. The answer is c. The patient has acute pancreatitis. **Lipase**, a pancreatic enzyme that hydrolyzes triglycerides, is the **most specific test** for pancreatitis. In the presence of pancreatic inflammation, it increases within 4 to 8 hours and peaks at 24 hours. At **five times the upper limits of normal,** lipase is **60% sensitive and 100% specific** for pancreatitis. The diagnosis is usually made with a lipase of two times the normal limit, thereby increasing its sensitivity.

The specificity of amylase (a) for pancreatitis is approximately 70%, making it less specific than lipase. The other laboratory values (b, d, and e) are used in the prognosis of pancreatitis, but are not necessary for the diagnosis.

86. The answer is a. Amebic abscesses are common in countries with tropical and subtropical climates and areas with poor sanitation. **Entamoeba histolytica** causes an intestinal infection, and the liver is seeded via the portal system. The clinical presentation includes abdominal tenderness in the RUQ, leukocytosis, and fever. Diagnosis is supported by identification of the pathogenic protozoan in the stool. Treatment includes metronidazole and supportive care measures. If medical therapy is unsuccessful, percutaneous catheter drainage is required.

Cholecystitis (**b**) presents with fever, leukocytosis, and RUQ pain, and a positive Murphy. Cryptosporidium (**c**) is the most common cause of chronic diarrhea in individuals with acquired immunodeficiency syndrome (AIDS) and presents with profuse watery diarrhea, abdominal cramping, anorexia, nausea, and flatulence. In immunocompetent individuals, the illness is self-limited, with symptoms persisting for 1 to 3 weeks. Patients with enterobiasis (**d**), also known as pinworms, complain of itching in the anal region, particularly at night, as the adult worm lays eggs in the anus. Pyogenic abscess (**e**) is the most common type of liver abscess; however, the history of travel and lack of primary source for the pyogenic abscess make it less likely a diagnosis. Most cases of pyogenic liver access occur in the setting of ascending cholangitis.

87. The answer is c. Any woman with abdominal pain, vaginal bleeding, and a positive pregnancy test needs to be ruled out for an **ectopic pregnancy.** Her vital signs are stable so she can undergo a **transvaginal ultrasound.** This is used to document the presence of an intrauterine pregnancy. If no intrauterine pregnancy is observed, this increases the likelihood of an ectopic pregnancy.

Laparoscopy is indicated in a patient with an equivocal ultrasound and/or unstable vital signs (**a**). If ultrasound confirms an intrauterine pregnancy and fails to reveal a cause of symptoms, yet the patient continues to have severe RLQ pain, then the risks of radiation exposure to the fetus from CT scan (**b**) must be weighed against the potential benefit of diagnosing another condition such as appendicitis. While a urinalysis (**d**) and swab for sexually transmitted infections (STIs) (**e**) is part of the general workup, ruling out ectopic pregnancy is the highest priority.

88. The answer is b. The patient's clinical presentation and abdominal radiograph are consistent with a diagnosis of **sigmoid volvulus.** A volvulus is kinking or twisting of the bowel that leads to intestinal obstruction and can lead to tissue ischemia or necrosis. Sigmoid volvulus occurs most commonly in elderly, debilitated, or institutionalized patients. The **classic triad** of symptoms includes **abdominal pain, abdominal distension, and constipation.** If the bowel becomes gangrenous, the mortality rate exceeds 50%. Percussive tympany may be present as well. Plain abdominal radiographs demonstrate distended large bowel loops without haustra and may resemble a bent inner tube. A contrast enema may help distinguish this from other causes of bowel obstruction.

Patients with an SBO present with diffuse, crampy abdominal pain. They may also report a lack of recent bowel movement or passage of flatus. However, on abdominal films you will see distended loops of small bowel and air-fluid levels in a stepladder appearance. **(a).** Gastric outlet obstruction **(c)** is a type of SBO and usually occurs at the pylorus or duodenum. Causes may include traumatic or spontaneous duodenal hematomas, pyloric stenosis (in children), or pancreatic malignancy. Patients present with vomiting and failure to thrive. Irritable bowel syndrome **(d)** is more common in younger patients and can present predominantly with diarrhea, predominantly with constipation, or alternating diarrhea and constipation accompanied by severe abdominal cramping that is relieved with defecation. Pneumoperitoneum **(e)** is a surgical emergency. Patient will have peritonitis on examination (eg, rebound tenderness, rigidity, involuntary guarding). Free intra-abdominal air under the diaphragm is best seen on an upright chest X-ray.

89. The answer is e. The patient has **ovarian torsion**. The differential diagnosis in a woman with RLQ pain is extensive and includes GI pathology such as appendicitis, inflammatory bowel disease, diverticulitis, hernia, and gynecologic pathology (ie, ectopic pregnancy, ruptured ovarian cyst, ovarian torsion, and PID). The report of sudden onset symptoms and **adnexal tenderness** raises suspicion for ovarian torsion; therefore, a Doppler ultrasound should be obtained. Ultrasound findings of ovarian torsion include a **unilateral enlarged ovary with decreased flow.** Ovarian torsion is a **gynecologic emergency. Patient should be taken to the OR for immediate laparoscopy or laparotomy.** Failure to surgically reduce the torsion and restore blood flow to the ovary in a timely manner results in ischemia and necrosis of the ovary.

Conservative management is not an option in suspected ovarian torsion **(a).** Antibiotic therapy **(b)** is the treatment for tubo-ovarian abscess and PID. Manual detorsion **(c)** is a temporizing measure for testicular torsion, the male counterpart of ovarian torsion. If pelvic ultrasound was normal and there is suspicion for GI pathology, then abdominal CT is warranted **(d).**

90. The answer is b. **PID** comprises a spectrum of infections of the female upper reproductive tract. Although *N. gonorrhoeae* and *C. trachomatis* are thought to cause the majority of infections, new evidence points to greater rates of polymicrobial infections. Most cases of PID are thought to start with a sexually transmitted disease of the lower genital tract, with subsequent ascension to the upper tract. Women typically present with lower abdominal pain and may have vaginal discharge, vaginal bleeding, dysuria, and fever. The examination typically reveals **lower abdominal tenderness** and **cervical motion tenderness** or **adnexal tenderness.** Many patients can be treated with outpatient antibiotics. Considerations for inpatient treatment include women who are pregnant, have failed outpatient therapy, are toxic appearing, have evidence for a tubo-ovarian abscess, or in whom a surgical emergency cannot be ruled out.

The onset of appendicitis is more insidious than what is presented in this case (**a**). Nausea and vomiting are common, and pain typically begins in the periumbilical area and migrates to the RLQ. Culdocentesis (**c**) is used to retrieve fluid in the cul-de-sac. The findings are limited and not specific to PID. Laparoscopy is used in the management of ovarian torsion, tubo-ovarian abscess, and other gynecologic pathology (**d**). Abdominal plain films are not useful in the diagnosis of PID (**e**).

91. The answer is b. The clinical scenario and radiograph are consistent with an **SBO.** Patients usually present with **diffuse, crampy abdominal pain that** is often episodic in nature. Typically, the patient reports no recent bowel movements or passage of flatus. The most common causes of SBO are **adhesions and hernias.** Abdominal films often reveal **distended loops of small bowel and air-fluid levels in a stepladder appearance.** However, abdominal films are not sufficiently sensitive to rule out SBO and a CT scan should be obtained if SBO is suspected and abdominal films are unremarkable.

Constipation (**a**) is a diagnosis of exclusion, although fecal impaction is a common problem in debilitated elderly patients and may present with symptoms of colonic obstruction. Cholelithiasis (**c**) typically presents with RUQ pain and fever. Ultrasound is diagnostic. The large bowel contains folds called *haustra* that do not cross the entire bowel width. In the figure mentioned previously, we see valvulae conniventes, folds of the small bowel that cross the entire width of the bowel, confirming this is a small, not large bowel obstruction (**d**). Neither the clinical scenario nor the plain film is consistent with inflammatory bowel disease (**e**).

92. The answer is a. An **obstructing stone in the presence of a UTI** is an acute **urologic emergency.** Bacteria in an obstructed collecting system can cause abscess formation, renal destruction, and severe systemic toxicity including septic shock. The patient requires **admission for IV antibiotics and urgent removal of the stone** and relief of the obstruction. In addition to an obstructing stone with infection, other indications for admission for kidney stones include uncontrolled pain, persistent nausea and vomiting, urinary extravasation, and hypercalcemic crisis.

Observation **(b)** is not recommended for several reasons. Most importantly, the patient requires IV antibiotics and removal of the stone due to the infection. A 9-mm large stone is unlikely to pass spontaneously. In general stones smaller than 4 mm pass 90% of the time, stones 4 to 6 mm pass 50% of the time, and stones larger than 6 mm pass 10% of the time. Discharge home is not appropriate in the case of an infected stone **(c, and e)**. Many patients with uninfected kidney stones can be discharged home with pain medications. Admission to a medical service without urologic consultation is not sufficient care as this patient will likely require emergent surgical intervention **(d)**.

93. The answer is b. Staphylococcal food poisoning is caused by foods contaminated by an enterotoxin-producing strain of *S. aureus*. Because symptoms are due to a preformed toxin, the onset of illness is **abrupt**, with symptoms typically beginning within **1 to 6 hours** of ingestion of the contaminated foods. Cramping abdominal pain and vomiting, often with forceful retching, are the predominant symptoms. Diarrhea is variable, and may be mild. Most **protein-rich foods** support the growth of staphylococci, particularly ham, eggs, custard, mayonnaise, and potato salad. Although often aggressive in onset, staphylococcal food poisoning is **short-lived** and usually **subsides in 6 to 8 hours,** rarely lasting more than 24 hours. Treatment is supportive. The **short incubation period** and **multiple cases** in people eating the same meal are highly suggestive of this disease.

Scombroid fish poisoning **(a)** results from the ingestion of heat-stable toxins produced by bacterial action on improperly stored fish. The symptoms occur within 20 to 30 minutes of ingestion and resemble histamine intoxication, consisting of facial flushing, diarrhea, throbbing headache, palpitations, and abdominal cramps. Treatment is supportive. *C. perfringens* **(c)** is a common cause of acute food poisoning in the United States. Symptoms usually appear within 6 to 12 hours but can occur up to 24 hours after ingestion of the contaminated food. Frequent, watery diarrhea and moderately severe abdominal cramping are the major symptoms. *Campylobacter* **(d)** is a common bacterial cause of diarrhea. The incubation period is approximately 2 to 5 days and symptoms include diarrhea, cramping abdominal pain, and fever. Salmonella **(e)** occurs most during the summer months and is acquired by the ingestion of contaminated food or drink. Poultry products, such as turkey, chicken, duck, and eggs, constitute the most common sources. The typical patient presents with fever, colicky abdominal pain, and loose, watery diarrhea, occasionally with mucus and blood.

94. The answer is b. The patient has mesenteric ischemia. **Acute mesenteric ischemia** is caused by lack of perfusion to the bowel. It primarily affects older patients, particularly those with significant cardiovascular or systemic disease. **Arterial occlusion** related to **atrial fibrillation** is the **most common cause** of mesenteric ischemia. Additional etiologies include venous thrombosis that is associated with a hypercoagulable state, or nonocclusive ischemia due to decreased cardiac output in the setting of severe congestive heart failure (CHF), acute MI, hypovolemia, or other causes of shock. Early in the disease course, patients may complain of severe pain but have minimal tenderness on examination (ie, the characteristic **pain out of proportion to examination**). As infarction manifests, abdominal distension and peritoneal signs develop. Sudden onset of pain suggests arterial vascular occlusion by emboli, whereas insidious onset is more suggestive of venous thrombosis or nonocclusive infarction. Radiographs may reveal dilated loops of bowel, air in the bowel wall (**pneumatosis intestinalis**), and thickening of the bowel wall, as seen in the CT scan. Management involves fluid resuscitation, antibiotics, and surgical intervention.

Classically, AAA **(a)** presents with constant abdominal pain, often with radiation to the back. Physical examination may reveal a pulsatile abdominal mass. Diverticulitis **(c)** usually presents with LLQ abdominal pain and low-grade fever. Patients with an SBO **(d)** present with crampy abdominal pain, abdominal distention, vomiting, and obstipation. Distended loops of bowel and air-fluid levels are seen on radiographs. Crohn's disease **(e)** may present with bloody diarrhea, abdominal pain, fever, anorexia, and weight loss.

95. The answer is e. When a sexual assault patient is evaluated in the ED, the emergency physician not only has the responsibility of addressing the patient's immediate physical and psychological health, but must also consider how the encounter may affect the patient's life once discharged from the ED. After life-threatening injuries are addressed, the physician is responsible for collecting physical evidence necessary for prosecuting the assailant by conducting a sexual assault examination with the patient's consent.

Medications should also be provided to sexual assault victims as prophylaxis against STIs, pregnancy, and tetanus. This includes prophylaxis against gonorrhea (**ceftriaxone**), *Chlamydia* (**azithromycin or doxycycline**), and trichomoniasis (**metronidazole**). The decision to provide **HIV postexposure prophylaxis (PEP)** after sexual assault must take into account the risks and benefits of treatment, the interval between exposure and treatment with antiretrovirals, and the likelihood of exposure to HIV. The average risk of HIV transmission per contact of unprotected receptive anal intercourse is approximately 1% to 5%. For unprotected receptive anal intercourse and receptive vaginal intercourse, the risk is approximately 0.1% to 1%. Some states mandate offering and providing HIV PEP to all sexually assaulted patients. The risk of pregnancy following sexual assault is approximately 5%. **Emergency contraception** is the use of hormone pills to prevent pregnancy. **Hepatitis B** vaccination should be administered to patients who never received the vaccine. Tetanus is administered to patients who have sustained tetanus-prone injuries.

All other answer choices (**a, b, c, and d**) do not provide adequate prophylaxis.

96. The answer is c. **Crohn's disease** is an autoimmune condition characterized by **chronic inflammation extending through all layers of the bowel wall**. The onset is generally between the ages of 15 and 40 years. Crohn's disease should be suspected in any patient whose symptoms show a picture consistent with chronic inflammatory colitis. Extraintestinal manifestations are seen in 25% to 30% of patients, and include aphthous ulcers, erythema nodosum, iritis or episcleritis, arthritis, gallstones, and thromboembolic disease. The incidence of these extraintestinal manifestations is similar for Crohn's disease and ulcerative colitis. **Nephrolithiasis** is seen as a result of hyperoxaluria because of increased oxalate absorption in patients with ileal disease.

Because ulcerative colitis affects only the large bowel, nephrolithiasis is seen only in patients with Crohn's disease. All other answer choices (**a, b, d, and e**) are seen in both conditions.

97. The answer is e. *C. trachomatis* **urethritis** accounts for 5% to 20% of cases of dysuria, and the diagnosis should be considered **when urine cultures are sterile**. If clinical symptoms and urinalysis point to a UTI, the urine culture is sterile, and standard antibiotic regimens fail, consider *Chlamydia* urethritis.

Although group A streptococcus is a possible pathogen (a), it would be very rare and would be susceptible to the antibiotics that the patient has taken. Initial episodes of herpes simplex virus (b) can result in symptoms that mimic true dysuria secondary to sensitivity of lesions on the external genital surface or near the urethra. Generally, these episodes are accompanied by fever, chills, systemic symptoms, and extremely painful and tender lesions. Although *T. vaginalis* (c) would not respond to the previous antibiotic therapy, trichomoniasis presents with a copious frothy vaginal discharge and would have been seen on wet mount preparation of the vaginal secretions. *E. coli* (d) accounts for 70% to 90% of community-acquired UTI in women. In a woman without recurrent UTI, the antibiotics taken by this patient would be appropriate. This pathogen should have also been grown on the standard culture medium.

98. The answer is e. GI bleeding is a common presenting complaint in the ED. **Upper GI bleeding**, defined as hemorrhage proximal to the ligament of Treitz (located at the junction of the duodenum and the jejunum), is more common than lower GI bleeding, representing approximately **75% of cases**. **Gastric and duodenal ulcers** are the most commonly identified sources of upper GI hemorrhage. Other common causes of upper GI hemorrhage include gastritis, Mallory-Weiss tears, and esophageal varices. Patients may present with hematemesis and/or melena. Hematochezia is usually associated with lower GI bleeding, though it may be seen in cases of a brisk upper GI bleed. Early aggressive resuscitation with large bore IV access, fluids, and blood products, if needed, is critical in reducing mortality from upper GI bleed. Endoscopy is diagnostic in determining the source of an upper GI bleed, and is often therapeutic as well, as bleeding vessels can be cauterized of ligated.

Esophageal varices, gastritis, and Mallory-Weiss tears (a, b, and c) are common causes of upper GI bleeding, but less common than peptic ulcer disease. Gastric adenocarcinoma (d) is a rare cause of upper GI hemorrhage.

99. The answer is a. The patient has an acute upper GI hemorrhage and is at risk for **esophageal varices** given his history of longstanding alcohol use. Management of acute upper GI bleeding involves maintaining a secure airway; administering blood products, antibiotics to cover gut flora, and PPI therapy (eg, omeprazole); emergency consultation with gastroenterology for diagnostic and therapeutic esophagogastroduodenoscopy (EGD) with vessel ligation or esophageal banding; and potentially balloon tamponade with a Minnesota tube or Sengstaken-Blakemore tube if endoscopy is not immediately available and the patient is exsanguinating. Patients with cirrhosis are at risk for esophagogastric varices. Variceal bleeds are one of the most common causes of deadly upper GI bleeding. Otherwise, exsanguination from upper GI bleeding is rare. **Octreotide** is a synthetic analog that causes splanchnic vasoconstriction and reduces portal venous hypertension. It is recommended in the management of upper GI bleeds in patients with varices as it reduces the risk of persistent bleeding, rebleeding, and need for blood transfusion. If it is unknown whether or not the patient has esophagogastric varices, **octreotide should be given empirically** if the patient has alcoholism, elevated liver enzymes, or other significant liver disease.

Ranitidine (b) or other antihistamines, while used in the management of peptic ulcer disease, are not used in the acute management of upper GI bleeding. Propranolol (c) and calcium carbonate (d) also do not play any role in managing acute upper GI bleeds. Patients with cirrhosis should be given empiric antibiotics to cover GI flora. Ciprofloxacin and ceftriaxone are currently recommended. Azithromycin (e) does not provide appropriate coverage.

100. The answer is c. NG tubes are commonly used for stomach decompression in the setting of GI obstruction, positive pressure ventilation, and to allow administration of medications and nutrition directly into the GI tract. However, **significant facial trauma** is an **absolute contraindication** for NG tube placement due to the risk of passage through the cribriform plate and resultant intracranial placement. Patients with facial injuries who need a NG tube should preferentially undergo orogastric (OG) tube placement. **Additional contraindications** for NG tube placement include alkali burns to the esophagus and esophageal strictures. Complications of NG tube placement include local bleeding, intracranial placement, pulmonary placement, perforation, and aspiration.

Neither infancy nor upper respiratory infections (a) are contraindications for NG tube placement. Although caution should be used in anticoagulated patients due to higher risk for bleeding (b), anticoagulated status alone is not an absolute contraindication for NG tube placement. An upper GI bleed (d) is not a contraindication for NG tube placement. Special caution should be exercised if esophageal varices are the cause of bleeding. However, several studies report that NG tube placement is safe in the setting of esophageal varices. NG and OG tube (e) placement are generally safe in intubated patients barring other contraindications.

101. The answer is e. This patient has **esophageal candidiasis**. A white coating on the oropharynx that can be scraped off is consistent with candidal pharyngitis, also known as thrush. However, the presence of severe odynophagia suggests that candidal esophagitis is also present. Candidal esophagitis is an **AIDS-defining illness** and is typically seen with CD4 counts below 100 cells/µL. The treatment for candidal esophagitis is **oral fluconazole**. If there is no clinical response within 5 to 7 days, a biopsy may be performed to assess for other causes of esophagitis associated with HIV, such as herpes simplex virus, cytomegalovirus, and deep aphthous ulcers.

Acyclovir **(a)** is the treatment for herpes esophagitis in immunocompromised individuals. White material coating the oropharynx suggests candida as the diagnosis. Amoxicillin and penicillin **(b and d)** are treatment options for streptococcal pharyngitis. Clotrimazole troches **(c)** are the treatment for oropharyngeal candidiasis, not esophageal candidiasis.

102. The answer is e. The patient has **choledocholithiasis**, defined as the presence of gallstones within the common bile duct. Most commonly, gallstones migrate from the gallbladder and become impacted within the common bile duct, creating acute biliary obstruction and biliary colic. Less commonly, gallstones originate from within the bile ducts. Nonobstructing stones do not cause symptoms, but when they obstruct the common bile duct, patients present with epigastric or RUQ abdominal pain that is steady and often postprandial, nausea, vomiting, and **jaundice**. Fever is usually absent unless acute cholecystitis or ascending cholangitis (biliary tract infection) is present. The normal diameter of the common bile duct on ultrasound is **less than 5 mm**. Dilatation greater than this suggests (but does not definitively diagnose) choledocholithiasis. Additional evaluation with magnetic resonance cholangiopancreatography (MRCP) or ERCP.

Ascending cholangitis **(a)** is infection of the biliary tract and is classically characterized by Charcot's triad of fever, RUQ pain, and jaundice or Reynold's pentad that includes the addition of altered mental status and hypotension. Gallstone pancreatitis **(b)** is pancreatitis caused by a gallstone. One-third to three-quarters of cases of pancreatitis are caused by gallstones. Pancreatitis does not present with jaundice. Additionally, a dilated common bile duct suggests an alternative diagnosis. Acalculous cholecystitis **(c)** is a gallbladder infection in the absence of gallstones. This usually occurs in critically ill patients with conditions such as burns, septic shock, or multisystem trauma; elderly patients; immunocompromised patients; and diabetics. Cholangiocarcinoma **(d)** is cancer of the biliary tree and is the second most common cause of hepatobiliary cancer after hepatocellular carcinoma. It is often diagnosed incidentally in asymptomatic patients upon routine imaging, or it may present with painless jaundice.

103. The answer is d. The patient has an adynamic (or paralytic) **ileus**, defined as a **functional** (rather than anatomic or mechanical) **bowel obstruction** as a result of abnormal peristaltic GI activity. Common causes include metabolic abnormalities (specifically **hypokalemia**), medications (eg, opioids), infections, recent abdominal trauma, or recent laparotomy. Patients may be dehydrated from poor oral intake or from vomiting. Adynamic ileus is most often transient and improves with rehydration, electrolyte correction, and treatment of the underlying cause.

Hypernatremia **(a)**, hypocalcemia **(b)**, hyperphosphatemia **(c)**, and hypermagnesemia **(e)** are not strongly associated with or causes of adynamic ileus.

Recommended Readings

Bessinger B, Stehman CR. Chapter 79. Pancreatitis and cholecystitis. In: Tintinalli JE, Ma O, Yealy DM, et al, eds. *Tintinalli's Emergency Medicine: A Comprehensive Study Guide.* 9th ed. New York, NY: McGraw-Hill, 2020.

Cole MA, Huang RD. Chapter 83. Acute appendicitis. In: Marx JA, Hockberger RS, Gausche-Hill M, eds. *Rosen's Emergency Medicine: Concepts and Clinical Practice.* 9th ed. Philadelphia, PA: Elsevier, 2018.

Colwell CB, Fox CJ. Chapter 76. Abdominal aortic aneurysm. In: Marx JA, Hockberger RS, Gausche-Hill M, eds. *Rosen's Emergency Medicine: Concepts and Clinical Practice.* 9th ed. Philadelphia, PA: Elsevier, 2018.

Germann CA, Holmes JA. Chapter 89. Selected urologic disorders. In: Marx JA, Hockberger RS, Gausche-Hill M, eds. *Rosen's Emergency Medicine: Concepts and Clinical Practice.* 9th ed. Philadelphia, PA: Elsevier, 2018.

Heaton HA. Chapter 98. Ectopic pregnancy and emergencies in the first 20 weeks of pregnancy. In: Tintinalli JE, Ma O, Yealy DM, et al, eds. *Tintinalli's Emergency Medicine: A Comprehensive Study Guide.* 9th ed. New York, NY: McGraw-Hill, 2020.

Kman NE, Werman HA, Greenberger SM. Chapter 73. Disorders presenting primarily with diarrhea. In: Tintinalli JE, Ma O, Yealy DM, et al, eds. *Tintinalli's Emergency Medicine: A Comprehensive Study Guide.* 9th ed. New York, NY: McGraw-Hill, 2020.

O'Mara SR, Wiesner L. Chapter 80. Hepatic disorders. In: Tintinalli JE, Ma O, Yealy DM, et al, eds. *Tintinalli's Emergency Medicine: A Comprehensive Study Guide.* 9th ed. New York, NY: McGraw-Hill, 2020.

Pour TR, Tibbles CD. Chapter 90. Selected gynecologic disorders. In: Marx JA, Hockberger RS, Gausche-Hill M, eds. *Rosen's Emergency Medicine: Concepts and Clinical Practice.* 9th ed. Philadelphia, PA: Elsevier, 2018.

Price TG. Chapter 83. Bowel obstruction. In: Tintinalli JE, Ma O, Yealy DM, et al, eds. *Tintinalli's Emergency Medicine: A Comprehensive Study Guide.* 9th ed. New York, NY: McGraw-Hill, 2020.

Trauma, Shock, and Resuscitation

Joshua Gauger, MD, MBA

Questions

104. A 58-year-old woman is brought to the emergency department (ED) by emergency medical service (EMS) after slipping on a patch of ice while walking to work and hitting her head on the cement pavement. Bystanders acknowledged that the patient was unconscious for approximately 1 minute. On arrival, her vital signs are blood pressure (BP) 155/75 mm Hg, heart rate (HR) 89 beats/minute, respiratory rate (RR) 18 breaths/minute, and pulse oxygenation 98% on room air. She has a 5-cm laceration to the back of her head that is actively bleeding. You ask the patient what happened, but she cannot remember. You inform her that she is in the hospital as a result of a fall. Over the next 10 minutes, she asks you repeatedly what happened and where she is. You do not find any focal neurologic deficits. As you bring the patient to the computed tomography (CT) scanner, she vomits once. CT results show a normal brain scan. Which of the following is the most likely diagnosis?

a. Cerebral concussion
b. Diffuse axonal injury
c. Cerebral contusion
d. Posttraumatic epilepsy
e. Trauma-induced Alzheimer disease

105. A 41-year-old restrained driver involved in a high-speed motor vehicle collision (MVC) is brought to the ED by EMS. The patient is breathing without difficulty and has bilateral and equal breath sounds. He has strong peripheral pulses. His HR is 121 beats/minute. His Glasgow Coma Scale (GCS) is 14. The secondary survey reveals bruising of the chest wall. You are concerned about a possible cardiac injury. Which area of the heart is most commonly involved in cardiac contusion?

a. Right atrium
b. Right ventricle (RV)
c. Left atrium
d. Left ventricle
e. Septum

106. A 25-year-old man is brought into the trauma resuscitation room after his motorcycle is struck by another vehicle. EMS reports that the patient was found 20 feet away from his motorcycle, which was badly damaged. His vital signs include a BP of 90/60 mm Hg, HR of 115 beats/minute, RR of 22 breaths/minute, and pulse oxygenation of 100% on 10 L of oxygen via face mask. In the adult population, what is the minimum percentage of blood loss necessary to cause a decrease in the systolic BP?

a. Loss of 5% of blood volume
b. Loss of 10% of blood volume
c. Loss of 15% to 30% of blood volume
d. Loss of 30% to 40% of blood volume
e. Loss of greater than 40% of blood volume

107. Paramedics bring a 17-year-old high school football player to the ED on a backboard and with a cervical collar. During a football game, the patient "speared" another player with his helmet and subsequently experienced severe neck pain. He denies paresthesias and is able to move all of his extremities. A cervical spine CT scan reveals multiple fractures of the first cervical vertebra. Which of the following best describes this fracture?

a. Odontoid fracture
b. Hangman fracture
c. Jefferson fracture
d. Clay shoveler's fracture
e. Teardrop fracture

108. A 20-year-old man presents to the ED with multiple stab wounds to his chest. His BP is 85/50 mm Hg and HR is 123 beats/minute. Two large-bore intravenous (IV) lines are established and IV fluids are running wide open. On examination, the patient is mumbling incomprehensibly, has good air entry on lung examination, and has jugular venous distension (JVD). As you are listening to his heart, the nurse calls out that the patient has lost his pulse and that she cannot get a BP reading. Which of the following is the most appropriate next step in management?

a. Atropine IV push
b. Epinephrine IV push
c. Placement of bilateral chest tubes
d. ED thoracotomy
e. Perform pericardiocentesis

109. A 22-year-old man calls the ED from a local bar. He was punched in the face 10 minutes ago and is holding his front incisor tooth in his hand. He wants to know what the best way is to preserve the tooth while coming to the ED. Which of the following is the most appropriate advice to give the caller?

a. Place the tooth in a napkin, and bring it to the ED
b. Place the tooth in a glass of water, and bring it to the ED
c. Place the tooth in a glass of beer, and bring it to the ED
d. Pour some water over the tooth, and place it back into the socket
e. Place the tooth in a glass of milk, and bring it to the ED

110. A 19-year-old man is brought into the trauma room by EMS after a head-on cycling accident. The patient was not wearing a helmet. Upon presentation, his BP is 125/75 mm Hg, HR is 105 beats/minute, RR is 19 breaths/minute, and oxygen saturation is 100% on 10 L of oxygen via face mask. His eyes are closed but he opens them to verbal command. He also moves his arms and legs on command. When you ask him questions, he is disoriented but able to converse. What is the patient's GCS score?

a. 11
b. 12
c. 13
d. 14
e. 15

111. A 61-year-old man presents to the ED with chest wall pain after a high-speed MVC. He is speaking in full sentences, breath sounds are equal bilaterally, and his extremities are well perfused. His BP is 150/75 mm Hg, HR is 92 beats/minute, and oxygen saturation is 97% on room air. Chest radiography reveals fractures of the seventh and eighth ribs of the right anterolateral chest. He has no other identifiable injuries. Which of the following is the most appropriate treatment for this patient's rib fractures?

a. Apply adhesive tape to the chest wall perpendicular to the rib fractures
b. Insert a chest tube into the right hemithorax
c. Send the patient to the operating room (OR) for surgical fixation
d. Provide analgesia and encourage incentive spirometry
e. Observe the patient in the ED for 6 hours

112. A 27-year-old man is brought to the ED by paramedics after a roll-over MVC. His BP is 85/55 mm Hg, HR is 112 beats/minute, RR is 45 breaths/minute, and oxygen saturation is 89% on 10 L via face mask. You auscultate his chest and hear decreased breath sounds on the left. Which of the following is the most appropriate next step in management?

a. Order a stat chest radiograph
b. Perform an emergent pericardiocentesis
c. Perform a diagnostic peritoneal lavage (DPL)
d. Perform an ED thoracotomy
e. Perform an emergent needle decompression

113. A 29-year-old man is brought to the ED by EMS after being stabbed in the back. His BP is 120/80 mm Hg, HR is 105 beats/minute, RR is 16 breaths/minute, and oxygen saturation is 98% on room air. On the secondary survey, you note motor weakness of his left lower extremity and the loss of pain sensation in the right lower extremity. Which of the following is the most likely diagnosis?

a. Spinal shock
b. Central cord syndrome
c. Anterior cord syndrome
d. Brown-Séquard syndrome
e. Cauda equina syndrome

114. A 33-year-old man, who was drinking heavily at a bar, presents to the ED after getting into a fight. A bystander informs paramedics that the patient was punched and kicked multiple times and sustained multiple blows to his head with a barstool. In the ED, his BP is 150/75 mm Hg, HR is 90 beats/minute, RR is 13 breaths/minute, and oxygen saturation is 100% on a nonrebreather mask. On examination, he opens his eyes to pain, and his pupils are equal and reactive. There is a laceration on the right side of his scalp. He withdraws his right arm to pain, but otherwise does not move. When you ask him questions, he is only able to moan. Which of the following is the most appropriate next step in management?

a. Perform rapid sequence induction and orotracheal intubation
b. Suture repair his scalp laceration
c. Administer IV mannitol
d. Perform bilateral burr holes of the cranium
e. Call a consult for emergent neurosurgical intervention

115. A 29-year-old man presents to the ED after being stabbed in his neck. The patient is speaking in full sentences. His breath sounds are equal bilaterally. His BP is 130/75 mm Hg, HR is 95 beats/minute, RR is 16 breaths/minute, and oxygen saturation is 99% on room air. The stab wound is located between the angle of the mandible and the cricoid cartilage and violates the platysma. There is blood oozing from the site although there is no expanding hematoma. Which of the following is the most appropriate next step in management?

a. Explore the wound and blindly clamp any sites of bleeding
b. Probe the wound with hemostats and look for injured vessels
c. Apply direct pressure and send the patient for operative exploration of a zone I injury
d. Apply direct pressure and send the patient for operative exploration of a zone II injury
e. Apply direct pressure and send the patient for operative exploration of a zone III injury

116. A 45-year-old man is brought to the ED after a head-on MVC. Paramedics who were at the scene report significant front-end damage to the vehicle. The patient's BP is 130/80 mm Hg, HR is 100 beats/minute, RR is 15 breaths/minute, and oxygen saturation is 98% on room air. Radiographs of the cervical spine reveal bilateral fractures of the C2 vertebra. The patient's neurologic examination is unremarkable. Which of the following best describes this fracture?

a. Colles' fracture
b. Boxer's fracture
c. Jefferson fracture
d. Hangman's fracture
e. Clay shoveler's fracture

117. A 71-year-old man is found lying on the ground one story below the balcony of his apartment. Paramedics bring the patient into the ED. He is cool to touch with a core body temperature of 96°F. His BP is 90/70 mm Hg and HR is 119 beats/minute. His eyes are closed, but they open when you call his name. He answers your questions but is confused. His limbs move to stimuli. On examination, you note clear fluid dripping from his left ear canal and an area of ecchymosis over his mastoid bone. Which of the following is the most likely diagnosis?

a. Le Fort fracture
b. Basilar skull fracture
c. Otitis interna
d. Otitis externa
e. Tripod fracture

The following scenario applies to questions 118-119.

A 34-year-old construction worker is brought to the ED by EMS after falling 30 feet from a scaffold. His vital signs include BP 80/40 mm Hg, HR 124 beats/minute, and oxygen saturation 93% on 100% oxygen via face mask. He has obvious head trauma with a scalp laceration overlying a skull fracture on his occiput. He does not speak when asked his name, his respirations are poor, and you hear gurgling with each attempted breath. Auscultation of the chest reveals diminished breath sounds on the right. There is no JVD or anterior chest wall crepitus. His pelvis is unstable with movement laterally to medially, and you note blood at the urethral meatus. His right leg is grossly deformed at the knee, and there is an obvious fracture of his left arm.

118. Which of the following is the most appropriate next step in management?

a. Insert a 32F chest tube into the right thoracic cavity
b. Perform a DPL to rule out intra-abdominal hemorrhage
c. Create two burr holes into the cranial vault to treat a potential epidural hematoma
d. Immediately reduce the extremity injuries and immobilize with splinting material
e. Plan for orotracheal intubation with in-line stabilization of the cervical spine

119. The patient is intubated and receives 1 L of IV crystalloid. His repeat vital signs are BP 84/42 mm Hg, HR 122 beats/minute, and oxygen saturation 92% on 100% fraction of inspired oxygen (FiO_2) via endotracheal (ET) tube. On repeat auscultation of the chest, you continue to hear diminished breath sounds of the right. What is the most appropriate next step in management of this patient?

a. Perform focused abdominal sonography for trauma (FAST) exam
b. Place a pelvic binder to stabilize the pelvis
c. Obtain CT scans of the patient's head and cervical spine
d. Perform need thoracostomy of the right chest
e. Administer 250 cc 3% hypertonic saline

120. Following need thoracostomy and chest tube placement, a pelvic binder is placed and the extremities are reduced and temporarily splinted. The patient has repeat vital signs of BP 88/52 mm Hg, HR 116 beats/minute, and oxygen saturation of 98%. Two units of packed red blood cells are given without improvement in vital signs. A FAST exam is performed and positive in the left upper quadrant. What is the most appropriate next step for this patient?

a. Send the patient for CT scans of the abdomen and pelvis
b. Consult orthopedic surgery to address bony injuries
c. Transfer the patient to the OR
d. Consult interventional radiology for embolization of bleeding pelvic vessels
e. Administer additional blood products until the vital signs are stable

121. A 20-year-old man was found on the ground next to his car after his vehicle struck a tree. Bystanders state that the man got out of his car after the collision, but collapsed within a few minutes. Paramedics subsequently found the man unconscious on the side of the road. In the ED, his BP is 175/90 mm Hg, HR is 65 beats/minute, RR is 12 breaths/minute, temperature is 99.2°F, and oxygen saturation is 97% on room air. His right pupil is fixed and dilated. His noncontrast head CT is shown in the figure. Which of the following is the most likely diagnosis?

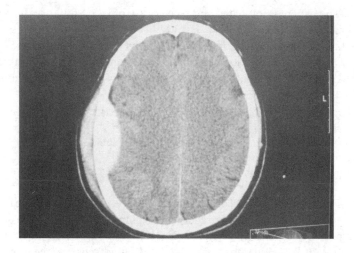

a. Epidural hematoma
b. Subdural hematoma
c. Subarachnoid hemorrhage (SAH)
d. Intracerebral hematoma
e. Cerebral contusion

122. An 81-year-old woman presents to the ED after tripping over the sidewalk curb and landing on her chin, causing hyperextension of her neck. She was placed in a cervical collar by paramedics. On examination, she has no sensorimotor function of her upper extremities. She cannot wiggle her toes, has 1/5 motor function of her quadriceps, and only patchy lower extremity sensation. Rectal examination reveals decreased rectal tone. Which of the following is the most likely diagnosis?

a. Central cord syndrome
b. Anterior cord syndrome
c. Brown-Séquard syndrome
d. Transverse myelitis
e. Exacerbation of Parkinson's disease

123. A 22-year-old woman presents to the ED after being ejected from her vehicle following a high-speed MVC. Upon arrival, her BP is 80/55 mm Hg and HR is 146 beats/minute. Two large-bore IVs are placed, and 2 L of IV fluids have been administered by EMS. Which of the following statements is most appropriate regarding management of this hypotensive trauma patient who fails to respond to initial volume resuscitation?

a. It is important to wait for fully cross-matched blood prior to transfusion
b. Begin an epinephrine infusion
c. Blood transfusion should not begin until after 4 L of crystalloid has been administered
d. Type O blood that is Rh-negative should be transfused
e. Type O blood that is Rh-positive should be transfused

124. A 24-year-old man is brought into the ED by paramedics after being run over by a car. His systolic BP is 90 mm Hg, HR is 121 beats/minute, RR is 28 breaths/minute, and oxygen saturation is 100% on a nonrebreather mask. The airway is patent and breath sounds are equal bilaterally. Large-bore access has been established and fluids are running wide open. Secondary survey reveals an unstable pelvis. Bedside FAST is negative for intraperitoneal fluid. Which of the following is the most appropriate immediate next step in management?

a. Bilateral chest tubes
b. Application of external fixator
c. Application of pelvic binder
d. Venographic embolization
e. Angiographic embolization

125. A 32-year-old man is brought to the ED by paramedics after a diving accident. The lifeguard on duty accompanies the patient and states that he dove head first into the shallow end of the pool and did not resurface. On examination, the patient is speaking clearly. He cannot move his arms or legs and cannot feel pain below his clavicle. He is able to feel light touch and position of his four extremities. A cervical spine radiograph does not reveal a fracture. Which of the following is the most likely diagnosis?

a. Spinal cord injury without radiographic abnormality (SCIWORA)
b. Central cord syndrome
c. Anterior cord syndrome
d. Cauda equina syndrome
e. Brown-Séquard syndrome

126. A 22-year-old man is brought to the ED 20 minutes after a head-on MVC in which he was the unrestrained driver. On arrival, he is alert and coherent but appears short of breath. His BP is 80/60 mm Hg, HR is 117 beats/minute, and oxygen saturation is 97% on a nonrebreather mask. Examination reveals bruising over the central portion of his chest. His neck veins are not distended. Breath sounds are present on the left but absent on the right, and his trachea is deviated to the left. Following administration of 2 L of IV fluid, his systolic BP remains at 80 mm Hg, and the patient has continued shortness of breath. Which of the following is the most appropriate next step in management?

a. Perform rapid sequence induction and orotracheal intubation
b. Perform a needle thoracostomy
c. Perform a DPL
d. Perform a FAST examination
e. Perform a pericardiocentesis

127. An 87-year-old man is brought to the ED on a long board and in a cervical collar after falling down a flight of steps. He denies losing consciousness. On arrival, his vital signs include a BP of 160/90 mm Hg, HR of 99 beats/minute, and RR of 16 breaths/minute. He is alert and speaking in full sentences. Breath sounds are equal bilaterally. Despite an obvious right arm fracture, his radial pulses are 2+ and symmetric. When examining his cervical spine, he denies tenderness to palpation and you do not feel any bony deformities. Which of the following is a true statement?

a. Epidural hematomas are more common than subdural hematomas in the elderly population
b. Cerebral atrophy in the elderly population is protective against subdural hematoma development
c. Increased lung elasticity allows elderly patients to recover from thoracic trauma more quickly than younger patients
d. The most common cervical spine fracture in this age group is a wedge fracture of the sixth cervical vertebra
e. Despite lack of cervical spine tenderness, imaging of his cervical spine is warranted

128. A 47-year-old man is brought into the ED after falling 20 feet from a ladder. His BP is 110/80 mm Hg, HR is 110 beats/minute, RR is 20 breaths/minute, and oxygen saturation is 100% on a face mask. He is able to answer your questions without difficulty. His chest is clear with bilateral breath sounds, abdomen is nontender, pelvis is stable, and the FAST examination is negative. You note a large scrotal hematoma and blood at the urethral meatus. Which of the following is the most appropriate next step in management?

a. Scrotal ultrasound
b. Kidney-ureter-bladder (KUB) radiograph
c. IV pyelogram
d. Retrograde cystogram
e. Retrograde urethrogram

129. A 24-year-old man is brought to the ED after being shot once in the abdomen. On arrival, his BP is 100/60 mm Hg, HR is 115 beats/minute, and RR is 22 breaths/minute. His airway is patent and you hear breath sounds bilaterally. On abdominal examination, you note a single ballistic wound approximately 1 cm to the right of the umbilicus. During the log roll, you see a single ballistic wound approximately 3 cm to the right of the lumbar spine. His GCS score is 15. The patient's BP is now 85/65 mm Hg and HR is 125 beats/minute after 2 L of fluid. Which of the following is the most appropriate next step in management?

a. Probe the entry wound to see if it violates the peritoneum
b. Perform a FAST examination
c. Perform a DPL
d. Obtain stat CT abdomen and pelvis
e. Transfer the patient to the OR

130. A 29-year-old man is brought to the ED with a gunshot wound (GSW) to his left thigh. Upon arrival, his BP is 140/80 mm Hg, HR is 95 beats/minute, RR is 18 breaths/minute, and oxygen saturation is 99% on room air. All of his distal pulses are 2+, and there is no gross deformity of his left leg. The patient is yelling that he is in pain. You turn to the nurse and say "Please give 50 mcg of fentanyl IV." The nurse repeats back to you, "I am going to give 50 mcg of fentanyl IV." You reply, "Yes, thank you." What type of communication is demonstrated between you and the nurse in this scenario?

a. Positive-feedback communication
b. Closed-loop communication
c. Redundant communication
d. Situation Background Assessment Recommendation (SBAR) communication
e. Team huddle communication

131. A 17-year-old adolescent boy is found unconscious in a swimming pool. He is brought into the ED by paramedics already intubated. In the ED, the patient is unresponsive with spontaneous abdominal breathing at a rate of 16 breaths/minute. His BP is 80/50 mm Hg and HR is 49 beats/minute. In addition to hypoxemia, what condition must be considered earliest in the management of this patient?

a. Cervical spine injury
b. Electrolyte imbalance
c. Metabolic acidosis
d. Severe atelectasis
e. Toxic ingestion

132. A 22-year-old man is brought to the ED after sustaining a single GSW to his right thigh. On arrival, his BP is 115/75 mm Hg and HR is 105 beats/minute. You note a large hematoma of his medial thigh. The patient complains of numbness in his right foot. On extremity examination, the right foot is pale. You cannot palpate a dorsalis pedis pulse in the right foot but can locate it by Doppler. In addition, the patient cannot move the foot. Which of the following is the most appropriate next step in management?

a. Angiography
b. Exploration of the wound in the OR
c. Fasciotomy to treat compartment syndrome
d. Place a long leg splint to the right lower extremity
e. CT scan of the right extremity

133. A 67-year-old woman is brought to the ED after being struck by a cyclist while crossing the street. On arrival to the ED, her eyes are closed and do not open to stimuli, she makes no verbal sounds, and withdraws only to painful stimuli. You assign her a GCS of 6. Her BP is 175/90 mm Hg and HR is 75 beats/minute. As you open her eyelids, you notice that her right pupil is 8 mm and nonreactive and her left is 4 mm and minimally reactive. Which of the following is the most common manifestation of increasing intracranial pressure (ICP) causing brain herniation?

a. Change in level of consciousness
b. Ipsilateral pupillary dilation
c. Contralateral pupillary dilation
d. Significantly elevated BP
e. Hemiparesis

134. A 34-year-old man is brought to the ED after being shot in the right side of his chest. The patient is awake and speaking. Breath sounds are diminished on the right. There is no bony crepitus or tracheal deviation. His BP is 95/65 mm Hg, HR is 121 beats/minute, RR is 23 breaths/minute, and oxygen saturation is 94% on a nonrebreather mask. Supine chest radiograph reveals a hazy appearance over the entire right lung field. You place a 36F chest tube into the right thoracic cavity and there is 1,200 mL of immediate blood output in the chest tube drainage system. Which of the following is an indication for thoracotomy?

a. 500 mL of initial chest tube drainage of blood
b. 1,200 mL of initial chest tube drainage of blood
c. Persistent bleeding from the chest tube at a rate of 50 mL/h
d. Chest radiograph with greater than 50% lung field whiteout
e. Evidence of a pneumothorax (PTX) on CXR or physical examination

135. A 36-year-old electrical worker presents to the ED after an electrical injury while working on a high-voltage line of over 1,200 V. The patient felt a shock in his left arm initially, but has no symptoms currently. The patient remembers the entire event and has no pain in his arm. His BP is 132/80 mm Hg and HR is 88 beats/minute. On physical exam, you are unable to visualize any signs of injury. You obtain an electrocardiogram (ECG) which shows normal sinus rhythm. Basic laboratory studies are normal. What is the most appropriate next step in management of this patient?

a. Admit the patient to the hospital for serial compartment checks of the left arm
b. Discharge the patient home with close primary care follow-up
c. Transfer the patient to the nearest burn center given the high-voltage exposure
d. Arrange for observation admission
e. Admit to the OR for immediate fasciotomy of the left arm

136. A 27-year-old pregnant woman, in her third trimester, is brought to the ED after being involved in a low-speed MVC. The patient was the restrained rear-seat passenger in a car that was struck head-on by another car. Her BP is 120/70 mm Hg and HR is 107 beats/minute. Her airway is patent, breath sounds are equal bilaterally, and skin is warm with 2+ pulses. FAST examination is negative for free fluid. Evaluation of the fetus reveals appropriate HR and movement. Repeat maternal BP is 120/75 mm Hg. Which of the following is the most appropriate next step in management?

a. Consult obstestrics for immediate cesarean section in the OR
b. Perform an immediate cesarean section in the ED
c. CT scan of the abdomen and pelvis to rule out occult injury
d. Discharge the patient if laboratory testing is normal
e. Monitor the patient and fetus for a minimum of 4 hours

137. A 61-year-old man presents to the ED with low back pain after slipping on an icy sidewalk the previous day. He states that the pain started on the left side of his lower back and now involves the right and radiates down both legs. He also noticed difficulty urinating since last night. On neurologic examination, he cannot plantar flex his feet. Rectal examination reveals diminished rectal tone. He has a medical history of chronic hypertension and underwent a "vessel surgery" many years earlier. Which of the following is the most likely diagnosis?

a. Abdominal aortic aneurysm (AAA)
b. Disk herniation
c. Spinal stenosis
d. Cauda equina syndrome
e. Osteomyelitis

138. Paramedics bring a 55-year-old woman to the ED after she was struck by a motor vehicle traveling at 30 miles per hour (mph). Her BP is 165/95 mm Hg, HR is 105 beats/minute, and RR is 20 breaths/minute. She does not open her eyes, is verbal but not making any sense, and withdraws to painful stimuli. You assign her a GCS score of 8. After you intubate the patient, a colleague notices that her left pupil has become dilated compared to the right. Which of the following most quickly reduces elevated ICP?

a. Cranial decompression
b. IV dexamethasone
c. IV furosemide
d. Hyperventilation
e. IV mannitol

139. A 79-year-old woman with a history of ischemic cardiomyopathy who underwent a coronary artery bypass graft (CABG) surgery 7 years ago is brought to the ED by her family for 2 days of worsening shortness of breath. She also has not gotten out of bed for 2 days and is confused. She denies chest pain, fever, or cough. Her BP is 85/50 mm Hg, HR is 125 beats/minute, RR is 26 breaths/minute, and oral temperature is 98.1°F. She is unable to follow commands and is oriented only to name. The cardiovascular examination reveals tachycardia with no murmurs. Her lungs have rales bilaterally at the bases. The abdomen is soft, nontender, and nondistended. Lower extremities have 2+ edema to the knees bilaterally. Which of the following is the most likely diagnosis?

a. Hypovolemic shock
b. Neurogenic shock
c. Cardiogenic shock
d. Anaphylactic shock
e. Septic shock

140. A 32-year-old man with no past medical problems presents to the ED with palpitations. For the past 2 days, he has been feeling weak. Over the last 6 hours, he has noticed that his heart is racing. He denies chest pain and shortness of breath. He has never felt this way before. His BP is 140/82 mm Hg, HR is 180 beats/minute, RR is 14 breaths/minute, and oral temperature is 98.9°F. His physical examination is normal. You obtain the following rhythm strip (Figure). What is your first-line treatment for this patient?

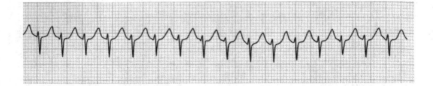

a. Synchronized cardioversion at 100 J
b. Adenosine 6 mg IV push
c. Adenosine 12 mg IV push
d. Valsalva maneuver
e. Verapamil 3 mg IV push

141. You are a passenger aboard an airplane when a 78-year-old woman starts complaining of chest pain and difficulty breathing. You are the only medical professional available and volunteer to help. Fortunately, the aircraft is well-equipped with basic medical equipment, advanced cardiac life support (ACLS) medications, and a cardiac monitor. On examination, the passenger's BP is 75/40 mm Hg, HR is 180 beats/minute, and RR is 24 breaths/min. On examination, the patient is in obvious distress, but able to answer basic questions. Her heart is tachycardic, regular, and without murmurs, rubs, or gallops. Physical examination is remarkable for a bounding carotid pulse. You attach the cardiac monitor and see a regular rhythm at 180 beats/min with wide QRS complexes and no obvious P waves. After asking the pilot to make an emergency landing, what is the most appropriate next step?

a. Administer IV amiodarone
b. Perform synchronized cardioversion
c. Administer IV verapamil
d. Administer IV lidocaine
e. Administer IV procainamide

142. A 75-year-old man complaining of chest pain is brought into the ED by paramedics. He is barely able to speak due to shortness of breath. The nurse immediately places him on the monitor, starts an IV, and gives him oxygen. His BP is 70/40 mm Hg, HR is 140 beats/minute, RR is 28 breaths/minute, temperature is 98.9°F, and oxygen saturation is 95% on room air. On examination, he is in mild distress. His heart is irregular and tachycardic. His lungs are clear to auscultation, with rales at the bases bilaterally. A rhythm strip is shown in the figure. What is your first-line treatment for this patient?

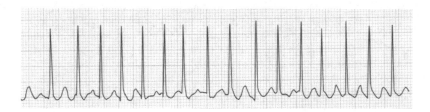

a. Heparin drip
b. Diltiazem 10 mg IV push
c. Metoprolol 5 mg IV push
d. Digoxin 0.5 mg IV
e. Synchronized cardioversion at 100 J

143. You are called to the bedside of a hypotensive patient with altered mental status. The nurse hands you an ECG which shows atrial flutter at 150 beats/minute with 2:1 arteriovenous (AV) block. Although the patient has a palpable pulse, you feel that the patient is unstable and elect to perform emergent cardioversion. You attach the monitor leads to the patient. What is the single most critical step in electrical cardioversion of a patient with a pulse?

a. Set the appropriate energy level
b. Position conductor pads or paddles on patient
c. Charge the defibrillator
d. Turn on the synchronization mode
e. Administer 25 mcg of fentanyl IV

144. Paramedics bring in a 54-year-old man who was found down in his apartment by his wife. He is successfully intubated in the field and paramedics are currently performing cardiopulmonary resuscitation (CPR). He is transferred to an ED gurney and quickly attached to the cardiac monitors. You ask the paramedics to hold CPR to assess the patient and the rhythm strip. The monitor shows sinus bradycardia, but no pulses are palpable. On examination, you appreciate bilateral breath sounds with mechanical ventilation, a soft abdomen, no rashes, and a left arm AV graft. In addition to CPR with epinephrine every 3 to 5 minutes, which intervention should be performed next?

a. Administer 1 ampule of sodium bicarbonate
b. Administer 1 ampule of calcium gluconate
c. Administer 1 ampule of D50 (dextrose)
d. Place a left-sided chest tube
e. Perform pericardiocentesis

145. A 72-year-old man is in the ED for the evaluation of generalized weakness over the previous 24 hours. He has a past medical history of coronary artery disease with a CABG performed 5 years ago, diabetes mellitus, and arthritis. The nurse places the patient on a cardiac monitor and begins to get his vital signs. While the nurse is obtaining the vital signs, he suddenly becomes unresponsive. You arrive at the bedside, look at the monitor, and see the following rhythm (Figure). Which of the following is the most appropriate next step in management?

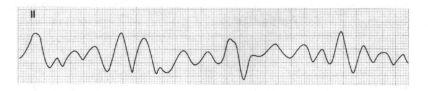

a. Wait 5 minutes to see if he wakes up on his own
b. Immediately defibrillate at 200 J (biphasic)
c. Perform synchronized cardioversion at 100 J
d. Immediately intubate the patient
e. Insert an IV line and administer amiodarone

146. An 82-year-old nursing home patient presents to the ED in septic shock. Her BP is 75/40 mm Hg, HR is 117 beats/minute, RR is 29 breaths/minute, temperature is 96.5°F, and oxygen saturation is 87% on room air. As you perform laryngoscopy to intubate the patient, you easily visualize the vocal cords and subsequently pass the orotracheal tube through the vocal cords. You place the colorimetric end-tidal carbon dioxide device over the tube and get appropriate color change. There are equal bilateral breath sounds on auscultation and you observe chest wall motion with ventilation. Which of the following is the most reliable method for verifying proper ET tube placement?

a. Chest radiograph
b. Visualization of the ET tube passing through the vocal cords
c. Observation of chest wall motion with ventilation
d. Hearing equal bilateral breath sounds on auscultation
e. End-tidal carbon dioxide color change

147. A 25-year-old man fell off his surfboard and landed on a large nearby rock. He was pulled from the water by lifeguards and brought to the ED in full spinal immobilization. He is alert and oriented to person, place, and time. He is complaining of weakness in all of his extremities. His BP is 85/50 mm Hg, HR is 54 beats/minute, RR is 20 breaths/minute, temperature is 98.4°F, and oxygen saturation is 98% on room air. On examination, he has no external signs of head injury. His heart is bradycardic without murmurs. The lungs are clear to auscultation and the abdomen is soft and nontender. He has grossly normal peripheral sensation but no motor strength in all four extremities. Which of the following is the most likely diagnosis?

a. Hypovolemic shock
b. Neurogenic shock
c. Cardiogenic shock
d. Anaphylactic shock
e. Septic shock

148. A 48-year-old man is brought to the ED by paramedics for generalized weakness. His medical history is significant for a CABG last month. He has been unable to get out of bed for the past day because of dizziness when changing position. He denies chest pain, shortness of breath, or syncope. His BP is 86/60 mm Hg, HR is 44 beats/minute, RR is 18 breaths/minute, temperature is 98.9°F, and oxygen saturation is 98% on room air. There is a well-healing midline sternotomy incision. Cardiac examination reveals a III/VI systolic ejection murmur. There are minimal rales at his lung bases. He is immediately attached to the cardiac monitor. His rhythm strip is shown in the figure. What is the most appropriate initial treatment?

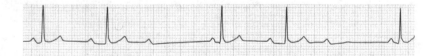

a. Observation on monitor
b. Transcutaneous pacing
c. Transvenous pacing
d. Atropine 0.5 mg IV
e. Epinephrine IV drip at 2 mcg/minute

149. You are caring for a 54-year-old woman with a history of schizophrenia and coronary artery disease who presents to the ED for chest pain. Her vital signs are within normal limits and her ECG is normal sinus rhythm with nonspecific ST/T-wave changes. Her first troponin is sent to the laboratory, and you are planning to admit her to the hospital for a complete acute coronary syndrome (ACS) evaluation. She receives aspirin and nitroglycerin and her chest pain resolves. A few minutes later, the nurse alerts you that the patient has become unconscious. You go to the bedside and find the patient awake and alert. You review the rhythm strip from during the unconscious episode (Figure). What is the most appropriate next step in management?

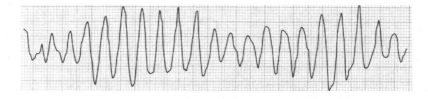

a. Observation of patient
b. IV magnesium sulfate
c. IV lidocaine
d. Placement of a transvenous pacemaker
e. IV isoproterenol

150. A 56-year-old woman is brought to the ED by EMS after being involved in an MVC. She was the restrained passenger in a head-on collision at approximately 55 mph. There was significant front-end damage to the vehicle including intrusion into the passenger compartment. The patient has normal vital signs and a GCS of 15. Her only complaint is right knee pain. An X-ray of the knee shows a posterior knee dislocation. Which of the following is a hard sign for vascular injury following a knee dislocation?

a. Severe knee pain
b. Paresthesia of the leg
c. Palpable popliteal thrill
d. Ankle-brachial index (ABI) more than 0.9
e. Nonexpanding hematoma of the affected calf.

151. An 82-year-old man with a history of chronic obstructive pulmonary disease (COPD) and hypertension presents with shortness of breath and fever. His medications include albuterol, ipratropium, prednisone, hydrochlorothiazide, and atenolol. His BP is 70/40 mm Hg, HR is 110 beats/minute, RR is 24 breaths/minute, temperature is 102.1°F, and oxygen saturation is 91% on room air. The patient is uncomfortable and mumbling incoherently. On chest examination, you appreciate rales on the left side of his chest. He is tachycardic, and auscultation reveals a regular rhythm with no murmurs, rubs, or gallops. His abdomen is soft and nontender. You believe this patient is in septic shock from pneumonia and start IV fluids, broad-spectrum antibiotics, and a dopamine drip. His BP remains at 75/50 mm Hg. Which of the following is the most appropriate next step in management?

a. D5 normal saline IV bolus
b. Phenylephrine IV drip
c. Fludrocortisone IV push
d. Hydrocortisone IV push
e. Epinephrine IV drip

152. A 64-year-old woman with a history of depression and hypertension was found down by her husband and brought in by EMS. She has recently been depressed and expressed thoughts of suicide. She usually takes fluoxetine atenolol. On arrival, the patient is obtunded but responds to pain and is maintaining her airway. Her BP is 70/40 mm Hg, HR is 42 beats/minute, RR is 12 breaths/minute, temperature is 98.1°F, and oxygen saturation is 94% on room air. On examination, her pupils are 3 mm and reactive bilaterally. Lungs are clear to auscultation. Heart is bradycardic, but regular, with no murmurs, rubs, or gallops. Extremities have no edema. An ECG shows first-degree AV block at 42 beats/min, but no ST/T-wave changes. Blood sugar is 112 mg/dL. What is the most specific treatment for this patient's ingestion?

a. IV fluid bolus
b. IV atropine
c. IV glucagon
d. IV epinephrine
e. Cardiac pacing

153. A 19-year-old man suffers a single GSW to the left chest and is brought in by his friends. He is complaining of chest pain. On examination, BP is 70/40 mm Hg, HR is 140 beats/minute, RR is 16 breaths/minute, temperature is 99°F, and oxygen saturation is 96% on room air. He has distended neck veins, but his trachea is not deviated. Lungs are clear to auscultation bilaterally. Heart sounds are difficult to appreciate, but you feel a bounding, regular pulse. Abdomen is soft and nontender. Extremity examination is normal. Two large-bore IV lines are placed and the patient is given 1 L normal saline and 1 unit of Type O+ packed red blood cells. Chest radiograph shows a globular cardiac silhouette but a normal mediastinum and no PTX. What is the definitive management of this patient?

a. Intubation
b. Tube thoracostomy
c. Pericardiocentesis
d. Thoracotomy
e. Blood transfusion

154. An 87-year-old woman with a history of dementia, arthritis, and hypertension presents to the ED for abdominal pain. Her caretaker reports that she is having midepigastric pain and had one episode of nonbloody, nonbilious vomiting prior to arrival. The patient is oriented to name only. Her vital signs include a BP of 80/44 mm Hg, HR of 110 beats/minute, RR of 16 breaths/minute, temperature of 99.8°F, and oxygen saturation 96% on room air. On examination, the abdomen is diffusely tender. Stool is brown and guaiac negative. You place two IV lines and begin fluid resuscitation. You send her blood to the laboratory and order an acute abdominal series including the following upright radiograph of her chest (Figure). Which of the following is the most appropriate next step in management?

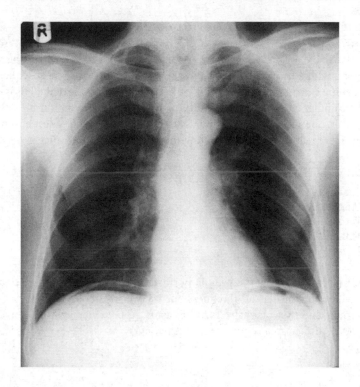

a. Start IV antibiotics
b. Order a CT scan of her abdomen
c. Emergent surgical consultation
d. Place a central venous line
e. Discharge home with an over the counter antacid

The following scenario applies to questions 155-156.

A 34-year-old woman is brought to the ED from a kitchen fire. She was cooking with a frying pan full of grease that caught fire, and subsequently the ceiling caught on fire. Upon arrival, her BP is 110/75 mmHg, HR is 115 beats/minute, RR is 18 breaths/minute, and pulse oxygenation is 98% on room air. She weighs 70 kg. She has tender blisters on her chest and both arms. Her breathing is nonlabored without stridor, and her voice is normal.

155. What classification of burns does this patient have?
a. Superficial
b. First degree
c. Partial thickness
d. Full thickness
e. Fourth degree

156. After the primary survey is performed, a complete examination of this patient reveals partial-thickness burns covering her anterior chest wall, abdomen, and the volar aspects of her arms. Approximately, what percentage body surface area is burned in this patient?
a. 1%
b. 4.5%
c. 9%
d. 18%
e. 27%

157. Which of the following is an indication for transfer to a burn center?
a. Severe sunburn, including the face with peeling skin
b. Greater than 5% body surface area with partial- and full-thickness burns
c. Greater than 20% body surface area with superficial-thickness burns
d. Greater than 50% body surface area with superficial-thickness burns
e. Burn patients with multiple comorbidities and poor social support

The following scenario applies to questions 158-159.

A 38-year old man presents to the ED with decreased vision in his right eye following an assault with head trauma. He has normal vital signs and a GCS of 15. On examination of the eye, you note proptosis and decreased extra-ocular movements. His right pupil is round and sluggishly reactive to light whereas the contralateral pupil reacts appropriately. There is no drainage from the eye. Visual acuity is 20/200 in the right eye and 20/20 in the left.

158. What is the most appropriate next step in evaluation of the patient's eye?

a. Fluorescein staining
b. Head CT
c. Perform and ultrasound to look for a retinal detachment
d. Consult ophthalmology
e. Obtain intraocular pressure

159. Intraocular pressure is 46 mm Hg in the right eye and 18 mm Hg in the left eye. What is the most appropriate next step in management?

a. Lateral canthotomy and cantholysis
b. Head CT with IV contrast
c. Decompression of the anterior chamber
d. Serial tonometry
e. IV mannitol

160. A 31 year-old man is brought in by EMS after being stabbed multiple times in the neck. The patient is able to speak, but his voice is muffled. There is no stridor with breathing. He has normal vital signs including pulse oximetry of 100% on room air. He is awake and alert with eyes open and is moving all four extremities. His radial pulses are intact. Examination of the neck reveals multiple small puncture wounds between his clavicles and mandible with no active bleeding. Which of the following would be an indication for immediate operative management?

a. Subcutaneous emphysema
b. Carotid bruit
c. Dyspnea
d. Nonexpanding hematoma
e. Dysphagia

Trauma, Shock, and Resuscitation

Answers

104. The answer is a. The patient sustained a **cerebral concussion.** This is caused by a head injury leading to a **brief loss of neurologic function**. These individuals are often amnestic to the event and frequently ask the same questions over and over again (perseveration). **Headache** with or without vomiting is generally present; however, there are **no focal neurologic findings** on examination. Loss of consciousness results from impairment of the reticular activating system (RAS). Patients show rapid clinical improvement. CT scan of the brain is normal.

Diffuse axonal injury **(b)** is the result of microscopic shearing of brain nerve fibers. Patients typically present unconscious and remain in a coma for a prolonged period of time. Initial CT scan is often insensitive for diffuse axonal injury and may lead to a false negative diagnosis. Patients with diffuse axonal injury have over a 33% mortality rate. The clinical features of a cerebral contusion **(c)** are similar to those of a concussion except that neurologic dysfunction is more profound and prolonged. Focal deficits may be present if contusion occurs in the sensorimotor area. Contusions occur when the brain impacts the skull and the lesion is typically seen on CT scan. Posttraumatic epilepsy **(d)** is associated with intracranial hematomas and depressed skull fractures. The seizures generally occur within the first week of the head injury. Some scientists believe that head trauma predisposes to Alzheimer disease **(e)**; however, this would take years to develop.

105. The answer is b. Blunt cardiac injury usually results from high-speed vehicular collisions in which the chest wall strikes the steering wheel. Although all forms are associated with potentially fatal complications, they should be viewed clinically as a continuous spectrum of myocardial damage: concussion (no permanent cell damage), contusion (permanent cell damage), infarction (cell death), tamponade (bleeding into the pericardium), and rupture (exsanguination). The mechanism of injury in a cardiac contusion involves a high-speed deceleration, which causes the heart to move forward, forcibly striking the sternum. In addition, the direct force of hitting an object (eg, the steering wheel) also can damage the heart. **The RV is most commonly injured** because it is the most anterior aspect of the heart and is closest to the sternum. The right atrium (**a**), left atrium (**c**), left ventricle (**d**), and the septum (**e**) are less commonly injured.

106. The answer is d. **Hypovolemia secondary to hemorrhage** is the most common cause of shock in the trauma patient. The earliest signs of hemorrhagic shock are tachycardia and cutaneous vasoconstriction. The amount of blood loss present can be estimated based on the individual's initial clinical presentation. Class I hemorrhage (**a and b**) is characterized by 0% to 15% blood loss (approximately 0-750 mL in an average adult). This stage exhibits minimal clinical signs and symptoms. Class II hemorrhage (**c**) is characterized by 15% to 30% blood loss (approximately 750-1,500 mL in an average adult). This stage exhibits tachycardia (HR > 100) with a narrow pulse pressure, delayed capillary refill, mild anxiety, tachypnea, and a slight decrease in urine output. **Class III hemorrhage** is characterized by **30% to 40% blood loss** (approximately 1,500-2,000 mL in an average adult). This stage exhibits **tachypnea, tachycardia (HR > 120), decrease in systolic BP, delayed capillary refill, decreased urine output, and a change in mental status**. Class IV hemorrhage (**e**) is characterized by blood loss greater than 40% (> 2 L in an average adult). This stage exhibits obvious shock, tachycardia (HR > 140), decreased systolic BP, extremely narrow pulse pressure, scant urine output, delayed capillary refill, confusion, and lethargy.

107. The answer is c. Spearing (hitting another player with the crown of the helmet) generates an axial loading force that is transmitted through the occipital condyles to the superior articular surfaces of the lateral masses of the first cervical vertebra (C1). This fracture is commonly referred to as a **Jefferson fracture** described as a **C1 burst fracture**. It is considered an **unstable** fracture and 40% have associated C2 fractures. On plain radiograph, it is best seen on the open-mouth odontoid view as the lateral masses are shifted laterally. It is associated with diving accidents, "spearing" in football, and other injuries in which there is an increased axial load to the cervical spine. Proper cervical spine precautions should remain in place throughout management in the ED.

Odontoid fractures (**a**) occur when there is a fracture through the odontoid process of the C2 vertebra, and it is considered an unstable cervical fracture. A hangman's fracture (**b**), or traumatic spondylolysis of C2, occurs when the cervico-cranium is thrown into extreme hyperextension secondary to abrupt deceleration (ie, head-on high-speed MVCs). This is also an unstable cervical fracture. A clay shoveler's fracture (d) occurs secondary to cervical hyperextension or direct trauma to the posterior neck, resulting in an avulsion fracture of the spinous process (ie, assault with a blunt object to the back of neck). A teardrop fracture (e) occurs from severe hyperflexion of the cervical spine and is commonly seen after diving accidents. This injury disrupts all of the cervical ligaments, facet joints, and causes a triangular fracture of a portion of the vertebral body and thus is an unstable cervical fracture. Teardrop fractures are associated with anterior cord syndrome.

108. The answer is d. The vignette describes a traumatic arrest after penetrating chest trauma. **ED thoracotomy** is the indicated therapeutic approach to the **penetrating trauma patient** who **has a witnessed loss of vital signs** en route to the ED or in the ED. The most likely cause in this vignette is **cardiac tamponade**, which occurs in approximately 2% of anterior penetrating chest traumas. Clinically, patients present with **hypotension, JVD**, and **muffled heart sounds**. The combination of these three signs is called **Beck's triad**. In addition, tachycardia is often present. JVD may not be present if there is marked hypovolemia. The most effective method for relieving acute pericardial tamponade in the trauma setting is via thoracotomy and incision of the pericardium with removal of blood from the pericardial sac. Patients with stab wounds are more likely to have a better outcome than the ones with ballistic wounds following thoracotomy.

The role of ACLS drugs **(a and b)** in traumatic arrest is unclear. However, patients in traumatic arrest typically require surgical rather than medical intervention. Chest tube placement **(c)** will not treat pericardial tamponade. If the patient had evidence of a tension PTX, then chest tubes would be the treatment of choice. Pericardiocentesis **(e)** may or may not be effective in acute traumatic tamponade because the pericardium is usually distended by clotted blood rather than by free blood. Pericardiocentesis is indicated for patients with suspected cardiac tamponade who have measurable vital signs.

109. The answer is d. The patient has an **avulsed tooth**, which is a **dental emergency**. Avulsed permanent teeth require prompt intervention. The **best environment for an avulsed tooth is its own socket. Reimplantation is most successful** if the tooth is returned to its socket **within 30 minutes** of the avulsion. A 1% chance of successful replantation is lost for every minute that the tooth is outside of its socket. The tooth should only be handled by the crown to prevent disruption of the root. If the patient cannot replant the tooth, he or she should keep the tooth under his or her tongue or in the buccal pouch so that it is bathed in saliva. If that cannot be achieved, then the tooth can be placed in a cup of milk (**e**) or in saline. The best transport solution is **Hank solution,** which is a buffered chemical solution. However, it is typically unavailable in this setting.

The worst option is to transport the tooth in a dry medium, such as a napkin (**a**). Water and beer (**b and c**) are less than ideal. Saliva, milk, or saline are better liquid transport mediums.

110. The answer is c. The GCS score, as shown later, may be used as a tool for classifying head injury and is an objective method for following a patient's neurologic status. The GCS assesses a person's **eye**, **verbal**, and **motor responsiveness.** Although the GCS was originally developed to assess head trauma at 6 hours postinjury, it is commonly used in the acute presentation. This patient received a score of 3 for eye opening to verbal command, 4 for being disoriented but conversant, and 6 for obeying verbal commands. This can be reported as **GCS 13 (E3, V4, M6).**

Glasgow coma scale	
Best eye response (E)	
4	Spontaneous—open with blinking at baseline
3	Opens to verbal command, speech, or shout
2	Open to pain, not applied to face
1	None
Best verbal response (V)	
5	Oriented
4	Confused conversation, but able to answer questions
3	Inappropriate responses, words discernible
2	Incomprehensible speech
1	None

Glasgow coma scale (Continued)	
Best motor response (M)	
6	Obeys commands for movement
5	Purposeful movement to painful stimulus (crosses midline)
4	Withdraws from pain
3	Abnormal (spastic) flexion, decorticate posture
2	Extensor (rigid) response, decerebrate posture
1	None

(Reproduced with permission from Adam J. Rosh, MD, and Rosh Review.)

All other answer choices (**a, b, d, and e**) are incorrect.

111. The answer is d. Simple rib fractures are the most common form of significant chest injury. Ribs usually break at the point of impact or at the posterior angle, which is structurally the weakest point. The fourth through ninth ribs are most commonly involved. Rib fractures occur more commonly in adults than in children due to the relative inelasticity of the adult chest wall compared to the more compliant pediatric chest wall. **The presence of two or more rib fractures at any level is associated with a higher incidence of internal injuries.** The treatment of patients with simple acute rib fractures includes **adequate pain relief** and **maintenance of pulmonary function.** Oral pain medications are usually sufficient for young and healthy patients. Older patients may require stronger analgesia with opioids, but care must be taken to avoid over sedation. Continuing daily activities and deep breathing are important to ensure ventilation and prevent atelectasis. **Incentive spirometry** assists the patient in taking routine deep breaths to prevent atelectasis and the development of pneumonia. If there is concern regarding the patient's ability to cough, breathe deeply, maintain activity, or if two or more ribs are fractured, it is preferable to admit the patient to the hospital for aggressive pulmonary care.

Attempts to relieve pain by immobilization or splinting (**a**) should be avoided. Although this may decrease pain, it also promotes hypoventilation, leading to atelectasis and pneumonia. A chest tube (**b**) is indicated only if a PTX or hemothorax is suspected. Simple acute rib fractures heal spontaneously and do not require surgical fixation (c). The main concern in treating rib fractures is preventing complications, such as atelectasis and pneumonia. Therefore, it is important that the patient be provided with adequate analgesia and ED observation alone is not sufficient treatment (e).

112. The answer is e. A PTX can be divided into three classifications—simple, communicating, and tension. A simple PTX occurs when there is no communication with the atmosphere or shift of the mediastinum and results from the accumulation of air within the pleural cavity. Communicating PTX is associated with a defect in the chest wall and is sometimes referred to as a "sucking chest wound." A tension PTX occurs when air enters the pleural cavity on inspiration, but cannot exit, leading to compression of the vena cava and subsequently decreased cardiac output and hypotension. The progressive accumulation of air under pressure in the pleural cavity may lead to a shift of the mediastinum to the contralateral hemithorax.

Patients with a traumatic PTX typically present with shortness of breath, chest pain, and tachypnea. The physical examination may reveal decreased or absent breath sounds over the involved side, as well as subcutaneous emphysema. Any **unstable patient** with respiratory symptoms in the **setting of a PTX** should be treated with **immediate needle decompression** in the **second intercostal space** in the **midclavicular line** on the affected side. Once stabilized, a definitive tube thoracostomy (chest tube) should be performed. The preferred site for insertion of a chest tube is the fourth or fifth intercostal space at the anterior or midaxillary line of the ipsilateral hemithorax. The tube should be positioned posteriorly and toward the apex so that it can effectively remove both air and fluid.

A chest radiograph (a) may be helpful in diagnosing a PTX; however, this patient is unstable and intervention should not be delayed for imaging. Pericardiocentesis (b) is a procedure used to remove fluid from the pericardial sac in the case of pericardial tamponade. DPL (c) is used to diagnose free fluid in the peritoneum. Although ultimately this may be necessary for this patient, it is important to address and follow the airway, breathing, and circulations (ABCs) (primary survey) of trauma resuscitation. In this patient, airway and breathing need to be addressed first. ED thoracotomy (d) is used in select circumstances, including penetrating trauma patients who have a witnessed loss of vital signs.

113. The answer is d. Brown-Séquard syndrome or hemisection of the spinal cord typically results from penetrating trauma, such as a gunshot or knife wound. Patients with this lesion have ipsilateral motor paralysis and contralateral loss of pain and temperature below the level of the injury. This syndrome has the best prognosis for recovery of all of the incomplete spinal cord lesions.

Spinal shock (a) is a clinical syndrome characterized by the bilateral loss of neurologic function and autonomic tone below the level of a spinal cord lesion. Patients typically exhibit flaccid paralysis with loss of sensory input, deep tendon reflexes, and urinary bladder tone. Patients in spinal shock are bradycardic, hypotensive, and hypothermic. Spinal shock generally lasts less than 24 hours, but may last several days. Central cord syndrome (b) most commonly occurs in a patient with degenerative arthritis of the cervical vertebrae and whose neck is forcibly hyperextended (ie, a forward fall onto the chin in an elderly person). Patients with central cord syndrome have greater sensorimotor neurologic deficits in the upper extremities compared to the lower extremities. Anterior cord syndrome (c) results in variable degrees of motor paralysis and absent pain sensation below the level of the lesion. Its hallmark is preservation of vibratory sensation and proprioception because of an intact dorsal column. Cauda equina syndrome (e) causes peripheral nerve injury rather than direct spinal cord damage. The presentation of cauda equina syndrome includes variable motor and sensory loss in the lower extremities, sciatica, bowel and bladder dysfunction, and saddle anesthesia.

Brown-Sequard syndrome

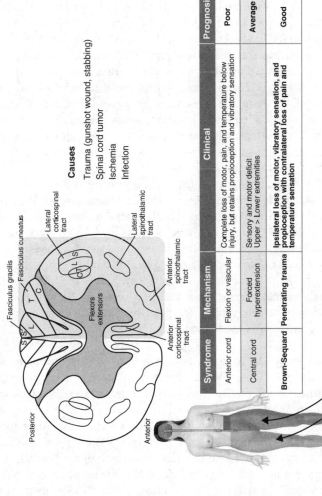

Causes

Trauma (gunshot wound, stabbing)
Spinal cord tumor
Ischemia
Infection

Syndrome	Mechanism	Clinical	Prognosis
Anterior cord	Flexion or vascular	Complete loss of motor, pain, and temperature below injury, but retains propioception and vibratory sensation	Poor
Central cord	Forced hyperextension	Sensory and motor deficit Upper > Lower extremities	Average
Brown-Sequard	Penetrating trauma	Ipsilateral loss of motor, vibratory sensation, and propioception with contralateral loss of pain and temperature sensation	Good

Ipsilateral loss of motor, vibratory, **and propioception**

Contralateral loss of pain **and temperature sensation**

(Reproduced with permission from Adam J. Rosh, MD, and Rosh Review.)

114. The answer is a. Head injury severity is assessed by the mechanism of injury and the initial neurologic examination. Although the GCS is currently used in multiple settings, it was initially developed for the clinical evaluation of hemodynamically stable, adequately oxygenated trauma patients with isolated head trauma. A score of 14 to 15 is associated with minor head injury, 9 to 13 with moderate head injury, and **8 or less** with **severe head injury.** This patient's **GCS score is 8** (2 points for eye opening to pain, 2 points for mumbling speech, 4 points for withdrawing from pain). He is classified as having a severe head injury. The overall mortality rate in severe head injury is almost 40%. In patients with a known or suspected severe head injury, it is recommended **to perform orotracheal intubation** patients with a **GCS score of 8 or less** for airway protection. These patients are at risk for increased ICP and herniation, which can lead to rapid respiratory decline. All patients with severe traumatic brain injury require an emergent CT scan and should be admitted to the intensive care unit in a hospital with neurosurgical capabilities.

Repairing his scalp laceration **(b)** is not a priority and can take place after diagnosing and stabilizing injuries that are more serious. If there is an active scalp bleed, staples can be rapidly placed to limit bleeding until definitive repair can take place. Mannitol **(c)** is an osmotic agent that is used to reduce ICP. It is administered if there are signs of impending or actual herniation (ie, fixed and dilated pupil). Bilateral ED cranial trephination (burr holes) **(d)** is rarely, if ever, performed and is considered when definitive neurosurgical care is not available. Although this individual may require neurosurgical intervention **(e)**, priority should be given to the primary surgery and his airway should be secured first.

115. The answer is d. Owing to its lack of bony protection, the neck is especially vulnerable to severe, life-threatening injuries. Neck trauma is caused by three major mechanisms—penetrating trauma, blunt trauma, and strangulation. All of these mechanisms can affect the airway, esophagus, vascular, and neurologic systems. The neck is divided into **three zones,** as seen in the following figure. Zone I extends superiorly from the sternal notch and clavicles to the cricoid cartilage. Injuries to this region can affect both neck and mediastinal structures. Zone II is the area between the cricoid cartilage and the angle of the mandible. Zone III extends from the angle of the mandible to the base of the skull. Zones I and III injuries typically pose a greater challenge to manage than zone II injuries because they are much less exposed than zone II. **Generally, zone II injuries are taken**

directly to the OR for surgical exploration. Injuries to zones I and III can be managed conservatively using a combination of angiography, bronchoscopy, esophagoscopy, and CT scanning.

Airway management is always given priority in trauma patients, particularly when neck structures are involved, because of the potential for rapid airway compromise. Active bleeding sites or wounds with blood clots should not be probed (**b**) because massive hemorrhage can occur. Blind clamping (**a**) should be avoided because of the high concentration of neurovascular structures in the neck. **Bleeding should be controlled by direct pressure.** The injury in this scenario involves zone II of the neck; therefore, the patient should be taken to the OR for surgical exploration. The injury is not in zone I (**c**) or zone III (**e**).

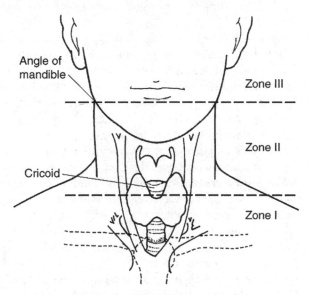

(Reproduced, with permission, from Doherty GM, Way LW. Current Surgical Diagnosis & Treatment. New York, NY: McGraw Hill, 2006: 210.)

116. The answer is d. **The hangman fracture**, or **traumatic spondylolysis of C2**, occurs when the head is thrown into **extreme hyperextension** because of **abrupt deceleration**, resulting in bilateral fractures of the C2 pedicles. This is considered an **unstable** cervical spine fracture. The name "hangman fracture" was derived from judicial hangings where the knot of the noose was placed under the chin, which caused extreme hyperextension of the head on the neck, resulting in a fracture at C2. However, many hangings resulted in death from strangulation rather than spinal cord damage. Today, the most common cause of a hangman fracture is **head-on automobile collisions**.

Colles' fracture (**a**) is the most common wrist fracture in adults. It is a transverse fracture of the distal radial metaphysis, which is dorsally displaced and angulated. These fractures usually occur from a fall on an outstretched hand. A boxer's fracture (**b**) is a fracture of the neck of the fifth metacarpal. It is one of the most common fractures of the hand and usually occurs from a direct impact to the hand (ie, punching a hard object with a closed fist). A fracture of C1 is called a Jefferson fracture (**c**), which is typically produced by a vertical compression force. A Clay shoveler's (**e**) fracture occurs secondary to cervical hyperextension or direct trauma to the posterior neck, resulting in an avulsion fracture of the spinous process.

117. The answer is b. The base of the skull base comprises the floors of the anterior, middle, and posterior cranial fossae. Fractures in this region typically do not have localized symptoms. However, indirect signs of injury may include visible evidence of bleeding from the fracture into surrounding soft tissue. Ecchymosis around the mastoid bone is referred to as **Battle sign** and periorbital ecchymosis is often described as "**raccoon eyes.**" The most common **basilar skull fracture** involves the petrous portion of the temporal bone, the external auditory canal, and the tympanic membrane. It is commonly associated with a dural tear, leading to **cerebrospinal fluid (CSF) otorrhea** or **rhinorrhea**. Other signs and symptoms of a basilar skull fracture include hemotympanum (blood behind the tympanic membrane), vertigo, decreased hearing or deafness, and seventh nerve palsy. Periorbital and mastoid ecchymosis develop gradually over hours after an injury and are often absent in the ED. If clear or pink fluid is seen from the nose or ear and a CSF leak is suspected, the fluid can be placed on filter paper and a "halo" or double ring may appear. This is a simple but insensitive test to confirm a CSF leak. Evidence of open communication, such as a CSF leak, mandates neurosurgical consultation and admission.

Le Fort fractures (**a**) typically result from high-energy facial trauma and are classified according to their location. A Le Fort I fracture involves a transverse fracture just above the teeth at the level of the nasal fossa, and allows movement of the alveolar ridge and hard palate. A Le Fort II fracture is a pyramidal fracture with its apex just above the bridge of the nose and extension laterally and inferiorly through the infraorbital rims allowing movement of the maxilla, nose, and infraorbital rims. A Le Fort III fracture represents complete craniofacial disruption and involves fractures of the zygoma, infraorbital rims, and maxilla. It is rare for these fractures to occur in isolation; they usually occur in combination. Otitis interna (**c**) and externa (**d**) are inflammation of the inner ear and outer ear, respectively. Both are commonly infectious and are not relevant in acute trauma. Tripod fractures (**e**) typically occur from blunt force applied to the lateral face causing fractures of the zygomatic arch, lateral orbital rim, inferior orbital rim, and anterior and lateral walls of the maxillary sinus. These fractures manifest clinically with asymmetric facial flattening, edema, and ecchymosis.

118. The answer is e. Based on the principles of advanced trauma life support (ATLS), injured patients are assessed and treated in a fashion that establishes priorities based on their presenting vital signs, mental status, and injury mechanism. The approach to trauma care consists of a **primary survey**, rapid resuscitation, and a more thorough secondary survey followed by diagnostic testing. The goal of the primary survey is to quickly identify and treat immediately life-threatening injuries. The assessment of the **airway, breathing, circulation, neurologic disability, exposure (ABCDEs)** is a model that should be followed in all trauma patients. **Airway patency is evaluated first** by listening for vocalizations, asking the patient to speak, and looking in the patient's mouth for signs of obstruction. Breathing is assessed by observing for symmetric rise and fall of the chest and listening for bilateral breath sounds over the anterior chest and axillae. The chest should be palpated for subcutaneous air and bony crepitus. The trachea should be palpated to ensure midline position. Circulatory function is assessed by noting the patient's BP, skin color, skin temperature, and central and distal pulses. The patient's neurologic status is assessed by noting level of consciousness and gross motor function. An initial GCS should be calculated. Last, the patient is completely undressed (exposed) to evaluate for otherwise hidden injuries (eg, bruises, lacerations, impaled foreign bodies, and open fractures). The secondary head-to-toe survey is undertaken only after the primary survey is complete, life-threatening injuries are addressed, and the patient is resuscitated and stabilized.

This patient will likely require a chest tube (**a**) for presumed hemothorax and/or PTX demonstrated by decreased breath sounds and oxygen saturation of 93%. However, the airway should be secured first. A DPL (**b**) or FAST examination is used to screen the abdomen for hemoperitoneum. However, airway and breathing take priority in this patient. Bilateral ED cranial trephination (burr holes) (**c**) is rarely, if ever, performed and should only be considered in the case of severe neurologic impairment when definitive neurosurgical care is not available. Extremity injuries (**d**) are typically not life threatening and are assessed after the ABC are evaluated.

119. The answer is d. In the ABCDEs of trauma, after the airway is secured attention should be turned to the patient's **breathing**. The patient remains hemodynamically unstable and hypoxic after endotracheal intubation and has decreased breath sounds on the right. **These are signs of tension PTX.** Tension PTX is a life-threatening condition that develops when air is trapped in the pleural cavity and expands to compress the mediastinum and compromises cardiopulmonary function. The diagnosis is based on clinical assessment and should not be delayed for further diagnostic testing. In the unstable patient, treatment for a tension PTX is accomplished by performing a **needle thoracostomy**.

Performing a FAST exam (**a**) is used to screen the abdomen for hemoperitoneum. This is an appropriate part of the trauma evaluation, however airway and breathing take priority in this patient. Pelvic binders (**b**) are a tamponade device used in trauma patients with suspected pelvic injury potentially associated with major hemorrhage. This intervention would take place after addressing the airway and breathing in this patient. CT scans of the patient's head and cervical spine (**c**) may play a role in evaluation of this patient, but the patient is too unstable and this point to be taken to CT scan. 3% hypertonic saline (**e**) is an osmotic agent given to patients with concern for increased intracranial pressure. This may be considered in this patient given the signs of head trauma and decreased mental status, but this is not the most immediate next action to be performed.

120. The answer is c. The patient remains hemodynamically unstable despite appropriate resuscitation with evidence of hemoperitoneum as determined by the positive FAST exam. This is an indication for **immediate operative intervention**.

If the patient were more stable, CT scans (**a**) could be helpful in determining the extent and location of the patient's injuries prior to operation, but this patient remains too unstable to undergo CT scans. Orthopedic surgery (**b**) will likely need to be involved in the care of this patient, but the immediate priority is to address the patient's life-threatening injuries. Occasionally, interventional radiology (**d**) can assist in embolization of bleeding vessels that cannot be addressed surgically, but this would take place after the patient is taken to the OR. Additional blood products (**e**) are likely to be required in this patient, but hemorrhage control is the priority at this time.

121. The answer is a. Epidural hematomas are the result of blood collecting in the potential space between the skull and the dura mater. Most epidural hematomas result from **blunt trauma** to the **temporal or temporoparietal area** with an associated skull fracture and **middle meningeal artery disruption**. The classic history of an epidural hematoma is a lucid period following immediate loss of consciousness in the setting of significant blunt head trauma. However, this clinical pattern occurs in a minority of cases. Most patients either never lose consciousness or never regain consciousness after the injury. On CT scan, epidural **hematomas appear lenticular or biconvex (football shaped)**, typically in the temporal region. The high-pressure arterial bleeding of an epidural hematoma can lead to herniation within hours after injury. Therefore, early recognition and evacuation are important to increase survival. Bilateral ED trephination (burr holes) is rarely, if ever, performed and should only be considered if definitive neurosurgical care is not available.

Subdural hematomas **(b)** appear as hyperdense, crescent-shaped lesions that cross suture lines. They result from a collection of blood below the dura and over the brain. To differentiate the CT finding from an epidural hematoma, think about the high pressure created by the arterial tear of an epidural that causes the hematoma to expand inward. In contrast, the low-pressure venous bleed of a subdural hematoma layers along the calvarium. Traumatic SAH **(c)** is probably the most common CT abnormality in patients with moderate to severe traumatic brain injury. Intracerebral hematomas **(d)** and contusions **(e)** occur secondary to traumatic tearing of intracerebral blood vessels. Contusions most commonly occur in the frontal, temporal, and occipital lobes. They may occur either at the site of the blunt trauma or on the opposite site of the brain, known as a contrecoup injury. Examples of each are shown in the figure (subdural, traumatic SAH, and cerebral hematoma/contusion, respectively).

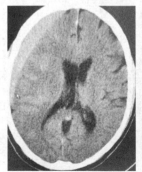 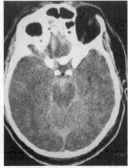 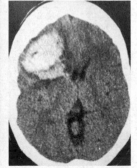

(Reproduced with permission from Adam J. Rosh, MD.)

122. The answer is a. **Central cord syndrome** is often seen in patients with degenerative arthritis of the cervical vertebrae, whose necks are subjected to **forced hyperextension**. Typically, this involves a forward fall onto the face in an elderly person. This causes the ligamentum flavum to buckle into the spinal cord, resulting in a contusion to the central portion of the cord. This injury affects the central gray matter and the most central portions of the pyramidal and spinothalamic tracts. Patients often have **greater neurologic deficits in the upper extremities, compared to the lower extremities**, since nerve fibers that innervate distal structures are located in the periphery of the spinal cord. In addition, patients with central cord syndrome usually have decreased rectal sphincter tone and patchy, unpredictable sensory deficits.

Anterior cord syndrome **(b)** results in variable degrees of motor paralysis and loss of temperature and pain sensation below the level of the lesion. Its hallmark is the preservation of vibratory sensation and proprioception because of an intact dorsal column. Brown-Séquard syndrome **(c)** results in ipsilateral loss of motor strength, vibratory sensation, proprioception, and contralateral loss of pain and temperature sensation. Transverse myelitis **(d)** is an inflammatory process that produces complete motor and sensory loss below the level of the lesion. Parkinson's disease **(e)** develops over years and does not result in paralysis.

Central cord syndrome

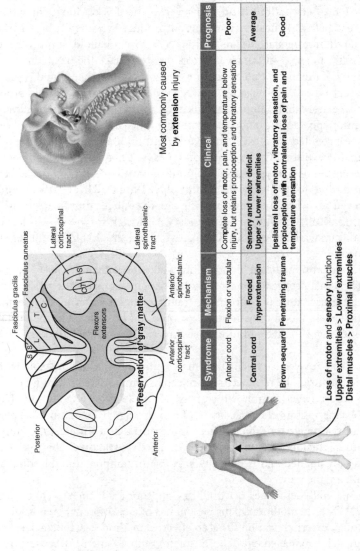

Most commonly caused by **extension** injury

Syndrome	Mechanism	Clinical	Prognosis
Anterior cord	Flexion or vascular	Complete loss of motor, pain, and temperature below injury, but retains proprioception and vibratory sensation	Poor
Central cord	Forced hyperextension	Sensory and motor deficit Upper > Lower extremities	Average
Brown-sequard	Penetrating trauma	Ipsilateral loss of motor, vibratory sensation, and proprioception with contralateral loss of pain and temperature sensation	Good

Loss of motor and sensory function
Upper extremities > Lower extremities
Distal muscles > Proximal muscles

(Reproduced with permission from Adam J. Rosh, MD, and Rosh Review.)

123. The answer is d. The decision to begin blood transfusion in a trauma patient is based on the initial response to crystalloid volume resuscitation. As directed in ATLS, **blood products should be administered if vital signs transiently improve or remain unstable despite resuscitation with 1 L of crystalloid fluid.** However, if there is obvious major blood loss, the patient is unstable, and blood product is available; blood transfusion should be started concomitantly with crystalloid administration. The main purpose in transfusing blood is to restore the oxygen-carrying capacity of the intravascular volume. Fully cross-matched blood is preferable (eg, type B, Rh-negative, antibody negative); however, this process may take more than 1 hour, which is inappropriate for the unstable trauma patient. Type-specific blood (eg, type A, Rh negative, unknown antibody) can be provided by most blood banks within 30 minutes. This blood is compatible with ABO and Rh blood types, but may be incompatible with other antibodies. If type-specific blood is unavailable, type O packed cells are indicated for patients who are unstable. **Type O, Rh-negative blood is reserved for women of childbearing age to reduce complications of Rh incompatibility in future pregnancies.** However, if type O, Rh-negative blood is unavailable, type O, Rh-positive blood should be administered to women.

Fully cross-matched blood **(a)** may take more than 1 hour to prepare, which is inappropriate for an unstable patient. Epinephrine **(b)** plays no role in resuscitation of hypotensive trauma patients suffering from hemorrhagic shock. Blood transfusion **(c)** should not be delayed in the unstable patient. Men should be administered type O, Rh-positive blood **(e)**.

124. The answer is c. This patient is hemodynamically unstable with a pelvic fracture. The retroperitoneum can accommodate up to 4 L of blood after severe pelvic trauma which may not be seen on FAST exam. There are several options in management of hemorrhage from an unstable pelvic fracture. A **pelvic binding garment** is the **initial and simplest** modality to use in the **unstable trauma patient with a pelvic fracture.** This device can be rapidly applied and is typically effective in tamponading bleeding and stabilizing the pelvis.

Bilateral chest tubes **(a)** would be appropriate if there were evidence for a PTX or hemothorax. This patient has bilaterally equal breath sounds. Although external fixation **(b)** is an effective method to stabilize the pelvis, it may delay management of an unstable trauma patient. Because a pelvic binding apparatus is quick and simple, it is preferred. The source of retroperitoneal bleeding with pelvic fractures is typically the pelvic venous plexus or smaller veins. However, venography is not useful in managing these patients; even when venous bleeding is localized, embolization **(d)** is ineffective because of the extensive anastomoses and collateral flow. Arterial angiography **(e)** is a major diagnostic and therapeutic modality for the patient with severe pelvic hemorrhage from arterial sources. Angiography is indicated when hypovolemia persists in a patient with a major pelvic fracture, despite control of hemorrhage from other sources. Since angiography typically takes place in the angiography suite, patients should have a pelvic binding device applied prior to being transferred.

125. The answer is c. **Anterior cord syndrome** results from **cervical flexion injuries** (eg, diving in shallow water) that cause cord contusion or protrusion of a bony fragment or herniated intervertebral disk into the spinal canal. It may also occur from vascular pathology, such as laceration or thrombosis of the anterior spinal artery. The syndrome is characterized by **different degrees of paralysis** and **loss of pain and temperature sensation** below the level of injury. **Its hallmark** is the **preservation of the posterior columns, maintaining position, touch, and vibratory sensation.**

SCIWORA **(a)** is a diagnosis that is reserved for the pediatric population because the spinal cord is less elastic than the bony spine and ligaments. The diagnosis is associated with paresthesias and generalized weakness. This syndrome is coming under scrutiny since the advent of the magnetic resonance imaging (MRI), in which spinal cord lesions are being identified in patients who otherwise had normal CT scans. Central cord syndrome **(b)** is often seen in patients with degenerative arthritis of the cervical vertebrae, whose necks are subjected to forced hyperextension. This is seen typically in a forward fall onto the chin in an elderly person. Patients often have greater sensorimotor neurologic deficits in the upper extremities compared to the lower extremities. Cauda equina syndrome **(d)** causes peripheral nerve injury rather than direct spinal cord damage. Its presentation may include variable motor and sensory loss in the lower extremities, sciatica, bowel and bladder dysfunction, and saddle anesthesia. Brown-Séquard syndrome **(e)** results in ipsilateral loss of motor strength, vibratory sensation, and proprioception, and contralateral loss of pain and temperature sensation (Table).

Syndrome	Neurologic Deficits
Anterior cord	B/L paralysis below lesion, loss of pain and temperature, and preservation of proprioception and vibratory function
Central cord	Upper extremity paralysis > lower extremity paralysis, some loss of pain and temperature with upper > lower
Brown-Séquard	*Ipsilateral:* Paresis, loss of proprioception, and vibratory sensation *Contralateral:* Loss of pain and temperature
Cauda equina	Variable motor and sensory loss in lower extremities, bowel/bladder dysfunction, saddle anesthesia

126. The answer is b. The treatment of a **tension PTX** involves immediate reduction in the intrapleural pressure on the affected side of the thoracic cavity. The simplest and quickest way to establish this is by inserting a **14-gauge catheter** into the **thoracic cavity in the second intercostal space in the midclavicular line.** After this procedure, a chest tube should be inserted as definitive management. **Needle thoracostomy** is necessary when a patient's vital signs are unstable; otherwise, direct insertion of a chest tube is adequate for suspicion of a PTX or hemothorax. A tension PTX is a life-threatening emergency caused by air entering the pleural space that is not able to escape secondary to the creation of a one-way valve. This increased pressure causes the ipsilateral lung to collapse, shifting the mediastinum away from the injured lung, and compromising vena caval blood return to the heart. The severely altered preload results in reduced stroke volume, increased cardiac output, and hypotension.

Airway management (**a**) is the first component addressed in the primary survey; however, the patient is breathing on his own and does not require intubation. Moreover, intubation would likely be avoided in this patient by appropriately addressing the PTX. If the BP does not improve with insertion of a chest tube, the next area to focus on is an intra-abdominal injury, which can be assessed either by a DPL (**c**) or FAST examination (**d**). A pericardiocentesis (**e**) is indicated in the trauma patient when there is suspicion for cardiac tamponade, which may present with tachycardia and Beck triad—hypotension, JVD, and muffled heart sounds.

127. The answer is e. The Canadian C-spine rule for radiography in alert and stable patients following blunt head or neck trauma identified **age older than 65 years as a risk factor for C-spine injury**, even among those with stable vital signs and a GCS score of 15. Therefore, C-spine imaging in all such elderly patients is warranted. Additionally, fall from approximately 3 feet or 5 stairs constitutes a dangerous mechanism requiring radiography per the Canadian C-spine rule.

It is thought that elderly patients experience a much lower incidence of epidural hematomas than the general population because of the relatively denser fibrous bond between the dura mater and the inner table of the skull in older individuals (**a**). There is, however, a high incidence of subdural hematomas (**b**) in elderly patients. As the brain mass decreases in size with age, there is greater stretching and tension of the bridging veins that pass from the brain to the dural sinuses, making them more susceptible to injury. In the elderly, diminished elasticity of the lungs (**c**) can lead to a reduction in pulmonary compliance and in the ability to cough effectively, resulting in an increased risk for nosocomial gram-negative pneumonia. Geriatric patients are thus more susceptible to the development of hypoxia and respiratory infections following trauma. The most common cervical spine fractures in this age group are upper cervical, particularly fractures of the odontoid, not lower C6 fractures (**d**).

128. The answer is e. Urethral injuries make up approximately 10% of genitourinary trauma. Anterior urethral injuries are most often attributed to falls with straddle injuries or a blunt force to the perineum. Approximately 95% of posterior urethral injuries are secondary to pelvic fractures. Signs and symptoms of urethral injury include **perineal pain, inability to void, gross hematuria, blood at the urethral meatus, perineal or scrotal swelling or ecchymosis, and an absent, high-riding, or boggy prostate**. A **retrograde urethrogram** is the study of choice when there is suspicion of a urethral injury. This procedure is performed by inserting an 8 F urinary catheter 2 cm into the urethral meatus and inflating the catheter balloon with 2 cc of saline to create a seal. Then 30 cc of radiopaque contrast is administered, and a radiograph is obtained looking for extravasation of contrast from the urethra.

A scrotal ultrasound (**a**) may be necessary later to evaluate for testicular injury, but it is not used to evaluate urethral injury. A KUB (**b**) is not useful to evaluate the urethra. Prior to CT scanning, it was commonly used to evaluate for kidney stones. An IV pyelogram (**c**) is an alternative to CT scanning for evaluating the kidneys and ureters. A retrograde cystogram (d) is a useful study to evaluate for bladder injury.

129. The answer is e. An important concern with **anterior abdominal GSWs** is to determine whether the missile traversed the peritoneal cavity. Nearly all patients with transabdominal GSWs have intraabdominal injuries requiring surgery. Most of the time, this can be determined by approximating the trajectory. Therefore, a hole in both the anterior and posterior abdomen highly suggests a transabdominal trajectory. If there are a single or odd number of holes, a plain film may help estimate the trajectory. In cases of tangential or multiple GSWs, it may be impossible to determine trajectory with any certainty. In a patient with evidence of peritoneal penetration, a missile tract that clearly enters the abdominal cavity, or has a positive diagnostic study (eg, DPL, FAST, or CT scan) in a tangential wound, he or she should undergo exploratory laparotomy. The standard algorithm for **penetrating abdominal trauma** recommends that any patient with **unstable** vital signs be taken **directly to the OR** to undergo an **exploratory laparotomy**. If their vital signs are stable, they should undergo further diagnostic studies, such as a FAST examination, DPL, or CT scan.

In general, penetrating abdominal wounds should not be probed (a). This may worsen the injury and disrupt hemostasis, resulting in uncontrolled hemorrhage. Instead, gently separate the skin edges to see if the base of the wound can be visualized. In the setting of penetrating abdominal trauma, further diagnostic tests (b, c, and d) should only occur if the patient has stable vital signs. Otherwise, patients should be taken directly to the OR to undergo exploratory laparotomy.

130. The answer is b. Closed-loop communication is a strategy in healthcare communication that is used to **minimize confusion and errors**. One person gives an order verbally, and the recipient of that information repeats the order back verbally to the person giving the order. Using this technique, **both parties** can **confirm** that they are **communicating the same message**.

Positive-feedback communication (a) and redundant communication (c) are not communication strategies used in healthcare. The SBAR method (d) is used in healthcare during transitions of care. It provides an organized way to give handoff from one provider to another. Team huddle communication (e) is a strategy that employs a quick meeting of a functional group to set the shift in motion via commentary with key personnel. Team huddles are microsystem meetings with a specific focus, based on the function of a particular unit and team.

131. The answer is a. Diving injuries must always be suspected in near-drowning patients. This patient presents with abdominal breathing and spontaneous respirations. This pattern provides an important clue to a **cervical spine injury**. The diaphragm is innervated by the phrenic nerve that originates from the spinal cord at the C3-C4 level, whereas the intercostal muscles of the rib cage are supplied by nerves that originate in the thoracic spine. Therefore, abdominal breathing in the absence of thoracic breathing indicates an injury below C4. His bradycardia in the presence of **hypotension** is suspicious for **neurogenic hypotension**, which is caused by loss of vasomotor tone and **lack of reflex tachycardia** from the disruption of autonomic ganglia. However, this is a diagnosis of exclusion and should only be made once all other forms of shock are ruled out. It is important to maintain **C-spine immobilization** to prevent further progression of an injury.

Electrolyte abnormalities **(b)** are typically not a concern in near-drowning injuries. Any patient with hypoxia and hypoperfusion generally also has a metabolic acidosis **(c)**. Treating the underlying pathology will also treat the acidosis. All near-drowning cases (fresh or saltwater) involve the loss of surfactant and subsequent atelectasis **(d)** with a high potential for hypoxia. Although a toxic ingestion **(e)** should always be considered, there are no specific indications for it in this patient.

132. The answer is b. Clinical manifestations of **penetrating arterial injury of the extremity** are generally divided into "hard signs" and "soft signs." Hard signs include pulsatile bleeding, expanding hematoma, palpable thrill or audible bruit, and evidence of distal ischemia (eg, pain, pallor, pulselessness, paralysis, paresthesia, and poikilothermia). Soft signs include diminished ankle-brachial indices, asymmetrically absent or weak distal pulse, history of moderate hemorrhage, wound close to a major artery, and a peripheral nerve deficit. **Emergent surgery** is generally necessary when there are **hard signs** of vascular injury. Although the management of penetrating extremity injury is evolving, whenever there is **evidence of distal ischemia**, the patient should be taken to the OR **for exploration and repair**. When severe ischemia is present, the repair must be completed within 6 to 8 hours to prevent irreversible muscle ischemia and loss of limb function. In the presence of hard signs without evidence of ischemia, some surgeons may prefer to first perform angiography to better define the injury.

Angiography (a) is a frequently used modality in penetrating extremity trauma and is the study of choice with some injuries that present with hard signs. However, when there is evidence of limb ischemia, the patient should undergo exploration and repair immediately. Fasciotomy (c) is the treatment for compartment syndrome. Although compartment syndrome can occur with blunt and penetrating extremity trauma, it is more common in crush injuries or fractures with marked swelling. It may be required, but should be performed in conjunction with and after the establishment of arterial blood flow. The patient may require a long leg splint (d) at some point during the course of treatment, but it is not an appropriate next step in the patient with limb ischemia. CT scanning (e) is not appropriate in the setting of limb ischemia. CT angiography may be indicated as an alternative to angiography in these cases.

133. The answer is b. Cerebral herniation occurs when increased ICP overwhelms the natural compensatory capacities of the central nervous system (CNS). Increased ICP may be the result of posttraumatic brain swelling, edema formation, traumatic mass lesion expansion, or any combination of the three. When increasing ICP cannot be controlled, the intracranial contents will shift and herniate through the cranial foramen. Herniation can occur within minutes or up to days after a traumatic brain injury. Once the signs of herniation are present, mortality approaches 100% without rapid reversal or temporizing measures. **Uncal herniation** is the most common clinically significant form of traumatic herniation and is often associated with traumatic extracranial bleeding. The classic signs and symptoms are caused by compression of the ipsilateral uncus of the temporal lobe. This causes **compression of cranial nerve III leading to anisocoria, ptosis, impaired extraocular movements, and a sluggish pupillary light reflex**. As herniation progresses, compression of the ipsilateral oculomotor nerve eventually causes ipsilateral pupillary dilation and nonreactivity.

An altered level of consciousness (a) is the hallmark of brain insult from any cause, not specifically for elevated ICP, and results from an interruption of the reticular activating system RAS or a global event that affects both cortices. Contralateral pupillary dilation (c) is a late manifestation in brain herniation and usually occurs after ipsilateral pupillary dilation. Progressive hypertension (d) associated with bradycardia and diminished respiratory effort is described as Cushing reflex and is a late manifestation of herniation. Contralateral hemiparesis (e) develops as herniation progresses.

134. The answer is b. **Hemothorax** is the accumulation of blood in the pleural space after blunt or penetrating chest trauma. It can lead to hypovolemic shock and can significantly reduce vital capacity if not recognized. It is associated with a PTX approximately 25% of the time. Hemorrhage from injured lung parenchyma is the most common cause of hemothorax, but this tends to be self-limiting unless there is a major laceration to the parenchyma. Specific vessels are less often the source of bleeding. A hemothorax is treated with **tube thoracostomy (chest tube)**, which is generally placed in the fourth or fifth intercostal space at the anterior or midaxillary line, over the superior portion of the rib. The tube should be directed **superior and posterior** to allow it to drain blood from the dependent portions of the chest. In an isolated PTX, the tube is positioned anteriorly to allow it to suction air. Once the tube is inserted, it is important to closely monitor blood output. **Indications for thoracotomy include the following:**

- Initial chest tube drainage of 1,000 to 1,500 mL of blood **(a and b)**
- 200 mL/h of persistent drainage **(c)**
- Persistent hypotension despite adequate blood replacement, and other sites of blood loss have been ruled out
- Decompensation after initial response to resuscitation
- Increasing size of hemothorax seen on serial chest x-ray studies **(d and e)**

135. The answer is d. Electrical burns can be caused by direct or indirect contact with electrical current. Morbidity and mortality increases are associated with both increased voltage and exposure time. High-voltage exposures are those over 1,000 V; whereas, low-voltage exposures are generally less than 240 V. Low-voltage exposures rarely are associated with significant injury. Due to the potential for serious injury, all patients with high-voltage exposures should undergo a complete skin examination. Furthermore, **regardless of symptoms and exam findings, all patients with high-voltage exposure should be observed for at least 12 hours** to allow for evaluation of cardiac dysrhythmias, renal damage, rhabdomyolysis, and electrolyte abnormalities. Electrical burns should also be evaluated for development of compartment syndrome given the potential for significant muscle damage that can occur. Significant electrical burns should be transferred to a burn center once stabilized.

The patient has no entrance or exit wounds from the electrical contact, therefore does not require admission for frequent compartment checks **(a).**

Patients with exposure to high-voltage should not be discharged with close follow-up (**b**). Because the patient does not have electrical burns, there is no indication for transfer to a burn center (**c**). The patient has no signs of compartment syndrome and does not require fasciotomy (**e**).

136. The answer is e. Trauma occurs in up to 7% of all pregnancies and is the leading cause of maternal death. It is important to **focus the primary examination on the patient and evaluate the fetus in the secondary examination**. The ABCs are followed in the usual fashion. Once the patient is deemed stable, the fetus should be evaluated. Fetal evaluation focuses on the HR and movement. Minor trauma to the patient does not rule out injury to the fetus. Therefore, it is important to monitor the fetus. **Cardiotocographic (cardio = fetal heartbeat, toco = uterine contractions, graphy = measuring) observation of the viable fetus of at least 24 weeks' gestation is recommended for a minimum of 4 hours** to detect any intrauterine pathology. The minimum should be extended to 24 hours if, at any time during the first 4 hours, there are more than three uterine contractions per hour, persistent uterine tenderness, a nonreassuring fetal monitor strip, vaginal bleeding, rupture of the membranes, or any serious maternal injury is present.

Cesarean section in the OR (**a**) may take place if the patient is stable, but the fetus is unstable and greater than 24 weeks' gestation. This decision should be made by an obstetrician. Cesarean section in the ED (**b**), or perimortem cesarean section, is performed if uterine size exceeds the umbilicus, fetal heart tones are present, and maternal decompensation is acute. Although radiation from CT scanning (**c**) in the setting of pregnancy is a concern, evaluation of the mother typically supersedes the radiation risk to the fetus. Shielding of the uterus in head and chest scans allows for an acceptable radiation exposure level. Abdominal and pelvic CT scanning incurs greater radiation exposure, and the risks and benefits of these studies should be discussed with the patient. Other diagnostic procedures can be used in the setting of blunt abdominal trauma such as ultrasound, DPL, and MRI. Minor trauma does not exempt the fetus from injury, and direct impact is not necessary for fetoplacental injury to occur. The mother with no obvious abdominal injury or normal laboratory values still requires monitoring (**d**).

137. The answer is d. Cauda equina syndrome is an injury to the lumbar, sacral, and coccygeal nerve roots, causing peripheral nerve injury that can lead to permanent neurologic deficits if not recognized and corrected rapidly. Because of the central location of the disk herniation, symptoms are often bilateral and involve **leg pain, saddle anesthesia, and impaired bowel and bladder function (retention or incontinence)**. On examination, patients may exhibit loss of rectal tone and display other motor and sensory losses in the lower extremities. Patients with suspected cauda equina syndrome require an emergent CT scan (CT myelogram) or MRI and neurosurgical consultation.

AAA **(a)** can present with low back pain and rarely a neurologic deficit if the aneurysm is large enough and impinges a nerve root. AAA should always be considered in patients over 50 years with hypertension and low back pain. A bedside ultrasound can usually identify large AAAs. If there is still concern for an AAA, a CT scan can rule out the diagnosis. Disk herniation **(b)** can result in peripheral nerve root compression and irritation leading to sensory and motor deficits. Patients with disk herniation, however, should not exhibit altered bowel and bladder function, or have decreased rectal tone. If so, the condition is likely cauda equina syndrome and is a neurologic emergency. Spinal stenosis **(c)** is narrowing of the spinal canal, which may cause spinal cord compression that typically is worse with back extension and relieved with flexion. Osteomyelitis **(e)** is an infection of the bone that typically presents with fever.

138. The answer is d. A **unilateral dilated pupil** in the setting of head trauma is an **indicator of increased ICP**. If ICP is not lowered immediately, the patient has little chance of survival. **Hyperventilation** to produce an arterial partial pressure of carbon dioxide (PCO_2) of 30 to 35 mm Hg will temporarily reduce ICP by promoting cerebral vasoconstriction and subsequent reduction in cerebral blood flow. The onset of action is **within 30 seconds**. In most patients, hyperventilation lowers the ICP by 25%. PCO_2 should not fall below 25 mm Hg because this may cause profound vasoconstriction and ischemia in both normal and injured areas of the brain. Hyperventilation is a **temporary maneuver** and should only be used for a brief period of time during the acute resuscitation and only in patients demonstrating neurologic deterioration.

ED cranial decompression (burr hole) **(a)** should only be performed under extreme circumstances when all other attempts at reducing ICP have failed. There is no evidence that steroids such as dexamethasone **(b)** lower ICP and are not recommended in head trauma. Furosemide **(c)** has no role in acute traumatic brain injury. Mannitol **(e)** is an osmotic agent to reduce

ICP. Its onset is within 30 minutes and lasts up to 6 to 8 hours. Mannitol has the additional benefit of expanding volume, initially reducing hypotension, and improving the blood's oxygen-carrying capacity.

139. The answer is c. This patient is in **cardiogenic shock** from **decreased cardiac output** producing inadequate tissue perfusion. Support for this diagnosis includes an older patient with a history of ischemic cardiomyopathy and coronary artery disease and new mental status changes coupled with signs of volume overload. Common causes of cardiogenic shock include **acute myocardial infarction (MI), pulmonary embolism, COPD exacerbation, and pneumonia.** This patient should be stabilized with IV vasopressors since there is already pulmonary congestion evident on examination. A rapid workup including 12-lead ECG, CXR, laboratory testing, echocardiogram, and hemodynamic monitoring should help confirm the etiology and direct specific treatment of the underlying cause.

Hypovolemic shock **(a)** occurs when there is inadequate volume in the circulatory system, resulting in poor oxygen delivery to the tissues. Neurogenic shock **(b)** occurs after an acute spinal cord injury, which disrupts sympathetic innervation resulting in hypotension and bradycardia. Anaphylactic shock **(d)** is a severe systemic hypersensitivity reaction, resulting in hypotension and airway compromise. Septic shock **(e)** is a clinical syndrome of hypoperfusion and multiorgan dysfunction caused by infection.

140. The answer is d. This patient has **supraventricular tachycardia (SVT)**, a narrow complex, regular tachycardia. It is caused by a reentry arrhythmia or ectopic pacemaker in areas of the heart above the bundle of His, usually the atria. Regular P waves will be present but may be difficult to discern owing to the very fast rate. The patient in this case has normal vital signs and physical examination, and is therefore stable. The first-line treatment for a patient with stable SVT is **vagal maneuvers** to **slow conduction and prolong the refractory period in the AV node.** The Valsalva maneuver can be accomplished by asking the patient to bear down as if they are having a bowel movement and hold the strain for at least 10 seconds. Other vagal maneuvers include carotid sinus massage (after auscultating for carotid bruits) and facial immersion in cold water.

If vagal maneuvers fail, the next step is adenosine, a very short-acting AV nodal blocking medication. Initially, adenosine 6 mg **(b)** is rapidly pushed through the IV in a site as close to the heart as possible. Patients may experience a few seconds of discomfort, including chest pain and facial flushing on receiving the adenosine. If the patient remains in SVT 2 minutes after receiving adenosine, a second dose of adenosine at 12 mg **(c)** is administered. If the second dose of adenosine fails and the patient remains stable, short-acting calcium channel blockers **(e)** (ie, verapamil), β-blockers, or digoxin can be administered. If at any time the patient is considered unstable (hypotension, pulmonary edema, severe chest pain, altered mental status, or other life-threatening concerns), synchronized cardioversion **(a)** should be performed immediately.

141. The answer is b. The patient is in **ventricular tachycardia (VT)**, a wide complex tachycardia. VT originates from ectopic ventricular pace-makers and is usually a regular rhythm with a rate greater than 100 beats/min and wide QRS complexes. Treatment of VT is primarily dependent on whether or not the patient is stable. Evidence of acute altered mental status, hypotension, continued chest pain, or other signs of shock are signs of instability. **Unstable patients**, such as the passenger on this airplane, should receive **immediate synchronized cardioversion**. It is critical that the cardioverter be placed in the synchronized mode, which permits a search for a large R wave and a corresponding shock around the incidence of such a wave. A shock administered outside of this constraint can induce ventricular fibrillation (VF).

Stable patients can be treated with antidysrhythmics. Amiodarone **(a)** lidocaine, **(d)** and procainamide **(e)** can all be administered. Verapamil **(c)** should not be used in VT as it may accelerate the HR and cause hypotension.

142. The answer is e. This rhythm strip shows **atrial fibrillation with rapid ventricular response (RVR)**. Normally, one area of the atria depo-larizes and causes uniform contraction of the atria. In atrial fibrillation, multiple areas of the atria continuously depolarize and contract, leading to multiple atrial impulses and an irregular ventricular response. Atrial fibril-lation reduces the effectiveness of atrial contractions and may lead to or worsen heart failure in patients with left ventricular failure. Treatment of atrial fibrillation is dependent on whether or not the patient is stable. This patient is clinically **unstable**; the atrial fibrillation with RVR has pushed him into heart failure, and he is hypotensive and tachypneic. Unstable patients like this should undergo **synchronized cardioversion**. Synchronized car-dioversion is performed at 100 J and then at 200 J if the first attempt fails.

The focus of emergency management in stable patients with atrial fibrillation with RVR is ventricular rate control. Diltiazem **(b)** or verapamil are excellent choices for rate control. Metoprolol (c) or digoxin (d) may also be used, but may depress BP. Recall that patients in atrial fibrillation for longer than 48 hours are at risk for atrial thrombus formation. If these patients are cardioverted (electrically or chemically), they have a 1% to 2% risk of arterial embolism. Since it is often difficult to determine time of onset, ED patients are generally only cardioverted if they are unstable or the timing of onset is known. Stable patients with atrial fibrillation should be anticoagulated with a loading dose of heparin (a) and oral warfarin for at least 1 month prior to elective cardioversion.

143. The answer is d. Low-energy cardioversion is very successful in converting atrial flutter to sinus rhythm. Remember, cardioversion is different than defibrillation. Cardioversion is performed on patients with organized cardiac electrical activity with pulses, whereas defibrillation is performed on patients without pulses (VT and VF without a pulse). **Patients with a pulse who receive electrical energy during their heart's relative refractory period are at risk for VF.** Therefore, cardioversion is a timed shock designed to avoid delivering a shock during the heart's relative refractory period. By activating **synchronization mode**, the machine will identify the patient's R waves and not deliver electrical energy during these times. **The key step, when cardioverting, is to activate the synchronization mode and confirm the presence of sync markers on the R waves prior to delivering electrical energy.**

It is important to set the appropriate energy level (a), position the conductor pads or paddles correctly on the patient (b), charge the machine (c), and premedicate the patient with an analgesic (e) and/or sedative if the patient's clinical condition will allow for it. But in this case, the most critical next step is to ensure that the synchronization mode is turned on since this patient has a pulse.

144. The answer is b. This patient has cardiac electrical activity (sinus bradycardia) but no detectable pulses. He is therefore in a state of **pulseless electrical activity** (PEA), and management should be directed by the American Heart Association's Advanced Cardiac Life Support (AHA's ACLS) PEA algorithm. Patients in PEA should be treated with **CPR** and **epinephrine** every 3 to 5 minutes, but a search for an underlying etiology with targeted interventions should still be performed. Common etiologies for PEA are shown in the following table along with their specific treatments. Many find the **H's** and **T's** in the table an easy way to remember the differential.

Each etiology should be considered for every patient with PEA and causes that are more likely given a patient's history and physical examination should be treated first. This patient has an AV graft indicating that he has a history of renal disease. Since patients with end-stage renal disease are at risk for **hyperkalemia** and since hyperkalemia can cause PEA, **calcium gluconate** should be given first to stabilize the cardiac membranes.

PEA Etiologies and Treatments			
H's	**Treatment**	**T's**	**Treatment**
Hypovolemia	IV fluids	Toxins	Antidotes
Hypoxia	Oxygen	Tamponade (cardiac)	Pericardiocentesis
Hydrogen ion (acidosis)	Sodium bicarbonate	Tension PTX	Needle decompression
Hypokalemia Hyperkalemia	KCl Calcium chloride or gluconate	Thrombosis (coronary)	Thrombolysis
Hypothermia	Warming	Thrombosis (pulmonary)	Thrombolysis

If the patient does not improve with calcium, sodium bicarbonate (a) could be given to treat for metabolic acidosis and 50% dextrose (c) can be given for suspected hypoglycemia. Cardiac tamponade is a possible etiology in a patient with renal disease and pericardiocentesis (e) can be attempted if the patient is not improving with the aforementioned treatments. A bedside ultrasound may also be helpful to look for signs of tamponade. PTX is a less likely etiology in this particular patient and is treated with a chest tube (d).

145. The answer is b. The rhythm is **VF**. Along with pulseless VT, these are **nonperfusing rhythms** that are treated identically because they are thought to be caused by the same mechanisms. The earlier a "shock" from a defibrillator is administered in cardiac arrest, the more likely the patient will return to spontaneous circulation with a perfusing rhythm. If there is a delay to defibrillation (> 4 minutes), CPR should be administered for 60 to 90 seconds before defibrillation. If after defibrillation (200 J biphasic or 360 J monophasic) the patient's rhythm is still VF or pulseless VT, assisted ventilation and chest compressions should be started. Intubation should be performed and IV access obtained for the administration of epinephrine or vasopressin. If the rhythm is unchanged after administration of vasopressor therapy, another attempt at defibrillation (360 J monophasic or 200 J biphasic) with subsequent administration of an antidysrhythmic (eg, amiodarone) is recommended. Of note, monophasic defibrillation delivers a charge in only one direction. Biphasic defibrillation delivers a charge in one direction for half of the shock and in the electrically opposite direction for the second half. Biphasic defibrillation significantly decreases the energy necessary for successful defibrillation and decreases the risk of myocardial damage.

There is no role for observation (a) with VF. Successful return of a perfusing rhythm is most likely to result with immediate defibrillation. Synchronized cardioversion (c) is energy delivered to match the QRS complex. This reduces the chance that a shock will induce VF. Synchronization is used to treat tachydysrhythmias (eg, rapid atrial fibrillation) in hemodynamically unstable patients who have a palpable pulse. It should not be used in VF or pulseless VT. The most beneficial intervention for this patient is immediate defibrillation. If this fails, the patient's airway management (ABCs) will require him to be intubated (d). Amiodarone (e), an antidysrhythmic, is used in patients with VF or pulseless VT after appropriate defibrillation and administration of vasopressor therapy.

146. The answer is b. The most serious complication of ET intubation is unrecognized esophageal intubation with resultant hypoxic brain injury. Esophageal placement is not always obvious. The best assurance that the tube is placed into the trachea is to **see it pass through the vocal cords during direct or video laryngoscopy**.

The chest radiograph (a) can be misleading and is essentially only useful to identify endobronchial intubation (ie, right main stem bronchus intubation). Although the chest wall (c) should expand with positive pressure and relax with expiration, this may not occur in patients with small tidal volumes or severe bronchospasm. You may hear normal breath sounds (d) if only the midline of the thorax is auscultated. In cardiac arrest situations, low exhaled carbon dioxide levels (e) are seen in both very-low-flow states and in esophageal intubation. In addition, colorimetric changes may be difficult to discern in reduced lighting situations, and secretions can interfere with color change.

147. The answer is b. This patient is in **neurogenic shock**. He suffered an acute cervical spine injury after his fall onto a rock and has **hypotension** and **bradycardia**. The pathophysiology behind neurogenic shock is still under investigation, but it is thought to be partially caused by **disrupted**

sympathetic outflow tracts and **unopposed vagal tone**. Note that all other forms of shock attempt to compensate for hypotension with tachycardia. Neurogenic shock lacks sympathetic innervation; therefore, bradycardia results. Given that this is a trauma patient, all other sources for hypotension must be ruled out. He should be treated with cervical spine immobilization and IV fluids. Vasopressors may be needed if the hypotension does not respond to fluids or fluid overload becomes a concern.

Hypovolemic shock (a) occurs when there is inadequate volume in the circulatory system, resulting in poor oxygen delivery to the tissues. Cardiogenic shock (c) is caused by decreased cardiac output producing inadequate tissue perfusion. Anaphylactic shock (d) is a severe systemic hypersensitivity reaction, resulting in hypotension and airway compromise. Septic shock (e) is a clinical syndrome of hypoperfusion, hypotension, or multiorgan dysfunction caused by infection.

148. The answer is d. Atropine is the initial treatment of choice for patients in second-degree, Mobitz I AV block. The majority of patients respond to atropine without further treatment. Mobitz I is associated with acute inferior MI, digoxin toxicity, myocarditis, and after cardiac surgery.

Observation alone (a) is appropriate for stable patients. However, this patient is hypotensive and needs more aggressive management. Transcutaneous (electrical pads are placed externally, most commonly on the anterior chest wall) (b) or transvenous (pacing wires are threaded into the RV through a central vein) (c) pacing is an appropriate treatment and should be attempted if atropine is unsuccessful. Finally, if all else fails, epinephrine (e) or dopamine drips can be started. These treatments should be applied judiciously as the resulting increased HR may worsen patients with active ischemia as the etiology for their bradycardia. Furthermore, patients with acute inferior wall MI may have right ventricular failure and may be hypotensive because of decreased preload, not bradycardia. IV fluids would be the therapy of choice in patients with inferior MI.

149. The answer is b. This patient had a run of **torsade de pointes**, an atypical VT where the QRS axis swings from positive to negative within a single ECG lead. This dysrhythmia is frequently seen in patients with significant heart disease who have a **prolonged QT interval**. There are many possible causes of prolonged QT; however, common etiologies include drugs (eg, antidysrhythmic and psychotropic medications), electrolyte abnormalities, and coronary heart disease. This patient was likely on a phenothiazine for her schizophrenia leading to prolonged QT syndrome and an episode of torsade de pointes. Administration of **magnesium sulfate** has been shown to decrease runs of torsades. If the patient has a pulse but his or her vital signs are unstable, you should perform immediate cardioversion.

Observation alone (**a**) is not adequate. Conventional VT treatments such as lidocaine (**c**) are often ineffective. Procainamide can actually further prolong the QT interval. If magnesium is unsuccessful, the next strategy involves increasing the HR from 90 to 120 beats/min, thereby reducing the QT interval and preventing recurrence of torsade de pointes. Increased HR is best achieved by placing a transvenous pacemaker (**d**); this technique is sometimes called overdrive pacing. During the time it takes for the transvenous pacemaker placement, unstable patients can be started on isoproterenol (**e**), a β-adrenergic receptor agonist, to medically increase the HR.

150. The answer is c. A knee dislocation is a very serious injury with potential for neurovascular complications. Knee dislocation involves disruption of the tibiofemoral joint and all of the ligamentous structures that comprise the joint. Posterior dislocations are caused by high-velocity direct trauma to a flexed knee, such as dashboard impact in an MVC. The most serious complication of a knee dislocation is a **popliteal artery injury**. A popliteal artery injury is a **true emergency** that requires immediate repair. Delayed repair greater than 8 hours is associated with an amputation rate more than 90%. There are both hard and soft signs of vascular injury in a knee dislocation. **Palpable thrill** or audible bruit as well as absent pulses, limp ischemia, observed pulsatile bleeding (in an open or penetrating injury), and a visible expanding hematoma are all hard signs of popliteal injury. The work-up for ruling out popliteal injury includes investigation such as ABI, CT or traditional angiography, or duplex ultrasonography.

Severe knee pain (**a**) is not a hard or soft sign of vascular injury. Paresthesia of the leg (**b**) is a soft sign of popliteal injury and should lead to further evaluation. ABI more than 0.9 (**d**) is a normal result. ABI less than 0.9 is concerning for vascular injury. A nonexpanding hematoma of the affected calf (**e**) is not a hard sign for vascular injury following knee dislocation.

151. The answer is d. This patient is in **septic shock** from pneumonia and also has **adrenal crisis**. Initial treatment with IV fluids, antibiotics, and dopamine is appropriate. **Continued hypotension** in a patient on **maintenance steroid therapy** should make you think of adrenal crisis, especially in this patient who was likely on chronic steroids for his COPD. Exogenous glucocorticoids suppress hypothalamic release of corticotropin-releasing hormone (CRH) and subsequently anterior pituitary release of adrenocorticotropic hormone (ACTH). The adrenals subsequently atrophy from lack of stimulation. The patient is now faced with an acute stress from pneumonia and sepsis. His adrenals have atrophied and are unable to respond with increased cortisol secretion. Laboratory clues to adrenal crisis include **hyponatremia** and **hyperkalemia** caused by a lack of aldosterone. The treatment of adrenal crisis in the face of septic shock is **hydrocortisone**.

Mineralocorticoids, such as fludrocortisone (c), are not needed. Additional fluids (a) and vasopressors, such as phenylephrine and epinephrine (b and e) are appropriate critical care management for sepsis and should be administered after glucocorticoids.

152. The answer is c. Toxic ingestions must always be considered, especially in suicidal patients. The patient regularly takes atenolol for hypertension and may have overdosed on this occasion. β-**Blocker toxicity** classically causes **bradycardia and hypotension**. Antidotes for β-blocker toxicity, such as **glucagon**, should be given to this patient immediately. Glucagon is thought to work through a separate receptor that is not blocked by β-adrenergic antagonists, ultimately enhancing inotropy and chronotropy. Patients who are hypotensive should receive IV fluids (normal saline) and be administered vasopressor agents, such as norepinephrine. Other medications that may be useful are phosphodiesterase inhibitors (eg, milrinone), which block cyclic adenosine monophosphate (cAMP) breakdown and maintain intracellular calcium levels. **High-dose euglycemic insulin** therapy is a promising treatment for β-blocker toxicity. Ultimately, the patient may require the other treatment options, but glucagon should be the first-line therapy.

You should administer an IV bolus of fluids (a), you may attempt to administer atropine (b), and you may place external cardiac pacers on the patient (e). However, because this is a β-blocker overdose, the administration of glucagon is necessary. Epinephrine (d) should be administered if the patient loses his pulse.

153. The answer is d. Patients with penetrating trauma to the chest with possible cardiac injury and signs of hemodynamic instability need immediate **operative thoracotomy**. This patient has signs of cardiac tamponade, a collection of blood surrounding the heart and interfering with the heart's ability to contract. He has **Beck's triad** of **hypotension, distended neck veins, and muffled heart sounds**. His CXR also shows an enlarged heart. An echocardiogram would be helpful in confirming the diagnosis, but, since this patient is unstable and echocardiogram may not be readily available, the treatment is immediate thoracotomy in the OR.

While pericardiocentesis (c) may help relieve tamponade, it is not the optimal procedure for traumatic tamponade, nor is it likely to be definite in this patient's care. Pericardiocentesis may be difficult when clots fill the pericardium and may therefore give false-negative results. The procedure may also injure the heart and delay definitive treatment. Some clinicians perform bilateral tube thoracostomies (b) prior to thoracotomy to rule out a hemothorax and PTX. However, with equal breath sounds, midline trachea, and no evidence of PTX or consolidation on radiograph, chest tubes are low yield in this patient. The patient is not in respiratory distress. Intubation (a) should be performed in the OR to prevent additional delays in definitive surgical care. IV fluids and blood transfusion (e) increase venous return to the heart and are excellent supportive measures prior to definitive thoracotomy.

154. The answer is c. Abdominal pain in the elderly can be challenging for many reasons, including poor histories and deviation from classic presentations of diseases. However, abdominal pain in patients over 65 must be taken seriously since 25% to 44% require surgical intervention and more than 50% require admission to the hospital. This CXR reveals **free air under the right diaphragm**, likely from a perforated viscous. This is a **surgical emergency** and the surgical service should be contacted.

Antibiotics (a) and a central venous line (d) are appropriate and can be started after the surgical team has been notified. It is important to obtain large-bore IV access for this patient. If peripheral lines are not obtained, a central venous line should be inserted. A CT scan (b) is not necessary in this patient, especially with her low BP. She should be taken directly to the OR for an exploratory laparotomy. Although the patient has a benign abdominal examination, the caretaker's report and her low BP are worrisome, and sending the patient home (e) prior to a complete workup would be a mistake.

155. The answer is c. Burns are classified into four major categories—superficial, partial thickness, full thickness, and fourth degree. **Partial-thickness burns (c)** involve both the **epidermis and the part of the dermis**. They present with **blister formation, tenderness, and local blanching**.

Superficial burns (a) are first-degree burns (b) and are limited to the epidermis and present with erythema, minimal swelling, and mild discomfort. Full-thickness burns (d) involve the epidermis, all layers of the dermis, and extend into the subcutaneous tissue. They appear dry, leathery, and are insensate. Fourth-degree burns **(e)** are full-thickness burns that extend to the muscle or bone.

156. The answer is e. The total body surface area involved is **27%**. The **"Rule of 9s"** can be used to quickly approximate the percentage body surface area burned. This calculation divides the major body parts into percentages that are multiples of 9. In an adult, the head is 9%, the anterior chest is 9%, the abdomen is 9%, the entire back is 18%, each entire arm is 9%, and each entire leg is 18%. The patient in this question has partial-thickness burns to her anterior chest (9%), abdomen (9%), and the volar surfaces of each arm (4.5% each), which totals 27%.

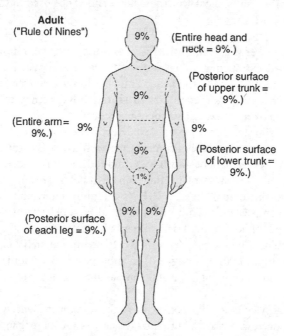

Adult
("Rule of Nines")

9% (Entire head and neck = 9%.)

(Posterior surface of upper trunk = 9%.)

9%

(Entire arm = 9%.) 9%

9%

9% (Posterior surface of lower trunk = 9%.)

1%

(Posterior surface of each leg = 9%.) 9% 9%

(Reproduced, with permission, from Tierney LM, McPhee SJ, Papadakis MA. Current Medical Diagnosis & Treatment. New York, NY: McGraw Hill, 2006.)

The palm of the patient's hand is estimated to be **1%** total body surface area. The calculation does not include superficial-thickness burns. All other answer choices **(a, b, c, and d)** are incorrect calculations for this patient's burn surface area.

157. The answer is e. The American Burn Association has identified criteria for burn injuries that require transfer to a **burn center**. Patients with **multiple trauma, comorbid conditions, or poor social support** require transfer to a burn center.

Additional transfer criteria include partial-thickness and full-thickness burns of greater than 10% of the BSA in any patient **(b)**, partial- and full-thickness burns involving the face, eyes, ears, hands, feet, genitalia and perineum, and overlying joints, full-thickness burns, significant electrical and chemical burns, those with inhalation injury, and patients with multisystem trauma, comorbidities, or poor social support. Superficial-thickness burns **(c and d)** are not used in the calculation of total body surface area burns and are not an indication for transfer to a burn center. Sunburn **(a)** is a superficial-thickness burn and is not used in the calculation of percent BSA.

158. The answer is e. This patient is presenting with eye trauma, proptosis, decreased extraocular movements, and decreased visual acuity after sustaining blunt trauma to the head. This should raise concern for **orbital compartment syndrome secondary to a retrobulbar hematoma**. This can be confirmed by **measuring intraocular pressure.**

Fluorescein staining **(a)** is used to detect corneal defects. While this is indicated in this patient, orbital compartment syndrome is a true emergency that can lead to permanent vision loss if not addressed rapidly. Therefore, evaluation and treatment of orbital compartment syndrome would take precedent in this case. A head CT **(b)** is useful to determine the cause of the orbital compartment syndrome, but should not delay treatment. Ultrasound **(c)** to look for a retinal detachment is a useful diagnostic tool in the right circumstance; however, it is unlikely to be immediately helpful in this case. Consulting ophthalmology **(d)** is appropriate, but should not delay recognition and treatment of orbital compartment syndrome.

159. The answer is a. The patient has orbital compartment syndrome as detected by decreased visual acuity, intraocular pressure more than 40 mm Hg, and proptosis. This is a true emergency that requires rapid treatment. **The treatment for orbital compartment syndrome is lateral canthotomy** and **cantholysis.** This will allow the orbital volume to expand and decrease intraocular pressure.

A head CT **(b)** is useful to determine the cause of the orbital compartment syndrome, but should not delay treatment. Although the anterior chamber **(c)** may have elevated pressure, orbital compartment syndrome is caused by increased pressure from the retrobulbar space. Anterior chamber pressure can be increased by conditions, such as hyphema and glaucoma. Serial tonometry (**d**) is employed after a lateral canthotomy and cantholysis is performed to relieve the intraocular pressure. IV mannitol (**e**) can be used as a temporizing agent to decrease intraocular pressure if definitive treatment is not immediately possible, but should not delay definitive treatment.

160. The answer is b. A **vascular bruit or thrill** is one for the hard signs of aerodigestive and neurovascular injury following penetrating neck trauma. Penetrative neck injuries are defined as disruption through the platysma muscle and are subdivided into **three distinct zones**. Zone I includes the portion of the neck from the sternum and clavicles to the cricoid cartilage. Zone II extends from the cricoid cartilage to the angle of the mandible. Zone III includes the area from the angle of the mandible to the base of the skull. Hard signs are physical exam findings that indicate evidence of major neurovascular or aerodigestive tract injury and require immediate operative management. Stable patients with soft signs should undergo CT angiogram of the neck to determine the extent of the injuries. Esophago-gastroduodenoscopy (EGD) and bronchoscopy should also be considered if there is concern for aerodigestive injury.

Subcutaneous emphysema (**a**), dyspnea (**c**), and dysphagia (**e**) are all soft signs of aerodigestive or neurovascular injury. Presence of a nonexpanding hematoma (**d**) is also a soft sign, however an expanding pulsatile hematoma is a hard sign.

Signs of Aerodigestive and Neurovascular Injury Following Penetrative Neck Trauma

Hard Signs	Soft Signs
Airway obstruction/stridor	Chest tube air leak
Cerebral ischemia	Dysphagia/dysphonia
Major hemoptysis/hematemesis	Dyspnea
Decreased or absent radial pulse	Minor hematemesis/hemoptysis
Expanding, pulsatile hematoma	Mediastinal emphysema
Fluid nonresponsive shock	Nonexpanding hematoma
Severe acute bleeding	Subcutaneous emphysema
Vascular bruit or thrill	
Focal neurologic deficit	

Recommended Readings

American College of Surgeons. *Advanced Trauma Life Support*. ATLS Student Course Manual. 10th ed. 2018.

American Heart Association. *Guidelines for CPR and ECC*. 2015.

Gorss EA, Martel ML. Chapter 33. Multiple trauma. In: Gausche-Hill M, Hockberger RS, Walls RM, et al, eds. *Rosen's Emergency Medicine: Concepts and Clinical Practice*. 9th ed. Philadelphia, PA: Elsevier, 2018.

Kaji AH, Hockberger RS. Chapter 36. Spine injuries. In: Gausche-Hill M, Hockberger RS, Walls RM, et al, eds. *Rosen's Emergency Medicine: Concepts and Clinical Practice*. 9th ed. Philadelphia, PA: Elsevier, 2018.

Kurz MC, Neumar RW. Chapter 8. Adult resuscitation. In: Gausche-Hill M, Hockberger RS, Walls RM, et al, eds. *Rosen's Emergency Medicine: Concepts and Clinical Practice*. 9th ed. Philadelphia, PA: Elsevier, 2018.

Mattox K, Moore E, Feliciano D. *Trauma*. 8th ed. New York, NY: McGraw-Hill, 2017.

Papa L, Goldberg SA. Chapter 34. Head trauma. In: Gausche-Hill M, Hockberger RS, Walls RM, et al, eds. *Rosen's Emergency Medicine: Concepts and Clinical Practice*. 9th ed. Philadelphia, PA: Elsevier, 2018.

Puskarich MA, Jones AE. Chapter 6. Shock. In: Gausche-Hill M, Hockberger RS, Walls RM, et al, eds. *Rosen's Emergency Medicine: Concepts and Clinical Practice*. 9th ed. Philadelphia, PA: Elsevier, 2018.

Williamson CA, Meurer WJ. Chapter 7. Brain resuscitation. In: Gausche-Hill M, Hockberger RS, Walls RM, et al, eds. *Rosen's Emergency Medicine: Concepts and Clinical Practice*. 9th ed. Philadelphia, PA: Elsevier, 2018.

Fever

Shannon M. Burke, MD and Aaron Kraut, MD

Questions

161. A 43-year-old man, with history of intravenous drug use (IVDU), presents to the emergency department (ED) with 2 weeks of fever, back pain, and progressive weakness in his legs bilaterally. He denies any history of trauma or prior surgery. His blood pressure (BP) is 130/75 mm Hg, heart rate (HR) is 106 beats/minute, respiratory rate (RR) is 16 breaths/minute, and temperature is 103°F. On physical examination, he has tenderness to palpation in the mid-lumbar spine, increased patellar reflexes, and decreased strength in the lower extremities bilaterally, with normal range of motion. Laboratory results reveal a white blood cell (WBC) count of 15,500/μL, hematocrit 40%, and platelets 225/μL. Urinalysis and lumbar spine X-rays are unremarkable. Which of the following is the most likely diagnosis?

a. Fibromyalgia
b. Ankylosing spondylitis
c. Spinal epidural abscess
d. Vertebral compression fracture
e. Spinal metastatic lesion

The following scenario applies to questions 162 and 163.

An 81-year-old woman is brought to the ED by her children who state that she is acting more tired than usual, has had fever for the last 2 days, and is more confused. Ordinarily, the patient is high functioning. She is ambulatory, cooks for herself, and walks on a treadmill 30 minutes a day. Her vital signs are BP 85/60 mm Hg, HR 125 beats/minute, RR 20 breaths/minute, temperature 101.3°F, and pulse oxygenation 97% on room air. On examination, the patient has dry mucous membranes. She is oriented to person and place but states that the year is 1925. Her laboratory results show a WBC 14,300/μL, hematocrit 31%, and platelets 350/μL. Her electrolytes are within normal limits. Blood glucose is 92 mg/dL. A chest radiograph does not show any infiltrates. Urinalysis reveals 2+ protein, trace ketones, WBC count of greater than 100/hpf, RBC 5 to 10/hpf, nitrite positive, and leukocyte esterase positive.

162. What is the most appropriate first step in management?

a. Administer 1 g intravenous (IV) ceftriaxone
b. Administer 0.3 mg 1:1,000 intramuscular (IM) epinephrine
c. Give 1 L IV fluid bolus and broad-spectrum antibiotics
d. Transfuse 1 unit of packed red blood cells (PRBCs)
e. Obtain a noncontrast computed tomography (CT) scan of the head

163. After administering a total of 3 L of normal saline and broad-spectrum antibiotics through her peripheral IV line, the patient's BP is 82/60 mm Hg. You suspect that the patient is in septic shock due to an acute urinary tract infection (UTI). Which of the following is the next most appropriate course of action to manage this patient?

a. Start a norepinephrine infusion
b. Transfuse 2 units of uncrossed matched packed RBCs
c. Place a central venous line into the right internal jugular vein to measure central venous pressure (CVP)
d. Start a dopamine infusion
e. Place a central venous line into the right internal jugular vein to measure mixed venous oxygen saturation (Svo_2)

164. A 40-year-old man with insulin-dependent diabetes mellitus (IDDM) presents to the ED with complaints of 2 days of increasingly severe perineal pain and subjective fevers. His BP is 95/55 mm Hg, HR is 118 beats/minute, RR is 24 breaths/minute, and temperature is 103.4°F. The point-of-care (POC) glucose reading is "high." Physical examination demonstrates crepitus over his medial thighs. There is widespread erythema and purple discoloration with sharp demarcation over his scrotum. His scrotum is markedly tender, warm, and edematous. Which of the following is the most likely diagnosis?

a. Cutaneous candidiasis
b. Fournier's gangrene
c. Phimosis
d. Paraphimosis
e. Testicular torsion

The following scenario applies to questions 165 and 166.

A 55-year-old man with a history of diabetes presents complaining of left knee pain several days following a fall from standing height. The patient was brought to the ED by ambulance after being found on a park bench stating he was unable to walk because of the pain. On physical examination, there are no rashes or external signs of trauma. His left knee is warm, diffusely tender, and swollen with a large effusion. He has pain on passive range of motion and is refusing to walk. His BP is 150/85 mm Hg, HR is 105 beats/minute, RR is 16 breaths/minute, and temperature is 102.7°F. POC glucose is 89 mg/dL.

165. Which of the following is the most definitive diagnostic test?

a. Knee radiographs
b. Magnetic resonance imaging (MRI)
c. Erythrocyte sedimentation rate (ESR) and C-reactive protein (CRP)
d. Arthrocentesis and synovial fluid analysis
e. Bone scan

166. Which of the following synovial fluid results is most indicative of a diagnosis of septic arthritis?

a. Clear appearance, 300 WBC/mm with 20% polymorphonuclear (PMN) cells, glucose 95
b. Turbid appearance, 5,000 WBC/mm with 80% PMNs, glucose 80
c. Turbid appearance, 40,000 WBC/mm with 80% PMNs, glucose 80
d. Turbid appearance, 80,000 WBC/mm with 90% PMNs, glucose 40
e. Turbid appearance, 40,000 WBC/mm with 50% PMNs, glucose 50

167. A 35-year-old woman with systemic lupus erythematosus (SLE) is brought to the ED by her brother for fever and confusion. Physical examination reveals fever, tachycardia, a waxing and waning mental status, petechiae over her oral mucosa, pallor, and mildly heme-positive stool. Her urinalysis is positive for blood, red cell casts, and proteinuria. Laboratory results reveal blood urea nitrogen (BUN) of 40 mg/dL and creatinine of 2 mg/dL. Her bilirubin is elevated (unconjugated > conjugated) and her international normalized ratio (INR) is 0.98. Her complete blood count reveals WBC 12,000/µL, hematocrit 29%, and platelet count 17,000/µL with schistocytes on the peripheral smear. Which of the following is the most appropriate next step in management?

a. Admit to the intensive care unit (ICU) for plasmapheresis
b. Admit to the ICU and begin platelet transfusion
c. Admit to the ICU for corticosteroid infusion, transfusion of platelets, and prompt surgical consultation for emergent splenectomy
d. Admit to the ICU for emergent hemodialysis
e. Perform a lumbar puncture (LP) for analysis of cerebrospinal fluid (CSF)

The following scenario applies to questions 168 and 169.

A 30-year-old woman presents to the ED with fever, headache, a "sunburn-like" rash, and confusion. A friend states that the patient has complained of nausea, vomiting, diarrhea, and a sore throat over the past few days. Her last menstrual period began 4 days ago. Vital signs are BP 80/45 mm Hg, HR 110 beats/minute, RR 18 breaths/minute, and temperature 103°F. On physical examination, you note an ill-appearing woman with a diffuse-blanching erythroderma. Her neck is supple without signs of meningeal irritation. On pelvic examination, you remove a tampon. You note a fine desquamation of her skin, especially over the hands and feet, and hyper-emia of her oropharyngeal, conjunctival, and vaginal mucous membranes. Laboratory results reveal a creatine phosphokinase (CPK) of 5,000, WBC 15,000/μL, platelets 90,000/μL, BUN 40 mg/dL, creatinine 2 mg/dL, and elevated liver enzymes. You suspect the diagnosis of toxic shock syndrome (TSS) and initiate IV fluids.

168. Your antibiotic coverage should target which of the following causative organisms?

a. *Staphylococcus aureus*
b. *Rickettsia rickettsii*
c. *Streptococcus pyogenes*
d. *Neisseria meningitidis*
e. *Neisseria gonorrhoeae*

169. Given your desire to halt rapidly proliferating bacteria and neutralize the inflammatory response of the body to the toxin released, which of the following antibiotics is added to the treatment regimen due to its important role against the toxins released by the bacteria?

a. Penicillin
b. Ceftriaxone
c. Metronidazole
d. Clindamycin
e. Amoxicillin-clavulanate

170. A 32-year-old diabetic man presents to the ED with a fever and 1 week of increasing right foot pain. He stepped on a nail while running in tennis shoes 2 weeks ago. The nail went through his shoe and punctured the bottom of his foot, but he did not seek treatment at that time. On physical examination, his heel is mildly erythematous with overlying warmth and edema and diffusely tender to palpation. There is a small amount of purulent drainage through the puncture hole in his heel. A plain radiograph of his foot demonstrates a slight lucency of the calcaneus. He has decreased range of motion, but you are able to passively dorsiflex and plantarflex his ankle without difficulty. His vital signs include BP 130/75 mm Hg, HR 98 beats/minute, RR 16 breaths/minute, and temperature 101.4°F. In addition to antibiotic coverage against *S. aureus*, therapy should include treatment against which of the following organisms?

a. *Salmonella*
b. *Pseudomonas aeruginosa*
c. Herpes simplex virus
d. *Listeria monocytogenes*
e. *Pasteurella multocida*

171. A 55-year-old man presents to the ED with fever, drooling, trismus, and a swollen neck. He reports a foul taste in his mouth caused by a tooth extraction 2 days ago. On physical examination, the patient appears anxious. He has bilateral submandibular swelling with elevation and protrusion of the tongue. He appears "bull-necked" with tense and markedly tender edema and brawny induration of the upper neck. He is tender over the lower second and third molars. There is no cervical lymphadenopathy. The lungs are clear to auscultation with good air movement. His vital signs are BP 140/85 mm Hg, HR 105 beats/minute, RR 26 breaths/minute, and temperature 102°F. Which of the following is the most appropriate management?

a. Administer IV antibiotics and obtain a soft tissue radiograph of the neck
b. Perform incision and drainage, obtain a sample for culture, and administer IV antibiotics
c. Administer IV antibiotics and obtain a CT scan of the neck
d. Administer IV antibiotics, obtain a CT scan of the neck, and obtain an emergent ENT consult
e. Secure his airway, administer IV antibiotics, and obtain an emergent ENT consult

172. A 37-year-old man presents to the ED with complaints of 2 days of a sore throat and subjective fever at home. He denies cough or vomiting. His BP is 130/75 mm Hg, HR is 85 beats/minute, RR is 14 breaths/minute, and temperature is 101°F. He has diffuse tonsillar swelling and bilateral exudates. His cervical lymph nodes are enlarged and tender bilaterally. Which of the following is the next best step in management?

a. Administer penicillin and discharge the patient without further testing
b. Perform a rapid antigen test; if negative, confirm with a throat culture
c. Perform a rapid antigen test; if negative, administer penicillin and discharge the patient
d. Perform a rapid antigen test; if positive, administer penicillin and discharge the patient
e. Discharge the patient without treatment or further testing

173. A 37-year-old man who just finished a full course of penicillin for pharyngitis presents to the ED. He reports taking the antibiotics exactly as prescribed by his primary care physician (PCP). Initially, he felt somewhat improved. He has had increased pain and progressive difficulty swallowing for the last 3 days. His vital signs include BP 130/65 mm Hg, HR 95 beats/minute, RR 16 breaths/minute, temperature 100.1°F, and oxygen saturation 99%. He is not in acute distress. There is swelling of his right tonsillar arch and deviation of his uvula to the left. Review of his records reveals a throat culture that was positive for *Streptococcus*. Which of the following is the most appropriate next step in management?

a. Perform needle aspiration, prescribe clindamycin, and have him return in 24 hours
b. Give IV morphine and IV ceftriaxone, and observe him in the ED for 6 hours
c. Admit him for incision and drainage in the operating room (OR) under general anesthesia
d. Prescribe clindamycin and have him return in 24 hours
e. Order a CT scan of the neck

174. A 45-year-old woman presents to the ED complaining of 3 days of fever, worsening throat pain, and odynophagia. She sits on a chair, leaning forward with her mouth slightly open. She is refusing to swallow and has a cup of saliva and a box of facial tissues at her side. Vitals are BP 110/70 mm Hg, HR 120 beats/minute, RR 22 breaths/minute, temperature 102.8°F, and oxygen saturation 99% on room air. You note a slight wheezing noise coming from her anterior neck. Her voice is hoarse and she is unable to open her mouth fully, making her examination quite difficult. From what you can visualize, her posterior oropharynx is moderately hyperemic, without exudates or tonsillar enlargement. You obtain the lateral cervical radiograph shown below. Which of the following is the most likely diagnosis?

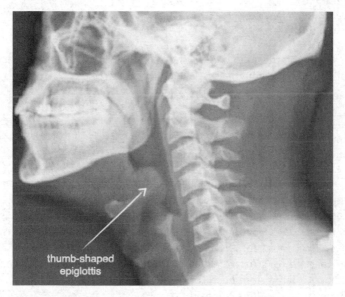

thumb-shaped
epiglottis

(Reproduced with permission from Adam J. Rosh, MD, and Rosh Review.)

a. Retropharyngeal abscess
b. Peritonsillar abscess
c. Epiglottitis
d. Pharyngitis
e. Laryngotracheitis

The following scenario applies to questions 175 and 176.

A 42-year-old man with a history of IV DU presents to the ED with fever, chills, pleuritic chest pain, myalgias, and general malaise. The patient's vitals include BP 110/65 mm Hg, HR 110 beats/minute, RR 18 breaths/minute, and temperature 103.4°F. Physical examination is notable for retinal hemorrhages, petechiae on the conjunctivae and mucous membranes, a faint systolic ejection murmur, and splenomegaly.

175. Which of the following is the most likely diagnosis?

a. Disseminated gonorrhea
b. Myocarditis
c. Pericarditis
d. Infectious mononucleosis
e. Endocarditis

176. Which of the following is the most sensitive diagnostic imaging modality for confirming the suspected diagnosis?

a. Transthoracic echocardiogram
b. CT angiography of the chest
c. Chest X-ray (CXR)
d. Ventilation–perfusion (VQ) scan
e. Transesophageal echocardiogram

177. A 51-year-old diabetic man complains of intense right ear pain and discharge. On physical examination, his BP is 145/65 mm Hg, HR 91 beats/minute, and temperature 101°F. He withdraws when you retract the pinna of his ear. The external auditory canal is erythematous, edematous, and contains what looks like friable granulation tissue. The tympanic membrane is partially obstructed, but appears to be erythematous. You make the presumptive diagnosis of necrotizing otitis externa. Which of the following statements regarding this condition is true?

a. This an uncommon complication of otitis media in otherwise healthy patients
b. The mainstay of treatment is outpatient oral antibiotics
c. Cranial nerve (CN) IX palsy is the most common complication
d. *P. aeruginosa* is the most common causative organism
e. Hearing loss is the most common complication

The following scenario applies to questions 178 and 179.

A 26-year-old woman presents to the ED with fever, malaise, and an evolving rash in the right axilla that she initially thought was an insect bite from hiking 1 week ago. She complains of generalized fatigue, nausea, headache, and joint pain over the past several days. Her vitals are BP 120/75 mm Hg, HR 75 beats/minute, RR 16 breaths/minute, and temperature 101°F. On physical examination, she is awake and alert, with a nonfocal neurologic examination. Her neck is supple, but she is diffusely tender over the shoulder, knee, and hip joints bilaterally without any distinct effusions. Her abdomen is soft and nontender. She has a 9-cm erythematous annular plaque with partial central clearing and a bright red outer border and a target center under her right axilla.

178. Which of the following is the most appropriate treatment plan?

a. Treat empirically with IV antibiotics and consult dermatology
b. Treat empirically with cephalexin for 10 days and arrange PCP follow-up
c. Treat empirically with doxycycline for 21 days and arrange PCP follow-up
d. Treat empirically with prednisone and diphenhydramine, and arrange PCP follow-up
e. Perform serologic testing for *Borrelia burgdorferi* and arrange PCP follow-up

179. Which of the following is a well-known and life-threatening complication of this disease?

a. Third-degree heart block
b. Endocarditis
c. Myositis
d. Pulmonary necrosis
e. Gastrointestinal (GI) hemorrhage

180. A 54-year-old man with a history of hepatitis C, alcohol abuse, and cirrhosis presents with increasing abdominal girth and pain. He complains of increasing difficulty breathing, especially when lying down, caused by worsening ascites. On physical examination, the patient is cachectic and appears older than his stated age. He has a diffusely tender abdomen and tense ascites. The liver is palpable 4 cm below the costal margin. Vitals include BP 110/65 mm Hg, HR 110 beats/minute, RR 22 breaths/minute, and temperature 102°F. Which of the following is the most common organism seen in spontaneous bacterial peritonitis (SBP)?

a. *P. aeruginosa*
b. *Enterococcus*
c. *Streptococcus pneumoniae*
d. Enterobacteriaceae
e. *Streptococcus viridans*

181. An otherwise healthy 3-year-old girl with a 3-day history of upper respiratory infection (URI) symptoms and 2 days of "barking cough" presents with fever and drooling. Patient's mother reports over the past 2 to 3 hours, the child has had a significant increase in fever and is now drooling and will not lie flat due to difficulty breathing. The child appears lethargic, however is sitting up, leaning forward, and drooling. She has inspiratory and expiratory stridor. Vitals include BP 90/60 mm Hg, HR 140 beats/minute, RR 40 breaths/minute, and temperature 104.1°F. What is the most likely diagnosis?

a. Croup
b. Retropharyngeal abscess
c. Peritonsillar abscess
d. Epiglottitis
e. Bacterial tracheitis

The following scenario applies to questions 182 and 183.

A 14-day-old neonate presents with his parents with a 4-hour history of fever. Parents report noticing that he "felt warm" and was having copious nasal secretions while feeding. His rectal temperature at home was 102.3°F. He was born via normal spontaneous vaginal delivery at term. The neonate appears lethargic and has mottled extremities, but is hot to the touch. Vitals include BP 74/48 mm Hg, HR 170 beats/minute, RR 40 breaths/minute, and temperature 102.9°F.

182. Which of the following is the most appropriate management?

a. Give a 20 cc/kg IV fluid bolus, administer broad-spectrum IV antibiotics, and admit the patient to the neonatal intensive care unit (NICU)
b. Obtain blood cultures, administer broad-spectrum IM antibiotics, and discharge home with close follow-up the next day
c. Give a 20 cc/kg IV fluid bolus, obtain blood and urine cultures, administer broad-spectrum IV antibiotics, and admit to the NICU
d. Give a 20 cc/kg IV fluid bolus, obtain blood and urine cultures, obtain CSF via LP and send for culture, administer broad-spectrum IV antibiotics, and admit to the NICU
e. Give a 20 cc/kg IV fluid bolus, obtain blood and urine cultures, administer broad-spectrum IV antibiotics, and discharge home with close follow-up the next day morning

183. Which pair of antibiotics is the most appropriate to empirically administer to this patient?

a. Ceftriaxone and azithromycin
b. Ampicillin and doxycycline

c. Cefotaxime and ampicillin
d. Piperacillin-tazobactam and vancomycin
e. Ceftriaxone and vancomycin

184. A 30-year-old man presents with fever, altered mental status, and involuntary movements. Patient's wife states he had a sore throat and fever several days prior, which resolved; however, the fever has returned and he now has writhing movements of his arms and torso. On examination, the patient is restless, warm to the touch, has an erythematous annular rash on his trunk and inner arms, and has writhing movements of his upper extremities. Vitals include BP of 110/70 mm Hg, HR of 120 beats/minute, RR of 30 breaths/minute, and temperature of 102.4°F. Which of the following is consistent with a presumptive diagnosis of rheumatic fever?

a. Positive antistreptolysin O (ASO) titer, chorea, fever, and elevated erythrocyte sedimentation rate (ESR)
b. Positive rapid strep antigen test, polyarthritis, and fever
c. Positive ASO titer, chorea, and elevated CRP
d. Positive rapid strep antigen test, subcutaneous nodules, and arthralgias
e. Positive ASO titer, fever, arthralgias, and elevated ESR

185. An otherwise healthy, sexually active, 32-year-old woman presents to the ED with fever, dysuria, and abdominal pain. She also had slight burning with urination over the past week. Her symptoms have continued to worsen and today she notes new nonradiating right-sided flank pain. She is nauseated, but has been tolerating food and drink. She denies any abnormal vaginal discharge or bleeding. Her BP is 120/82 mm Hg, HR is 87 beats/minute, RR is 16 breaths/minute, pulse oximetry is 99%, and temperature is 101.2°F. She has right cerebrovascular accident (CVA) and suprapubic tenderness. Pelvic exam reveals no vaginal discharge, no cervical motion tenderness (CMT), and no adnexal tenderness. Serum laboratory studies reveal a WBC count of 11,500 cells/μL, creatinine of 0.7 mg/dL, and BUN of 20 mg/dL. Urinalysis shows 1+ protein, WBC count greater 50/hpf, no RBCs, positive leukocyte esterase, positive nitrites, with bacteria present on microscopy. Her pregnancy test is negative. Which of the following includes the correct diagnosis and treatment?

a. She has pyelonephritis and should be discharged home on trimethoprim/sulfamethoxazole
b. She has pyelonephritis and should undergo CT scan of the abdomen to assess for an abscess
c. She has cystitis and should be discharged home on nitrofurantoin
d. She has pyelonephritis and should be admitted for IV ceftriaxone
e. She has pelvic inflammatory disease (PID) and should be given a single dose of IM ceftriaxone and discharged with a prescription for doxycycline

186. A 45-year-old woman with history of depression on escitalopram presents to the ED via emergency medical services (EMS) after her boyfriend found her altered at their home this morning. Her boyfriend states she has had an URI over the past few days and has been taking over-the-counter (OTC) medications to help with her symptoms. Patient's BP is 145/82 mm Hg, HR is 122 beats/minute, RR is 22 breaths/minute, pulse oximetry is 97%, and temperature is 103°F. She appears tired, but is easily arousable and becomes agitated when awakened. Her physical exam reveals clear lungs, bilateral lower extremity clonus, and significant diaphoresis. Which of the following is the most appropriate management of her condition?

a. IV fluid resuscitation and empiric broad-spectrum antibiotics
b. Lorazepam
c. Ibuprofen
d. Acetaminophen
e. Dantrolene

The following scenario applies to questions 187 and 188.

An otherwise healthy 20-year-old university student presents to the ED in January via EMS after his roommate had trouble waking him this morning. His roommate states that the patient had been complaining that he did not feel well over the past few days and has not gone to class. BP is 110/90 mm Hg, HR is 101 beats/minute, RR is 20 breaths/minute, and temperature is 102°F. He is sleepy, but is arousable to voice. He is able to answer questions appropriately. When you passively flex the patient's neck, he winces and draws his knees up toward his abdomen. You perform a full neurologic exam and you note that the patient has a left-sided facial nerve palsy.

187. In addition to administering broad-spectrum IV antibiotics, which of the following is the next most appropriate step in management?

a. Perform endotracheal intubation
b. Perform an LP
c. Obtain a neurology consult
d. Obtain a CT of the head without contrast
e. Obtain Lyme's disease titers

188. The patient's roommate asks if there is anything that he should do to avoid getting sick. Which of the following is the best course of action?

a. Admission for observation so he can be treated if he develops symptoms
b. Cleaning their dorm room thoroughly with antibiotic wipes
c. No treatment with close monitoring at home for the development of symptoms
d. Rifampin prophylaxis
e. Amoxicillin prophylaxis

189. A 45-year-old man with history of acquired immunodeficiency syndrome (AIDS) previously complicated by esophageal candidiasis presents to the ED with complaint of fatigue, fever, dry cough, and dyspnea. He does not always remember to take his antiretroviral medications due to a constantly changing work schedule. His most recent CD4+ T-cell count 2 weeks ago was 150 cells/mm^3. His symptoms have developed over the past few weeks and have been progressively worsening. He denies any other associated symptoms such as rhinorrhea, nasal congestion, headache, vomiting, or diarrhea. BP is 115/75 mm Hg, HR is 95 beats/minute, RR is 24 breaths/minute, pulse oximetry is 88% on room air, and temperature is 101°F. His lungs are diffusely coarse to auscultation. His CXR is shown below. What is the most likely cause of the patient's symptoms?

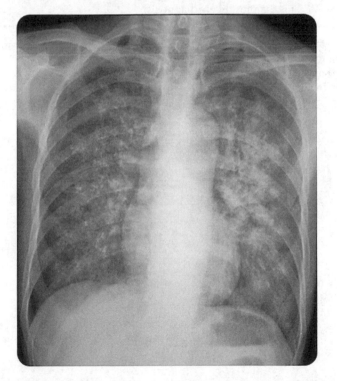

a. Influenza
b. *Pneumocystis jirovecii*
c. *S. aureus*
d. *S. pneumoniae*
e. *Mycoplasma pneumoniae*

190. A 65-year-old woman with history of obesity, hypertension, and hyperlipidemia presents to the ED with complaints of fever, nausea, left-sided abdominal pain, and constipation. These symptoms developed over the past 3 days and she first noticed decreased bowel movements. Her fever started this morning and the pain in her left lower abdomen worsened, so she came to the ED for evaluation. She had a "normal" colonoscopy performed 5 years ago. BP is 134/82 mm Hg, HR is 90 beats/minute, RR 18 breaths/minute, pulse oximetry is 95%, and temperature is 100.8°F. Her exam is overall reassuring except for tenderness to palpation in the left lower quadrant. She has no rebound, guarding, or rigidity on exam. Laboratory studies reveal leukocytosis. She underwent a CT of her abdomen and pelvis that showed inflammation of the sigmoid colon along with a 2-cm abscess. What is the most likely diagnosis?

a. Diverticulitis
b. Ischemic colitis
c. Crohn's disease
d. Appendicitis
e. *Clostridium difficile* infection

Fever

Answers

161. The answer is c. Epidural abscesses are most commonly found in **immunocompromised patients**, **IV DU**, and the **elderly**. Signs and symptoms of epidural abscess usually develop over 1 to 2 weeks and include fever, localized pain, and progressive weakness, often localized to the lower extremities. An elevated WBC count, along with elevated inflammatory markers (ESR and CRP), are also commonly seen. MRI is the most useful diagnostic test. Unfortunately, X-ray and even CT may lack appropriate sensitivity for the diagnosis. *S. aureus* is the most common causative organism, followed by gram-negative bacilli and tuberculosis bacillus.

Fibromyalgia **(a)** is a common cause of chronic back pain, but one would not expect the physical findings (weakness and/or hyperreflexia) or laboratory abnormalities. Fibromyalgia should be a diagnosis of exclusion after other more emergent conditions are ruled-out. Inflammatory conditions, including ankylosing spondylitis **(b)**, may cause back pain. The key findings in this disease include gradual onset of morning stiffness improved with exercise in a patient younger than 40 years. On physical examination, these patients may have limited back flexion, reduced chest expansion, and sacroiliac joint tenderness, all of which are nonspecific. Fever and weakness would not be expected. Back pain may result from vertebral compression fractures **(d).** These may be secondary to trauma or may be atraumatic in a patient with osteoporosis. Osteoporotic compression fractures usually involve patients older than 70 years or patients with acquired bone weakness (eg, prolonged steroid use). X-ray may miss some compression fractures. CT is a more sensitive diagnostic modality. Metastatic lesions **(e)** invade the spinal bone marrow, leading to compression of the spinal cord. Most common primary tumors include the breast, lung, thyroid, kidney, prostate (easily remembered by the acronym "BLT with Kosher pickles"), as well as lymphoma and multiple myeloma. Maintain a high level of suspicion for any cancer patient who develops back pain; these patients must be investigated for spinal metastases. Although this patient does have symptoms of spinal cord compression, his fever, tachycardia, and leukocystosis make an infectious cause more likely.

162. The answer is c. The treatment for sepsis has evolved considerably over the past 10+ years with emphasis on the early recognition and aggressive therapy. Early goal direct therapy (EGDT) initiated the practice of rapid recognition and treatment of sepsis in the ED. The extensive monitoring of EGDT, such as the monitoring of CVP, has been shown to be unnecessary by several recent trials [Protocolized Care for Early Septic Shock (**ProCESS**) trial, etc.]. However, the key tenants of resuscitation in sepsis **remain early fluid resuscitation and broad-spectrum antibiotics.**

This patient is exhibiting signs of sepsis and should receive IV fluid boluses and broad-spectrum antibiotics. Ceftriaxone (**a**) may be an appropriate agent; however, it would be advisable to start broad given evidence of sepsis and then narrow the antibiotic choice as the patient stabilizes and cultures/susceptibilities return. Epinephrine at a dose of 0.3 mg of 1:1,000 IM (**b**) is the appropriate treatment for anaphylaxis. PRBCs (**d**) can be transfused if there is evidence of poor oxygen delivery to the tissues and if the hemoglobin is less than 7. Overall, this recommendation was a standard part of EGDT and transfusions are not usual practice currently unless significant anemia exists. A CT scan (**e**) is not indicated at this time as the most reasonable explanation for the patient's change in mental status is the acute infection and hemodynamic changes and there is a great deal of risk involved in moving a hemodynamically unstable patient to the CT scanner.

163. The answer is a. Vasopressor therapy should be started after the patient receives a total of 2 to 3 L of IV normal saline fluid boluses and remains hypotensive with a mean arterial pressure (MAP) of less than 65 mm Hg in order to improve BP and end-organ/tissue perfusion. **Norepinephrine is the vasopressor of choice in septic shock.**

Packed RBCs (**b**) were previously recommended in EGDT protocols if there was evidence of poor oxygen delivery to the tissues as measured by the central venous oxygen saturation ($ScvO_2$) or if hematocrit was less than 30%. $ScvO_2$ monitoring is invasive and recent trials [ProCESS, PRogesterone In Spontaneous Miscarriage Trial (PRISM), etc.] have shown no mortality benefit for patients when invasive testing and historical protocols such as EGDT are utilized. A central line (**c**) is indicated in this patient for administration of vasopressors—not for measurement of CVP as it has been shown in the recent literature that such close monitoring is not useful in directing ED resuscitation of septic patients. Dopamine (**d**) used to be the vasopressor of choice in sepsis; however, it has fallen out of favor as it has been shown to increase mortality when compared to norepinephrine. Monitoring of central Svo_2 **(e)** has also fallen out of favor as it was also shown in recent literature to not convey a benefit in patients with septic shock.

164. The answer is b. **Fournier's syndrome** (also known as **Fournier's gangrene**) is a **polymicrobial necrotizing fasciitis** of the **perineal subcutaneous tissue**. It is more common in male patients and usually begins as a simple abscess or cellulitis that quickly spreads, especially in an immunocompromised patient (eg, diabetics). If not promptly diagnosed, it can lead to end-artery thrombosis in the subcutaneous tissue and widespread necrosis. While laboratory and imaging studies can be suggestive of Fournier's, the diagnosis is made clinically. Treatment includes aggressive fluid resuscitation; broad-spectrum antibiotics to cover gram-positive, gram-negative, and anaerobic bacteria; wide surgical debridement; and, in some instances, hyperbaric oxygen therapy.

Cutaneous candidiasis **(a)** is common in diabetics with poorly controlled blood sugar and may be a presenting complaint in new-onset diabetes. However, this rash is nontoxic, without systemic signs and symptoms, and often limited to moist areas such as between skin folds. Phimosis **(c)** is a chronic condition in which the foreskin cannot be retracted from the glans penis and can lead to urinary retention. Paraphimosis **(d)** is an emergency condition where there is an inability to reduce the proximal foreskin over the glans penis (the foreskin becomes "stuck" behind the glans penis). It may lead to decreased arterial flow and eventual gangrene. Testicular torsion **(e)** is the twisting of a testicle on the spermatic cord that usually occurs during strenuous activity or following trauma, but can occasionally occur during sleep. It is most common in infants and young adults.

165. The answer is d. This patient is exhibiting the common signs and symptoms of **septic arthritis**, an infection of a joint space. The knee is the most commonly involved joint, followed by the hip, shoulder, and wrist. Preexisting arthritis (eg, osteoarthritis or rheumatoid arthritis), immunocompromised states (eg, alcoholism, diabetes, or cancer), and sexually transmitted infections are risk factors for the development of septic arthritis. Patients present with a warm, tender, erythematous, swollen joint and pain with passive range of motion. Fever and chills are common. **Arthrocentesis** is diagnostic with joint fluid demonstrating a WBC count greater than 50,000/μL with more than 75% neutrophils. *S. aureus* remains the predominant pathogen for all age groups. However, in young adults, gonococcal septic arthritis is common and should also be considered when selecting empiric antibiotic coverage.

Patients with sickle cell disease are also at increased risk for septic arthritis due to salmonella. Patients with septic arthritis should receive a **first dose of antibiotics in the ED** prior to admission. If a coincident cellulitis is present over the involved joint, arthrocentesis may need to be delayed, though this decision should be made in consultation with an orthopedic surgeon, as delay in diagnosis of a septic joint can lead to significant morbidity.

Plain radiographs (**a**) should be obtained to identify any underlying osteomyelitis or joint disease, but are often nondiagnostic in acute septic arthritis. MRI (**b**) plays no role in the diagnosis of acute septic arthritis but may be useful in evaluating for chronic disease, osteomyelitis, and other musculoskeletal injuries involving the knee. The ESR and CRP (**c**) are often elevated in septic arthritis and can be trended to assess treatment success, but neither is specific or diagnostic. A bone scan (**e**) is useful in the detection of osteomyelitis that may not be immediately apparent on a plain radiograph, but is not sensitive in the diagnosis of septic arthritis.

166. The answer is d. In septic arthritis, the synovial fluid is typically cloudy, has a **high WBC (> 50,000 WBC/mm), a predominance of PMNs, and a low glucose** when compared to serum. In this question, the fluid that is turbid in appearance has a WBC more than 50,000 per mm with 90% PMNs and a low glucose level.

The following table demonstrates what the synovial fluid from arthrocentesis should look like for various joint problems.

Condition	Appearance	WBCs/mm*	% PMNs*	Glucose % of Serum Level*	Crystals
Normal	Clear	<200	<25	95-100	None
Degenerative (noninflammatory)	Clear	<400	<25	95-100	None
Acute gout	Turbid	2000-5000	>75	80-100	Negatively birefringent, needle-like
Pseudogout	Turbid	5000-50,000	>75	80-100	Positively birefringent, rhomboid
Septic arthritis	Purulent/turbid	> 50,000	>75	<50	None
Inflammatory arthritis	Turbid	5000-50,000	50-75	75	None

*Note: These values represent common laboratory findings in each condition and may not be present in all instances.

Degenerative joint disease is reflected in the synovial fluid of choice (a). Choice(b) represents gout. Choice (c) represents pseudogout. Choice (e) represents inflammatory arthritis.

167. The answer is a. This patient has **thrombotic thrombocytopenic purpura (TTP)**, caused by increased platelet destruction. In TTP, platelet-fibrin thrombi deposit in vessel and cause injury to RBCs and platelets, resulting in microangiopathy hemolytic anemia and thrombocytopenia. Patients tend to be females who are 10 to 45 years of age. Risk factors include pregnancy, autoimmune disorders (eg, SLE), infection, allogeneic bone marrow transplantation, malignancy, and medications (eg, quinine, clopidogrel, and ticlopidine). The **pentad** includes **fever** (microangiopathic hemolytic), **anemia, thrombocytopenia, renal failure**, and **neurologic changes** (fluctuating symptoms with a waxing and waning mental status). Unfortunately, only 40% of patients presents with the classic pentad. Untreated, TTP carries a mortality rate up to 80%. Although steroids, splenectomy, anticoagulation, and exchange transfusion have been attempted, daily **plasmapheresis** until platelet count normalizes is the current initial treatment of choice. In addition, RBCs may be transfused in patients with symptomatic anemia. All patients with TTP should be admitted to an ICU for close monitoring of acute bleeds.

The initial therapy for TTP generally does not include platelet transfusion (b), as this could worsen the condition and increase mortality. However, platelets should be administered in patients with a life-threatening bleed. Corticosteroids and splenectomy (c) are used in refractory cases, but are not considered appropriate initial treatments. Fever and altered mental status may indicate meningitis, but this patient has other signs and symptoms consistent with TTP. An LP (e) could be dangerous given the very low platelet count and presumptive treatment should be provided if there is concern for meningitis. Hemodialysis (d) is not a treatment for TTP.

168. The answer is a. This patient suffers from **TSS**, a toxin-mediated systemic inflammatory response that results in a severe, rapidly progressive, life-threatening syndrome of high fevers, diffuse macular erythroderma, profound hypotension, desquamation, and multisystem dysfunction (including vomiting or diarrhea, severe myalgias, mucous membrane hyperemia, renal or hepatic dysfunction, decreased platelets, and disorientation). TSS was initially recognized as a disease of young, healthy, menstruating women, in which tampon use increased the risk 33 times. With increased awareness and changes in tampon composition, cases of TSS have declined over the past 20 years. An **exotoxin** produced by *S. aureus* is the presumed cause in menstrual-related TSS (MRTSS) and two endotoxins have been implicated in non–menstrual-related TSS (NMRTSS). **TSS should be considered in any unexplained febrile illness associated with erythroderma, hypotension, and diffuse organ dysfunction.** Patients with MRTSS usually present between the third and fifth day of menses. In severe cases, headache is the most common complaint. The rash is a diffuse, blanching erythroderma, often described as painless "sunburn" that fades within 3 days and is followed by desquamation, especially of the palms and soles. For severe cases, treatment includes aggressive IV fluid resuscitation, IV antibiotics, and hospital admission in a monitored setting.

Rocky Mountain spotted fever (RMSF) **(b)** is caused by *R. rickettsii*, which is transmitted by ticks. The organism multiplies in endothelial cells lining small vessels, causing generalized vasculitis as well as headache, fever, confusion, rash, myalgias, and shock. The rash usually appears on days 2 to 3, initially on the wrists, ankles, palms, and soles, spreading rapidly to the extremities and trunk. Lesions begin as small, erythematous blanching macules that become maculopapular and petechial. The location and type of rash, along with the history distinguish RMSF from TSS. Serologic tests are confirmatory, but treatment with doxycycline or chloramphenicol should be started prior to confirmation. Streptococcal scarlet fever **(c)** is an acute febrile illness primarily affecting young children, caused by *S. pyogenes* [group A streptococci (GAS)]. The "sandpaper" rash of scarlet fever differs from the macular sunburn rash of TSS. The treatment is penicillin or macrolide in penicillin-allergic patients. While *S. aureus* is the causative organism of TSS, a less common, but more aggressive, TSS-like syndrome, streptococcal TSS (STSS), has also been identified. The treatment is similar to that of TSS, with aggressive fluid management along with IV penicillin and clindamycin. These patients may progress to a necrotizing fasciitis or myositis, requiring surgical intervention. Meningococcemia **(d)** is an infectious vasculitis caused by disseminated *Neisseria meningitides*, a gram-negative diplococcus. Fever, headache, arthralgias, altered mental status, and abnormal vitals may also be found, along with neck stiffness. There is no indication of meningeal irritation in this patient. Furthermore, the rash of meningococcemia is distinctly different from that of TSS, involving petechial, hemorrhagic vesicles, macules, and papules with surrounding erythema, especially on the trunk and extremities. The treatment is IV ceftriaxone. Disseminated gonococcemia (e), usually seen in young, sexually active female patients, is caused by *N. gonorrhoeae*. The rash of gonococcemia is pustular with an erythematous base, rather than petechial and hemorrhagic, as are the lesions of RMSF and meningococcemia. It can also be associated with fever and arthralgias. The treatment is IV ceftriaxone or oral ciprofloxacin.

169. The answer is d. The treatment for TSS centers around treating the bacteria causing the infection, as well as mediating the body's response to the toxins. Antibiotic recommendations are based off local resistance patterns. Therefore, patients should be treated with vancomycin or linezolid if there is concern for methicillin-resistant *S. aureus*. The antibiotic of choice to help halt the body's response to the bacterial toxin is **clindamycin.** Clindamycin is effective against rapidly proliferating *Staphylococcus* and *Streptococcus* species and works by inhibiting protein synthesis and toxin production.

Both penicillin (a) and ceftriaxone (b) are effective against gram-positive bacteria; however, clindamycin is the antibiotic that is most effective against the particular species involved in TSS, which proliferate rapidly and release potent endotoxins and exotoxins. Metronidazole (c) is particularly effective against anaerobes; however, the organisms that most commonly cause TSS are aerobes. Amoxicillin-clavulanate (e) is often used to treat skin or HEENT (head, eyes, ears, nose, and throat) infections by the oral route. In this instance, an IV medication is needed in order to rapidly deliver a drug to target the rapidly proliferating *Staphylococcus* and *Streptococcus* and the associated potent toxin within the bloodstream.

170. The answer is b. Osteomyelitis is an infection or inflammation of a bone with an incidence following plantar puncture wounds of 0.1% to 2%. Pain, swelling, fever, redness, and drainage may all occur, but pain is the presenting complaint in most cases. Risk factors include trauma, surgery, soft tissue infections, and being immunocompromised [(eg, human immunodeficiency virus (HIV), diabetes, IVDU, sickle-cell disease, and alcoholism]. Overall, *S. aureus* is the leading cause of osteomyelitis, followed by various *Streptococcus* species. *Pseudomonas* is implicated in specific subpopulations (eg, someone who **steps on a nail and suffers a puncture wound through footwear**, those with implanted orthopedic prosthetic devices, and IV drug abusers). *Pseudomonas* does not appear to grow on puncture objects but rather appears to grow on the footwear and may be inoculated into the wound when an object punctures through the footwear as is seen in this question. Definitive diagnosis is made by bone scan, which will demonstrate osteomyelitis within 72 hours of symptom onset. Radiographs may be normal early on but will demonstrate periosteal elevation within 10 days. ESR and CRP are often elevated, but normal or slightly elevated levels do not rule out the diagnosis. They are most valuable in following response to treatment, as levels should fall as the infection resolves. Blood cultures, which are positive in 50% of cases, should be used to guide antibiotic treatment. All patients with puncture wounds should receive tetanus prophylaxis.

Patients with sickle-cell disease and asplenism are at higher risk for *Salmonella* (**a**) osteomyelitis, although *S. aureus* remains the most common cause. Herpes simplex virus (**c**) does not cause osteomyelitis. *L. monocytogenes* (**d**) is associated with immunocompromised individuals (particularly neonates and the elderly) and can cause meningitis and sepsis. *P. multocida* (**e**) is a common etiology of cellulitis following a cat bite.

171.   The answer is e. Secure his airway, administer IV antibiotics, and obtain an emergent ENT consult. **Ludwig angina** is a potentially life-threatening cellulitis of the connective tissue of the floor of the mouth and neck that **begins in the submandibular space** and is **commonly caused by an infected or recently extracted tooth**. Typically, it is a **polymicrobial** infection involving aerobic and anaerobic bacteria of the mouth. The most common physical findings are bilateral submandibular swelling and tongue protrusion or elevation. A tense edema and brawny induration of the neck above the hyoid may be present and is described as a **"bull neck."** Marked tenderness to palpation of the neck and subcutaneous emphysema may be noted. Trismus and fever are often present but usually no palpable fluctuance or cervical lymphadenopathy. The involved teeth may be tender to palpation. Appropriate regimens include high-dose penicillin with metronidazole, or cefoxitin used alone. Clindamycin, ticarcillin-clavulanate, piperacillin-tazobactam, or ampicillin-sulbactam may also be used. Oral antibiotics are not adequate. Importantly, this is considered an **unstable airway** regardless of the initial examination and the patient **should never**

be left alone because airway impairment can suddenly occur. Signs of impending airway compromise include stridor, tachypnea, dyspnea, drooling, and agitation. Patients should be seated in an upright position to increase airway diameter and aid with airway protection. Of note, the upper airway may be severely distorted making endotracheal intubation difficult or impossible. Cricothyrotomy may also be difficult due to the swelling and increases the risk of spreading infection into the mediastinum. Therefore, **fiberoptic nasotracheal intubation** is preferred.

This is a clinical diagnosis. Soft tissue radiographs **(a)** and CT scans **(c and d)** of the neck confirm the diagnosis by demonstrating edema of the affected area, airway narrowing, and gas collections. However, imaging must *not delay treatment*, compromise the patient's ability to protect their airway (ie, by lying supine for CT scan), or place the patient in an area where emergent airway management is difficult (eg, radiology suite). Therefore, these studies should be delayed until the airway is stabilized. Prior to broad-spectrum antibiotics, incision and drainage **(b)** was the treatment of choice. Today, surgery is used only for those patients who fail to respond to antibiotic therapy or those with purulent collections. In these rare cases, surgery, including incision and drainage, followed by excision of facial planes, would best be performed in an OR, not at the bedside. Additionally, cultures are often of little utility given the polymicrobial nature of the infection.

172. The answer is a. The patient has a **modified Centor** score of 4 (history of fever, tender adenopathy, no cough, exudates, age 15-45 years) (see following figure). The Centor criteria are used for predicting streptococcal pharyngitis and whether or not to treat the patient with antibiotics. Because of his high score, it is likely that the patient has group A β-hemolytic streptococcal infection and that he should receive **empiric antibiotics**. In addition, he should be treated symptomatically with fluids, topical anesthetics, and acetaminophen or ibuprofen.

Patients with a Centor criterion of 2 or 3 should have a rapid antigen test and a throat culture performed. If the rapid antigen test is negative, a confirmatory throat culture may be sent **(b)**, but antibiotics **(c)** should not be initiated. If the rapid antigen test is positive, patients should be treated with an antibiotic **(d)**. A patient with many predictive signs and symptoms should be treated with antibiotics rather than discharged **(e)**.

Centor criteria	Points
Presence of tonsillar exudates	+1
Tender anterior cervical adenopathy	+1
Fever by history	+1
Absence of cough	+1
Age <15 years	+1
Age >45 years	−1

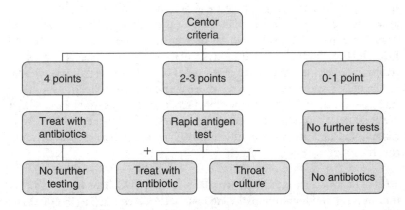

173. The answer is a. The patient's presentation is typical for a **peritonsillar abscess**. Signs and symptoms include a sore throat, muffled voice, trismus, fluctuant mass, deviation of the uvula, odynophagia, and drooling. Many of these patients have a history of being recently treated for strep throat. The abscess is **usually unilateral** and in the **superior pole of the tonsil**. Airway patency must be assessed because of the obstructing potential of an abscess. As with most abscesses, **drainage** (through needle aspiration or incision and drainage) is the most important factor in treating these patients. However, **antibiotics** are useful adjunctive medications and should be prescribed.

The abscess will not resolve without an attempt at drainage. Antibiotics and pain control alone **(b)** are not sufficient. Incision and drainage of the abscess may be performed in the OR (c) if the abscess is large, complicated, or the patient's airway shows signs of compromise. However, this is not necessary in the patient described. Drainage of the abscess is the most important factor in treating these patients. Antibiotics alone (d) are not sufficient. A CT scan (e) may aid in the diagnosis of a peritonsillar abscess in patients with severe trismus. In this patient, it would be an unnecessary radiation as he could be examined adequately.

174. The answer is c. Epiglottitis is a life-threatening inflammatory condition, usually infectious, of the epiglottis and the aryepiglottic and periglottic folds. Because most children are immunized against *Haemophilus influenzae* type B (Hib), **most cases of epiglottitis are now seen in adults**, with an average age of 46 years. Signs and symptoms include a prodromal period of 1 to 2 days consisting of constitutional symptoms, and then the patient exhibits high fever, dysphagia, odynophagia, drooling, inspiratory stridor, and dyspnea. The **"thumbprint sign,"** as seen in on this patient's lateral cervical radiograph, demonstrates a swollen epiglottis obliterating the vallecula.

Retropharyngeal abscess (a) can present with similar signs and symptoms as epiglottitis. Cervical lymphadenopathy is prominent and inflammation may be so severe that patients develop an inflammatory torticollis, causing the patient to rotate the head toward the affected side. Soft tissue cervical radiograph may demonstrate excess prevertebral swelling. Treatment is IV hydration and antibiotics, which should be started in the ED, and drainage in the OR. Peritonsillar abscess (b) presents with a unilaterally swollen and erythematous tonsil and uvula deviation toward the unaffected side. It is most common during the second and third decades of life. CT scan or ultrasound easily makes the diagnosis, but aspiration of purulent material is sufficient for diagnosis. Treatment is incision and drainage or needle aspiration, followed by high-dose penicillin or clindamycin. Pharyngitis (d) is an infection of the pharynx and tonsils that occur in adults, but has a peak incidence in children aged 4 to 7 years. The etiology is most often viral. *S. pyogenes* (group A β-hemolytic strep) is the most common cause of bacterial pharyngitis (5% to 15%) in adults. Patients present with erythematous tonsils, tonsillar exudates, and enlarged and tender anterior cervical lymph nodes. Laryngotracheitis, or croup, (e) presents with stridor but lacks the other oropharyngeal findings and is generally seen in children aged 6 months to 3 years.

175. The answer is e. Symptoms of **endocarditis** are nonspecific and vary widely, but the most common include fever (85%) and malaise (80%). In IVDU, fever is present 98% of the time. Other symptoms include weakness, myalgias, dyspnea, chest pain, cough, headache, and anorexia. Neurologic signs and symptoms (eg, confusion, personality changes, decreased level of consciousness, and focal motor deficits) are seen in 30% to 40% of patients. Vasculitic lesions, including petechiae, splinter hemorrhages, tender fingertip nodules (Osler nodes), and nontender palmar plaques (Janeway lesions), are seen in 35% of patients. Splenomegaly, new heart murmur, and retinal hemorrhages may also be detected on physical examination. Risk factors for infective endocarditis include rheumatic or congenital heart disease, calcific degenerative valve disease, prosthetic heart valve, mitral valve prolapse, a history of IV drug use, or a history of endocarditis. Although any valve can be affected, IV drug use is the most common cause of right-sided endocarditis. The recurrence rate in these patients is 41%, significantly higher than the rate of less than 20% in non-IV DU.

Disseminated gonorrhea **(a)** often presents with the arthritis-dermatitis syndrome of fevers/chills, arthralgias, a rash, and tenosynovitis. One would not expect splenomegaly or vasculitic lesions. Myocarditis **(b)** is often infectious and results from inflammatory damage to the myocardium and presents with flu-like complaints, including fever, fatigue, and myalgias. Tachycardia out of proportion to the patient's temperature or clinical picture may be present, but vasculitic lesions are not expected. Bacteria and Enteroviruses, especially Coxsackie B virus and adenovirus, predominate as causative agents in the United States while Chagas disease is the leading cause, worldwide. Pericarditis **(c)** is caused by inflammation of the pericardial sac. The etiology is broad, including infection, trauma, metabolic diseases (ie, uremia), medications, systemic autoimmune diseases, and most often the cause is idiopathic. The diagnosis of infectious mononucleosis **(d)**, a syndrome caused by the Epstein-Barr virus, is often made based on the triad of fever and chills, pharyngitis, and tender cervical lymphadenopathy.

176. The answer is e. Transesophageal echocardiogram is the **most sensitive test** to diagnose vegetations on the valves, especially the mitral valve. This is one of the most essential tests for making the diagnosis of endocarditis.

Transthoracic echocardiogram **(a)** can be used to diagnose vegetations; however, this is less sensitive test and transesophageal echocardiogram is considered the gold standard for this reason. CT angiography of the chest (b) is highly sensitive for vascular pathology such as aortic dissection; however, it is not sensitive for valvular vegetations characteristic of endocarditis. CXR (c) would potentially show septic emboli; however, it is not sensitive for valvular vegetations and cannot aid in definitively diagnosing endocarditis. VQ scan (d) is a second-line test for pulmonary embolism and is not useful in diagnosing endocarditis.

177. The answer is d. Necrotizing otitis externa is an uncommon complication of otitis externa that occurs primarily in adult **diabetics** and other **immunocompromised** individuals. It is primarily caused by a very aggressive *P. aeruginosa* infection and is associated with a **high mortality rate**. The infection typically starts in the external ear canal and then progresses through the tissues into the bony junction of the external auditory meatus, base of the skull, and adjacent soft tissues. Thus, the condition is actually better described as an osteitis of the bone of the external auditory canal. It is distinguished by fever, intense ear pain, erythema, edema, and granulation tissue in the external canal. CN palsies (CN VII, IX, X, and XI) and trismus can also occur. These patients require **hospitalization and treatment with broad-spectrum, antipseudomonal IV antibiotics**. Patients also require emergent ENT consultation for possible surgical debridement.

Malignant otitis externa is rare in immunocompetent adults (a). Patients are usually diabetics, debilitated, or immunocompromised. Owing to its high morbidity and mortality, this condition requires in-patient management with IV antibiotics (b). Although hearing loss (e) is a possibility, the most common CN involved is the facial nerve (CN VII), but CNs IX, X, and XI can also be involved (c).

178. The answer is c. **Lyme's disease** is the most common vector-borne disease in the United States and is particularly prevalent in the Northeast and upper Midwest during the late spring and early summer. It is caused by the spirochete *B. burgdorferi* that is spread through the bite of the *Ixodes* tick. Lyme's disease has three stages—early localized, early disseminated, and late. It typically begins with a **target rash** [known as **erythema migrans (EM)**] and associated flu-like symptoms. EM is the most characteristic clinical manifestation of Lyme's disease and is recognized in 90% or more of patients. However, if untreated, neurologic, joint, or cardiac symptoms develop weeks to months later. These are followed by chronic arthritic and neurologic abnormalities weeks to years later. Recommended treatment for early Lyme's disease includes doxycycline, amoxicillin (for children < 8 years or for pregnant or lactating women), or cefuroxime for a period of 3 weeks. The same drugs can be used for the second stage of disease, but their course of therapy needs to be longer. Neurologic disease requires long-term IV antibiotics.

Unfortunately, routine laboratory studies are nonspecific and nondiagnostic. This patient has early localized Lyme's disease, and should be treated empirically based on the presence of the rash. Serologic testing may be positive weeks after inoculation, but a biopsy of the rash (a) would neither be necessary nor informative. Although the patient presents with an erythematous rash surrounding a purported bug bite, the classic appearance indicates EM and treatment for cellulitis with cephalexin (b) is inappropriate. It would also be inappropriate to mistake this for an urticarial rash and thus treat the patient with prednisone and diphenhydramine for a cutaneous allergic reaction (d). Confirmatory serologic testing should be performed (e), but empiric treatment based on the presumptive diagnosis should not be delayed.

179. The answer is a. Lyme's disease has three distinct phases—the early localized phase, the early disseminated phase, and the late disseminated phase. **Second- or third-degree AV blocks** are part of the **early disseminated phase** of Lyme's disease. This phase can also be characterized by meningitis and diffuse rash of erythema chronicum migrans. The early disseminated phase occurs several days to weeks after initial infection. It is most often noted approximately 1 to 6 weeks after the initial rash. Approximately 10% to 15% of patients will progress to have the serious complications of Lyme's disease mentioned previously during the early disseminated phase. Patients who progress to having second- or third-degree AV block can have pauses or such profound bradycardia that, in rare cases, they can suffer a cardiac arrest and death.

The other answer choices (**b, c, d, and e**) are not complications associated with Lyme's disease.

180. The answer is d. SBP is a common complication of cirrhotic ascites and should be suspected in all patients with a history of cirrhosis who present with fever, abdominal pain or tenderness, worsening ascites, or encephalopathy. **Paracentesis** should be performed to confirm the diagnosis. Ascitic fluid should be tested for glucose, total protein, lactate dehydrogenase (LDH), Gram stain, WBC count, and sent for culture. **Total WBC count greater than 1000/μL or neutrophil count greater than 250/μL is**

diagnostic for SBP. Gram-negative **Enterobacteriaceae** (such as *Escherichia coli* and *Klebsiella*) account for up to 65% of all cases. Empiric treatment for suspected SBP includes third-generation cephalosporins, ticarcillin-clavulanic acid, piperacillin-tazobactam, or ampicillin-sulbactam.

Other causes of SBP include *S. pneumoniae* and *S. viridans* (15%), enterococci (6% to 10%), and anaerobes (1%) (**a, b, c, and e**).

181. The answer is e. Bacterial tracheitis will typically present with findings similar to both croup and epiglottitis. The patient will usually present with a history of **2 to 3 days of barking cough** and potentially with stridor with activity but without significant fever. The patient will **then become toxic in** appearance **with a high fever and drooling**, characteristic of epiglottitis. Thus, bacterial tracheitis has features of both croup and epiglottitis at different phases of the disease process and that is the clue to make this diagnosis. Patients with bacterial tracheitis will also often have an inspiratory and expiratory stridor as well as a productive cough.

Croup (**a**) presents with barking cough and potentially with stridor (at rest if severe). The patient may be febrile, but is usually nontoxic in appearance (as opposed to the patient in the question who now acutely appears toxic). Retropharyngeal abscess (**b**) is often seen in young children (< 2 years of age) and presents with the child sitting up and forward, drooling, and toxic in appearance. There is usually not a prodrome of barking cough or other viral symptoms. Peritonsillar abscess (**c**) often presents with sore throat, muffled voice, trismus, and fever. There is significant peritonsillar swelling with uvula deviation. Epiglottitis (**d**) often presents with stridor, toxic-appearance, drooling, and high fever. There is usually not a prodrome of barking cough or other viral symptoms.

182. The answer is d. A febrile neonate is a child 28 days and younger who presents with a fever. These neonates are at very high risk of serious bacterial infections including UTI, pneumonia, meningitis, and bacteremia. These neonates, therefore, need to receive a **fluid bolus at 20 cc/kg and broad-spectrum antibiotics** to cover for the most common pathogens in this age group (discussed later). The workup must also include **blood and urine cultures** and an **LP** in order to obtain CSF for culture. These patients then need to be admitted to the hospital for IV antibiotics and observation until cultures have returned.

The other answer choices are incorrect for various reasons. Choice (**a**) does not include blood, urine, or CSF cultures. Choice (**b**) does not include urine or CSF culture and involves discharging the patient home. Choice **(c)** does not include the LP with CSF culture. Choice **(d)** does not include LP and CSF culture and involves discharging the patient home.

183. The answer is c. The **appropriate antibiotics to use in neonates** with fever to cover for the bacteria of concern (*L. monocytogenes*, group B *Streptococcus*, and *E. coli*) are **ampicillin** and **cefotaxime**.

Choices **(a)** and **(e)** include ceftriaxone. Ceftriaxone is typically not utilized in the neonatal period due to hepatic and biliary immaturity, leading to biliary sludging and increased risk of kernicterus. There is also a very high risk of precipitation of this drug if used with other calcium-containing drugs or supplements in this age group. Choice **(b)** includes doxycycline, which is not used in children under the age of 8 due to risk of discoloration of the teeth (yellow, gray). It is also useful to treat atypical organisms, but not those organisms that commonly cause serious bacterial infections in the neonate. Choice **(d)** is the typical combination used to treat sepsis in adults as opposed to neonates.

184. The answer is a. The Jones Criteria are used to diagnose rheumatic fever. There are required criteria, major criteria, and minor criteria. You must have **EITHER**:

- **One required criteria, two major criteria, and zero minor criteria**

  OR
- **One required criteria, one major criteria, and two minor criteria**

The *required criteria* is evidence of antecedent Strep infection by positive ASO titer, positive Strep group A throat culture or rapid antigen testing, or recent scarlet fever.

The *major criteria* include the following:

- Carditis
- Polyarthritis
- Chorea
- Erythema marginatum
- Subcutaneous nodules

The *minor criteria* include the following:

- Fever
- Arthralgia
- Previous rheumatic fever or rheumatic heart disease
- Elevated ESR, CRP, or WBC
- Prolonged PR interval

Choice (a) includes the required criteria of positive ASO titer, one major criteria (chorea), and two minor criteria (fever and/or elevated ESR).

Choices (b, c, d) include one required criteria, one major criteria, and one minor criteria. Choice (e) includes one required criteria and three minor criteria.

185. The answer is a. With a urinalysis supporting a UTI along with systemic symptoms including fever and CVA tenderness, the patient's presentation is consistent with **pyelonephritis**. Since she is otherwise young, healthy, able to tolerate oral intake, and does not have signs of severe infection such as hypotension or altered mental status, she may be discharged home with appropriate outpatient antibiotic treatment, such as trimethoprim/sulfamethoxazole.

Imaging to evaluate for renal abscess, infected ureteral stone, or emphysematous pyelonephritis is indicated if the patient is severely ill, has a known urinary tract obstruction, or does not appropriately respond to initial therapy (b). As mentioned above, the patient's flank pain and fever are more consistent with pyelonephritis than cystitis. Further, nitrofurantoin does not have adequate renal penetration to treat pyelonephritis (c). As mentioned above, as this patient is otherwise young, healthy, able to tolerate oral intake, and is not severely systemically ill, she does not require admission for treatment of pyelonephritis (d). Although PID should be considered in sexually active women complaining of abdominal pain, lack of vaginal discharge, CMT, and the location of her abdominal pain and tenderness to the right flank make PID a less likely diagnosis (e).

186. The answer is b. This patient has a history of depression and is on a **selective-serotonin reuptake inhibitor (SSRI)**, escitalopram. **Dextromethorphan** is commonly used in many OTC URI medications and can precipitate serotonin syndrome in patients taking SSRIs. **Serotonin syndrome** is the cause of this patient's clinical presentation, and is characterized by fever, altered mental status, muscle rigidity, hyperreflexia, and clonus. Benzodiazepines such as **lorazepam** are typically utilized in the treatment of agitation associated with serotonin syndrome.

Fluid resuscitation and broad-spectrum antibiotics are appropriate for sepsis, but are not indicated in the management of serotonin syndrome (a). This patient's fever and tachycardia is most likely related to serotonin syndrome in the setting of the neurologic findings on her physical exam and known escitalopram use with dextromethorphan. There is no role for acetaminophen (**d**) or ibuprofen (**c**) or other antipyretics in the treatment of hyperthermia associated with serotonin syndrome. Dantrolene (e) is used in the treatment of severe neuroleptic malignant syndrome (NMS) and malignant hyperthermia. NMS is related to the use of antipsychotic medications and is not related to SSRI use. This patient does not have known antipsychotic use. Malignant hyperthermia is a rare condition triggered by the use of inhaled anesthetics and paralytics such as succinylcholine in susceptible individuals who have a particular genetic defect. This patient has not received any inhaled anesthetics or paralytics.

187. The answer is d. This patient is presenting with signs and symptoms concerning for **bacterial meningitis**. Given that he is a college student living in a dorm and has a petechial rash, *N. meningitidis* (meningococcal meningitis) is the most likely cause. A focal neurologic deficit, such as an asymmetric smile in a patient with signs and symptoms of meningitis should prompt a **CT of the head without contrast** before performing a LP (**b**). CT is indicated for patients such as this in whom there is a concern for increased intracranial pressure. This CT will also help rule out other causes of altered mental status and focal neurologic deficits, such as an intracranial hemorrhage or mass. Other indications for performing a CT of the head before an LP include altered mental status or deteriorating level of consciousness, new seizure, papilledema, immunocompromised state, malignancy, history of focal CNS disease (eg, stroke, tumor), concern for mass CNS lesion, and age greater than 60 years. An LP in a patient with increased intracranial pressure carries a theoretical risk of brain herniation.

As with all patients in the ED, the ABCs must always be assessed first. Although this patient is fatigued, he can participate in the exam and answer questions appropriately. Therefore, he does not require intubation at this time (**a**). Neurology consults are appropriate in patients with new-onset seizures; however, this patient's seizure is most likely related to his infection. Therefore, a neurology consult (**c**) does not need to be obtained immediately. The most common neurological manifestation of the second stage of Lyme's disease is a unilateral or bilateral facial nerve palsy. However, this patient's overall history, rapid onset of symptoms, high fever, and meningeal signs point more toward a diagnosis of a bacterial meningitis than Lyme's disease (**e**).

188. The answer is d. Chemoprophylaxis is recommended for **close contacts** of patients diagnosed with *N. meningitidis*. This includes housemates, those exposed to secretions (through kissing, etc.), and providers who intubated patients without a facemask. Recommended medications include oral **rifampin** for four doses, a single dose of oral **ciprofloxacin**, or a single dose of IM **ceftriaxone**.

Amoxicillin is not among the recommended antibiotics for close-contact prophylaxis for meningococcal meningitis (**e**). Admission for an asymptomatic person to monitor for the onset of symptoms (**a**) would not be indicated or appropriate. Although things such as cleaning their dorm room (**b**) and monitoring for symptoms are reasonable actions (**c**), chemoprophylaxis would be the most appropriate recommendation as it has been shown to decrease the rate of transmission of *N. meningitidis* by 89% in close contacts.

189. The answer is b. A CD4+ T-cell count less than 200 cells/mm^3 puts a patient with HIV at risk for opportunistic infections and is also a diagnostic criterion for AIDS. This patient's presentation and CXR are most consistent with a diagnosis of pneumocystis pneumonia caused by *P. jirovecii pneumonia (PCP)*. PCP is often the opportunistic infection that leads to a diagnosis of AIDS and about 70% of patients with HIV will develop this infection during the course of their disease. Although diffuse interstitial infiltrates are often described as a **"bat wing" pattern** are typical, normal radiographic findings can exist in 15% to 25% of patients. Initial treatment is with **trimethoprim-sulfamethoxazole**. Oral **prednisone** should be added if there is partial pressure of arterial oxygenation less than 70 mm Hg or alveolar-arterial gradient less than 35 mm Hg.

Although bacteria are still the most common causes of respiratory infections in patients with AIDS, the insidious onset of the patient's symptoms, CXR findings, and previously diagnosed opportunistic infections and low CD4+ count make PCP more likely. *S. pneumoniae* (**d**) usually causes a lobar infiltrate on CXR. CXR findings in *S. aureus* (**c**) pneumonia include multilobar consolidation, cavitation, pneumatoceles, and possibly pneumothorax. *Mycoplasma pneumoniae* (e) is a common cause of atypical pneumonia and may have similar CXR findings to PCP. However, it is often associated with upper respiratory tract symptoms. Influenza (a) can cause a viral pneumonia; however, it is also commonly associated with upper respiratory tract symptoms. Influenza is also unlikely to progress slowly over a period of weeks such as PCP.

190. The answer is a. Diverticulitis is inflammation of small herniations of the colon known as diverticula. The most common bacterial pathogens are anaerobes such as *Bacteroides, Peptostreptococcus,* and *Clostridium* as well as gram-negative bacteria such as *E. coli.* Uncomplicated diverticulitis accounts for approximately 75% of the cases and is managed in the outpatient setting, often with oral antibiotics. Complicated diverticulitis includes translocation of the bacteria, microperforation, and **abscess** or phlegmon formation. These patients generally require **admission** for treatment tailored to their specific complication including IV antibiotics and possible drainage.

Ischemic colitis (b) can present with similar pain to diverticulitis, however, this patient's fever, leukocytosis, and lack of risk factors for bowel ischemia make this less likely. Risk factors for bowel ischemia include hypercoagulable states, strenuous exercise, and poor perfusion of the colon caused by systemic illness such as shock. Although Crohn's disease (c) can cause abdominal abscesses, this patient has no history of Crohn's disease. Crohn's disease classically presents by the time patient is in their 20s to 30s and therefore this patient would be expected to already have a known diagnosis. Appendicitis (d) can also be complicated by abscess formation; however, the appendix is located near the cecum on the right side of the colon. *C. difficile* infection (e) can lead to perforation of the colon, but it is unlikely in this patient as she has no risk factors such as recent hospitalization, antibiotic use, or recent bowel surgery. *C. difficile* infection is also associated with diarrhea as opposed to the constipation that this patient is experiencing.

Recommended Readings

Anderson E, French S, Maloney G. Chapter 65. Community-acquired pneumonia, aspiration pneumonia, and non-infectious pulmonary infiltrates. In: Tintinalli JE, Ma OJ, Yealy DM, et al, eds. *Tintinalli's Emergency Medicine: A Comprehensive Study Guide.* 9th ed. New York, NY: McGraw-Hill, 2019.

Askew K. Chapter 91. Urinary tract infections and hematuria. In: Tintinalli JE, Ma OJ, Yealy DM, et al, eds. *Tintinalli's Emergency Medicine: A Comprehensive Study Guide.* 9th ed. New York, NY: McGraw-Hill, 2019.

Brady WJ, Pandit AK, Sochor MR. Chapter 249. Generalized skin disorders. In: Tintinalli JE, Ma OJ, Yealy DM, et al, eds. *Tintinalli's Emergency Medicine: A Comprehensive Study Guide.* 9th ed. New York, NY: McGraw-Hill, 2019.

Kelly EW. Chapter 152. Toxic shock syndromes. In: Tintinalli JE, Ma OJ, Yealy DM, et al, eds. *Tintinalli's Emergency Medicine: A Comprehensive Study Guide.* 9th ed. New York, NY: McGraw-Hill, 2019.

Kitch BB, Meredith JT. Chapter 161. Zoonotic infections. In: Tintinalli JE, Ma OJ, Yealy DM, et al, eds. *Tintinalli's Emergency Medicine: A Comprehensive Study Guide.* 9th ed. New York, NY: McGraw-Hill, 2019.

Marco CA, Balhara KS, Rothman R. Chapter 155. Human immunodeficiency virus infection. In: Tintinalli JE, Ma OJ, Yealy DM, et al, eds. *Tintinalli's Emergency Medicine: A Comprehensive Study Guide.* 9th ed. New York, NY: McGraw-Hill, 2019.

Mouncey PR, Osborn TM, Power GS, et al. Trial of early, goal-directed resuscitation for septicshock. *New Engl J Med.* 2015;372:1301-1311.

PROCESS Investigators, Yealy DM, Kellum JA, et al. A randomized trial of protocol-based carefor early septic shock. *New Engl J Med.* 2014;370(18):1683-1693.

Puskarich MA, Jones AE. Chapter 151. Sepsis. In: Tintinalli JE, Ma OJ, Yealy DM, et al, eds. *Tintinalli's Emergency Medicine: A Comprehensive Study Guide.* 9th ed. New York, NY: McGraw-Hill, 2019.

Rodriguez DM, Nesiama JO, Wang VJ. Chapter 119. Fever and serious bacterial illness in infants and children. In: Tintinalli JE, Ma OJ, Yealy DM, et al, eds. *Tintinalli's Emergency Medicine: A Comprehensive Study Guide.* 9th ed. New York, NY: McGraw-Hill, 2019.

Surviving Sepsis Campaign. Available at: http://www.survivingsepsis.org/Pages/default.aspx. Accessed March 30, 2020.

Tanski M, Ma OJ. Chapter 174. Central nervous system and spinal infections. In: Tintinalli JE, Ma OJ, Yealy DM, et al, eds. *Tintinalli's Emergency Medicine: A Comprehensive Study Guide.* 9th ed. New York, NY: McGraw-Hill, 2019.

Poisoning and Overdose

Bram A. Dolcourt, MD

Questions

The following scenario applies to questions 191-193.

You are on duty in the emergency department (ED) when you are notified that an explosion and mass casualty event has occurred. The first patient, an approximately 30-year-old man, arrives poorly responsive and confused. He is sweating profusely and vomiting, with an episode of diarrhea. Vital signs include a blood pressure of 170/90 mm Hg, respiratory rate (RR) of 22 breaths/minute, heart rate (HR) of 55 beats/minute, temperature 37.0°C, and pulse oximetry 93% on room air. He requires frequent suctioning of his airway. His pupils are pinpoint and he has prominent rales on lung exam.

191. After you clear and control the patient's airway, what is the most appropriate initial pharmacologic therapy?

a. Atropine
b. Flumazenil
c. Methylene blue
d. Naloxone
e. Sodium bicarbonate

192. In the setting of this exposure, which agent should be avoided due to its metabolism and mechanism of action?

a. Diazepam
b. Levetiracetam
c. N-acetylcysteine (NAC)
d. Rocuronium
e. Succinylcholine

193. Once the patient's initial symptoms have been treated, what is the recommended treatment to try to reverse the effects of this exposure?

a. Hemodialysis
b. High-dose insulin
c. Intravenous (IV) fat emulsion
d. Physostigmine
e. Pralidoxime (2-PAM)

194. A 19-year-old man is brought to the ED by emergency medical services (EMS) after he was found lying on the floor at a dance club. EMS states that the patient seemed unconscious at the dance club, but as soon as they transferred him onto the gurney, he became combative. Upon arrival in the ED, his BP is 120/65 mm Hg, HR is 75 beats/minute, RR is 12 breaths/minute, temperature is 98.9°F, and oxygen saturation is 98% on room air. On physical examination, his pupils are midsized, equal, and reactive to light. His skin is warm and dry. Lung, cardiac, and abdominal examinations are unremarkable. As you walk away from the bedside, you hear the monitor alarm signaling zero respirations and the oxygen saturation starts to drop. You perform a sternal rub and the patient sits up in bed and starts yelling at you. As you leave him for the second time, you hear the monitor alarm again signal zero respirations. You administer naloxone, but there is no change in his condition. Which of the following substances did the patient most likely ingest?

a. γ-Hydroxybutyrate (GHB)
b. Diazepam
c. Cocaine
d. Phencyclidine (PCP)
e. Heroin

195. A 43-year-old woman presents to the ED with a 3-week history of intermittent headache, nausea, and fatigue. She was seen at her private doctor's office 1 week ago along with her husband and children, who also have similar symptoms. They were diagnosed with a viral syndrome and told to increase their fluid intake. She states that the symptoms began approximately when it started to get cold outside. The symptoms are worse in the morning and improve while she is at work. Her BP is 123/75 mm Hg, HR is 83 beats/minute, temperature is 98.9°F, and oxygen saturation is 98% on room air. Physical examination is unremarkable. You suspect her first diagnosis was incorrect. Which of the following is the most appropriate next step to confirm your suspicion?

a. Order a Mono spot test
b. Perform a nasal pharyngeal swab to test for influenza
c. Consult psychiatry to evaluate for malingering
d. Order a carboxyhemoglobin (COHb) level
e. Order a lead level

196. An 18-year-old woman is brought to the ED by her mother. Her mother thinks she tried to commit suicide. The patient admits to ingesting a few handfuls of acetaminophen (APAP) approximately 3 hours ago. Her BP is 105/70 mm Hg, HR is 92 beats/minute, RR is 17 breaths/minute, temperature is 99.1°F, and oxygen saturation is 99% on room air. She is diaphoretic and vomiting. She is mildly tender in her right upper quadrant, but there is no rebound or guarding. Bowel sounds are normoactive. She is alert and oriented and has no focal deficits on neurologic examination. You administer 50 g of activated charcoal. At this point, she appears well and has no complaints. Her serum APAP concentration 4 hours after the reported time of ingestion is 350 mg/mL. You plot the level on the nomogram seen in the figure. Which of the following is the most appropriate next step in management?

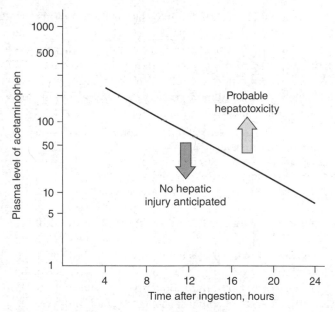

(Reproduced, with permission, from Brunton LL, et al. Goodman and Gilman's The Pharmacological Basis Therapeutics. New York, NY: McGraw Hill, 2006, 694.)

a. Discharge home with instructions to return if symptoms worsen
b. Observe for 6 hours and if the patient remains asymptomatic, discharge her home
c. Repeat the APAP level 4 hours after the patient arrived in the ED and treat only if this level is above the line
d. Admit to the psychiatry unit and keep on suicide watch while performing serial abdominal examinations
e. Begin NAC and admit to the hospital

197. A 47-year-old man is brought to the ED by EMS after being found wandering in the street mumbling. His BP is 150/75 mm Hg, HR is 110 beats/minute, RR is 16 breaths/minute, temperature is 100.5°F, oxygen saturation is 99% on room air, and point-of-care glucose is 98 mg/dL. On examination, the patient is confused with mumbling speech. His pupils are dilated and face is flushed. His mucous membranes and skin are dry. Which of the following toxic syndromes is this patient exhibiting?

a. Sympathomimetic syndrome
b. Anticholinergic syndrome
c. Cholinergic syndrome
d. Opioid intoxication
e. Ethanol intoxication

198. A 25-year-old man is carried into the ED by two of his friends who state that he is not breathing. The patient has a history of heroin abuse. His vital signs are BP 115/70 mm Hg, HR 99 beats/minute, RR 3 breaths/minute, temperature 98.9°F, and oxygen saturation 87% on room air. You notice fresh needle marks and miotic pupils. You begin bag-valve-mask ventilation and his oxygen saturation increases to 99%. Which of the following is the most appropriate next step in management?

a. Continue bag-valve-mask ventilation until he breathes on his own
b. Perform endotracheal intubation of the patient
c. Evaluate response to administration of naloxone
d. Put the patient on supplemental oxygen
e. Place a nasogastric tube and administer activated charcoal

The following scenario applies to questions 199 and 200.

199. A 42-year-old man who is actively seizing is brought to the ED by EMS after a massive ingestion of an unknown substance. The man is known to have a history of acquired immunodeficiency syndrome (AIDS). An IV line is established and anticonvulsant therapy is administered. After high doses of diazepam, phenobarbital, and phenytoin, it is determined that the seizures are refractory to standard anticonvulsant therapy. Which of the following substances did this patient most likely ingest?

a. Cocaine
b. Diphenhydramine
c. Amitriptyline
d. Haloperidol
e. Isoniazid (INH)

200. Which of the following additional treatments should be given to control this patient's seizures?

a. Doxylamine
b. Folinic acid
c. Levetiracetam
d. Ketamine
e. Pyridoxine

201. A 60-year-old woman with a history of diabetes is brought into the ED by EMS workers who state that the patient was found on a bus in a lethargic and diaphoretic condition. Her point-of-care glucose level at the scene was 35 mg/dL. EMS workers quickly administered dextrose through an IV line. The patient became alert and responsive, stating that she just took her normal medication. Her blood sugar went up to 110 mg/dL and she remained this way throughout her trip to the ED. However, in the ED you notice that the patient is again diaphoretic and is mumbling her speech. Her point-of-care glucose is now 47 mg/dL. You administer dextrose and she improves. Which of the following diabetes medications commonly causes hypoglycemia for which the patient is likely to require hospital admission?

a. Regular insulin
b. Metformin
c. Glyburide
d. Sitagliptin
e. Acarbose

202. A 23-year-old woman presents to the ED complaining of abdominal pain, nausea, and vomiting. She has a history of depression but is not currently taking any antidepressant medications. Upon further questioning, the patient states that she ingested a bottle of pills in her medicine cabinet approximately 3 hours ago. Her BP is 115/65 mm Hg, HR is 101 beats/minute, RR is 29 breaths/minute, temperature is 100.1°F, and oxygen saturation is 100% on room air. Physical examination is unremarkable except for mild diffuse abdominal tenderness. Laboratory results reveal a white blood cell (WBC) count of 10,300/μL, hematocrit (Hct) 46%, platelets 275/μL, aspartate transaminase (AST) 70 U/L, alanine transaminase (ALT) 85 U/L, alkaline phosphatase 75 U/L, sodium 143 mEq/L, potassium 3.7 mEq/L, chloride 98 mEq/L, bicarbonate 8 mEq/L, blood urea nitrogen (BUN) 22 mg/dL, creatinine 0.9 mg/dL, and glucose 85 mg/dL. Arterial blood gas values on room air are pH 7.51, P_{CO_2} 11 mm Hg, and P_{O_2} 134 mm Hg. Which of the following substances did this patient most likely ingest?

a. Diphenhydramine
b. Ibuprofen
c. APAP
d. Aspirin
e. Pseudoephedrine

203. A 35-year-old agitated man presents to the ED in police custody. He denies any past medical history and takes no medication. He admits to using some drugs today. His BP is 195/90 mm Hg, HR is 121 beats/minute, RR is 18 breaths/minute, temperature is 100.1°F, and oxygen saturation is 99% on room air. On examination, he is diaphoretic, and has pupils that are 8 mm in diameter, along with 3+ patella reflexes bilaterally. Electrocardiogram (ECG) reveals sinus tachycardia with a rate of 123 beats/minute. Which of the following toxic syndromes is this patient exhibiting?

a. Anticholinergic
b. Cholinergic
c. Sympathomimetic
d. Opioid
e. Sedative hypnotic

204. A 27-year-old man presents to the ED extremely agitated complaining of mild chest pain and dyspnea. He states that he was snorting cocaine all afternoon. You place him on a monitor and get his vital signs. His BP is 215/130 mm Hg, HR is 112 beats/minute, RR is 17 breaths/minute, temperature is 100.1°F, and oxygen saturation is 98% on room air. An ECG reveals sinus tachycardia at a rate of 116 beats/minute. Which of the following is the most appropriate medication to administer?

a. Haloperidol
b. Labetalol
c. Esmolol
d. Diltiazem
e. Diazepam

205. A 30-year-old man is brought to the ED by police officers. The patient is agitated, vomiting, and complaining of body aches. He states that he is withdrawing from his medication. His vital signs are BP 160/85 mm Hg, HR 107 beats/minute, RR 20 breaths/minute, and temperature 99.7°F. On examination he is diaphoretic, has rhinorrhea, piloerection, and hyperactive bowel sounds. Which of the following substances is this patient most likely withdrawing from?

a. Ethanol
b. Cocaine
c. Nicotine
d. Methadone
e. Clonidine

206. A 25-year-old man is brought into the ED by two police officers because of suspected drug use. The patient is extremely agitated and is fighting the police officers. It takes three hospital staff members and the two police officers to keep him on the stretcher. His vital signs are BP 150/80 mm Hg, HR 107 beats/minute, RR 18 breaths/minute, temperature 99.7°F, and oxygen saturation 99% on room air. Physical examination is unremarkable except for cool, diaphoretic skin, persistent vertical and horizontal nystagmus, and occasional myoclonic jerks. Which of the following is the most likely diagnosis?

a. Cocaine intoxication
b. Cocaine withdrawal
c. Anticholinergic toxidrome
d. PCP intoxication
e. Opiate withdrawal

207. A 49-year-old man presents to the ED with altered mental status. His BP is 149/75 mm Hg, HR is 93 beats/minute, RR is 18 breaths/minute, temperature is 97.5°F, and oxygen saturation is 99% on room air. Physical examination reveals an unkempt man with the odor of "alcohol" on his breath. His head is atraumatic and pupils are 4 mm, equal, and reactive. The neck is supple. Cardiovascular, pulmonary, and abdominal examinations are unremarkable. There is no extremity edema and his pulses are 2+ and symmetric. Neurologically, he withdraws all four extremities to deep stimuli. ECG is sinus rhythm. Laboratory results reveal:

Sodium 141 mEq/L	Arterial blood pH 7.26
Potassium 3.5 mEq/L	Lactate 1.7 mEq/L
Chloride 101 mEq/L	Ethanol level undetectable
Bicarbonate 14 mEq/L	Measured serum osmolarity 352 mOsm/L
BUN 15 mg/dL	Calculated serum osmolarity 292 mOsm/kg
Creatinine 0.7 mg/dL	Urinalysis: no blood, ketones, or protein
Glucose 89 mg/dL	

Which of the following statements best describes the laboratory findings?

a. Anion gap metabolic acidosis and osmolar gap
b. Anion gap metabolic acidosis without osmolar gap
c. Nonanion gap metabolic acidosis and osmolar gap
d. Nonanion gap metabolic acidosis without osmolar gap
e. Metabolic alkalosis with secondary acidosis

208. A 26-year-old woman with a history of depression is brought into the ED. She was found lying on the floor of her apartment next to an unlabeled empty pill bottle. Her BP is 95/65 mm Hg, HR is 117 beats/minute, RR is 14 breaths/minute, and oxygen saturation is 97% on 2 L nasal cannula. On examination, the patient appears obtunded, and her pupils are 3 mm and reactive. Her oropharynx is dry and there is no gag reflex to pharyngeal stimulation. Her neck is supple. The heart is tachycardic without murmurs, the lungs are clear to auscultation, and the abdomen is soft. There is normal rectal tone and brown stool that is heme negative. Her skin is cool and moist with no signs of needle tracks. Neurologically, she is unresponsive but withdraws all extremities to deep palpation. Point-of-care blood glucose is 85 mg/dL. Her ECG is below. Which of the following is the most appropriate next step in management?

a. Orotracheal intubation and IV naloxone
b. Orotracheal intubation and IV sodium bicarbonate
c. Orotracheal intubation and IV NAC
d. Orotracheal intubation and administer syrup of ipecac through orogastric tube
e. Orotracheal intubation and administer activated charcoal through orogastric tube

The following scenario applies to questions 209 and 210.

A 31-year-old man is brought to the ED by EMS after he was found lying on the floor of his garage. He is rousable in the ED, speaks with slurred speech, and vomits. His BP is 140/85 mm Hg, HR is 94 beats/minute, RR is 24 breaths/minute, temperature is 98.8°F, and oxygen saturation is 99% on room air. You place an IV line, draw blood, and start a liter of normal saline running through the line. Laboratory results reveal serum sodium 139 mEq/L, potassium 3.5 mEq/L, chloride 101 mEq/L, bicarbonate 5 mEq/L, BUN 15 mg/dL, creatinine 1 mg/dL, glucose 105 mg/dL, arterial blood pH 7.05, COHb 4%, and lactate 2.8 mEq/L. Urinalysis shows 1+ protein, trace ketones, WBC 4/hpf (high-power field), red blood cell (RBC) 2 to 3/hpf, and multiple envelope-shaped and needle-shaped crystals.

209. Which of the following conditions would best explain his metabolic acidosis?

a. Ibuprofen toxicity
b. Ethylene glycol poisoning
c. Diabetic ketoacidosis (DKA)
d. Lactic acidosis
e. Isopropyl alcohol poisoning

210. What is the most appropriate initial treatment for this condition?

a. Fomepizole
b. Hemodialysis
c. Sodium bicarbonate infusion
d. Methylene blue
e. Pyridoxine

211. A 51-year-old man presents to the ED complaining of nausea and abdominal pain after drinking some "bitter stuff." He is considered one of the "regulars" who is usually at triage with ethanol intoxication. His BP is 130/65 mm Hg, HR is 90 beats/minute, RR is 16 breaths/minute, temperature is 97.9°F, and oxygen saturation is 97% on room air. Physical examination is unremarkable, except for slurred speech and the smell of acetone on the patient's breath. Laboratory results reveal serum sodium 138 mEq/L, potassium 3.5 mEq/L, chloride 105 mEq/L, bicarbonate 23 mEq/L, BUN 10 mg/dL, creatinine 2.1 mg/dL, glucose 85 mg/dL, arterial blood pH 7.37, and lactate 1.4 mEq/L. Serum ethanol is undetectable. Serum osmolarity is measured at 330 mOsm. Urinalysis shows moderate ketones. Which of the following is the most likely diagnosis?

a. DKA
b. Promethazine intoxication
c. Methanol intoxication
d. Isopropyl alcohol intoxication
e. Ethylene glycol intoxication

212. A 55-year-old man presents to the ED 6 hours after ingesting two bottles of his baby aspirin. He complains of nausea, vomiting, dizziness, and tinnitus. His BP is 140/80 mm Hg, HR is 105 beats/minute, RR is 30 breaths/minute, temperature is 100.3°F, and oxygen saturation is 94% on room air. Arterial blood gas on room air reveals a pH of 7.52, Pco_2 10 mm Hg, and Po_2 129 mm Hg. The blood salicylate level is 90 mg/dL. While waiting for his labs, he complains worsening of shortness of breath. A chest radiograph shows pulmonary edema. Which of the following is the most definitive step in management?

a. Administer activated charcoal, begin IV hydration, and administer IV sodium bicarbonate
b. Prepare to intubate the patient for respiratory failure
c. Administer activated charcoal, begin IV hydration, and administer NAC
d. Arrange for immediate hemodialysis
e. Gastric lavage, IV hydration, and repeat levels before beginning therapy

213. A 19-year-old woman presents to the ED with abdominal pain, nausea, vomiting, diarrhea, and hematemesis after ingesting an unknown substance in a suicide attempt. Which of the following is the correctly paired toxic overdose and antidote for this clinical scenario?

a. Organophosphate overdose and physostigmine
b. Iron overdose and deferoxamine
c. Aspirin overdose and NAC
d. APAP overdose and naloxone
e. Anticholinergic overdose and fomepizole

214. You receive notification from EMS that they are bringing in a 17-year-old adolescent. A police officer snuck up on a group of three kids that he thought were using drugs. Two of kids ran away and patient fell to the ground seconds after standing up. Three plastic bags were found on the ground near where the kids were found. According to the emergency medical technician (EMT), the patient was in ventricular fibrillation on scene. He was defibrillated and is now in a sinus rhythm. The EMT also administered IV dextrose, thiamine, and naloxone without any change in mental status. Which of the following substances was the patient most likely abusing?

a. Butane
b. Ethanol
c. Heroin
d. Cocaine
e. PCP

215. A 22-year-old woman presents to the ED by ambulance from a dance club. The paramedics report that the patient was agitated in the club and had a generalized seizure. Her BP is 165/100 mm Hg, HR is 119 beats/minute, RR is 17 breaths/minute, temperature is 101.9°F, oxygen saturation is 98% on room air, and point-of-care glucose is 92 mg/dL. On examination, the patient is hyperactive and appears to be hallucinating. Her pupils are dilated to 6 mm bilaterally and reactive. Her neck is supple. Examination of the heart is unremarkable except for tachycardia. Her lungs are clear and abdomen is soft and nontender. The patient moves all four extremities. Laboratory results are as follows:

Sodium 109 mEq/L   WBC 12,000/mm³
Potassium 3.5 mEq/L   Hct 49%
Chloride 83 mEq/L   Platelets 350/µL
Bicarbonate 20 mEq/L
BUN 10 mg/dL
Creatinine 1 mg/dL
Glucose 103 mg/dL

Which of the following substances did this patient most likely consume?

a. Cocaine
b. Heroin
c. 3,4-Methylenedioxymethamphetamine (MDMA)
d. Ketamine
e. PCP

216. An asymptomatic young adult was brought to the ED by a police officer after his home was raided. The patient swallowed five small packets of an unknown substance before being arrested. His BP is 125/75 mm Hg, HR is 85 beats/minute, RR is 16 breaths/minute, and temperature is 98.7°F. Physical examination is unremarkable. An abdominal radiograph confirms intraluminal small bowel densities. Which of the following is the most appropriate treatment?

a. Magnesium citrate
b. Gastric lavage
c. Activated charcoal and polyethylene glycol
d. Syrup of ipecac
e. NAC

The following scenario applies to questions 217 and 218.

A 55-year-old farmer presents to the ED for a complaint of shortness of breath. He is mildly tachycardic and appears cyanotic. His oxygen saturation via oximeter reads at 85% on room air and does not change with the addition of supplemental oxygen. His chest X-ray appears normal. An arterial blood gas measurement shows a measured oxygen saturation of 100%.

217. Which of the following laboratory tests will provide the correct diagnosis?

a. COHb percentage
b. Cyanide concentration
c. D-dimer
d. Methemoglobin percentage
e. Aspirin concentration

218. Which of the following is the most appropriate treatment for this condition?

a. Enoxaparin
b. Hyperbaric oxygen
c. Hydroxocobalamin
d. Methylene blue
e. Sodium bicarbonate

219. Which of the following medication classes is associated with the most accidental poisoning deaths in the United States?

a. Anticoagulants
b. Antihypertensive medications
c. Hypoglycemic medications
d. Nonsteroidal anti-inflammatory drugs (NSAIDs)
e. Opioids

220. A 34-year-old man with a history of severe asthma presents to the ED with sudden onset difficulty in breathing. Vital signs include RR 36 breaths/minute, temperature 37°F, and oxygen saturation of 85% on room air. Despite aggressive treatment, he requires emergent endotracheal intubation. He is given etomidate and succinylcholine for rapid sequence induction. Shortly after intubation, he develops muscle rigidity and a temperature of 40.0°F. Which of the following is the most appropriate next step in treatment?

a. Administer bromocriptine
b. Administer dantrolene
c. Administer IV antibiotics and order a chest X-ray
d. Administer IV fluids
e. Administer physostigmine

221. A 45-year-old man presents to the ED. According to his family, he has been depressed, but recently stated he "was trying to get his life back together" and has been actively adopting healthy lifestyle habits. They witnessed him having a 1-minute seizure before arrival. He currently complains of a headache, a feeling of pins and needles in his hands and feet, and flashes of light in his eyes. Vitals signs show a BP of 160/80 mm Hg, HR of 110 beats/minute, RR of 14 breaths/min, temperature of 37.0°C, and oxygen saturation of 99% on room air. On examination, he appears to fidget and thinks the date is 2 days prior. He is noticeably diaphoretic and has fine tremor. Which of the following is the most reasonable first line for treatment?

a. Endotracheal intubation with rapid sequence induction
b. Oral chlordiazepoxide
c. IV haloperidol
d. IV phenobarbital
e. IV phenytoin

222. You are treating a 32-year-old man for a shoulder dislocation sustained during a football game. To reduce the shoulder and provide ongoing pain relief, you perform an intrascalene block. After the reduction, the patient starts to complain of a metallic taste in his mouth and the cardiac monitor shows the QRS duration has increased from 80 ms to 140 ms. You look at the bottle and realize you have 0.5% bupivacaine, rather than the 0.25% you requested. What is next most appropriate treatment?

a. Amiodarone
b. Sodium bicarbonate
c. IV phenytoin
d. IV lipid emulsion therapy
e. Hemodialysis

223. A 25-year-old man is bitten on the foot by a snake while walking around local nature park. He states the injury is painful and has become very swollen over the last hour. Vital signs show a BP of 140/70 mm Hg, pulse of 130 beats/minute, RR of 20 breaths/minute, temperature of 37.0°C, and a saturation of 100% on room air. On examination, there are two puncture wounds on the dorsal foot. There is slow, venous bleeding from the site that does not stop with pressure. The limb is markedly swollen from the site of the wound up to the knee, with tense, firm skin, and diminished sensation in the foot. Laboratory studies show hemoglobin of 13.5 gm/dL, platelet count of 6000/μL, a fibrinogen of 10 mg/dL, and international normalized ratio of 2.0. What is the next best step in treatment?

a. Apply a tourniquet above the level of the swelling to prevent the venom from spreading further
b. Attempt venom extraction with a Sawyer extractor or other similar suction device
c. Consult general surgery for fasciotomy
d. Administer polyvalent crotalid (rattlesnake) antivenin
e. Transfuse blood platelets, cryoprecipitate, and fresh frozen plasma

224. Which of the following medication combinations have the potential to result in a fatal drug-drug interaction?

a. Estrogen and rifampin
b. Ceftriaxone and ethanol
c. Amlodipine and warfarin
d. Phenelzine and meperidine
e. Valproic acid and levocarnitine

Poisoning and Overdose

Answers

191. The answer is a. The patient was exposed to an **organophosphate**. Organophosphates **inhibit acetylcholinesterase**, the enzyme responsible for the breakdown of acetylcholine. The patient is having a "cholinergic crisis." Overstimulation of muscarinic and nicotinic receptors leads to his symptoms, commonly remembered by the mnemonics **SLUDGE** [salivation, lacrimation, urination, defecation, gastrointestinal (GI) upset, emesis] or **DUMBBELS** (defecation, urination, miosis, bronchospasm, bronchorrhea, emesis, lacrimation, salivation). The initial pharmacologic treatment for organophosphate toxicity is to administer **atropine** until the patient no longer has significant secretions and the mucous membranes appear slightly dry. Atropine is an anticholinergic; therefore, it competitively inhibits the excess acetylcholine, both peripherally and in the central nervous system (CNS).

Flumazenil (**b**) is a mixed agonist/antagonist that can be used to reverse benzodiazepine effects. Due to a risk of seizures and limited benefit, it is used infrequently. Methylene blue (**c**) is used to reverse methemoglobinemia. Naloxone (**d**) is used to reverse opiate (eg, heroin) overdoses. Sodium bicarbonate (**e**) has a number of uses in overdose, but is primary used to treat the cardiac effects of tricyclic antidepressant (TCA) overdose and to enhance the elimination of aspirin through urinary alkalization.

192. The answer is e. Succinylcholine is a depolarizing neuromuscular blocker, often used in rapid sequence induction for endotracheal intubation. It is metabolized by plasma cholinesterase. **Organophosphates inhibit plasma cholinesterase and will significantly prolong the duration of action of succinylcholine.** Organophosphate exposure leads to excess acetylcholine and a depolorizing neuromuscular block in much the same fashion as succinylcholine. The use of succinylcholine can potentially worsen the toxic effects of an organophosphate and result in prolonged muscle paralysis.

Diazepam (**a**) is a benzodiazepine and is indicated, in the setting of severe organophosphate exposure, for seizure prophylaxis. Seizures in organophosphate exposure are associated with increase mortality. Diazepam is the best most studied medication for this indication. Levetiracetam (**b**) is a novel antiepileptic medication. Its use in the setting of organophosphate exposure has not been well evaluated but would not be contraindicated as an additional treatment. NAC (**c**) is used for APAP exposure and may be of use for other toxic hepatitis. While it is not indicated for organophosphate exposure, there is no contraindication to its use if there are other indications for its use. Rocuronium (**e**) is a short acting, nondepolarizing neuromuscular blocker used for rapid sequence induction. It will antagonize the acetylcholine excess seen in organophosphate toxicity. It is hepatically metabolized and metabolism should be minimally affected by organophosphate exposure.

193. The answer is e. In the United States, 2-PAM is used to regenerate acetylcholine esterase by binding to and removing a linked organophosphate molecule. Oximes used in other countries include Obidoxime and HI-6 (dimethanesulfonate).

Organophosphates are not amenable to hemodialysis (**a**). High-dose insulin (**b**) is typically used to treat the cardiovascular effects of β-blocker and calcium blocker overdose. IV fat emulsion (**c**) is used to treat local anesthetic overdose. Physostigmine (**d**) is a reversible cholinesterase inhibitor. Its effect is to increase acetylcholine in the pre- and postsynaptic junctions. This will worsen the patient's condition by exacerbating the cholinergic syndrome.

194. The answer is a. GHB is a natural neurotransmitter that induces sleep. GHB has been sold as a muscle builder (sleep increases release of growth hormone), diet aid, and a sleep aid. Patients with GHB overdose generally have a decreased level of consciousness. In contrast to other sedative/hypnotic overdoses, the level of consciousness tends to fluctuate quickly between agitation and depression. A distinctive feature of GHB intoxication is **respiratory depression with apnea, interrupted by periods of agitation and combativeness**, especially following attempts at intubation.

Diazepam (**b**), a benzodiazepine, also depresses mental and respiratory function but typically patients remain sedate. Any respiratory depression from diazepam will occur early in the ingestion. Cocaine (**c**) is a stimulant that increases HR, BP, and usually causes the pupils to dilate. PCP (**d**) intoxication may cause bizarre behavior, lethargy, agitation, confusion, or violence. Unlike GHB, this drug acts more as a stimulant than a depressant. Heroin (**e**) intoxication can cause respiratory depression. Patients usually present with miotic pupils and a decreased RR and depth.

195. The answer is d. The most useful diagnostic test in suspected **CO poisoning** is a **COHb level**. Normal levels are less than 5% in nonsmokers as CO is a natural by-product of the metabolism of porphyrins. COHb levels may be slightly more elevated in smokers and those who live in large cities. CO poisoning should be suspected when multiple patients (usually in the same family) present with flu-like symptoms, and were exposed to products of combustion (ie, home heaters/generators). The level may not be elevated if they have not been exposed recently (<12 hours). This most commonly occurs in colder, winter months. The mainstay of treatment is the delivery of oxygen. Hyperbaric oxygen is usually used for patients with COHb levels greater than 25%. The patient's house should be evaluated by the fire department or a heating and cooling specialist.

A Mono spot test **(a)** can be helpful in detecting acute mononucleosis. Without pharyngitis, lymphadenopathy and given the duration of symptoms, this choice is not likely. CO poisoning is often confused for a viral syndrome **(b)**. Patients with influenza usually present to the ED with high fever. The duration of symptoms also makes this less likely. Malingering **(c)** is the intentional production of false or exaggerated symptoms motivated by external incentives. It is unlikely to happen in entire families. Lead toxicity **(e)** is mainly a disease of children resulting from ingestion of lead-based paints. Adults can be exposed to lead in a variety of occupational circumstances, such as welders, glassmakers, and scrap metal workers. There is no classic presentation of lead toxicity. Therefore, high suspicion and a thorough history are critical. The diagnosis is made by an elevated whole-blood lead level.

196. The answer is e. APAP is one of the most commonly used analgesic-antipyretic medications and causes more hospitalizations after overdose than by any other pharmaceutical agent. It also is the **single most common drug that leads to death in overdose**. In the case of a single acute ingestion, risk of hepatotoxicity is best established by plotting the APAP concentration on the APAP nomogram. APAP concentration must be measured between 4 and 24 hours after ingestion and then plotted on the nomogram. Patients with APAP concentrations on or above the treatment line should be treated. This patient has a 4-hour APAP concentration of 350 μg/mL. According to the nomogram, at 4 hours, any concentration above 150 μg/mL (200 mg/mL outside of the United States) should be treated. Therefore, the **patient should be started on NAC** and **admitted to the hospital**. During her admission, she should be evaluated by a psychiatrist regarding her attempted suicide.

The patient is at risk for APAP toxicity and meets criteria for treatment with NAC. Without treatment with NAC, she is at risk of developing liver failure and possible death. The patient is in first phase of an APAP poisoning. This phase usually lasts 0.5 to 24 hours. Patients are usually asymptomatic or exhibit findings, such as nausea, vomiting, anorexia, malaise, and diaphoresis.

All other answer choices (**a, b, c, and d**) are incorrect.

197. The answer is b. The term **toxidrome** refers to **a constellation of physical findings** that can provide important clues in a toxic ingestion. This is particularly useful in patients who cannot provide an adequate history. The **anticholinergic syndrome** typically presents with delirium, mumbling speech, tachycardia, elevated temperature, flushed face, dry mucous membranes and skin, dilated pupils, and hypoactive bowel sounds. The anticholinergic syndrome can be remembered by the phrase **"blind as a bat (mydriasis), red as a beet (flushed skin), hot as a hare (hyperthermia secondary to lack of sweating), dry as a bone (dry mucous membranes), and mad as a hatter (mental status changes)."**

The sympathomimetic syndrome (**a**) is usually seen after ingestion of cocaine, amphetamines, or decongestants. It typically presents with delirium, paranoia, tachycardia, hypertension, hyperpyrexia, diaphoresis, mydriasis, seizures, and hyperactive bowel sounds. Sympathomimetic and anticholinergic syndromes are frequently difficult to distinguish. The main difference is that sympathomimetics usually cause diaphoresis whereas anticholinergics cause dry skin. The cholinergic syndrome (**c**) is commonly remembered by the mnemonics SLUDGE or DUMBBELS. Opioids (**d**) and ethanol (**e**) are part of the sedative-hypnotic syndrome. It typically presents with sedation, miosis, respiratory depression, hypotension, bradycardia, hypothermia, and decreased bowel sounds.

198. The answer is c. The patient presents to the ED with central nervous and respiratory depression and miotic pupils. Along with his history of heroin abuse and fresh needle marks, this is most likely a **heroin overdose**. Opioid toxicity is associated with the toxidrome of **CNS depression, respiratory depression, and miosis**. Attention is always first directed at **airway and breathing management** in emergency medicine. The first action for this patient is to provide oxygen via bag-valve-mask ventilation. Because his respiratory depression is most likely secondary to opioid overdose, an **opioid antagonist** should be administered. **Naloxone** is the antidote most frequently used to reverse opioid toxicity. The goal of naloxone therapy is not necessarily complete arousal; rather, it is to reinstitute adequate spontaneous respiration, while attempting to avoid inducing acute opioid withdrawal. The duration of action for naloxone is between 30 and 60 minutes. A patient like this may need more than one dose. If he does, consideration should be given to a naloxone drip.

Theoretically, one can continue bag-valve-mask ventilation until the effects of the drug wear off; however, this is not practical (a). If the patient overdosed on a long-acting opioid, respiratory depression can last for more than 24 hours. Similar to continued bag-valve-mask ventilation, the cause of this patient's respiratory depression is theoretically reversible with the administration of naloxone. If there is a delay to administration of naloxone or it is unsuccessful in restarting his respirations, the patient can be intubated (b). His hypoxia is a result of central respiratory depression. As breathing is composed of both oxygenation and ventilation, administration of oxygen to this patient will mask his hypoventilation (d). In an otherwise healthy patient, hypoxia will only occur with hypoventilation and should not be addressed by supplemental oxygen without either end-tidal CO_2 monitoring or checking a blood gas. Activated charcoal should not be administered in patients with CNS depression who are not intubated owing to the risk of emesis and aspiration (e).

199. The answer is e. An overdose of any of these agents can lead to seizures. However, **INH** is notorious for causing **seizures that are refractory to standard therapy**. Marked lactic acidosis and respiratory compromise may also be present. INH is used for the treatment of tuberculosis, which is seen with a greater incidence in patients with AIDS. The pathophysiology of these seizures is complex but related to decreased γ-aminobutyric acid (GABA) synthesis from pyridoxine deficiency.

All of the other substances listed as answer choices should respond to standard therapy with benzodiazepines (a, b, c, and d). There are many seizure-inducing substances that may be poorly responsive to benzodiazepines. Some of them include ipecac (a proemetic compound previously recommended for ingestions), camphor, false morel mushrooms (*Gyromitra* species), lindane (scabicide), theophylline [used for refractory chronic obstructive pulmonary disease (COPD)], and caffeine.

200. The answer is e. Pyridoxine **(vitamin B₆)** is the treatment of choice for INH overdose. Typically, 70 to 100 mg/kg, up to 5 grams, is given for refractory INH-induced seizures. Pyridoxine replacement should **return GABA synthesis to normal and allow normal activation of the GABA receptor**. Pyridoxine can cause peripheral neuropathy in overdose, so repeated, large doses should be avoided.

Doxylamine (**a**) is a common over-the-counter sleep aid and is often paired with pyridoxine for the treatment of nausea and vomiting in pregnancy. It is an antihistamine and has no roll in treatment of refractory seizures. Folinic acid (**b**) is the activated form of folic acid. It is used to treat methotrexate overdose and can be used as adjuvant treatment of methanol poisoning. Levetiracetam (**c**) and ketamine (**d**) are increasingly being used in refractory seizures; however their role in INH-induced seizures is limited.

201. The answer is c. Glyburide is a commonly prescribed **sulfonylurea**. Sulfonylureas are oral agents that stimulate the β cells of the pancreas to secrete insulin. Many of the sulfonylureas have relatively **long durations of action**. Glyburide can act up to 24 hours after ingestion. Hypoglycemia secondary to sulfonylureas generally **requires hospital admission** to monitor for **recurrent hypoglycemia**. The antidote to this toxicity is octreotide. High serum glucose levels are what stimulate the pancreas to secrete insulin; therefore, **glucose boluses are likely to lead to large releases of insulin and a subsequent hypoglycemia**.

Excess insulin (**a**) is the most common cause of hypoglycemia in patients who present to the ED. Often hypoglycemia results from the unintentional overdose of short- or intermediate-acting insulin. After correcting the initial hypoglycemia, a meal and observation are usually enough for patients to be discharged. Very large injections of insulin, such as what can occur in suicide attempts, can lead to recurrent hypoglycemia, but this was not the scenario here. Metformin (**b**), a biguanide, acts by increasing peripheral sensitivity to insulin and suppressing gluconeogenesis. Metformin should not produce hypoglycemia. Sitagliptin (**d**) is in the class of drugs known as dipeptidyl peptidase-4 inhibitors. It should not lead to hypoglycemia. Acarbose (**e**) is an α-glucosidase inhibitor that acts to decrease GI absorption of carbohydrates. It does not cause hypoglycemia.

202. The answer is d. The patient most likely ingested **aspirin**. Patients with an acute salicylate overdose may present **with nausea, vomiting, tinnitus, fever, diaphoresis, and confusion**. Salicylates are capable of producing several types of acid-base disturbances. Acute respiratory alkalosis, without hypoxia, is caused by salicylate stimulation of the respiratory center in the brainstem. The next stage of acid base disorders is a **mixed respiratory alkalosis and metabolic acidosis.** This is because of interference with the Krebs cycle, uncoupling oxidative-phosphorylation, and increased fatty acid metabolism as well as increasing amounts of exogenous acid. The next stage is a metabolic and respiratory acidosis.

The more acidotic the serum becomes, the more the equilibrium shifts toward the protonated form of the salicylate. The protonated form is more lipophilic, crosses the blood-brain barrier, and may lead to seizures. This shift may cause the serum levels to fall but heralds impending collapse. If the patient is hypoxic, salicylate-induced noncardiogenic pulmonary edema should be considered and is one of the indications for dialysis. If these patients need to be intubated, the vent settings must match or exceed the patient's minute ventilation.

Diphenhydramine (**a**) is a common decongestant that has antihistaminergic and anticholinergic properties. Overdoses may present as an anticholinergic toxidrome, including altered mental status, mydriasis, flushed skin, hyperthermia, and dry mucous membranes. The antihistaminergic properties may cause sedation. Ibuprofen (**b**) overdose includes GI symptoms (nausea, vomiting, and epigastric pain), mild CNS depression, renal failure, and an elevated anion gap acidosis. Most of these effects are seen only in extremely high doses (>100 mg/kg). APAP (**c**) overdose usually lacks clinical signs or symptoms in the first 24 hours. Patients may have nonspecific GI complaints. Pseudoephedrine (**e**) is a commonly used decongestant. An overdose may present with CNS stimulation, hypertension, tachycardia, and dysrhythmias.

203. The answer is c. The **sympathomimetic syndrome** usually is seen after acute abuse of cocaine, amphetamines, or decongestants. Patients are usually **hypertensive, tachycardic,** and have **mydriatic pupils.** In massive overdoses, cardiovascular collapse can result in shock and wide-complex dysrhythmias. CNS effects include seizures. Sympathomimetic syndrome is sometimes difficult to distinguish from anticholinergic syndrome. The difference is that patients usually present with dry mucous membranes with an anticholinergic overdose, whereas patients are **diaphoretic** with sympathomimetics.

The anticholinergic syndrome (**a**) typically presents with delirium, mumbling speech, tachycardia, elevated temperature, flushed face, dry mucous membranes and skin, dilated pupils, and hypoactive bowel sounds.

The cholinergic syndrome **(b)** is commonly remembered by the mnemonics SLUDGE or DUMBBELS. Opioids **(d)** typically present with sedation, miosis, respiratory depression, hypotension, bradycardia, hypothermia, and decreased bowel sounds. Sedative hypnotic toxidrome **(e)** is characterized by a relatively normal set of vitals and a normal examination except for CNS depression.

204. The answer is e. Benzodiazepines such as **diazepam** should be used as the first-line agent for nearly all cocaine toxicities. Many effects of cocaine are thought to be mediated through CNS stimulation via catecholamine release or inhibition of catecholamine reuptake. The effects that acute cocaine intoxication has on the heart include coronary vasoconstriction with increasing myocardial oxygen demand. Benzodiazepines restore the CNS inhibitory tone on the peripheral nervous system. The use of β-adrenergic antagonists should be avoided with acute cocaine toxicity because of unopposed α adrenergic receptor stimulation and coronary artery vasoconstriction.

Although haloperidol **(a)** can be used for sedation, its anticholinergic and pro-seizure effects can limit cooling by impeding diaphoresis and may increase morbidity. It is best to avoid β-adrenergic antagonists, such as labetalol and esmolol **(b and c)** in the setting of cocaine intoxication. Their use leads to unopposed α-adrenergic stimulation that results in vasoconstriction. Although labetalol is an α- and β-adrenergic receptor blocker, it has substantially more β-adrenergic antagonism than α-adrenergic antagonist effects and is still not recommended as first-line treatment for this patient. Calcium channel blockers such as diltiazem **(d)** are not recommended for the treatment of cocaine-induced chest pain.

205. The answer is d. Opioid withdrawal initially presents with drug craving, yawning, rhinorrhea, and **piloerection**, and progresses to nausea, vomiting, diarrhea, hyperactive bowels, diaphoresis, myalgias, arthralgias, anxiety, fear, and mild tachycardia. **Methadone withdrawal** starts approximately 24 hours after the last dose and persists for 3 to 7 days. Heroin withdrawal begins about 6 hours after the last dose and usually fully manifests at 24 hours. Opioid withdrawal is not a life-threatening condition as long as adequate hydration and nutritional support are maintained.

Ethanol withdrawal **(a)** is a life-threatening condition that develops 6 to 24 hours after the reduction of ethanol intake. It is characterized by autonomic hyperactivity, including nausea, anorexia, coarse tremor, tachycardia, hypertension, hyperreflexia, sleep disturbances, hallucinations, and seizure. To meet the definition of being in "delirium tremens (DTs)," the patient must be both delirious and tremulous. Treatment for this withdrawal state is benzodiazepines and very large doses may be required. When cocaine (b) use is stopped or when a binge ends, a crash follows almost immediately. This is accompanied by a strong craving for more cocaine, fatigue, lack of pleasure, anxiety, irritability, sleepiness, and sometimes agitation or extreme suspicion. Patients withdrawing from cocaine may be extremely difficult to wake up. Nicotine withdrawal (c) manifests largely as cigarette craving and subjective dysphoric symptoms. There are some symptoms of irritability and restlessness. Discontinuation of clonidine (e) leads to hypertension, headache, flushing, sweating, hallucinations, anxiety, and reflex tachycardia. There is no piloerection in these patients and this is usually over within 24 hours.

206. The answer is d. PCP intoxication is characterized by a wide spectrum of findings. Behavior may be bizarre, agitated, confused, or violent. The hallmark of PCP toxicity is the **recurring delusion of superhuman strength and invulnerability** resulting from both the anesthetic and dissociative properties of the drug. Patients have broken police handcuffs, fracturing bones in doing so. The major cause of death or injury from PCP is behavioral toxicity leading to suicide and provoked homicide. Typical neurologic signs include **nystagmus** (horizontal, vertical, or rotary), ataxia, and altered gait. Pupils are usually midsized and reactive but can be mydriatic or miotic. Bizarre posturing, grimacing, and writhing may be seen. Management is conservative. To prevent self-injury, the patient must be safely restrained. Antipsychotics or benzodiazepines are frequently administered for chemical sedation. PCP intoxication usually ranges from 8 to 16 hours but can last longer in chronic users.

Cocaine and amphetamines are sympathomimetics (a) that can be confused with PCP intoxication. However, the hallmark to PCP intoxication that is not usually observed in sympathomimetic intoxication is the recurring delusion of superhuman strength and nystagmus. When cocaine (b) use is stopped or when a binge ends, a crash follows almost immediately. This is accompanied by a strong craving for more cocaine, fatigue, lack of pleasure, anxiety, irritability, sleepiness, and sometimes agitation or extreme suspicion. While in the anticholinergic toxidrome (c), there may be an altered mental status and tachycardia, nystagmus is not classically associated with the anticholinergic toxidrome. Additionally, the skin would be dry. Opioid withdrawal (e) initially presents with drug craving, yawning, rhinorrhea, and piloerection, and progresses to nausea, vomiting, diarrhea, hyperactive bowel, diaphoresis, myalgias, arthralgias, anxiety, fear, and mild tachycardia.

207. The answer is a. This patient has an **anion gap metabolic acidosis and an osmolar gap.** An **anion gap** is the difference between unmeasured anions (proteins and organic acids) and unmeasured cations (potassium, calcium, and magnesium). The anion gap can be calculated from the formula:

$$\text{Anion gap} = [Na^+] - [HCO_3^- + Cl^-]$$

The normal anion gap is approximately 6 to 10 mEq/L.

The cause of increased anion gap is frequently remembered by the mnemonic **MUD PILES**:

M: methanol, metformin   **P:** paraldehyde
U: uremia   **I:** iron, INH
D: DKA   **L:** lactate
   E: ethylene glycol, ethanol
   S: salicylate

Our patient's anion gap is $(141) - (101 + 14) = 26$.

The **measured serum osmolarity** performed by the laboratory is measured by a depression in the freezing point or an elevation in the boiling point of the solution. If there is an increase in low-molecular-weight molecules (ie, acetone, methanol, ethanol, mannitol, isopropyl alcohol, or ethylene glycol), the osmolarity increases more than what is calculated from the regular serum molecules.

The formula to calculate serum osmolarity is as follows:

$$\text{Serum Osm (mOsm/kg)} = 2[Na^+] + \text{glucose}/18 + \text{BUN}/1.8 + \text{EtOH}/4.6$$

The difference between the actual measured osmolarity and the calculated osmolarity is as follows:

$$\text{osmolar gap} = (\text{measure} - \text{calculated})$$

Our patient's osmol gap is $(352) - (292) = 60$.

When the osmol gap is greater than 50 mOsm/L, it should be considered nearly diagnostic of **toxic alcohol** ingestion. However, a normal or even negative osmol gap does not exclude the presence of toxic alcohols. The patient's clinical presentation of altered mental status, anion gap metabolic acidosis, and osmol gap is consistent with toxic alcohol ingestion. In this case, the ingested substance was methanol.

All other answer choices **(b, c, d, and e)** are incorrect.

208. The answer is b. For young patients with altered mental status, toxic ingestion should be high on the differential. This clinical scenario is most consistent with toxic ingestion of a **TCA**. Treatment of all toxic ingestions should begin with assessment of airway, breathing, and circulation. As a result of this patient's obtunded mental status and loss of gag reflex, **orotracheal intubation** is indicated for airway protection.

Acute cardiovascular toxicity is responsible for most of the mortalities from TCA overdose. The characteristic features are conduction delays, dysrhythmias, and hypotension. The sodium-blocking activity of TCAs leads to a **widened QRS and rightward axis**. It is believed that there is an increased chance of cardiac dysrhythmias, if the QRS is greater than 100 milliseconds. It is recommended that you treat this condition with **IV sodium bicarbonate** until the QRS narrows to 100 milliseconds or the serum pH increases to 7.55. In addition, the patient is hypotensive and should receive a fluid bolus of normal saline and be placed in the Trendelenburg position. If the hypotension does not resolve after these maneuvers and administration of bicarbonate, the patient should receive norepinephrine. TCA overdose may progress rapidly and while frequently difficult to predict, most fatalities occur before 4 to 6 hours of the onset of hypotension. It is common for a patient to present to the ED awake and alert and then develop life-threatening cardiovascular and CNS toxicity within a couple of hours.

Activated charcoal **(e)** can be administered but is not likely to affect the outcome in this already very symptomatic patient. Routine administration is no longer recommended in the undifferentiated toxic ingestion. In an obtunded patient, it is important to first secure an airway, if charcoal administration is indicated, to prevent aspiration in the event of vomiting. Narcan **(a)** is the antidote for opioid toxicity; this patient requires sodium bicarbonate for a TCA overdose. Additionally, you should not give naloxone to an intubated patient. NAC **(c)** is the antidote for APAP overdose. Syrup of ipecac **(d)** cannot be administered to a patient who is intubated and is not recommended generally.

209. The answer is b. **Ethylene glycol** is a colorless, odorless, slightly sweet-tasting liquid that is found in some antifreeze compounds. Ingestions of antifreeze are either accidental, suicidal, or in substitute of ethanol. Ethylene glycol is metabolized to glycolic acid, which results in a profound **anion gap metabolic acidosis**.

In this case: $(Na) - ([Cl] + [HCO_3^-]); (139 - [101 + 5]) = 33.$

Glycolic acid is subsequently metabolized to oxalic acid, which combines with calcium to form calcium oxalate crystals, which then precipitate in renal tubules, brain, and other tissues. The finding of **crystalluria** is considered the **hallmark of ethylene glycol ingestion**; however, its absence does not rule out the diagnosis. Another test that can be done in the ED involves examining freshly voided urine for fluorescence with a Wood lamp. Sodium fluorescein is added to most antifreeze products to aid in the detection of radiator leaks. This test may not be positive if the ingestion was not recent (<4 hours). Ingestion of ethylene glycol is associated with neurologic, cardiopulmonary, and renal abnormalities.

Ibuprofen (**a**) can cause an elevated gap acidosis but would not give you crystalluria and should give you some GI symptoms or renal insufficiency in doses that would give you this degree of acidosis. DKA (**c**) can cause a metabolic acidosis. Patients usually have a history of diabetes, elevated blood glucose (>200 mg/dL), and ketones in their urine. Lactic acidosis (**d**) can cause a metabolic acidosis. This patient's lactate is within normal limits. Isopropyl alcohol (**e**) (rubbing alcohol) is less toxic than methanol and ethylene glycol but more toxic than ethanol. Patients typically present with CNS depression. Isopropanol also causes a hemorrhagic gastritis. Unlike the other toxic alcohols, it is not usually associated with a high anion gap metabolic acidosis.

210. The answer is a. Ethylene glycol and methanol are metabolized to their toxic components by the enzyme **alcohol dehydrogenase**, which is the rate limiting step. Initial treatment of toxic alcohol ingestion involves blocking alcohol dehydrogenase with either **ethanol or fomepizole** to prevent further formation of the toxic metabolites. A single 15 mg/kg dose provides effective enzyme inhibition for 12 hours, after which time it must be redosed. A serum ethanol concentration of greater than 100 mg/dL must be maintained in order to prevent methanol and ethylene glycol metabolism.

Hemodialysis (**b**) is an effective treatment and removes methanol and ethylene glycol from the serum; however, effective removal requires several hours of treatment. If alcohol dehydrogenase is not blocked with either fomepizole or ethanol, the patient will continue to metabolize the toxic alcohol into the toxic metabolites while undergoing hemodialysis. Sodium bicarbonate (**c**) infusion will start to treat the acidosis; however, it does not prevent the formation of the toxic metabolites. Methylene blue (**d**) treats methemoglobinemia and facilitates reduction of iron (III) to iron (II). Pyridoxine (**e**) is an adjuvant treatment for ethylene glycol poisoning. It is a cofactor that facilitates the metabolism of the toxic metabolites. It cannot treat the poisoning without blocking metabolism.

211. The answer is d. **Isopropyl alcohol** is one of the **toxic alcohols** (ethylene glycol, methanol, and isopropyl alcohol). It is a clear, colorless liquid with a **bitter taste**. It is commonly used as a **rubbing alcohol** and as a solvent in hair care products, skin lotion, and home aerosols. It is ingested as an inexpensive and convenient substitute for ethanol. Clinically, GI and CNS complaints predominate. Its GI irritant properties cause patients to complain of abdominal pain, nausea, and vomiting. Pupillary size varies but miosis is commonly observed. Large ingestions can result in coma. Hypotension, although rare, signifies severe poisoning. Characteristically, metabolic acidosis, unlike the other **toxic alcohols**, is not present. This is because isopropyl alcohol is metabolized to **acetone**, a ketone, not an acid. It is also the cause for the presence of urinary ketones and the odor on the patient's breath. Isopropyl alcohol intoxication is often remembered by **ketosis without acidosis**. Another unique finding is the presence of "pseudo renal failure" or isolated false elevation of creatinine with a normal BUN. This results from interference of acetone and acetoacetate by the colorimetric method used to measure the creatinine level.

If the patient had a history of diabetes with an elevated blood sugar and ketones present in the urine, DKA would be highly suspected **(a)**. Differentiating between ethanol and isopropyl alcohol ingestion can be very difficult, without an undetectable measurement of ethanol. Ethanol can also cause measurable ketones. This patient's clinical presentation of drinking a bitter liquid, abdominal pain, nausea, vomiting, odor of acetone, and ketosis without acidosis and a negative ethanol level is most consistent with isopropyl alcohol intoxication. Methanol and ethylene glycol intoxications **(c and e)** are typically associated with an anion gap metabolic acidosis. Promethazine **(b)**, both with and without codeine, is used as cough syrup, but has been popularized as a drug of abuse. It has some dopamine antagonism and antihistamine effects. It has been known to result in seizures in overdose. It presents with sedation and anticholinergic effects—dry mouth, dry skin, decreased bowel sounds, and miotic pupils. It should not cause an elevated osmolar gap.

212. The answer is d. The treatment of **salicylate toxicity** has three objectives—(1) prevent further salicylate absorption, (2) correct fluid deficits and acid-base abnormalities, and (3) reduce tissue salicylate concentrations by increasing excretion. When initial treatment fails or the patient is showing significant signs of toxicity, extracorporeal removal of aspirin with **hemodialysis** is recommended. The EXtrip guidelines for initiation of hemodialysis include a (1) salicylate level greater than 100 mg/dL, (2) a salicylate level greater than 90 mg/dL with impaired renal function, (3) elevated salicylate levels and altered mental status, or (4) elevated salicylate levels and new hypoxemia requiring oxygen. **In this case, the patient has a significantly elevated level aspirin level and requires oxygen.** Definitive treatment with hemodialysis is indicated. His chest X-ray shows pulmonary edema (likely from aspirin-induced basement membrane dysfunction), and it is unlikely he would tolerate the large volumes of sodium bicarbonate needed for serum and urinary alkalinization.

Generally, **activated charcoal** should be administered as soon as possible to reduce salicylate absorption. Dehydration occurs early in salicylate intoxication and should be treated with **IV hydration**. **Sodium bicarbonate** alkalizes both the serum and, with some effort, the urine. Because salicylic acid is a weak acid, it is ionized in an alkaline environment and gets "trapped," limiting the amount that crosses the blood-brain barrier and increasing urinary excretion. **Serum alkalization** is done to keep the salicylic acid out of the brain and **urine alkalization** is done to keep the salicylate in the urine (prevent reabsorption in the distal tubule and collecting duct). Alkalization should be considered in patients with salicylate levels greater than 30 mg/dL. This is performed by administering IV sodium bicarbonate to maintain a serum pH between 7.45 and 7.55 and a urine pH greater than 7.5. Potassium supplementation is usually needed to achieve urinary alkalization. Choice (a) would be correct earlier in the patient's course or with a less severe intoxication; however this patient is significantly intoxicated and needs more definitive treatment.

Endotracheal intubation (b) may be necessary in respiratory failure; however, in a salicylate-poisoned patient, it is important to maintain or exceed the patient's minute ventilation. An alkaline serum is needed to keep salicylic acid ionized, which limits it from crossing the blood-brain barrier. It is difficult to maintain an appropriate level of hypocarbia and hyperventilation through assisted ventilation. NAC (c) is the antidote for APAP poisoning. It is important, however, to obtain an APAP and salicylate level in every overdose patient because they are common, deadly, and treatable. (e) Gastric lavage is rarely indicated in any overdose. Gastric lavage should be done on intubated patients within the first hour after an ingestion and only in very specific circumstances. The use of gastric lavage has fallen out of routine use. There is no need to repeat any levels before beginning therapy on this patient.

213. The answer is b. Deferoxamine is a specific chelator of **ferric iron (Fe^{3+})**. It binds with iron to form a water-soluble compound, ferrioxamine, which can be excreted by the kidneys. Deferoxamine has a half-life of 1 hour, so continuous infusion is the preferred method of administration. The patient's clinical presentation is consistent with **acute iron poisoning**. Initial presentation reflects the corrosive effects of iron on the gut and includes nausea, vomiting, diarrhea, and sometimes GI bleeding. Patients with severe overdose may present with shock or coma. In acute iron toxicity, there can be a brief quiescent period when the patient feels better.

Deferoxamine can cause hypotension; therefore, correction of the patient's lost fluid from vomiting and diarrhea should be done quickly when deferoxamine is considered.

The treatment for organophosphate toxicity (a) is atropine and 2-PAM. Physostigmine (a) is an antidote for the anticholinergic syndrome. Aspirin overdose (c) is treated with decontamination, alkalinization, and sometimes dialysis. NAC (c) is the antidote for APAP (d) overdose. Naloxone (d) is the antidote for opioid overdose. Anticholinergic overdose (e) can be treated with physostigmine. Fomepizole (e) is the treatment for toxic alcohol ingestion.

214. The answer is a. Butane is a **hydrocarbon (HC)** family, a diverse group of organic compounds that contain hydrogen and carbon. Some common products containing HCs are household polishes, glues, paint remover, and industrial solvents. Acute HC toxicity usually affects three main target organs—the lungs, CNS, and heart. The lungs are most commonly affected by aspiration of ingested HCs. Pulmonary toxicity is associated with cough, crackles, bronchospasm, pulmonary edema, and pneumonitis on chest radiograph. Certain HCs (ie, toluene, benzene, gasoline, butane, and/or chlorinated HCs) can have sedative/opioid-like effect and cause euphoria, disinhibition, confusion, and obtundation. HCs can also cause **sudden cardiac death**, particularly after sudden physical activity after intentional inhalation. It is thought that the HCs produce **myocardial sensitization** of endogenous and exogenous catecholamines, which precipitates ventricular dysrhythmias and myocardial dysfunction. One scenario is the solvent-abusing person. EMS workers often describe an individual who has used inhaled solvents, performed some type of physical activity, and then suddenly collapsed. In this scenario, the patient inhaling **butane** was approached by a police officer and tried to run away. This sudden exertion most likely led to a cardiac dysrhythmia. Paraphernalia is often found at the scene, including plastic bags used for "bagging" (pouring HCs in a bag, then deeply inhaling) or HC-soaked cloths used for "huffing" (inhaling through a saturated cloth). Other paraphernalia includes gasoline containers, multiple butane lighters, and spray paint cans.

Ethanol intoxication (**b**) typically does not lead to ventricular fibrillation. In patients with heroin overdose (**c**) who become hypoxic, ventricular fibrillation is possible. However, in this scenario, the patient's mental status did not change in response to naloxone, the reversal agent for opioids. Cocaine intoxication (**d**) may lead to ventricular fibrillation due to its cardiac effects; however, this scenario is more consistent with HC abuse. PCP (**e**) generally does not lead to cardiac dysrhythmias.

215. The answer is c. MDMA is currently one of the most widely abused **amphetamines** by college students and teenagers. It is commonly known as "ecstasy," "E," "XTC," and "M&M." MDMA is an entactogen, a substance capable of producing euphoria, inner peace, and a desire to socialize. Negative effects include ataxia, restlessness, confusion, poor concentration, and memory problems. MDMA, although classified as an amphetamine, is also a potent stimulus for the release of serotonin. MDMA can also cause significant **hyponatremia**. The increase in serotonin results in the excessive release of vasopressin [antidiuretic hormone (ADH)]. Moreover, large free-water intake (increased thirst) combined with sodium loss from physical exertion (dancing) certainly contributes to the development of hyponatremia.

Cocaine (**a**) use can cause agitation and seizures but should not cause significant hyponatremia. Heroin (**b**) intoxication usually causes people to be more sedate rather than agitated. It should not cause seizures or hyponatremia. Ketamine and PCP (**d and e**) can cause agitation and hallucinations; however, significant hyponatremia is not usually present.

216. The answer is c. Patients who swallow bags of drugs can be classified into two large categories—**"body stuffers"** and **"body packers."** Patients being arrested who swallow illicit drugs to conceal the evidence are referred to as **"body stuffers."** They commonly tend to ingest any and all the drugs they possess, potentially resulting in a polypharmaceutic overdose. Body stuffers are usually seen in the ED before symptoms have developed. **Activated charcoal** should be administered immediately and **whole-bowel irrigation** may be indicated. Sometimes, there is radiographic evidence of the swallowed substances as seen in crack vials or staples on the packaging materials. Whole-bowel irrigation uses a **polyethylene glycol electrolyte solution (eg, GoLYTELY)**, which is not absorbed and flushes drugs or chemicals through the GI tract. This procedure seems to be most useful when radiopaque tablets or chemicals, swallowed packets of street drugs, or sustained-released drugs have been ingested. **"Body packers"** are people who transport large amounts of drugs in very tightly wrapped packages. This takes pre-planning and is not done as the police are raiding. "Packers," if symptomatic, may need to go to the operating room (OR). Cocaine can lead to bowel perforation.

Magnesium citrate (**a**) is a cathartic whose action begins 4 to 6 hours after ingestion. It is contraindicated in patients with renal failure. Gastric lavage (**b**) is not indicated for this patient. Syrup of ipecac (**d**) is also ineffective for the packets in the small bowel. NAC (**e**) is the antidote for APAP toxicity.

217. The answer is d. Methemoglobinemia occurs when an oxidative stress causes the iron in hemoglobin to go from iron (II) to the iron (III) oxidation state. Once oxidized, it can no longer carry oxygen and a functional anemia is created. Patients develop a distinct cyanotic appears when methemoglobin levels reach 10% to 15%. Patients without anemia and no underlying cardiopulmonary disease may be asymptomatic until levels reach 30%. Methemoglobin is read as deoxyhemoglobin by pulse oximeters, but is read correctly with co-oximetry. This leads to the "saturation gap" in which the pulse oximeter indicates a lower saturation than a measured saturation. In this case, the oxidative stress is most likely from fertilizer nitrites contaminating the farm's drinking water.

Carbon monoxide (**a**) prevents oxygen unloading from hemoglobin and cyanide (**b**) prevents oxygen from being used by the electron transport chain. Patients do not appear cyanotic and may actually appear quite pink. The saturation will be high on pulse oximetry and when measured. Additionally, cyanide levels are technically very difficult to obtain and rarely return in a timely fashion for diagnostic use in the ED. D-dimer (**c**) is used to screen for venous thromboembolism. An abnormal A-a gradient (the difference between alveolar oxygen tension and the measured hemoglobin oxygen tension) rather than saturation gap, suggests a possible pulmonary embolism. An abnormal D-dimer suggests a possible pulmonary embolism, but is not diagnostic or confirmatory. Aspirin (**e**) causes acidosis, but does not affect the pulse oximeter reading or cause cyanosis.

218. The answer is d. Methylene blue is the antidote for symptomatic methemoglobinemia. It takes an electron from NADPH, generated through the pentose phosphate pathway, and reduces iron (III) to iron (II). Very large doses can actually cause the reaction to run in reverse and cause methemoglobinemia.

Enoxaparin **(a)** treats venous thromboembolism. Hyperbaric oxygen **(b)** is used to treat carbon monoxide poisoning. It has been proposed as a "last ditch" treatment for refractory, moribund patients with very high (>80% to 90%) methemoglobinemia, although it is experimental for this purpose. Hydroxocobalamin **(c)** treats cyanide poisoning by combining with cyanide to form cyanocobalamin (vitamin B_{12}). Sodium bicarbonate **(e)** is used to treat TCA and aspirin poisoning.

219. The answer is e. Accidental drug overdose has overtaken motor vehicle collision as the number one cause of accidental death in the United States. **Opioid-based medications and drugs** are the most common cause.

The other medication types **(a, b, c, and d)** have significant potential for mortality; however, cause less accidental deaths than opioid medications.

220. The answer is b. This patient has **malignant hyperthermia** (MH), a rare reaction associated with some inhaled anesthetics and **succinylcholine**. It is caused by an abnormality in the ryanodine receptor on the sarcoplasmic reticulum on skeletal muscle. Abnormal triggering results in increased muscle metabolic activity. The diagnosis can be challenging, but the clinical findings include **muscle rigidity, hyperthermia, and hypercarbia**. Treatment is with **dantrolene**, which sequesters calcium back into the sarcoplasmic reticulum. Succinylcholine and other triggers must be scrupulously avoided in potentially susceptible individuals.

Bromocriptine **(a)** is a dopamine agonist and can be used to treat neuroleptic malignant syndrome (NMS). While there are some similarities between MH and NMS, MH is caused by succinylcholine and some inhaled anesthetics, while NMS is caused by dopamine antagonist medications such as antipsychotics. IV antibiotics and a chest X-ray **(c)** should be considered in the treatment of bacterial pneumonia. While the fever in the setting of respiratory failure could be related to pneumonia, the muscle rigidity and the association with succinylcholine suggest MH. IV fluids **(d)** may be of benefit to help prevent circulatory collapse, however will not treat the underlying pathology. Physostigmine **(e)** is used to treat central and peripheral antimuscarinic syndrome.

221. The answer is d. Altered mental status can be a challenging diagnosis. Detailed history and exam are critical to find the cause and to initiate appropriate treatment. In this case, the patient presents in a hyperadrenergic state with auditory, visual, and tactile hallucinations. He also was witnessed having a seizure. This constellation of findings is consistent with **alcohol withdrawal**. Alcohol withdrawal is caused by an abrupt cessation of alcohol use. The pathophysiology is complex, but involves a maladaptive upregulation of NMDA receptors in response to consistent background amounts of alcohol. With abrupt cessation of alcohol consumption, the inhibitory effect of alcohol is removed, resulting in an unbalanced, excitatory state. Untreated, this can lead to seizures, DTs, and death.

The degree of alcohol withdrawal symptoms can be scored and followed using the CIWA-Ar tool. This tool assesses a variety of symptoms including orientation, agitation, sweating, anxiety, agitation, tremor and visual, auditory, and tactile hallucinations. A score is then summed with a range of 0 to 62. Patients with scores above 9 generally need medication to treat withdrawal. Those with scores above 20 often need intensive care unit (ICU) level care. In this case, the patient has a score in the mid to high 20s and is at significant risk for the development of DT. Patients in severe alcohol withdrawal should be treated and brought under control with IV GABAnerigic agents such as a benzodiazepine or phenobarbital. Adjuvant thiamine with thiamine should considered, if there is concern for Wernicke's encephalopathy. Pyridoxine deficiency is also associated with alcohol abuse. IV **phenobarbital** is the correct answer as it is the **only parenteral GABA agent listed**.

Endotracheal intubation with RSI (**a**) may be needed if the patient is at risk of airway compromise, after high doses of sedative agents, but it should not be performed prophylactically. Chlordiazepoxide (**b**) is a benzodiazepine commonly used for alcohol withdrawal; however it is an oral medication and takes hours to reach peak effect. It is difficult to titrate in a severely ill patient. Once a patient's symptoms have been controlled, transitioning to an oral benzodiazepine can be considered. It is not the best choice for initial, in patient treatment. Neuroleptics such as haloperidol (**c**) as monotherapy for alcohol withdrawal are associated with increased mortality. Phenytoin (**e**) is used to treat epileptic seizures but is a poor choice for the control of toxic seizures and does little to control the pathophysiology of alcohol withdrawal.

222. The answer is d. The patient developed **local anesthetic toxicity** from an accidental double dose of bupivacaine. The overdose occurred due to use of an unexpected concentration. It is important to double check medication dosage and concentration, prior to administering medications. **Bupivacaine** is an amide type local anesthetic and is Type 1b antidysrhythmic, like lidocaine. In overdose, it can cause **QRS widening, arrhythmia, seizures, and cardiac arrest.** A **metallic taste** is a frequently reported prodrome to seizures in the setting of local anesthetic toxicity. **Intravenous fat emulsion** (IFE) was developed to treat local anesthetic toxicity, specifically with bupivacaine. Treatment involves giving a large bolus of 20% fat emulsion (typically 1-1.5 mL/kg). The exact mechanism is not known, but its suspected mechanism is to absorb the local anesthetic into lipid micelles in the blood and pull the medication away from vulnerable tissue. There is some evidence that IFE may be useful for other overdoses; however, the data is limited. If a patient goes into cardiac arrest from local anesthetics, in addition to other advanced cardiovascular life support (ACLS) and IFE, cardiopulmonary resuscitation (CPR) should be performed for a prolonged period of time to assist with medications redistribution. It is recommended that IFE a readily available treatment anywhere regional anesthesia is performed.

Amiodarone (**a**) is used to treat refractory arrhythmias. This patient is showing some cardiac toxicity, but no arrhythmias. Amiodarone could potentially worsen the situation by affecting cardiac repolarization. Sodium bicarbonate (**b**) therapy is a potential choice to treat local anesthetic toxicity, due to the type 1b sodium channel effect; however, IFE is the first line treatment. Phenytoin (**c**) is a weak type 1b sodium channel blocker and would not be expected to be of benefit. Hemodialysis (**e**) is usually effective at removing medications if they have a low volume of distribution (1 L/kg or less) and are not protein bound. Bupivacaine is highly protein bound and not amenable to removal by hemodialysis.

223. The answer is d. This patient was bitten and envenomated by a **rattlesnake**. In North America, the vast majority of snake envenomation in the wild are from snakes in the Crotalinae family (pit vipers). The venom from these snakes usually present with **swelling and hematologic abnormalities.** A few members of this family, namely the canebrake (*Crotalus horridus*) and the majove (*Crotalus scutulatus*), may have some neurotoxic effects, similar to the venom of a Cobra. The patient is presenting with **clear signs of envenomation**, namely soft tissue swelling beyond local effect (crossing a joint line), changes in vital signs, and laboratory findings of a consumptive coagulopathy. The treatment is **polyvalent crotalid**

antivenin. Currently, there is an equine-derived and ovine-derived antivenin on the market. These antivenins are made with the venoms of several different snakes and approved for the treatment of moderate to severe envenomation from rattlesnakes. The products are administered, typically in doses of 4 to 6 vials, until the patient no longer shows progression of symptoms and the coagulation profile improves.

While applying loose fitting, gentle compression bandage on the extremity can be used in the field to slow progression of an elapid envenomation, the use of compression bandages or tourniquets (a) is not recommended for crotalid bites. Venom extraction (b) has not been shown to be effective at reducing the severity of an envenomation and care should not be delayed attempting to perform the procedure. Snake bite can mimic compartment syndrome; however, fasciotomy (c) is potentially harmful, especially if the coagulation abnormalities have not been controlled. Venom-induced compartment like-syndrome can almost always be managed with antivenin alone. A fasciotomy should only be performed in rare circumstances, after adequate antivenin has been administered to control the envenomation and after compartment pressure measurements confirm elevated muscle pressures. Crotalid envenomation results in consumptive coagulopathy. Blood products (e) that are administered, without first obtaining control with antivenin, will just be consumed and will not improve coagulation.

224. The answer is d. Drug-drug interactions are of significant concern, especially as the U.S. population ages. Patients on five medications or more are at high risk of a clinically significant medication interaction. Medications that are metabolized by or affect the P450 CYP3A4 and/or CYP2D6 are of significant risk; however, there are multiple other potential interactions. In this question, the administration of the synthetic opioid **meperidine** results in excess serotonin, which then cannot be broken down by the enzyme monoamine oxidase due to inhibition by the monoamine oxidase inhibitor (MAOI), **phenelzine**. This combination can result in a **potentially fatal serotonin syndrome**, as illustrated in the famous case of Libby Zion.

Rifampin is a P450 3A4 inducer and will result in lower levels of estrogen (a). While this is a clinically relevant interaction and may reduce the effectiveness of hormonal contraception, the interaction is unlikely to be fatal. Ceftriaxone has been implicated in disulfiram-like reactions with ethanol (b), however this interaction is rarely reported and not-fatal. Of all medications on the market, warfarin has one of the highest reported incidences of serious and fatal drug-drug and drug-food interactions; however, there is no clinically relevant interaction between warfarin and amlodipine (**c**). The combination is generally regarded as safe. As part of its metabolism, valproic acid binds to levocarnitine. This process results in a relative loss of levocarnitine, which is also necessary to shuttle ammonia into the mitochondria for conversion to urea and ultimate excretion. Levocarnitine deficiency leads to hyperammonemia. Levocarnitine given with valproic acid (**e**) prevents this side effect and levocarnitine supplementation is used to treat hyperammonemia from valproic acid overdose.

Recommended Readings

Brunton LL, Hilal-Dandan R, Knollmann BC. *Goodman and Gilman's The Pharmacological Basis Therapeutics.* New York, NY: McGraw-Hill, 2006: 694.

EXtracorporeal Treatments in Poisoning Working Group (EXTRIP). Blood Purification in Toxicology: Reviewing the Evidence and Providing Recommendations—Executive Summary of Recommendations. 2019. Available at: https://www.extrip-workgroup.org/recommendations. Accessed June 19, 2020.

Nelson LS, Howland MA, Lewin NA, et al. Initial evaluation of the patient: vital signs and toxic syndromes. *Goldfranks' Toxicologic Emergencies.* 11th ed. New York, NY: McGraw-Hill, 2019.

Nelson, LS Howland MA, Lewin NA, et al. Principles of managing the acutely poisoned or overdosed patient. *Goldfranks' Toxicologic Emergencies.* 11th ed. New York, NY: McGraw-Hill, 2019.

Rachel L, LoVecchio F. Salicylates. In: Tintinalli JE, Stapczynski JS, Ma OJ, et al, eds. *Tintinalli's Emergency Medicine: A Comprehensive Study Guide.* 9th ed. New York, NY: McGraw-Hill, 2020.

Rachel SW, Nelson LS. Acetaminophen. In: Tintinalli JE, Stapczynski JS, Ma OJ, et al, eds. *Tintinalli's Emergency Medicine: A Comprehensive Study Guide.* 9th ed. New York, NY: McGraw-Hill, 2020.

Altered Mental Status

Benjamin R. Parva, MD and Jonah Gunalda, MD

Questions

225. A 69-year-old woman with a past medical history of hypertension, hypercholesterolemia, diabetes mellitus type 1, and alcohol abuse is brought to the emergency department (ED) by her daughter who states that her mom has been acting funny over the last hour. The patient did not know where she was despite being in her own house. She also did not recognize her family and was speaking incomprehensibly. Her blood pressure (BP) is 150/80 mm Hg, heart rate (HR) is 90 beats/minute, respiratory rate (RR) is 16 breaths/minute, and temperature is 98.9°F. On physical examination she is diaphoretic, agitated, and tremulous. Electrocardiogram (ECG) is sinus rhythm with normal ST segments and T waves. Which of the following is the most appropriate course of action for this patient?

a. Administer a benzodiazepine for ethanol withdrawal
b. Activate the stroke team and obtain a stat computed tomographic (CT) scan of the head
c. Obtain a stat point-of-care glucose
d. Request a psychiatric consult for probable sundowning
e. Administer haloperidol for sedation

226. A 74-year-old woman is brought to the ED by her family. Her daughter states that the patient has been progressively somnolent over the last week and could not be woken up today. The patient takes medications for diabetes, hypertension, hypothyroidism, and a hydrocodone/acetaminophen combination for a recent ankle sprain. In the ED, the patient is profoundly lethargic, responsive only to pain, and has periorbital edema and delayed relaxation of the deep tendon reflexes. Her BP is 145/84 mm Hg, HR is 56 beats/minute, RR is 12 breaths/minute, and temperature is 94.8°F. Which of the following is the most likely diagnosis?

a. Hypoglycemia
b. Opioid overdose
c. Stroke
d. Myxedema coma
e. Depression

227. An 18-year-old woman is brought in by her roommate for confusion. Over the last 24 hours, her roommate says the patient became progressively confused, saying she was the president. On examination, she is somnolent, but arouses to pain. She is not oriented to person, place, or time. Her initial vital signs are BP 90/40, HR 120, temperature 101.1°F, and RR 20 breaths/minute. She has a flat, round, pinpoint rash on her abdomen that does not blanch when pressed. After fluid resuscitation, what is the next best step for this patient?

a. Call her parents for permission to treat
b. Obtain urine drug screen
c. Perform a lumbar puncture (LP)
d. Administer antibiotics
e. Admit the patient to the ICU

228. A 21-year-old college student is brought to the ED by her roommate who states that the patient has been very sleepy today. She has a history of diabetes and has not refilled her medication in over a week. Her BP is 95/61 mm Hg, HR is 132 beats/minute, RR is 30 breaths/minute, and temperature is 99.7°F. Her point-of-care glucose is 530 mg/dL. Which of the following choices most closely matches what you would expect to find on her arterial blood gas (ABG) with electrolytes and urinalysis?

a. pH 7.38, anion gap 5, normal urinalysis
b. pH 7.57, anion gap 21, presence of glucose and leukocytes in urine
c. pH 7.47, anion gap 12, presence of glucose and ketones in urine
d. pH 7.26, anion gap 12, presence of glucose and ketones in urine
e. pH 7.26, anion gap 21, presence of glucose and ketones in urine

229. A 59-year-old man is brought into the ED accompanied by his son who states that his father is acting irritable and occasionally confused. The son states that his father has a history of hepatitis from a transfusion he received many years ago. Over the past 5 years, his liver function slowly deteriorated. His vital signs include BP of 145/80 mm Hg, HR of 78 beats/minute, RR of 16 breaths/minute, temperature of 98°F, and oxygen saturation of 98%. Laboratory results are all within normal limits, except for a significantly elevated ammonia level. Which of the following is the best therapy?

a. Vancomycin and gentamycin
b. Lactulose and neomycin
c. Ampicillin and gentamycin
d. Levofloxacin
e. Ciprofloxacin

230. A 57-year-old man is brought to the ED after a seizure. His partner reports that the patient has a known seizure disorder and currently takes levetiracetam, but may have missed his last few doses due to a stressful work schedule. On examination, the patient is lying in the stretcher, not oriented. Thirty seconds later, the patient begins jerking and loses control of his bladder. You establish IV access and ask for a medication to be drawn up. Which is the most appropriate initial medication you should administer in this actively seizing patient?

a. Phenytoin
b. Lorazepam
c. Phenobarbital
d. Valproic acid
e. Levetiracetam

231. A 32-year-old G1P1 woman, who gave birth by normal vaginal delivery at term 2 days ago, presents to the ED complaining of bilateral hand swelling and severe headache that started 2 hours ago. Her BP is 187/110 mm Hg, HR is 85 beats/minute, RR is 15 breaths/minute, and temperature is 97.5°F. Urinalysis reveals 3+ protein. When you are examining the patient, she proceeds to have a generalized tonic-clonic seizure. Which of the following is the most appropriate next step in management?

a. Administer intravenous (IV) magnesium sulfate
b. Administer IV labetalol and morphine sulfate
c. Administer IV sumatriptan
d. Administer an IV loading dose of phenytoin
e. Administer IV diazepam and normal saline

232. An unconscious 51-year-old woman is brought to the ED by emergency medical services (EMS). A friend states that the patient was complaining of feeling weak. She vomited and subsequently "blacked out" in the ambulance. The friend states that the patient has no medical problems and takes no medications. She also states that the patient smokes cigarettes and uses cocaine, and that they were snorting cocaine together prior to her blacking out. The patient's BP is 195/80 mm Hg, HR is 50 beats/minute, RR is 7 breaths/minute, and temperature is 98.6°F. What is the eponym associated with her vital signs?

a. Cushing's syndrome
b. Cushing's reflex
c. Cullen's sign
d. Charcot's triad
e. Chvostek's sign

233. A 47-year-old man is brought to the ED by EMS after being persistently agitated at a business meeting. His coworkers state that he has been working nonstop for a day and a half. They report that he always seemed like a healthy guy and frequents bars every night. EMS administered 25 g of dextrose and thiamine with no symptom improvement. In the ED, the patient is anxious, confused, tremulous, and diaphoretic. He denies any medical problems, medications, or drug ingestions. His BP is 182/92 mm Hg, HR is 139 beats/minute, RR is 18 breaths/minute, temperature is 100.4°F, and point-of-care glucose is 103 mg/dL. An ECG reveals sinus tachycardia. Which of the following is the next best step?

a. Administer acetaminophen
b. Administer folate
c. Administer lorazepam
d. Recheck point-of-care glucose
e. Administer labetalol

234. A 65-year-old man presents to the ED with a headache, drowsiness, and confusion. He has a history of long-standing hypertension. His BP is 230/120 mm Hg, pulse is 87 beats/minute, RR is 18 breaths/minute, and oxygen saturation is 97% on room air. On examination, you note papilledema. A head computed tomography (CT) scan is performed and there is no evidence of ischemia or hemorrhage. Which of the following is the most appropriate method to lower his BP?

a. Administer propofol for rapid reduction in BP
b. Administer mannitol for rapid reduction in BP and intracranial pressure (ICP)
c. Administer a high-dose diuretic to reduce preload
d. Administer labetalol until his BP is 140/80 mm Hg
e. Administer labetalol until his BP is 180/100 mm Hg

The following scenario applies to questions 235 and 236.

A 74-year-old woman is brought to the ED by EMS from a nursing home for altered mental status. She is currently being treated for breast cancer. Her BP is 138/72 mm Hg, HR is 90 beats/minute, RR is 17 breaths/minute, and temperature is 100.9°F. A head CT is normal. LP results revealed the following:

White blood cell (WBC) count: 1020/mm^3 with 90% polymorphonuclear cells (PMNs)
Glucose: 21 mg/dL
Protein: 225 g/L

235. Which of the following is the most likely diagnosis?

a. TB meningitis
b. Bacterial meningitis
c. Viral meningitis
d. Fungal meningitis
e. Encephalitis

236. Which antibiotic regimen should be initiated?

a. Vancomycin and ceftriaxone
b. Vancomycin, ceftriaxone, ampicillin
c. Vancomycin
d. Ceftriaxone and valacyclovir
e. Amphotericin B

237. A 67-year-old man presents to the ED for worsening confusion. His wife states that he received his first dose of chemotherapy for lung cancer 2 days ago. Over the last 24 hours, the patient became confused. His BP is 130/70 mm Hg, HR is 87 beats/minute, and temperature is 98.9°F. While in the ED, the patient seizes. You administer an antiepileptic and the seizure immediately stops. You compare his current electrolyte panel to one taken 2 days ago.

	Two Days Prior	Today
Sodium (mEq/L)	139	113
Potassium (mEq/L)	4.1	3.9
Chloride (mEq/L)	105	98
Bicarbonate (mEq/L)	23	20
Blood urea nitrogen (BUN) (mg/dL)	13	17
Creatinine (mg/dL)	0.4	0.7
Glucose (mg/dL)	98	92

Which of the following is the most appropriate treatment?

a. 0.45% saline
b. 0.9% saline
c. 3% saline
d. 5% dextrose
e. 50% dextrose

The following scenario applies to questions 238 and 239.

A 31-year-old woman with a history of schizophrenia presents to the ED for altered mental status. A friend states that the patient is on multiple medications for her schizophrenia. Her BP is 150/80 mm Hg, HR is 122 beats/minute, RR is 20 breaths/minute, and temperature is 104.5°F. On examination, the patient is diaphoretic with distinctive "lead-pipe" rigidity of her musculature. You believe the patient has neuroleptic malignant syndrome (NMS).

238. After basic stabilizing measures, which of the following medications is most appropriate to administer?

a. Haloperidol
b. Droperidol
c. Dantrolene
d. Diphenhydramine
e. Acetaminophen

239. Which of the following abnormalities associated with this condition leads to the greatest morbidity and mortality?

a. Elevated creatine phosphokinase (CPK)
b. Muscle rigidity
c. Hypertension
d. Hyperpyrexia
e. Tachycardia

240. A 56-year-old man is brought in from the homeless shelter for strange, irrational behavior, and unsteady gait for 1 day. A worker at the shelter reports that the patient is a frequent abuser of alcohol. On examination, the patient is alert but oriented to name only and is unable to give a full history. He does not appear clinically intoxicated. You note horizontal nystagmus and ataxia. What is the most likely diagnosis?

a. Wernicke encephalopathy
b. Korsakoff syndrome
c. Normal pressure hydrocephalus
d. Central vertigo
e. Alcohol withdrawal

241. You are called to evaluate a 57-year-old woman brought in by EMS for abdominal pain and altered mental status. Her initial vital signs are BP 80/40 mm Hg, HR 117 beats/minute, RR 18 breaths/minute, oxygen saturation 97%, and temperature of 38.4°C. On examination, she grimaces when you palpate her right upper quadrant (RUQ) and her sclerae appear icteric. She is notably confused and only oriented to person. What antibiotic is the best monotherapy for her condition?

a. Vancomycin
b. Ciprofloxacin
c. Gentamicin
d. Metronidazole
e. Piperacillin-tazobactam

242. A 78-year-old woman is transferred from a nursing home with altered mental status and fever. The nursing home reports that the patient was febrile to 102.3°F, disoriented, confused, and incontinent of urine. Her past medical history includes hypertension, a stroke with residual right-sided weakness, and nighttime agitation for which she was started on haloperidol 3 days ago. Her BP is 215/105 mm Hg, HR is 132 beats/minute, and temperature is 102.8°F. On examination, the patient is oriented to name only, tremulous, diaphoretic, and has marked muscular rigidity and three out of five right upper- and lower-extremity strength. What is the most likely diagnosis?

a. Urinary tract infection (UTI)
b. Malignant hyperthermia
c. NMS
d. Recurrent stroke
e. Meningoencephalitis

243. A 54-year-old man is brought to the ED by his wife for bizarre behavior. The wife complains that her husband has not been acting like his usual self over the last several months. He has seemed increasingly irritable and has started spending all of their savings without warning. The patient's father died at a young age from a chronic illness. The patient's BP is 135/87 mm Hg, HR is 76 beats/minute, RR is 14 breaths/minute, and temperature is 98.9°F. During his examination, he repeatedly flails his left arm in the air, seemingly uncontrollably. Which of the following is most likely to be seen on CT scan?

a. Enlargement of ventricles
b. No identifiable pathology
c. Hyperintense signal in the basal cistern
d. Cerebral edema surrounding mass that crosses the gray-white matter
e. Atrophy of the caudate nucleus

244. A 46-year-old woman is brought to the ED by her husband for 1 day of worsening confusion. The patient has a history of systemic lupus erythematosus (SLE) and takes chronic oral steroids. She has not been feeling well for the last few days. Her BP is 167/92 mm Hg, HR is 95 beats/minute, RR is 16 breaths/minute, and temperature is 100.3°F. On examination, the patient is oriented to name and has diffuse petechiae on her torso and extremities. Laboratory results reveal hematocrit 23%, platelets 17,000/mL, BUN 38 mg/dL, and creatinine 1.9 mg/dL. Which of the following is the most likely diagnosis?

a. Henoch-Schönlein purpura (HSP)
b. Disseminated intravascular coagulopathy (DIC)
c. von Willebrand's disease
d. Idiopathic thrombocytopenic purpura (ITP)
e. Thrombotic thrombocytopenic purpura (TTP)

245. A 58-year-old woman is brought into the ED after a witnessed syncopal event. Upon arrival, the patient appears confused and agitated. Her vitals include a BP of 145/70 mm Hg, HR of 89 beats/minute, RR of 16 breaths/minute, and oxygen saturation of 98% on room air. Within a few minutes, the patient is more alert and oriented. She denies any chest pain, headache, abdominal pain, or weakness preceding the event and is currently asymptomatic. She also states that she has not taken her antiepileptic medications in 2 days. The patient's examination is unremarkable including a nonfocal neurologic examination. Given this patient's history and evolving examination, what is the most likely etiology of this patient's syncopal event?

a. Cerebrovascular accident (CVA)
b. Transient ischemic attack (TIA)
c. Seizure
d. Aortic dissection
e. Pulmonary embolus

The following scenario applies to questions 246 and 247.

A 75-year-old woman presents to the ED with complaints including abdominal pain, nausea and vomiting, frequent urination, and achy pain in her extremities. According to her family, she became confused over the last week, does not remember her family member's names, and has been more fatigued than usual. She has a history of breast cancer and was recently told it had metastasized. On examination, her vital signs are normal. She has diffuse pain in her extremities without swelling or point tenderness. She is mildly confused without lateralizing signs. Urinalysis does not show leukocyte esterase or nitrites; however, calcium oxalate crystals are present.

246. Which of the following tests is likely to confirm your suspected diagnosis?

a. Cancer antigen-125 (CA-125)
b. CT of the head
c. Serum calcium
d. Urine culture
e. Urine drug screen

247. Which of the following treatments provides the best long-term treatment of this patient's condition?

a. IV normal saline and IV furosemide
b. Thalidomide
c. Parathyroidectomy
d. Phenoxybenzamine
e. Zoledronic acid

The following scenario applies to questions 248 and 249.

A 3-year-old boy presents with confusion and lethargy that has been progressive over the last 2 days. He lives with his parents in home that was built in the early 1920s. According to his parents, he has been complaining that his stomach hurts for the last 2 weeks and has been constipated. He has been eating and drinking normally, but also tries to eat things that are not food. The abdominal examination shows no tenderness. Laboratory results are as follows:

WBC: 8.0 (4.1-11.3) mL

Hemoglobin: 8.0 g/dL (11.6-15.1)

Hematocrit: 22.3% (34.2-44.6)

Platelets: 281 (130-450) mL

An abdominal X-ray shows no obstruction; however, there are radiopaque flecks in the small bowel. A representative X-ray of the knee is shown in the figure.

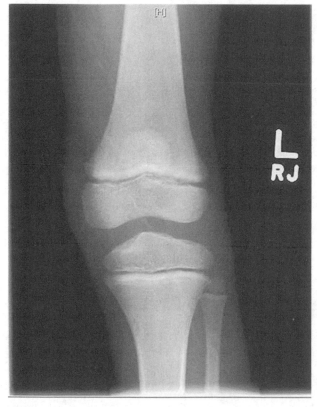

(Reproduced with permission from Bram A. Dolcourt, MD.)

248. Which of the following laboratory tests is most likely to reveal the definitive diagnosis?

a. Point-of-care glucose
b. Serum calcium level
c. Serum lead level
d. Serum thyroid-stimulating hormone (TSH) level
e. Urine organic acids

249. Which of the following therapies is most appropriate for his condition?

a. Deferoxamine
b. Dimercaprol (British anti-Lewisite)
c. Folinic acid
d. N-acetylcysteine
e. Lorazepam

The following scenario applies to questions 250 and 251.

A 48-year-old man presents with personality changes and ataxia that have been progressive over the course of a month. He complains of shooting "electric shocks" down his legs. He has also had episodes of urinary incontinence. He walks with a wide-based, high-stepping gait. Pupillary examination shows small, nonreactive pupils that accommodate. Patellar reflexes are absent.

250. Which of the following findings confirms the most likely diagnosis?

a. Abnormal prions on brain biopsy
b. Gram-positive cocci in pairs on cerebrospinal fluid (CSF) gram stain
c. Plaques in the white matter on magnetic resonance imaging (MRI) of brain
d. Positive fluorescent treponemal antibody absorption on CSF
e. Positive polymerase chain reaction for herpes simplex virus (HSV) in the CSF

251. Which of the following is the most appropriate therapy for his condition?

a. Hospice consultation
b. Monthly B_{12} injections and with daily oral folic acid supplementation
c. IM interferon beta daily
d. IV acyclovir
e. IV penicillin

252. A 34-year-old woman presents to the ED with confusion, lethargy, and episodes of syncope upon standing. She has been vomiting for most of the day. The point-of-care glucose on presentation was 55 mg/dL; however, her mental status did not improve with IV dextrose administration. She recently ran out of her medications, but cannot remember her medical history. Her BP is 80/40 mm Hg and unresponsive to 2 L of normal saline, HR is 80 beats/minutes, RR is 12 breaths/minute, temperature is 100.8°F, and oxygen saturation is 99% on room air. Physical examination reveals no nuchal rigidity. The skin of her palms and buccal mucosa appear darkened. A basic metabolic panel is sent and results are as follows:

> Sodium: 128 mMol/L (135-145)
> Potassium: 5.8 mMol/L (3.5-5.0)
> Chloride: 96 mMol/L (98-106)
> Bicarbonate: 20 mMol/L (23-27)
> Glucose: 120 mg/dL (80-120)
> Calcium: 10.4 mg/dL (8.5-10.3)
> BUN: 10 mg/dL (5-12)
> Creatinine: 1.0 mg/dL (0.6-1.2)

An LP is performed and CSF analysis is shown as follows:

> WBC: 3/mm^3 (<5)
> Red blood cell (RBC): 0/mm^3 (0)
> Protein: 30 mg/dL (15-45)
> Glucose: 75 mg/dL (40-80)

Which of the following treatments should be initiated immediately?

a. Vancomycin
b. Diphenhydramine
c. Hydrocortisone
d. Norepinephrine
c. Propylthiouracil (PTU)

The following scenario applies to questions 253 and 254.

A 64-year-old man with a history of chronic obstructive pulmonary disease (COPD) comes into the ED for difficulty breathing. He smokes 2 packs of cigarettes and drinks a 12 pack of beer each day. His vital signs include BP of 140/90 mm Hg, HR 100 beats/minute, RR 20 breaths/minute, and oxygen saturation of 93%. On initial examination, he is somnolent, with shallow breathing. He awakens to sternal rub and groans when you ask him his name. He has diffuse, coarse, shallow breath sounds heard throughout all lung fields. The rest of the physical examination is normal.

253. What test will confirm the diagnosis?

a. ABG
b. LP
c. CT head without contrast
d. Carboxyhemoglobin level
e. Ammonia level

254. What is the next best step in the care of this patient?

a. Draw blood cultures and administer broad-spectrum antibiotics
b. Initiation of Bi-level positive airway pressure (BiPAP) therapy
c. Administer lactulose
d. Endotracheal intubation
e. Arrange hyperbaric oxygen therapy

Altered Mental Status

Answers

225. The answer is c. The patient never received a **point-of-care glucose** at triage. **Hypoglycemia** can mimic a CVA or seizure. Therefore, it is critical that all patients who present with altered mental status get a point-of-care glucose. Glucose level should be considered a vital sign. Hypoglycemia is a common problem in patients with type 1 diabetes. The clinical presentation of hypoglycemia is caused by increased secretion of epinephrine, as well as central nervous system (CNS) dysfunction. Symptoms include diaphoresis, nervousness, tremor, tachycardia, hunger, and neurologic symptoms ranging from confusion and bizarre behavior to seizures and coma.

Ethanol withdrawal **(a)** can present in a similar fashion as hypoglycemia because both include symptoms of an adrenergic state (eg, tachycardia, hypertension, diaphoresis, and/or agitation). Even if you suspect ethanol withdrawal, it is mandatory to check a glucose. The stroke team **(b)** should be activated in patients who present with signs and symptoms of a stroke that are not caused by hypoglycemia. Sundowning **(d)** refers to people who become increasingly confused at the end of the day and into the night. Sundowning is not a disease but a symptom that often occurs in people with dementia such as Alzheimer's disease. It is more commonly observed on the hospital wards than in the ED. Haloperidol **(e)** is commonly used as a sedative for agitated patients. However, this patient is agitated because of an organic cause, hypoglycemia. By treating the underlying cause (administering glucose), the agitation will resolve.

226. The answer is d. Myxedema coma is a life-threatening **complication of hypothyroidism**. Mortality in myxedema coma approaches 20% to 50% even with appropriate management. The patient exhibits classic signs and symptoms of the disease—lethargy or coma, hypothermia, bradycardia, periorbital and nonpitting edema, and a delayed relaxation phase of deep tendon reflexes (areflexia in more severe cases). Myxedema coma can be triggered by sepsis, trauma, surgery, congestive heart failure, prolonged cold exposure, or use of sedatives or narcotics (as seen in this example).

It is critical that a point-of-care glucose is checked (**a**). However, myxedema coma differs from the early stages of hypoglycemia in that myxedema coma results in the progressive slowing of all bodily functions; by contrast, in early hypoglycemia, the body is stimulated by the release of adrenergic hormones. The classic findings in opioid toxicity (**b**) include miotic pupils and respiratory depression. Stroke (**c**) should be on the differential in this case, but the patient's signs and symptoms are more consistent with an abnormal metabolic state than with purely neurovascular change. Depression (**e**) is an often-forgotten diagnosis in the elderly and may present with a wide variety of signs and symptoms. Severe depression may appear as lethargy. It is unlikely, however, to have associated hypothermia and abnormal reflexes.

227. The answer is d. This patient presents with signs and symptoms of **meningitis**, as evidenced by altered mental status, fever, and a petechial rash. Initial management is to stabilize the patient by attempting fluid resuscitation. The next step should be blood cultures, antibiotics, and an LP, typically in that order. Even delaying antibiotic initiation by 1 hour can increase mortality by 3% to 7%. Therefore, antibiotics (**d**) would be the correct first step out of the available answer choices.

This patient will need an LP, but since antibiotic delay can increase mortality and it takes up to an hour for antibiotics to enter CSF and alter test results, antibiotics should always be administered prior to obtaining an LP (**c**). The patient will require hospitalization, most likely in the ICU (**e**), but first needs further stabilization and treatment in the ED. Not only is this patient 18, and allowed to make her own decisions, but in any emergent or altered state, patients should be administered life-saving treatments and thus, contacting her parents (**a**) is not immediately indicated. While a urine drug screening (UDS) (**b**) may be obtained as part of the altered mental status workup, in the setting of fever and hypotension, meningitis is much more likely and therefore treating the infection is a higher priority at the moment.

228. The answer is e. This patient presents with an anion gap metabolic acidosis, glucosuria, and ketonuria, which is consistent with **diabetic keto-acidosis (DKA)**. DKA is an acute, life-threatening disorder occurring in patients with insulin insufficiency. It results in hyperglycemia, ketosis, and osmotic diuresis, and clinically presents with gastrointestinal (GI) distress, polyuria, fatigue, dehydration, mental confusion, lethargy, or coma.

When the diagnosis of DKA is clinically suspected and hyperglycemia is confirmed by elevated point-of-care glucose, the results of blood gas and urinalysis confirm the diagnosis. In DKA, the liver metabolizes free fatty acids into ketone bodies for alternative fuel in the setting of cellular glucose underutilization. The result is **ketonuria** and **anion gap metabolic acidosis (pH < 7.4 and HCO$_3^-$ < 24)**. **Glucosuria**, the result of hyperglycemia-related osmotic diuresis, is another manifestation of DKA.

The anion gap is calculated by subtracting Cl$^-$ and HCO$_3^-$ from Na$^+$

Anion gap (AG) = [Na$^+$] − ([Cl$^-$] + [HCO$_3^-$])

A normal anion gap is 8 to 12 mEq/L. An elevated gap is a result of an increased concentration of unmeasured anions. In DKA, the elevated anion gap is caused by the production of ketones.

Other answers (**a, b, c, and d**) are incorrect choices in the DKA presentation.

229. The answer is b. The patient has **hepatic encephalopathy**, which is a clinical state of disordered cerebral function occurring secondary to acute or chronic liver disease. Laboratory tests may be normal in patients, but the serum ammonia level is usually elevated. **Lactulose and neomycin** represent the main therapeutic agents. Lactulose is a poorly absorbed sugar metabolized by colonic bacteria that traps ammonia and helps excrete it in the stool. Neomycin is a poorly absorbed aminoglycoside that is believed to act by reducing colonic bacteria responsible for producing ammonia.

No other antibiotics (**a, c, d, and e**) are indicated in the management of hepatic encephalopathy.

230. The answer is b. Generally, the **first-line** pharmacologic treatment in an actively seizing patient is a parental **benzodiazepine**, such as diazepam (Valium), lorazepam (Ativan), or midazolam (Versed). Benzodiazepines are effective in terminating seizure activity in 75% to 90% of patients. Diazepam can be administered intravenously, intramuscularly, or down an endotracheal tube. Lorazepam and midazolam can be given intravenously or intramuscularly. According to the ACEP clinical policy on seizures, midazolam or lorazepam should be used first-line, and IV lorazepam has been found to be clinically superior in terminating seizures when compared to IV diazepam.

Phenytoin (**a**) is a second-line agent that can be administered intravenously. Although the cause of the patient's seizure may be because of subtherapeutic levels of phenytoin, benzodiazepines are still the first-line therapy owing to their rapid onset. The onset of diazepam is 2 to 5 minutes while phenytoin is 10 to 30 minutes. In addition, phenytoin requires at least 20 minutes for administration because of its potential to cause hypotension and cardiac dysrhythmias. Phenobarbital (c) is a third-line agent. Its onset of action is 15 to 30 minutes. Valproic acid (d) is rarely used in the acute seizure setting. Levetiracetam (e) may be used in acute seizure management; however, it is currently not first-line therapy for acute seizure abortion or status epilepticus.

231. The answer is a. This patient has **postpartum eclampsia**, which needs to be managed with IV **magnesium sulfate** and admission to the obstetrical service. Preeclampsia is defined as new-onset hypertension (>140/90 mm Hg) and proteinuria (1 g/L in random specimen or >3 g/L over 24 hours). Some clinicians also use generalized edema as a requirement. Preeclampsia is most common in the third trimester. Eclampsia occurs with the development of seizures or coma in a patient with preeclampsia. A preeclamptic woman may worsen after delivery and develop late postpartum eclampsia, which usually occurs in the first 24 to 48 hours postpartum but may present several weeks after delivery. Management of eclamptic seizures in the ED involves administering magnesium sulfate, which is believed to act as a membrane stabilizer and vasodilator, reducing cerebral ischemia. Although magnesium sulfate is not a direct antihypertensive, the hypertension associated with eclampsia is often controlled adequately by treating the seizure.

Treating the seizure will most likely also lower the patient's BP. Fewer than 10% of eclamptic patients require specific antihypertensive therapy (b). Sumatriptan is the treatment for migraines (c), which this patient does not have. This patient's seizure is secondary to eclampsia. The first-line treatment is with magnesium sulfate. If the seizure is not treated despite appropriate magnesium sulfate, a benzodiazepine can be administered and etiologies of seizure other than eclampsia should be sought and treated (d and e).

232. The answer is b. The patient has a triad of **hypertension, bradycardia**, and **respiratory depression**, which is called **Cushing's reflex**. This is observed in one-third of patients with a potentially lethal **increase in ICP**. Increased ICP may result from traumatic brain injury or, as in this patient's case, from hemorrhagic stroke and subsequent brain edema. Tobacco and

cocaine use are known risk factors for **hemorrhagic stroke**. Increasing ICP can result in cerebral herniation, which has a mortality rate close to 100%. For any chance of survival, it must be rapidly controlled by intubation, elevation of the head of the bed, hyperventilation, mannitol, and definitive neurosurgical intervention.

Cushing's syndrome (a) describes the hyperadrenal state associated with increased production of cortisol, leading to hypertension, truncal obesity, abdominal striae, and hirsutism. Cullen's sign (c) is purplish discoloration around the umbilicus that results from intraperitoneal hemorrhage. Charcot's triad (d) constitutes fever, RUQ pain, and jaundice, and is associated with cholangitis. Chvostek's sign (e), associated with hypocalcemia, is twitching of the nose or lips with tapping of the facial nerve.

233. The answer is c. This patient presents with **alcohol withdrawal**. Signs and symptoms of this condition occur along a continuum ranging from simple shakes to delirium tremens (DTs) following a reduction or cessation of alcohol. Early symptoms usually appear 6 to 8 hours after cessation of drinking and involve tremulousness, anxiety, mild hypertension, and tachycardia. In more severe withdrawal, these symptoms worsen and paranoia, auditory, and visual hallucinations may develop proceeding to DTs with severe autonomic hyperactivity and profound altered mental status. DTs usually occur 3 to 5 days after alcohol cessation and carry 5% to 15% mortality even with supportive care. Additionally, alcohol withdrawal seizures may occur anywhere from 6 to 48 hours after cessation of alcohol. **Benzodiazepines** are the mainstay of therapy in alcohol withdrawal, as well as in sympathomimetic overdose and sedative-hypnotic withdrawal.

Acetaminophen (a) and labetalol (e) would treat the symptoms of low-grade fever and hypertension/tachycardia, respectively, without addressing the underlying etiology. Folate (b) should be given to all potentially undernourished patients, especially alcoholics, to prevent folate-deficient anemia. Dextrose was just administered by EMS without symptom improvement; however, point-of-care glucose (d) levels are important to check in all patients with altered mental status.

234. The answer is e. The patient has **hypertensive encephalopathy**, which is defined by a rapid rise in BP that is accompanied by **neurologic changes**. Patients typically present with a systolic BP greater than 220 mm Hg and diastolic BP greater than 110 mm Hg. Neurologic findings include severe headache, vomiting, drowsiness, confusion, seizure, blindness, focal neurologic deficits, or coma. Hypertensive emergency is a medical emergency. The goal of therapy is to stop and reverse the progression of end-organ dysfunction while maintaining organ perfusion and avoiding complications. Reduction in BP should be done rapidly but carefully. It is important to avoid dropping the pressure too low as this may lead to cerebral ischemia. **The immediate goal is to reduce the mean arterial BP by 20% to 30% of pretreatment levels over the first hour of therapy.** This can be accomplished by **labetalol,** a β_1-, β_2-, and α_1-receptor blocker. Another useful medication is nitroprusside, which is a better choice if the patient's BP is being monitored through an intraarterial line. Nitroprusside can cause a reflex tachycardia.

Propofol **(a)** is an excellent sedating agent that has a rapid onset of action and metabolizes quickly. It is also known to cause hypotension and apnea as side effects. However, it should not be used as an antihypertensive because of its unpredictable properties. Mannitol **(b)** is an osmotic agent that is used to lower ICP in patients with impending or actual brain herniation. It is not appropriate as an antihypertensive agent. Diuretics **(c)** are not useful to acutely lower BP but may be started as a maintenance antihypertensive. Lowering the BP to 140/80 mm Hg can cause cerebral ischemia **(d)**. The mean arterial pressure should only be lowered by 20% to 30% in the first hour.

235. The answer is b. The CSF analysis in **bacterial meningitis** typically shows an **elevated WBC count** with predominant **PMNs. Protein is elevated and glucose is low.** A Gram stain may show bacteria. The most specific marker for the diagnosis is a positive culture. Tests that evaluate the presence of antigen in the CSF (ie, latex agglutination studies) are particularly useful in the diagnosis of partially treated bacterial meningitis.

Tuberculosis meningitis **(a)** typically presents with less than 1000 WBC/μL with monocytic predominance. Symptoms are generally insidious in nature, typically not appearing until after a week has passed. In viral meningitis **(c)**, the CSF WBC count is made up of lymphocytes or monocytes, but early in the disease PMNs may predominate. CSF glucose is normal and protein is elevated in viral meningitis. A Gram stain will be negative and culture will show no growth. Fungal meningitis **(d)** is rare and generally presents in immunocompromised patients. LP usually reveals less than 500/μL WBCs. Encephalitis **(e)** is diagnosed by CSF culture or serology. CSF analysis that reveals blood is suspicious for herpes encephalitis.

Test	Normal	Bacterial	Viral	Fungal	TB
Protein	<50	>200	<200	>200	>200
Glucose	>40	<40	>40	<40	<40
WBCs	<5	>1000	<1000	<500	<1000
Cell type	Monos	>50% Polys	Monos	Monos	Monos
Gram stain	Negative	Positive	Negative	Negative	Positive (Acid-fast bacillus)

236. The answer is b. Bacterial meningitis is caused by different organisms in different age groups. Therefore, the empiric antibiotic therapy for suspected bacterial meningitis varies based on age. This older (>50-year-old) woman, who is immunocompromised and resides in a nursing home, needs coverage for *Listeria, Neisseria meningitidis,* and *Staphylococcus aureus.* **Vancomycin** covers methicillin-resistant Staphylococcus aureus (MRSA), **ampicillin** covers Listeria, and **ceftriaxone** is the best option to cover Neisseria. This regimen is also acceptable for neonates, who need covered for Group B streptococcus (GBS).

Vancomycin only or vancomycin and ceftriaxone (**c** and **a**) will not cover Listeria, which is needed in this elderly, immunocompromised patient. Valacyclovir and amphotericin B (**d, e**) would be indicated if the patient was suspected of having Herpes simplex or fungal meningitis, both of which are not indicated by this clinical presentation and LP results.

237. The answer is c. Hyponatremia is defined as a measured serum sodium less than 135 mEq/L. However, **the development of symptoms secondary to hyponatremia is related more to the rate of change in the serum sodium than to the absolute value.** Levels less than 120 mEq/L tend to cause symptoms regardless of the rate to reach this value. Symptoms can include confusion, lethargy, nausea, vomiting, anorexia, muscle cramps, and **seizures.** There are many causes of hyponatremia, including renal or GI losses, third-spacing, endocrine abnormalities, syndrome of inappropriate antidiuretic hormone (SIADH) release, cirrhosis, congestive heart failure (CHF), and nephrotic syndrome. Many medications cause SIADH, in addition to pulmonary and CNS disease. This patient, in particular, just started chemotherapy for lung cancer. The treatment for hyponatremia is guided by the cause of the process. If a patient is symptomatic (ie, seizing),

hypertonic saline (3%) should be carefully administered to raise the serum sodium to 120 mEq/L. A known complication of hypertonic saline is the development of central pontine myelinolysis.

0.45% and 0.9% **(a and b)** do not provide adequate amounts of sodium to raise the serum level and can actually cause a decrease serum sodium in certain conditions. Dextrose **(d and e)** is the treatment of choice for hypoglycemic patients.

238. The answer is c. NMS is a rare but potentially fatal reaction commonly associated with the use of **antipsychotic drugs**. The classic triad for its clinical presentation includes **altered mental status, hyperthermia, and muscle rigidity**. The cornerstone of treatment is supportive care with rapid cooling, fluid and electrolyte repletion, and monitoring. **Dantrolene**, a nonspecific skeletal muscle relaxant, generally used in the treatment of malignant hyperthermia, is also effective for NMS. In addition, benzodiazepines are useful in the treatment of NMS. The offending agent should be discontinued.

Haloperidol and droperidol are both antipsychotic medications **(a and b)** that can worsen the symptoms of NMS and should not be administered. Diphenhydramine **(d)**, an anticholinergic, should be avoided as it is ineffective and may worsen the reaction by interfering with temperature regulation. Acetaminophen **(e)**, an antipyretic, may help in lowering the temperature. However, NMS is a centrally mediated process. External cooling is more effective.

239. The answer is d. Hyperpyrexia is the symptom of NMS that is most associated with **severe morbidity and mortality**. The patient's temperature must be controlled and frequently with active cooling in addition to pharmacologic agents.

Muscle rigidity and an elevated CPK **(a and b)** go hand in hand NMS and may be markers of severity, but are not independently associated with mortality in NMS. NMS can cause hypertension and tachycardia **(c and e)**; however, hypotension and autonomic instability would be the greater concern. The presence of these are concerning, but not predictors of mortality.

240. The answer is a. This patient exhibits the classic triad of **Wernicke's encephalopathy (WE)—confusion, ataxia, and ophthalmoplegia**. WE is the result of **thiamine deficiency** leading to decreased glucose metabolism and neuronal destruction, primarily in the cerebellum, hypothalamus, vestibular system, and memory. It is typically found in **chronic alcoholics** caused by nutritional deficiency but can also occur in other malnutrition states, pregnancy, persistent vomiting, or dialysis. WE can mimic acute stroke symptoms and can lead to permanent nystagmus and ataxia. It carries 10% to 20% mortality if untreated. Eye examination findings in WE include horizontal nystagmus, vertical gaze palsy, or cranial nerve VII palsy. Cerebellar destruction presents with ataxic, wide-based gait. WE is a clinical diagnosis. Thiamine deficiency can also lead to the development of high-output cardiac failure and Korsakoff syndrome. The treatment is **parenteral thiamine supplementation**.

Korsakoff syndrome (**b**) is another sign of thiamine deficiency and involves disorientation and confabulation. Normal pressure hydrocephalus (**c**) presents with dementia, ataxic gait, and urinary incontinence. Head CT shows large ventricles. Central vertigo (**d**) is caused by lesions in the brainstem or cerebellum. It is associated with vertical or rotary nystagmus and nausea and vomiting. Alcohol withdrawal (**e**) typically presents with sympathetic and CNS overactivity.

241. The answer is e. This patient has **ascending cholangitis** as suggested by the presence of **Charcot's triad** of RUQ pain, jaundice, and fever. When these three symptoms are present with altered mental status and hypotension—known as **Reynaud's Pentad**—this is the classic picture of ascending cholangitis. In cholangitis, a stone blocks the common bile duct and allows bacteria to infect the biliary tree. The "classic" findings in Charcot's triad occur in 50% of patients; however, Reynaud's pentad, as seen in this patient, occurs in less than 5% of patients. When deciding on antibiotics for cholangitis, coverage is aimed at gram negatives (*Escherichia coli*, Enterococcus, Bacteroides) and anaerobes (Clostridium). Possible options for monotherapy include piperacillin-tazobactam (**e**), meropenem, imipenem, or doripenem.

Metronidazole (**a**) alone would not be sufficient monotherapy as it has poor action against gram-negative bacteria; a physician would need to add ciprofloxacin (**b**) to provide sufficient coverage. Likewise, gentamicin has poor activity against some of the anaerobes and would need at least metronidazole added. Vancomycin (**d**) would need to be added if there was a suspicion for MRSA, but would not be indicated otherwise and is a poor choice for monotherapy in this patient.

242. The answer is c. The patient presents with a rare but potentially life-threatening **NMS**. **Antipsychotic drugs** (ie, **haloperidol**) are the most common offending agents in the development of NMS, causing **central dopamine depletion**. The disorder is typically characterized by **hyperthermia, muscle rigidity, altered mental status**, and **autonomic instability**. Because NMS carries a high mortality, it is important to aggressively treat it with muscle relaxers, such as IV benzodiazepines, dantrolene, and dopamine agonists.

UTI (**a**) in a debilitated or nursing home patient can easily lead to altered mental status and sepsis. The patient's muscular rigidity, however, does not fit this diagnosis. The presentation of malignant hyperthermia (**b**) is similar to NMS, also involving hyperthermia and muscle rigidity. It is caused by anesthetic agents, which this patient did not receive. Dantrolene is also used for muscle relaxation in malignant hyperthermia. Recurrent stroke (**d**) is unlikely in this presentation with hyperthermia and muscle rigidity. Right-sided motor findings on examination are residual deficits from the old stroke. Meningoencephalitis (**e**) is certainly high on the differential in this patient but is unlikely to cause generalized muscular rigidity. It typically presents with fever, headache, nuchal rigidity, altered mental status, and focal neurologic signs.

243. The answer is e. The most likely diagnosis in this patient is Huntington's disease. Huntington's disease is a genetic, neurodegenerative disorder involving neurons, primarily in the caudate nucleus and the putamen. The hallmark imaging is **atrophy of the caudate**, causing enlargement of the ventricles with preserved cortex volume. Inheritance is an autosomal dominant pattern, causing a repeat of CAG trinucleotide on Chromosome 4. The disease process is characterized by uncontrollable, jerky, and random movements, called **chorea**, and **personality changes**, including irritability, depression, apathy, and impairment of executive functions.

Enlargement of the ventricles (**a**) is a nonspecific finding that can be seen in Alzheimer's disease, normal pressure hydrocephalus, and Huntington's. The distinguishing factors in these conditions are the way the ventricles affect the rest of the brain, notably the cortex, gyri, sulci, and caudate nucleus. Altered mental status can be caused by a variety of things that would result in a normal CT scan (**b**), but in this patient with chorea and personality changes, Huntington's is much more likely. Hyperintense signal in the basal cisterns (**c**) is indicative of a subarachnoid hemorrhage (SAH). SAH typically presents with severe headache of acute onset, classically described as "the worst headache of my life," with associated nausea and vomiting. Cerebral edema surrounding a mass that crosses the gray-white border (d) is indicative of a brain mass, most likely glioblastoma multiform (GBM). It is relatively uncommon to see masses on CT scan, as they are much better evaluated on MRI.

244. The answer is e. This patient presents with four of the five symptoms classically associated with **TTP**. These include **thrombocytopenia, hemolytic anemia, neurologic deficits, renal impairment, and fever.** TTP develops with fibrin-strand deposition in small vessels that attract platelets leading to platelet thrombi and thrombocytopenia. Passing RBCs get sheared in occluded vessels, resulting in microangiopathic hemolytic anemia. Renal and neurologic impairments occur because of the lodging of thrombi in respective circulations. Plasmapheresis decreases TTP mortality from 90% to 10%. Adjunct therapies include fresh frozen plasma infusion and steroids. It is important to realize that although patients may be severely thrombocytopenic, platelet infusion is contraindicated because it exacerbates the underlying cycle of thrombogenesis. **Risk factors for TTP** include pregnancy, **autoimmune disorders**, drugs, infection, and malignancy. Hemolytic uremic syndrome (HUS) is a closely related entity usually seen in children. There is pronounced renal dysfunction without altered mentation.

HSP (a) is a small-vessel vasculitis mostly seen in children and associated with a preceding upper respiratory illness in about 50% of patients. It is characterized by purpura (usually lower extremities), abdominal pain, and hematuria. Disseminated intravascular coagulation (DIC) (b) is a coagulopathic state triggered by major trauma, infection, malignancy, drugs, or pregnancy complications. The underlying process activates the coagulation cascade that leads to diffuse thrombosis and coagulopathy as platelets and coagulation factors are consumed. Patients with DIC have profuse GI or puncture site bleeding, markedly prolonged prothrombin time/partial thromboplastin time (PT/PTT) times, thrombocytopenia, and elevated fibrin split products. DIC management involves treatment of the underlying disorder and replacement of depleted coagulation cascade components. von Willebrand's disease (c) is the most common bleeding disorder and involves deficiency or defect in von Willebrand's factor, which normally aids in platelet adherence and carries factor VIII in plasma. von Willebrand's disease presents clinically with GI bleeding, epistaxis, easy bruising, and prolonged bleeding. ITP (d) is a disorder of antibody-mediated platelet destruction. It is acute in children, usually following a viral infection, and is chronic in adults who often require splenectomy for definitive treatment.

245. The answer is c. The emergency medicine physician is often faced with differentiating whether the cause of a patient losing consciousness is a result of syncope or a **seizure**. The most likely etiology of this patient's symptoms is in the history that she gives. She tells you that she has **not taken her antiseizure medications** in 2 days. Also, given her evolving mental status and improvement in alertness, this patient most likely presented in a **postictal state** after she has seized. Without any focal deficit and further improvement in her mental status, one might be comfortable with this diagnosis. Serum testing of her antiepileptic drug levels must be performed to further investigate this suspicion. A CT of the head, ECG, and further investigation is warranted if these levels are normal and do not explain her loss of consciousness.

Other neurologic causes, such as a CVA (**a**) and TIA (**b**) should also be in the differential. Typical TIA symptoms include any neurologic symptom, which improves within 30 minutes. In this case, however, the patient's history and presentation most likely precludes this diagnosis. The possibility of her having a stroke is further diminished by her normal neurologic examination. This patient did not complain of any chest or abdominal symptoms (**d and e**), which place aortic dissection and pulmonary embolus further down on the differential list.

246. The answer is c. This patient has **hypercalcemia**. She has the **classic symptoms** of "bones" (deep skeletal pains), "stones" (calcium oxalate crystals in the urine), "moans" (abdominal pain), and "psychiatric overtones" (confusion), in the setting of metastatic cancer. This is likely from metastatic lesions to the bones.

CA-125 (**a**) can be used to track progression in several types of cancer, most notably ovarian, but is not diagnostic and an elevated level will not explain altered mental status. While a CT of the head (**b**) is useful in the setting of altered mental status to evaluate for stroke or a space-occupying lesion, the lack of lateralizing signs or seizure and the other symptoms makes the head CT a lower yield study. Urine culture (**d**) would be confirmatory for a UTI; however, the urinalysis does not suggest a UTI as the cause. Urine drug screen (**e**) is unlikely to provide a diagnosis in this scenario.

247. The answer is e. **Zoledronic acid** is a bisphosphonate that is approved for the treatment of hypercalcemia and pain associated with metastatic cancer. The medication reduces bone reabsorption by inhibiting osteoclast activity and proliferation.

IV fluids and furosemide (a) are the initial treatment for hypercalcemia. Treatment is continuous and not suitable for long-term therapy. Thalidomide (b) is used for treatment of multiple myeloma. While multiple myeloma is a cause of hypercalcemia, this is not this patient's diagnosis. Parathyroidectomy (c) is used to treat hyperparathyroidism, a leading cause hypercalcemia. Phenoxybenzamine (d) is an irreversible α-receptor blocker used in the treatment of pheochromocytoma.

248. The answer is c. This child has **lead poisoning** which can lead to encephalopathy. Homes built before 1978 may have been painted with **lead-based paint**. The leading cause of lead poisoning in children is eating lead-based paint chips. Pica is a risk factor. He has severe **anemia**, caused by lead disrupting the formation of heme. Abdominal pain without physical findings **(lead colic)** and **peripheral neuropathy** are symptoms of lead poisoning. Abdominal X-rays may show **lead chips** in the stomach or intestines. Long bone X-rays may show dense bands **(lead lines)**, caused by osteoclast inhibition and increased calcium deposition. Lead is a potent neurotoxin and lead encephalopathy has high morbidity and potential for mortality.

A blood sugar (a) is recommended for evaluation of anyone with altered mental status; however, this child has been eating well and his symptoms have been progressive. Hypercalcemia (b) is a consideration given the altered mental status and abdominal pain; however, the other notable elements, such as pica, anemia, and lead lines on X-ray suggest lead poisoning. TSH (d) is for diagnosing hypothyroidism and myxedema coma. The typical presentation is an elderly patient with hypoglycemia, hypotension, hypothermia, hyponatremia, and bradycardia. Urine organic acids (e) are used for diagnosing in born errors of metabolism.

249. The answer is b. Dimercaprol is a chelating agent. It is given every 4 hours by a deep intramuscular (IM) injection. It is used for **lead and arsenic poisoning**. Other lead chelators include calcium disodium ethylenediamine tetraacetic acid (EDTA) and succimer.

Deferoxamine (a) is used for iron poisoning. Folinic acid (c) is the activated form of folic acid. It has many uses and is used to treat methotrexate overdose. N-acetylcysteine (**d**) is used for treating acetaminophen overdose. Lorazepam (**e**) is a benzodiazepine. It has many uses including acute control of seizure and intoxication with sympathomimetic agents.

250. The answer is d. This patient has **tertiary syphilis with tabes dorsalis**. He has personality change, ataxia, incontinence, Argyll Robertson pupil, and posterior spinal column signs (eg, wide-based, high-stepping gait). Diagnosis of neurosyphilis requires finding *Treponema pallidum* in a CSF sample.

Abnormal prions (**a**) would be found in Creutzfeldt-Jakob disease (CJD). Most cases (~85% are sporadic); however, it can be passed through exposure to implants, transplants, or neural tissue from infected individuals. CJD can be difficult to diagnose. Patients typically develop early dementia. Other neurologic manifestation may present based on which parts of the brain are most affected. MRI may be suggestive of the diagnosis. Biopsy may show abnormal prions or vacuolization of the brain. Gram-positive cocci in pairs in the CSF (**b**) would suggest meningitis from *Streptococcus pneumoniae*. The patient does not have the other symptoms of meningitis and the time frame is too long. White matter plaque on MRI would suggest multiple sclerosis (**c**). The typical eye-related findings include optic neuritis leading to visual loss, rather than accommodation without reactivity to light. HSV PCR (polymerase chain reaction) of the CSF (**e**) would diagnose herpes encephalitis. HSV typically affects the temporal lobe. Patients will present with altered mental status or personality changes, but will not have the dorsal spinal column findings.

251. The answer is e. Despite newer antibiotics, **penicillin** remains the treatment of choice for syphilis. A single dose of 2.4 million units of IM benzathine treats primary and secondary syphilis. A weekly dose of benzathine penicillin for 3 weeks treats latent syphilis. **Neurosyphilis is typically treated with 3 to 4 million units of IV penicillin every 4 hours for 10 to 14 days.**

Hospice would be the best treatment for CJD (**a**), as there is no known treatment. Vitamin B_{12} is (**b**) used to treat pernicious anemia and subacute combined degeneration of the spinal cord. Folic acid is used for a number of deficiencies. Interferon-β (**c**) is one of the first-line treatments for relapsing-remitting multiple sclerosis. IV acyclovir (**d**) treats herpes simplex infection.

252. The answer is c. This patient has **Addison's disease** and is having a crisis, most likely from running out of her medications. The typical presentation includes abdominal pain, nausea, vomiting, and altered mental status. The examination shows the characteristic skin finding from elevated adrenocorticotropic hormone (ACTH) levels. **Hyponatremia, hyperkalemia, and hypercalcemia** are characteristic. The treatment is to replace glucocorticoids and mineralocorticoids as soon as possible. **Hydrocortisone and fludrocortisone** are typically administered.

Addisonian crisis can be triggered by an infectious etiology; however, the first treatment is cortisone replacement. The CSF studies are not suggestive of meningitis. Meningitis typically presents with WBC count greater than 1000 mm^3, low CSF glucose, and high protein. Therefore, antibiotics such as vancomycin **(a)** are not warranted at this time. Diphenhydramine **(b)** would be used for anaphylactic shock. The skin findings are typically erythema or urticarial. Norepinephrine **(d)** may be necessary to bring up the patient's BP until there is a response to the hydrocortisone; however, steroids should be administered as soon as the diagnosis is made. PTU **(e)** treats hyperthyroidism. It decreases thyroid hormone production and decreases thyroid hormone release.

253. The answer is a. In this patient with known COPD, who is not moving air well on exam (shallow breaths), it is reasonable to assume this is a COPD exacerbation and **CO_2 narcosis**, a condition where patients can develop depressed mental status, lethargy, and somnolence due to a toxic level of CO_2 in the blood. This condition is caused by hypoventilation or underlying lung disease where not enough oxygen enters circulation and not enough carbon dioxide is emitted on expiration. Therefore, an **ABG** would be most reasonable to assess this patient's clinical status and confirm an abnormally high CO_2 level.

An LP **(b)** would be best to evaluate meningitis as a cause of altered mental status, however, this patient displays no signs of meningitis, such as shock, fever, or rash, making it a much less likely diagnosis. In the absence of hypertension, anticoagulation, known family history, focal neurologic deficits, or other risk factors, an intracranial hemorrhage—which is best detected by CT head without contrast **(c)**—is much less likely and not the first step in evaluation. Carbon monoxide (CO) poisoning is first detected by carboxyhemoglobin saturation **(d)**. CO poisoning can present with "flu-like" symptoms including headache, dizziness, weakness, vomiting, and/or chest pain, but also can present as confusion, altered mental status, or seizures in severe cases. Risk factors for CO poisoning include fires, faulty furnaces, and cigarette smoking. While this patient smokes, his physical exam and history make CO poisoning less likely. An ammonia (e) level would be useful if the patient had a known history of liver disease, or clinical signs of decompensated liver failure, such as telangiectasias, abdominal distention, ascites, or palmar erythema.

254. The answer is d. In this patient, the most appropriate step is **endotracheal intubation**. When a patient is altered from CO_2 intoxication, the treatment is to provide assistance in breathing off the gas, either by ventilation (endotracheal intubation) or by BiPAP.

Patients must be awake to be safely treated with BiPAP (**b**), as the risk of aspiration is high for those who cannot protect their own airway. This patient is far too somnolent to tolerate BiPAP and therefore requires endotracheal intubation. Blood cultures and broad-spectrum antibiotics (**a**) would be the appropriate step, if the patient was suspected to be altered due to septic shock; however, the patient is not febrile or hypotensive on examination. If the patient had a history of liver disease, elevated ammonia level, or physical exam findings suspicious for decompensated cirrhosis, lactulose (**c**) would be the appropriate treatment. Lastly, hyperbaric oxygen (**e**) would be the appropriate treatment for CO poisoning, not CO_2 narcosis.

Recommended Readings

ACEP Now. Best Practices for Seizure Management in the Emergency Department. Available at: www.acepnow.com/article/best-practices-seizure-management-emergency-department. Accessed June 15, 2020.

Bassin BS, Cooke JL. Chapter 16. Depressed consciousness and coma. In: Marx JA, Hockberger RS, Walls RM, et al, eds. *Rosen's Emergency Medicine: Concepts and Clinical Practice.* 8th ed. Philadelphia, PA: Saunders, 2014.

Feller-Kopman DJ, Schwartzstein RM. The Evaluation, Diagnosis, and Treatment of the Adult Patient with Acute Hypercapnic Respiratory Failure. In: Stoller JK. UpToDate. 2019. Available at: www.uptodate.com/contents/the-evaluation-diagnosis-and-treatment-of-the-adult-patient-with-acute-hypercapnic-respiratory-failure. Accessed June 15, 2020.

Han JH, Wilber ST. Altered mental status in elderly patients. *Clin Geriatr Med.* 2013;29(1):101-136.

Huff JS. Chapter 17. Confusion. In: Marx JA, Hockberger RS, Walls RM, et al, eds. *Rosen's Emergency Medicine: Concepts and Clinical Practice.* 8th ed. Philadelphia, PA: Saunders, 2014.

Lung DD, Catlett CL, Tintinalli JE. Chapter 165. Emergencies after 20 weeks of pregnancy and the postpartum period. In: Tintinalli JE, Stapczynski J, Ma O, eds. *Tintinalli's Emergency Medicine: A Comprehensive Study Guide.* 7th ed. New York, NY: McGraw-Hill, 2011.

Solomkin JS, Mazuski JE, Bradley JS, et al. Diagnosis and management of complicated intra-abdominal infection in adults and children: guidelines by the Surgical Infection Society and the Infectious Diseases Society of America. *Clin Infect Dis.* 2010;50:133.

van de Beek D, Brouwer MC, Thwaites GE, et al. Advances in treatment of bacterial meningitis. *Lancet.* 2012;380(9854):1693-1702.

Gastrointestinal Bleeding

Nicole A. Bonk, MD

Questions

255. A 45-year-old woman presents to the emergency department (ED) with 1 day of painful rectal bleeding. Review of systems is negative for weight loss, abdominal pain, nausea, and vomiting. On physical examination, you note an exquisitely tender area of swelling with engorgement and a bluish discoloration distal to the anal verge. Her vital signs are blood pressure (BP) 140/70 mm Hg, heart rate (HR) 105 beats/minute, respiratory rate (RR) 18 breaths/minute, and temperature 99°F. Which of the following is the next best step in management?

a. Recommend warm sitz baths, topical analgesics, stool softeners, high-fiber diet, and arrange for surgical follow-up
b. Incision and drainage under local anesthesia followed by packing and surgical follow-up
c. Obtain a complete blood count (CBC), clotting studies, type and cross, and arrange for emergent colonoscopy
d. Excision under local anesthesia followed by sitz baths and analgesics
e. Surgical consult for immediate operative management

256. A 20-year-old man presents to the ED with fever and severe right lower quadrant (RLQ) pain for 1 day. Prior to this episode, he reports 2 months of crampy abdominal pain, generalized malaise, a 10-lb weight loss, and occasional bloody diarrhea. On examination, his BP is 125/70 mm Hg, HR is 115 beats/minute, RR is 18 breaths/minute, and temperature is 100.8°F. His only significant past medical history is recurrent perirectal abscesses. He appears uncomfortable and has a tender mass in the RLQ, without guarding or rebound. Rectal examination is positive for trace heme-positive stool. An abdominal computed tomographic (CT) scan reveals no periappendiceal fat stranding. There is inflammation of the distal ileum and several areas of the colon. There are no rectal inflammatory changes. Which of the following is the most likely diagnosis?

a. Crohn's disease
b. Ulcerative colitis
c. Appendicitis
d. Pseudomembranous enterocolitis
e. Diverticulitis

257. A 62-year-old woman with known history of coronary artery disease on aspirin and clopidogrel presents to the ED with bright red blood per rectum. Patient reports that she has had intermittent blood in her stool for the past 2 days. Just prior to arrival, she had two episodes of large volume bright red bloody stools. Her temperature is 98.6°F, HR is 98 beats/minute, and BP is 115/74 mm Hg. She reports mild cramping that resolved and is not having any pain at this time. A hemoglobin in the ER is 8.6 mg/dL (hematocrit 26%) and white blood cell (WBC) count 7000/µL. Previous colonoscopy records show colonic diverticula. She does not have any bloody bowel movements during her stay in the emergency room (ER). Which is the most appropriate diagnostic work-up for this patient?

a. CT abdomen and pelvis
b. Admit for bowel clean out and colonoscopy
c. Discharge for outpatient gastrointestinal (GI) follow-up
d. Tagged red blood cell (RBC) scan
e. Small bowel capsule endoscopy

258. A 62-year-old man with a history of hypertension presents to the ED with severe constant mid-epigastric pain for the past hour. Over the last several months, he has had intermittent pain shortly after eating, but never this severe. He states he now has generalized abdominal pain that began suddenly about 15 minutes ago. He denies trauma, has never had surgery, and takes no medications. His vitals include BP of 170/105 mm Hg supine, falling to 145/85 mm Hg when sitting up with HR of 115 beats/minute lying supine, increasing to 135 beats/minute when sitting up. He appears pale. His abdomen is rigid and diffusely tender with guarding and rebound. Bowel sounds are absent and stool hemoccult is positive. The WBC count is 8500/µL, hemoglobin 8.5 mg/dL, hematocrit 27%, and platelets 255/µL. Which of the following is the most likely diagnosis?

a. Boerhaave syndrome
b. Perforated gastric ulcer
c. Abdominal aortic aneurysm (AAA)
d. Inflammatory bowel disease (IBD)
e. Diverticulosis

259. A 60-year-old man with a history of alcohol abuse presents to the ED with hematemesis for 1 day. He denies abdominal or chest pain. On physical examination, his eyes appear reddened which he attributes to having drunken heavily the night before. He also reports vomiting several times after this recent binge. Vital signs are BP 130/85 mm Hg, HR 115 beats/minute,

RR 18 breaths/minute, and temperature 99.5°F. Chest radiograph is unremarkable. Laboratory results reveal a WBC 10,000/μL, hemoglobin 14 mg/dL, hematocrit 40%, and platelets 210/μL. Which diagnosis is endoscopic evaluation most likely to confirm?

a. Esophageal varices
b. Boerhaave syndrome
c. Curling ulcer
d. Perforated gastric ulcer
e. Mallory-Weiss tear

The following scenario applies to questions 260 and 261.

A 50-year-old man is brought to the ED by ambulance with significant hematemesis. In the ambulance, paramedics placed two large-bore IVs and began infusing normal saline. In the ED, his BP is 79/45 mm Hg, HR is 127 beats/minute, RR is 24 breaths/minute, temperature is 97.9°F, and oxygen saturation is 92%. His abdomen is nontender, but you note spider angiomata, palmar erythema, and gynecomastia. The patient continues to have large volume hemoptysis in the ED. Laboratory results reveal WBC 9000/μL, hematocrit 28%, platelets 40/μL, aspartate transaminase (AST) 675 U/L, alanine transaminase (ALT) 325 U/L, alkaline phosphatase 95 U/L, total bilirubin 14.4 mg/dL, conjugated bilirubin 12.9 mg/dL, sodium 135 mEq/L, potassium 3.5 mEq/L, chloride 110 mEq/L, bicarbonate 26 mEq/L, blood urea nitrogen (BUN) 40 mg/dL, creatinine 1.1 mg/dL, and glucose 150 mg/dL.

260. Which of the following is the most likely diagnosis?

a. Perforated gastric ulcer
b. Diverticulosis
c. Splenic laceration
d. Esophageal varices
e. Ruptured AAA

261. What are the most appropriate next steps in management?

a. Emergent gastroenterology (GI) consultation for esophagogastroduodenoscopy (EGD) and sclerotherapy
b. Transfusion of two units of packed red blood cells (PRBCs)
c. IV norepinephrine for vasopressor support
d. Endotracheal intubation for airway protection
e. Pantoprazole bolus followed by continuous pantoprazole infusion

262. Which of the following medications can assist in temporizing the bleeding associated with esophageal varices?

a. Octreotide
b. Glucagon
c. Insulin
d. Phenylephrine
e. Epinephrine

263. If the adverse event rate of performing endoscopy with sclerotherapy alone is 50% and the adverse event rate of administering octreotide followed by endoscopy with sclerotherapy is 30%, what is the number of patients you need to treat with octreotide to prevent one bad outcome?

a. Four patients
b. Seven patients
c. Ten patients
d. Five patients
e. Two patients

264. A 70-year-old woman presents to the ED with dark stool for 3 weeks. She occasionally notes bright red blood mixed with the stool. Review of systems is positive for decreased appetite, constipation, and a 10-lb weight loss over 2 months. She denies abdominal pain, nausea, vomiting, and fever, but feels increased weakness and fatigue. She also describes a raspy cough with white sputum production over the previous 2 weeks. Examination reveals she is pale, with a supine BP of 115/60 mm Hg and HR of 90 beats/minute. Standing BP is 100/50 mm Hg and HR is 105 beats/minute. Which of the following is the most likely diagnosis?

a. Hemorrhoids
b. Diverticulitis
c. Mallory-Weiss tear
d. Diverticulosis
e. Adenocarcinoma

The following scenario applies to questions 265 and 266.

A 76-year-old woman with a history of congestive heart failure, coronary artery disease, and an "irregular heart beat" is brought to the ED by her family. She has been complaining of increasing abdominal pain over the past several days. She denies nausea or vomiting and bowel movements remain unchanged. Vitals are BP of 110/75 mm Hg, HR of 114 beats/minute, and temperature of 98°F. She appears to be in significant pain. Her HR is irregular with no murmur detected. The abdomen is soft, nontender, and nondistended. The stool is heme-positive.

265. What is the most likely diagnosis?
a. Perforated gastric ulcer
b. Diverticulitis
c. Acute cholecystitis
d. Mesenteric ischemia
e. Sigmoid volvulus

266. What is the gold standard utilized to diagnose this condition?
a. Serum lactate levels
b. Abdominal radiograph (supine and upright)
c. CT scan
d. Angiography
e. Barium contrast study

The following scenario applies to questions 267 and 268.

A 27-year-old man presents to the ED with significant epigastric abdominal pain. He is generally healthy, but did recently sustain an ankle sprain playing soccer. He reports that he has been having worsening heartburn for the past several days, but tonight it became severe and he was nauseous. He had one episode of coffee ground emesis prior to arrival. On further questioning, he admits his stools have become black and tarry over the past few days as well. He has an HR of 110 beats/minute and BP of 110/75 mm Hg. His hemoglobin is 9.8 mg/dL. You start IV fluids and call for a GI consult as you think he may need an upper endoscopy.

267. Which medication should you consider starting in the ED?
a. Octreotide
b. Calcium carbonate
c. Famotidine
d. Pantoprazole
e. Acetaminophen

268. The upper endoscopy confirms a diagnosis of peptic ulcer disease (PUD). Use of which of the medications likely contributed to the development of his ulcer?

a. Acetaminophen
b. Naproxen
c. Cetirizine
d. Zolpidem
e. Fluoxetine

269. A 55-year-old man with hypertension and end-stage renal disease requiring hemodialysis presents with 2 days of painless hematochezia. He reports similar episodes of bleeding in the past, which were attributed to angiodysplasia. He denies abdominal pain, nausea, vomiting, diarrhea, and fever. His vitals include BP of 145/95 mm Hg, HR of 90 beats/minute, RR of 18 breaths/minute, and temperature of 98°F. His abdomen is soft and nontender, and his stool is grossly positive for blood. Which of the following are true regarding angiodysplasia?

a. Cause of greater than 50% of acute lower GI bleeding
b. More common in younger patients
c. Angiography is the most sensitive method for diagnosis
d. Less common in patients with end-stage renal disease
e. Majority are located on the right side of the colon

The following scenario applies to questions 270 and 271.

A 68-year-old man presents to the ED 4 hours after an upper endoscopy was performed for evaluation of progressive dysphagia. During the procedure, a 1-cm ulcerated lesion was found and biopsied. Now, the patient complains of severe neck and chest pain. His vitals are BP 135/80 mm Hg, HR 123 beats/minute, RR 26 breaths/minute, and temperature 101°F. On physical examination, he appears diaphoretic and in moderate distress with crepitus in the neck and a crunching sound over the heart.

270. Which of the following can confirm the suspected diagnosis?

a. Bronchoscopy
b. Electrocardiogram (ECG)
c. Repeat endoscopy
d. Thoracotomy
e. Esophagram with water-soluble agent

271. Which of the following medications should be administered as soon as the diagnosis is suspected?

a. Octreotide
b. Clindamycin
c. Piperacillin-tazobactam
d. Glucagon
e. Atropine

272. An 11-month-old baby presents with her mother due to complaints of blood in the baby's stool. Her mother reports that the past three diapers had blood in them. The patient was recently transitioned from breast milk to formula. She started solid foods 3 months ago and has been varying her diet. She previously had 5 to 6 soft bowel movements daily, now has been having a hard stool every other day and appears to be in pain while passing the stool. What should be done next?

a. Allergy testing
b. Change formula
c. Colonoscopy
d. Abdominal X-ray
e. Physical exam

273. A 75-year-old man with a history of AAA status post repair presents with a complaint of cramping abdominal pain and one episode of bright red blood per rectum. He notes approximately 1 cup of blood with his last bowel movement. He has some mild abdominal cramping and a sense that "I am about to die." Vitals include BP 100/70 mm Hg, HR 110 beats/minute, RR 22 breaths/minute, and temperature 97.8°F. What is the most important first step in management?

a. Secure the airway by performing endotracheal intubation
b. Order two units of crossmatched blood from the blood bank
c. Performing a digital rectal examination to evaluate for guaiac positive stool
d. Placing two large bore IVs
e. Performing a bedside, point-of-care ultrasound of the patient's abdomen

274. An otherwise healthy 23-year-old woman presents with diffuse abdominal cramping, fever, and multiple episodes of bloody diarrhea throughout the day. She has had fevers despite taking Tylenol at home. She and her friends ate a spinach salad at a restaurant the previous night. Her friends are also ill. On physical examination, she appears ill, pale, and has dry mucous membranes. Her vitals include BP 100/70 mm Hg, HR 140 beats/minute, RR 24 breaths/minute, and temperature 102.1°F. Which of the following is the most likely etiology of the patient's symptoms?

a. *Salmonella*
b. *Shigella*
c. *Vibrio cholerae*
d. *Campylobacter*
e. *Escherichia coli* O157:H7

The following scenario applies to questions 275 and 276.

A previously healthy 14-month-old child presents with his parents for complaints of abdominal pain and lethargy. Parents note that over the past several days, he has seemed to have intermittent abdominal pain that involves him pulling his legs into his chest and screaming. He is normal between these episodes. They also note he has had some squishy red stools on the day of presentation, has vomited twice, and has become more lethargic over the past several hours. Examination reveals a child who is difficult to arouse, warm to the touch, and pale. Vitals include BP 90/60 mm Hg, HR 150 beats/minute, RR 30 breaths/minute, and temperature 102.4°F.

275. Which of the following is the most likely diagnosis?

a. Intussusception
b. Meckel diverticulum
c. Malrotation
d. Appendicitis
e. Pyloric stenosis

276. What is the most appropriate management for this condition?

a. Consult surgery for immediate operative intervention
b. Consult GI for immediate endoscopy
c. Begin a high-dose proton-pump inhibitor (PPI) infusion
d. Start IV fluids, broad-spectrum antibiotics, and admit to the pediatric intensive care unit
e. Consult radiology for immediate air enema decompression

The following scenario applies to questions 277 and 278.

A 78-year-old woman with a known history of hypertension controlled on hydrochlorothiazide presents to the ED with bright red blood per rectum and crampy abdominal pain. She reports fevers, chills, body aches, nausea, vomiting, and diarrhea 2 days prior to presentation. The fevers have resolved, but she has still been quite fatigued with no appetite. The morning of presentation, she developed crampy pain and frequent stools with bright red blood. She appears pale and reports lightheadedness when she sits up. On examination, she is found to have a BP of 85/40 mm Hg, HR is 110 beats/minute, temperature of 98.6°F, and tenderness in the left lower quadrant (LLQ) of her abdomen.

277. Which of the following is the next best step?

a. Nasogastric (NG) tube lavage
b. Start IV crystalloid infusion
c. Transfuse 2 units of packed RBCs
d. Computed tomography (CT) angiography of abdomen and pelvis
e. Stool studies

278. What is the most likely cause of her bright red blood per rectum?

a. Ischemic colitis
b. Diverticulitis
c. *Shigella*
d. Appendicitis
e. Adenocarcinoma

Gastrointestinal Bleeding

Answers

255. The answer is d. This patient is suffering from an acutely **thrombosed external hemorrhoid**. **Hemorrhoids** are dilated venules of the hemorrhoidal plexuses. They are associated with constipation, straining, increased abdominal pressure, pregnancy, increased portal pressure, and a low-fiber diet. Hemorrhoids can be either internal or external. Those that arise above the dentate line are internal and painless. Those below the dentate line are external and painful. Individuals commonly present with thrombosed external hemorrhoids. On examination, there is a tender mass at the anal orifice that is typically bluish-purple in color. **If pain is severe and the thrombosis is less than 48 hours, the physician should excise the thrombus under local anesthesia followed by a warm sitz baths.** If not excised, symptoms will most often resolve within several days when the hemorrhoid ulcerates and leaks the dark accumulated blood. Residual skin tags may persist. Excision provides both immediate- and long-term relief and prevents the formation of skin tags.

The symptoms of nonthrombosed external and nonprolapsing internal hemorrhoids can be improved by the **WASH** regimen **(a)**. **Warm water**, via sitz baths or by directing a shower stream at the affected area for several minutes, reduces anal pressures; mild oral **analgesics** relieve pain; **stool softeners** ease the passage of stool to avoid straining; and a **high-fiber diet** produces stool that passes more easily. **Incision** of a hemorrhoid (as opposed to **excision**) leads to incomplete clot evacuation, subsequent rebleeding, and swelling of lacerated vessels **(b)**. This patient has a thrombosed external hemorrhoid. It is recommended that she have a colonoscopy as she is over 40 and has had rectal bleeding, however it does not need to be done on an emergent basis **(c)**. Hemorrhoids rarely require immediate operative management, unless there is evidence of thrombus formation with progression to gangrene **(e)**.

256. The answer is a. IBD refers to chronic inflammatory disease of the GI tract. There are two major types—**Crohn's disease and ulcerative colitis. Crohn's disease** can involve any part of the GI tract, from mouth to anus, and is characterized by segmental involvement. The distal ileum is involved in the majority of cases; therefore, acute presentations can mimic appendicitis. Crohn's disease spares the rectum in 50% of cases. There is a bimodal age distribution, with the first peak occurring in patients 15 to 22 years of age and a second in patients 55 to 60 years of age. Definitive diagnosis is by upper GI series, air-contrast barium enema, and colonoscopy. Segmental involvement of the colon with rectal sparing is the most characteristic feature. Other findings on colonoscopy include involvement of all bowel wall layers, **skip lesions** (ie, interspersed normal and diseased bowel), **aphthous ulcers**, and **cobblestone** appearance from submucosal thickening interspersed with mucosal ulceration. Extraintestinal manifestations are seen in 25% to 30% of patients with Crohn's disease.

Ulcerative colitis **(b)** primarily involves the mucosa only with formation of crypt abscesses, epithelial necrosis, and mucosal ulceration. Rectal pain and bloody diarrhea are more common in ulcerative colitis than in Crohn's disease. Ulcerative colitis begins in the rectum, and fails to progress beyond this point in one-third of patients. Colonoscopy demonstrates inflammation of the mucosa only and continuous lesions of the GI tract. Although blood loss from sustained bleeding may be the most common complication, toxic megacolon must not be missed. While appendicitis **(c)** may be in the differential diagnosis, the acute chronic nature of this disease and a normal-appearing appendix on abdominal CT rules it out. Pseudomembranous enterocolitis **(d)** is an IBD that results from toxin-producing *Clostridium difficile*, a spore-forming obligate anaerobic bacillus. The disease typically begins 7 to 10 days after the institution of antibiotic therapy, most often in hospitalized patients. However, incidence in the community is rising. Diverticulitis **(e)** is an acute inflammatory disease caused by bacterial proliferation within existing colonic diverticula. The most common presentation is pain, often in the LLQ. Abdominal CT demonstrates inflammation of pericolic fat, presence of diverticula, bowel wall thickening, or peridiverticular abscess.

257. The answer is b. This patient should be **admitted for bowel clean out and colonoscopy**. Patient likely has bleeding from diverticulosis. Diverticula are small outpouchings in the wall of the colon. They can become inflamed and cause diverticulitis which is painful and typically associated with an elevated inflammatory marker (WBC). Diverticulitis does not usually cause painless bleeding.

The patient is hemodynamically stable and does not have any active bleeding therefore might be eligible for outpatient follow-up (**c**). However, she is anemic and on aspirin and clopidogrel, therefore it would not be safe for her to be discharged without further evaluation. A CT abdomen and pelvis (**a**) would be more useful in the setting of acute abdominal pain or concern for inflammation, such as colitis or diverticulitis. A tagged RBC scan (**d**) is useful when a patient is continuing to have active bleeding. Evaluation of the small bowel with capsule endoscopy (**e**) may ultimately be necessary if no other source is identified but is not the first step in evaluation.

258. The answer is b. This patient had an untreated **gastric ulcer** that just **perforated**. The history of epigastric pain related to eating points to a gastric ulcer, whereas pain 2 to 3 hours after eating is more likely caused by a duodenal ulcer. The sudden onset of generalized abdominal pain associated with a rigid abdomen is concerning for a perforated viscus (ie, perforated gastric ulcer). This is a **surgical emergency**. An abdominal and upright chest radiograph can be performed quickly to look for **free air under the diaphragm** on the chest radiograph. This is useful for the majority of perforations, which are anterior, but may miss posterior perforations because the posterior duodenum is retroperitoneal. The treatment includes IV hydration, antibiotics, and immediate surgical correction.

Boerhaave syndrome (**a**) is a full-thickness tear of the left posterolateral aspect of the distal esophagus. It is typically associated with epigastric and retrosternal chest pain that often radiates to the back, neck, left chest, or shoulders. Although it may present similar to a perforated ulcer, in general the pain is more focused in the chest. While the history of untreated hypertension is concerning for a ruptured AAA (**c**), the history clearly points to previously undiagnosed PUD. IBD (**d**) is a chronic condition affecting the GI tract. The abdominal pain is usually crampy, while GI bleeding is generally associated with bloody diarrhea. Diverticula (**e**) are saclike herniations of colonic mucosa that occur at weak points in the bowel wall. They may bleed (diverticulosis) or become filled with fecal matter and lead to inflammation (diverticulitis). Diverticulosis is most commonly associated with substantial painless rectal bleeding but not with significant abdominal pain.

259. The answer is e. A **Mallory-Weiss tear** usually follows a **forceful bout of retching** and vomiting and involves a 1- to 4-cm tear of the **mucosa or submucosa of the GI tract**; 75% of cases occur in the stomach with the remainder near the gastroesophageal (GE) junction. Bleeding is usually mild and self-limited. However, 3% of deaths attributed to upper GI bleeding result from Mallory-Weiss tears.

Esophageal varices **(a)** are dilated submucosal veins found in 50% of patients with cirrhosis of the liver. They usually develop as a result of portal hypertension. Up to 30% of patients with esophageal varices develop massive upper GI bleeding. Patients are often asymptomatic until the varices rupture and bleed. Although this patient is certainly predisposed to varices secondary to his ethanol abuse, his acute presentation of pain after vomiting is more consistent with a Mallory-Weiss tear. Boerhaave syndrome **(b)** involves a spontaneous full-thickness perforation of the esophagus—80% involving the posterolateral aspect of the distal esophagus—that usually results from violent retching. Alcohol ingestion is a risk factor. Because the overlying pleura is torn, esophageal contents can spill into the mediastinum and thorax, leading to severe epigastric and retrosternal chest pain, with radiations to the back, neck, or shoulders. Characteristic findings on chest radiograph include a left pneumothorax, a left pleural effusion, mediastinal emphysema, and a widened mediastinum, all of which the individual in the question does not exhibit. Boerhaave syndrome represents a surgical emergency, with mortality approaching 50%, if surgery is not performed within 24 hours. A Curling ulcer **(c)** is an ulcer or erosion caused by stress gastritis because of patients with severe burn injuries. The most common finding is painless GI bleeding. There is no evidence of severe burn injury in this patient. A perforated gastric ulcer **(d)** is a complication of chronic gastritis, which is usually associated with severe, acute abdominal pain. Perforations occur when an ulcer erodes through the wall and leaks air and digestive contents into the peritoneal cavity. Often, pain initially begins in the epigastrium but becomes generalized shortly thereafter. Patients usually lie still and avoid movement that might disturb the peritoneal cavity. An upright chest radiograph may demonstrate air under the diaphragm.

260. The answer is d. Esophageal varices develop in patients with **chronic liver disease** in response to **portal hypertension**. Approximately 60% of patients with portal hypertension will develop varices. Of those who develop varices, 25% to 30% will experience hemorrhage. Patients who develop varices from alcohol abuse have an even higher risk of bleeding, especially with ongoing alcohol consumption. This patient has evidence of chronic liver disease with thrombocytopenia and elevated bilirubin and liver enzymes. In alcoholic hepatitis, the AST is greater than the ALT by a factor of 2. Spider angiomata, palmar erythema, and gynecomastia further suggest underlying liver disease.

A perforated gastric ulcer (**a**) typically presents with severe sudden abdominal pain in a patient with a history of PUD. Diverticulosis (**b**) results from saclike herniations in the colonic mucosa (diverticula) that occurs at weak points in the bowel wall, usually where arteries insert. Diverticulosis is most commonly associated with painless rectal bleeding. Splenic laceration (**c**) generally results from trauma. The most common symptom with rupture of an AAA (**e**) is sudden and severe abdominal pain. Back pain, also sudden and severe, is noted by half of patients. Incidence of AAA increases with age in both men and women and is typically associated with a history of hypertension.

261. The answer is d. The management of critical patients in emergency medicine should start with the ABCs. In a patient with severe hematemesis, the patient is often in jeopardy of losing his or her airway and/or aspirating blood. **Frank recurrent hematemesis in a critically ill patient is an indication for endotracheal intubation to protect the airway**.

The definitive management is emergent GI consultation for EGD and sclerotherapy or banding (**a**) of patient's esophageal varices. Transfusing blood (**b**) is also indicated in this instance; however, this falls under the "C" of ABCs and should be done after the airway is secured. Norepinephrine (**c**) is often used for vasopressor support; however, in this instance, the patient needs volume (ie, blood) as opposed to vasoconstriction in order to improve his or her BP. A pantoprazole bolus and infusion (**e**) would be indicated in an upper GI bleed; however, this is secondary to the ABCs and can be started after the patient has been intubated and received blood.

262. The answer is a. Octreotide is a somatostatin analog that is used in esophageal varices to **reduce portal venous pressure**, which is thought to reduce bleeding.

Glucagon (**b**) is a peptide secreted from α cells in the pancreas that acts as an antagonist to insulin. It is released when blood glucose is low. Its primary responsibility is to mobilize glucose by acting in the liver and causing stored glycogen to be converted to glucose. Glucagon can also be used in β-blocker overdose and in patients with anaphylaxis who take β-blockers. It has no use in GI bleeding secondary to esophageal varices. Insulin (**c**) is a peptide secreted from β cells in the pancreas that acts to reduce blood glucose levels. It does this by stimulating the uptake and storage of glucose by liver and adipose tissue. Insulin has no use in GI bleeding secondary to esophageal varices. Phenylephrine (**d**) is an α-adrenergic receptor agonist that acts to vasoconstrict blood vessels. Phenylephrine works primarily on peripheral circulation as opposed to portal venous circulation. Epinephrine (**e**) is a nonselective α- and β-agonist that causes increased inotropy, bronchodilation, and peripheral vasoconstriction. Epinephrine has not been shown to work in the portal venous system and would likely have adverse effects of increasing portal venous pressure if it did have any cross-over effects on portal venous pressure.

263. The answer is d. To calculate **number needed to treat (NNT)**, you must first devise the **absolute risk reduction (ARR)**. In order to do this, you must subtract the experimental event rate (EER) from the control event rate (CER). The CER is 50% (0.5) and the EER 30% (0.3) in this question. Thus, the **ARR is 20%** or 0.2 (0.5 − 0.3 = 0.2). **The NNT is 1/ARR;** in this question it is 1/0.2 = 5. Thus, the NNT is five patients.

All other answer choices (**a, b, c, and e**) are incorrect based on the previous calculation.

264. The answer is e. The combination of lower GI bleed with weight loss and decreased appetite points toward carcinoma, most likely **adenocarcinoma of the colon**. The lack of esophageal, abdominal, or rectal pain makes the other choices unlikely, as does the lack of associated symptoms (nausea, vomiting, or fever). Anemia or rectal bleeding in an elderly person should be assumed to be malignancy until proven otherwise.

Bleeding with defecation is the most common complaint with hemorrhoids (**a**), and unless the hemorrhoids are thrombosed, the bleeding is usually painless. Patients usually report bright red blood on the toilet paper or in the toilet bowl. Weight loss would not be expected, and only in rare circumstances is the blood loss substantial. Diverticulitis (**b**) occurs with inflammation of a diverticulum and is the most common complication of diverticulosis. Patients typically present with persistent abdominal pain. Initially, the pain may be vague and generalized, but it often becomes localized to the LLQ. Most patients can be managed medically with bowel rest, hydration, analgesics, and antibiotics. A Mallory-Weiss tear (**c**) is a partial tear of the esophagus that usually results from significant vomiting or retching. Diverticulosis (**d**) is the presence of diverticula with massive painless lower GI bleeding. It is one of the most common causes of massive GI bleeding in this population. In most instances, the bleeding stops spontaneously.

265. The answer is d. Patients with coronary artery disease, valvular heart disease, and arrhythmias, particularly **atrial fibrillation**, are at high risk for **mesenteric ischemia**. In addition, age greater than 50 years, congestive heart failure, recent myocardial infarction, critically ill patients with sepsis or hypotension, use of diuretics or vasoconstrictive medications, and hypercoagulable states place patients at higher risk. The most common cause of acute mesenteric ischemia is **arterial embolus**, which accounts for 50% of cases. The classic finding is "**pain out of proportion to examination findings**"; that is, a patient complains of severe pain but is not particularly tender on examination. A high degree of suspicion for mesenteric ischemia in an elderly patient with abdominal pain is warranted.

Perforated gastric ulcer (**a**) presents with acute onset of severe epigastric pain and bleeding, generally in someone with PUD. Diverticulitis (**b**) presents as LLQ pain that is usually described as dull and constant. Acute cholecystitis (**c**) occurs with an obstruction of the cystic duct with gallstones and is often accompanied by fever, chills, nausea, and a positive Murphy sign. It is the most common surgical emergency in elderly patients. The classic triad for sigmoid volvulus (**e**) includes abdominal pain, abdominal distention, and constipation. Nausea and vomiting are often present, and diagnosis can be made on plain radiograph in 80% of cases.

266. The answer is d. Angiography remains the "gold standard" in the diagnosis of **mesenteric ischemia**. Unlike any other diagnostic tools, it is capable of both **diagnosing and treating** the problem. It is capable of identifying all four types of acute mesenteric ischemia: (1) arterial embolus, (2) arterial thrombosis, (3) venous thrombosis, and, under most circumstances, (4) nonocclusive mesenteric ischemia. Angiography should be obtained without delay when the last diagnosis is suspected.

With the exception of angiography, the results of all other studies are most useful in ruling out other diagnoses or finding out baseline levels. Abdominal radiographs (**b**) should be performed on any patient with suspected mesenteric ischemia to rule out bowel obstruction or free air. However, in the early stages, plain radiographs are most often normal in patients with mesenteric ischemia and should not be used to rule out this entity. Positive findings include intraluminal gas or gas in the portal venous system, usually coincide with the development of necrotic bowel, and signify a grim prognosis. Because of its availability, speed, and improved quality, CT is often used in the ED for assessing abdominal pain of unclear etiology in high-risk patients. CT (**c**) may identify indirect signs of ischemia—including edema of the bowel wall or mesentery, abnormal gas patterns, intramural gas, and ascites. Occasionally, CT may accurately identify direct evidence of mesenteric venous thrombosis. As with abdominal radiographs, many patients may have normal or nonspecific findings on CT, so it cannot be used to rule out the diagnosis of mesenteric ischemia. While a few studies have found CT to be as sensitive as angiography, it is not currently the study of choice. The sensitivity of serum lactate is high (a), nearly 100%, in the presence of mesenteric ischemia, but the specificity is low, ranging from 42% to 87%. Elevated serum lactate may best be used as a predictor of mortality. Some studies suggest that the presence of an unexplained acidosis should prompt a search for reversible causes of mesenteric ischemia. Intraluminal barium contrast studies (e) are contraindicated with suspected mesenteric ischemia because residual contrast material can limit visualization of the vasculature during diagnostic angiography.

267. The answer is d. Pantoprazole is a **PPI** and should be given as he has an upper GI bleed most likely due to PUD or gastritis. Acutely, pantoprazole **decreases the pH of the stomach and improves the ability of clotting**. PPIs have also been shown to decrease the chance of rebleeding after endoscopy.

Octreotide (a) is a somatostatin analog and should be given for suspected variceal hemorrhage. Esophageal variceal hemorrhages can be very dangerous and should be considered in patients with liver disease. Calcium carbonate (b) is an antacid and although it is useful to treat symptoms of heartburn, it is not useful in acute GI bleeding. Famotidine (c) is an H2 blocker and would also decrease the pH of the stomach. However, it has not been shown to decrease the risk of rebleeding after endoscopy; therefore, PPIs are preferred. Acetaminophen (e) is a nonopioid analgesic and antipyretic that would not have a role in acute management of upper GI bleeds.

268. The answer is b. Naproxen is a nonsteroidal anti-inflammatory drug (NSAID). Overuse can cause **damage to the gastric mucosa**. It works by inhibiting cyclooxygenase (COX) activity. This decreases prostaglandin formation and ultimately impacts the ability of the gastric mucosa to protect itself from acid.

The other medications do not have an impact on the gastric mucosa. Acetaminophen (a) is a nonopioid analgesic. Cetirizine (c) is a histamine (H1) antagonist. Zolpidem (d) is a hypnotic sleep aid. Fluoxetine (e) is a selective serotonin reuptake inhibitor.

269. The answer is e. An **angiodysplasia**, also known as an **arteriovenous malformation**, is a group of small ectatic blood vessels in the submucosa of the GI tract. More than half of angiodysplasias are located on the **right side of the colon**.

Angiodysplasias are responsible for 3% to 20% of acute lower GI bleeds **(a)**. Although angiodysplasia accounts for the most common cause of lower GI bleeding in younger patients, its incidence overall increases with age over 50 years **(b)**. While angiography may identify angiodysplasias **(c)**, colonoscopy remains the most sensitive diagnostic modality. On colonoscopy, angiodysplasias appear as red, flat lesions, measuring approximately 2 to 20 mm in diameter. Angiodysplasias are associated with many medical problems, including end-stage renal disease, aortic stenosis, and von Willebrand disease, among others **(d)**.

270. The answer is e. The patient most likely has an **esophageal perforation**, a serious, life-threatening **complication of endoscopy** that must be identified and treated quickly. Although sometimes reported as a result of forceful vomiting (ie, Boerhaave syndrome), the **most common cause is iatrogenic**. These usually occur as a complication of GI procedures, including upper endoscopy, dilation, sclerotherapy, and even nasogastric tube placement or endotracheal intubation. The signs and symptoms may include chest pain near the rupture site, fever, respiratory distress, hoarseness, or dysphagia. Most patients have **mediastinal or cervical emphysema,** which may be noted by palpation or by a **crunching sound** heard during auscultation **(ie, Hamman sign). An immediate esophagram with a water-soluble agent (eg, gastrografin) is indicated.**

Bronchoscopy **(a)** is used to evaluate a patient with suspected bronchial obstruction or endobronchial disease. It is not indicated in a case of suspected esophageal perforation. While an ECG should be obtained **(b)**, the likelihood that this patient's chest pain is cardiac in origin is fairly small. Repeating the endoscopy may be useful **(c)**, especially in cases of trauma; however, small perforations may be difficult or impossible to detect. An esophagram is better to evaluate for a suspected perforation. A chest radiograph and an upright abdominal radiograph are usually obtained first and may detect abnormalities in up to 90% of patients. These findings may include subcutaneous emphysema, pneumomediastinum, mediastinal widening, pleural effusion, or pulmonary infiltrate, but radiographic changes may not be present in the first few hours after the perforation. Thoracotomy **(d)** is the treatment for an esophageal perforation; however, an immediate esophagram with a water-soluble agent should be performed to confirm the diagnosis.

271. The answer is c. In a patient with esophageal perforation, it is imperative to start **broad-spectrum antibiotics** as soon as the diagnosis is suspected in order to prevent necrotizing mediastinitis and sepsis, which can result secondary to contamination of the mediastinum with gastric contents. **Piperacillin-tazobactam** is an appropriate agent because it is broad-spectrum and will cover all potential pathogens that can result from gastric contents entering the mediastinum (gram positive and negative organisms).

Clindamycin (**b**) is a less optimal choice on its own as its spectrum of action is less broad than that of piperacillin-tazobactam. It can be added as a second agent to cover anaerobes if desired. Octreotide (**a**) is a somatostatin analogue utilized to lower portal venous pressure in the treatment of bleeding esophageal varices. Glucagon (**d**) is a peptide secreted from α cells in the pancreas that acts as an antagonist to insulin. It is released when blood glucose is low. Its primary responsibility is to mobilize glucose by acting in the liver and causing stored glycogen to be converted to glucose. Glucagon can also be used in β-blocker overdoses and in patients with anaphylaxis who take β-blockers. Atropine (**e**) is an anticholinergic agent that acts to dry up secretions, increase HR, and dilate pupils. It has no antimicrobial action and is often used in patients with symptomatic bradycardia or cholinergic toxicity.

272. The answer is e. The **physical exam** is the most important step in the evaluation of this infant as she most likely has an **anal fissure**. **Anal fissures** result from linear tears of the anal canal at or just inferior to the dentate line and extend along the anal canal to the anal verge. This area has a rich supply of somatic sensory never fibers. Consequently, anal fissures are exquisitely painful and represent the **most common cause of painful rectal bleeding** in the first year of life and in adults. They are usually produced by the passage of a large, hard stool but may also occur with severe diarrhea.

Milk-protein allergies occur in 2% to 3% of infants and can cause blood-streaked stools as well. These are typically related to diarrhea, not hard stools. Allergy testing (**a**) and changing formulas (**b**) could be important if there were concern for a milk-protein allergy. A colonoscopy (**c**) and abdominal X-ray (**d**) are not indicated as the source of bleeding can be identified without imaging.

273. The answer is d. This patient is at risk of **aortoenteric fistula**. He has had a **prior AAA** repair, putting him at risk of a fistula forming between his aortic graft and his bowel, resulting in a massive, life-threatening GI bleed. As always in emergency medicine, assess the ABCs. In this instance, the patient is protecting his airway and is breathing spontaneously. His greatest risk is the "C" in ABCs—circulation. The first step in assessing circulation is **to place two large-bore IVs** for access in order to **transfuse un-crossmatched blood.**

This patient is currently protecting his airway (**a**) and is not experiencing hematemesis; thus, you do not need to intubate immediately. If his mental status were to change, you should reconsider intubation—this is why you should be continuously reassessing your critically ill patients. You should be calling for un-crossmatched blood in this critically ill patient, not waiting for crossmatched blood (**b**). The patient had an episode of gross blood by rectum and is at risk for aortoenteric fistula. It is imperative to get good access before performing a rectal examination as the bleed described likely represents a sentinel event before the patient's life-threatening bleed (**c**). Bedside ultrasound to evaluate for free fluid or a new AAA is appropriate; however, getting good access should be your top priority in this instance (**e**).

274. The answer is b. The most likely etiology of this patient's symptoms (fever, bloody diarrhea, and diffuse abdominal cramping) is *Shigella*. *Shigella* is often found in **leafy greens (eg, spinach or alfalfa sprouts)**. *Shigella* releases a toxin that causes sloughing and hemorrhage of the bowel mucosa as well as fever and significant abdominal cramping. It can lead to significant dehydration and even bacteremia and sepsis.

Salmonella (**a**) is often contracted from eggs or from contact with pet reptiles. *V. cholerae* (**c**) is typically contracted from eating oceanic seafood or drinking unclean water and results in prolific watery diarrhea, not dysentery. *Campylobacter* (**d**) is often contracted from eating undercooked poultry. *E. coli O157:H7* (**e**) is often contracted from eating raw hamburger meat.

275. The answer is a. Intussusception is most commonly seen between 6 and 18 months of age. It often presents with reported **colicky abdominal pain** that results in the child **pulling the knees up and screaming**, interspersed with **periods of normal** activity and absence of pain. It is typically accompanied by vomiting. There can be a palpable sausage-shaped mass in the right abdomen; however, this is often not felt. **Currant jelly stool** is a late finding and the child will often look septic at this point.

Meckel diverticulum (**b**) is often seen at age 2 months and represents GI bleeding secondary to ectopic gastric mucosa producing gastric acid within the bowel. This gastric acid results in erosion within the bowel and often painless rectal bleeding. Malrotation (**c**) is often seen under the age of 1 and results in vomiting and abdominal distension. This can be diagnosed on ultrasound or upper GI series. Appendicitis (**d**) will often result in fever, abdominal pain, and vomiting; however, it should not involve rectal bleeding. Pyloric stenosis (**e**) often results in projectile vomiting in infants at approximately 2 months of age. There can be a palpable olive-shaped mass at the site of the hypertrophied pylorus. The patient is typically afebrile and without rectal bleeding.

276. The answer is e. The proper management of intussusception is to consult radiology for immediate **air or barium enema decompression.** General surgery should also be consulted should the radiology decompression be unsuccessful, as the patient will then require emergent operative intervention.

General surgery (**a**) should be consulted as a back-up for operative intervention should air enema decompression be unsuccessful. GI (**b**) should be consulted for endoscopy if you suspect ingested foreign body. High-dose PPI therapy (**c**) should be used for upper GI bleed, especially if thought to be due to PUD. IV fluids (**d**) should be started in this patient and IV antibiotics should also be given as this patient appears to be developing symptoms of sepsis; however, the air enema is the definitive management in this condition.

277. The answer is c. Start **IV crystalloid infusion**. Patient is hypotensive and tachycardic likely from volume depletion and dehydration due to 2 days of vomiting and diarrhea. Fluid resuscitation is the most important first step while further evaluation is starting.

An NG tube lavage (**a**) can be used to evaluate for upper GI bleeding but is rarely indicated as the risks often outweigh the potential benefits. She may ultimately require a transfusion of PRBCs (**c**), but in the initial treatment crystalloid fluids are appropriate. CT angiography of the abdomen and pelvis (**d**) can be useful to help identify the source but the patient needs to be stabilized before being sent for any imaging. Stool studies (**e**) might be appropriate to evaluate for infectious causes of her diarrhea, however they are not the most urgent step.

278. The answer is a. This is a common presentation of **ischemic colitis.** The patient most likely developed significant hypotension from dehydration due to her GI illness in combination with the hydrochlorothiazide she takes for BP management. Hydrochlorothiazide is a diuretic and therefore may have exacerbated the problem. Ischemic colitis is the most common form of GI ischemia. Nonocclusive ischemic colitis is often **precipitated by an event that causes hypotension or low blood flow to the colon.** This results in transient ischemia to the mucosal and submucosal lining of the colon. This can be managed conservatively as long as it does not become necrotic.

Diverticulitis **(b)** is inflammation of diverticula and although it does commonly cause crampy abdominal pain and diarrhea, it does not typically cause bleeding. *Shigella* **(c)** is a possibility but the timing of the bleeding starting after the acute diarrhea illness makes this less likely. Appendicitis **(d)** does not typically cause bright red blood per rectum. Adenocarcinoma **(e)** could cause bright red blood per rectum but would not commonly be preceded by an acute episode of fever, nausea, vomiting, and diarrhea.

Recommended Readings

Goralnick E, Meguerdichian DA. Chapter 27. Gastrointestinal bleeding. In: Marx JA, Hockberger RS, Walls RM, eds. *Rosen's Emergency Medicine: Concepts and Clinical Practice.* 9th ed. Philadelphia, PA: Elsevier Saunders, 2018.

Kurz MC, Neumar RW. Chapter 8. Adult resuscitation. In: Marx JA, Hockberger RS, Walls RM, eds. *Rosen's Emergency Medicine: Concepts and Clinical Practice.* 9th ed. Philadelphia, PA: Elsevier Saunders, 2018.

Lo BM. Chapter 76. Lower gastrointestinal bleeding. In: Tintinalli JE, Stapczynski J, Ma O, et al, eds. *Tintinalli's Emergency Medicine: A Comprehensive Study Guide.* 9th ed. New York, NY: McGraw-Hill, 2020.

Maloney P. Chapter 171. Gastrointestinal disorders. In: Marx JA, Hockberger RS, Walls RM, eds. *Rosen's Emergency Medicine: Concepts and Clinical Practice.* 9th ed. Philadelphia, PA: Elsevier Saunders, 2018.

Reid SM. Chapter 134. Gastrointestinal bleeding in infants and children. In: Tintinalli JE, Stapczynski J, Ma O, et al, eds. *Tintinalli's Emergency Medicine: A Comprehensive Study Guide.* 9th ed. New York, NY: McGraw-Hill, 2020.

Silen W. *Cope's Early Diagnosis of the Acute Abdomen.* 22nd ed. Oxford, New York: Oxford University Press, 2010.

Ziebell C, Kittowski A, Welch J, Friesen P. Chapter 75. Upper gastrointestinal bleeding. In: Tintinalli JE, Stapczynski J, Ma O, et al, eds. *Tintinalli's Emergency Medicine: A Comprehensive Study Guide.* 9th ed. New York, NY: McGraw-Hill, 2020.

Musculoskeletal Injuries

Kaitlin Ray, MD

Questions

The following scenario applies to questions 279 and 280.

While playing in his family's annual Thanksgiving Day touch-football game, a 41-year-old man fell onto his outstretched hand upon attempting to make the game winning catch. He presents to the emergency department (ED) complaining of right wrist pain.

279. Which of the following carpal bones is most frequently fractured during a fall on an outstretched hand (FOOSH)?

a. Triquetrum
b. Lunate
c. Capitate
d. Scaphoid
e. Pisiform

280. On examination of the patient's right wrist, you note tenderness at the anatomic snuffbox and pain with axial loading of his thumb. You suspect he has a scaphoid fracture. A series of wrist radiographs are performed and are negative for fracture. Which of the following is the most appropriate next step in management?

a. Place an ACE wrap around the hand and wrist and advise him to wear this until the pain resolves
b. Immobilize in a thumb spica splint and discharge home with outpatient follow-up with an orthopedist for repeat radiographs in 10 to 14 days
c. Advise him to ice the wrist and take ibuprofen for the next 24 to 48 hours
d. Order a computed tomography (CT) scan to evaluate for an occult fracture
e. Place him in a short arm cast and discharge him home with outpatient follow-up with an orthopedist for repeat radiographs in 2 days

281. A 64-year-old man presents to the ED complaining of knee pain since yesterday. He denies trauma or similar presentation in the past. On examination, you note an erythematous, tender, and swollen knee. Radiographs do not reveal a fracture, but do show calcium deposits. Fluid collected from an arthrocentesis demonstrates 20,000/μL white blood cells (WBCs) with a predominance of neutrophils, a negative Gram stain, and rhomboid-shaped crystals that are positively birefringent under polarized light. Which of the following is the most likely diagnosis?

a. Pseudogout
b. Gout
c. Septic arthritis
d. Rheumatoid arthritis
e. Osteoarthritis

282. A 22-year-old soccer player presents to the ED complaining of right knee pain and swelling. Earlier in the day, during a soccer match, he was running for the ball and stopped abruptly and tried to run in a new direction. Immediately thereafter, he felt intense pain in his knee with instant swelling. Which of the following is the most commonly injured major ligament of the knee?

a. Anterior cruciate ligament (ACL)
b. Posterior cruciate ligament (PCL)
c. Medial collateral ligament (MCL)
d. Lateral collateral ligament (LCL)
e. Patellar ligament

283. A 45-year-old man is on his way to work and loses his footing while walking up a flight of stairs. He feels excruciating pain at the back of his ankle and felt a snap. He cannot ambulate. He has a past medical history of hypertension and hypercholesterolemia. He spends most of his free time playing video games. On examination, you note swelling of the distal calf. Which of the following is likely to be positive in this individual?

a. Homans sign
b. Lachman test
c. McMurray test
d. Ballotable patella
e. Thompson test

The following scenario applies to questions 284 and 285.

A 32-year-old construction worker reports standing on scaffolding before it suddenly gave way beneath him. In an attempt to catch his fall, he quickly grabbed and hung on to an overhead beam for approximately 30 seconds. Two hours later, he presents to the ED with left shoulder pain and decreased range of motion. Vital signs are within normal limits, except for the patient's pain scale of 10/10. He is holding his left arm with the contralateral hand. On physical examination, the patient's shoulder appears swollen with no skin breakage. The upper extremity is otherwise without obvious deformity. The patient has palpable brachial, radial, and ulnar pulses with capillary refill that is less than 2 seconds. He can wiggle his fingers but cannot internally rotate his shoulder or raise his left arm above his head. Pinprick testing reveals decreased sensation along the lateral deltoid of the affected arm.

284. What is the most likely etiology of this patient's symptoms?

a. Acromioclavicular joint sprain
b. Posterior shoulder dislocation with axillary nerve impingement
c. Anterior shoulder dislocation with axillary nerve impingement
d. Anterior shoulder dislocation with median nerve impingement
e. Posterior shoulder dislocation with ulnar nerve impingement

285. A radiograph of the shoulder is obtained and is shown in the following figure. What is the most common fracture associated with the patient's diagnosis?

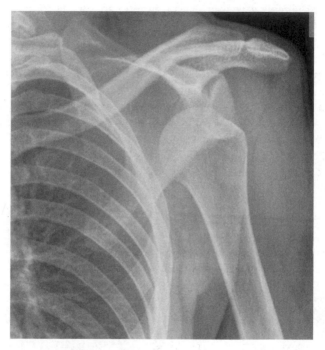

(Reproduced with permission from Adam J. Rosh, MD.)

a. Bankart fracture
b. Hill-Sachs deformity
c. Clavicle fracture
d. Coronoid process fracture
e. Scapula fracture

286. A 35-year-old man presents to the ED with right hand swelling, pain, and erythema that began 3 days ago. He denies any trauma, sick contacts, insect bites, or recent travel. The patient's vitals are significant for an oral temperature of 101°F. Upon physical examination, you note an area of erythema surrounding multiple small lacerations over the right third and fourth metacarpophalangeal (MCP) joints with localized tenderness. The patient is neurovascularly intact with limited flexion caused by the swelling and pain. Given this presentation, what is the most appropriate disposition for this patient?

a. Suture and close follow-up with a hand surgeon
b. Suture and prescription for oral antibiotics
c. Wound irrigation and prescription for oral antibiotics
d. Wound irrigation and tetanus prophylaxis
e. Admission for intravenous (IV) antibiotics

287. A 23-year-old man presents to the ED complaining of right hand pain. He was mad at a friend and punched his bedroom wall. Immediately after he had punched the wall, he felt intense pain in his right hand. On physical examination, you note swelling and tenderness over the fifth metacarpal. When you ask him to make a fist, his fifth finger rotates to lie on top of his fourth finger. The radiograph is shown in the next figure. What is the name of this type of fracture?

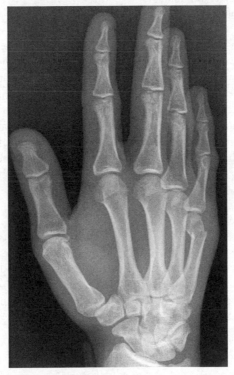

(Reproduced with permission from Adam J. Rosh, MD.)

a. Colles' fracture
b. Smith fracture
c. Scaphoid fracture
d. Galeazzi fracture
e. Boxer fracture

288. A 41-year-old man is brought into the ED after having a witnessed tonic-clonic seizure. He is alert and oriented, and he states that he has not taken his seizure medication for the last week. His blood pressure (BP) is 140/75 mm Hg, heart rate (HR) is 88 beats/minute, respiratory rate (RR) is 16 breaths/minute, and temperature is 99.7°F. On examination, you notice that his arm is internally rotated and adducted. He cannot externally rotate the arm and any movement of his shoulder elicits pain. Which of the following is the most likely diagnosis?

a. Humerus fracture
b. Clavicle fracture
c. Scapula fracture
d. Posterior shoulder dislocation
e. Anterior shoulder dislocation

289. A 54-year-old man presents to the ED with 2 days of right foot pain that suddenly worsened at night. The touch of his bed sheets on his foot made the pain worse while he was trying to sleep. The pain is burning in nature without radiation. He denies fever or trauma. His medical history is significant for chronic kidney disease. He believes the pain is due to a gout flare. Pain began after he recently celebrated his birthday at a local gastro-pub known to have the best steak and craft beers in town. Which of the following is indicated in the treatment of this patient's condition?

a. Indomethacin
b. Dexamethasone
c. Naproxen
d. Topical triamcinolone ointment
e. Ketorolac

290. A 31-year-old homebuilder is cutting a piece of wood when the table saw backfires and amputates his left thumb at the base. You stabilize the patient and call the plastic surgeon. What is the best method of preserving the amputated digit?

a. Cleanse it with 10% povidone-iodine solution to remove gross contamination, wrap it in sterile gauze moistened with normal saline, and place it between two ice packs

b. Cleanse it with normal saline to remove gross contamination, wrap it in sterile gauze moistened with normal saline, and then place it on ice

c. Cleanse it with normal saline to remove gross contamination, wrap it in sterile gauze moistened with normal saline, place it in a sterile watertight container, and store this container on ice water

d. Place it in a container of 10% povidone-iodine solution and store this container on ice water

e. Attempt reimplantation of the amputated part with 3-0 nylon sutures until the vascular surgeon arrives

291. A 33-year-old carpenter was building a new house and using a high-pressure paint gun when he inadvertently injected his left index finger. On arrival to the ED, he complains of intense hand pain. On examination, you note a 2 mm wound over the second proximal phalanx. He has full range of motion and brisk capillary refill. Radiographs of the finger show soft tissue swelling, a small amount of subcutaneous air, but no fracture. His tetanus is up to date. Which of the following is the most appropriate disposition for this patient?

a. Place the hand in a radial gutter splint and have the patient follow-up with a hand surgeon in 1 week

b. Discharge home with pain medication and have the patient return for repeat radiographs in 1 week

c. Order a CT scan of the finger to confirm that there is no occult fracture before discharging the patient home

d. Place the hand in a radial gutter splint, prescribe a 10-day course of antibiotics, and have the patient follow-up with a hand surgeon in 1 week

e. Place the hand in a radial gutter splint, administer broad-spectrum antibiotics, and consult the hand surgery service for operative debridement

The following scenario applies to questions 292 and 293.

A 24-year-old man reports that he was working on a scaffolding 15 feet above the ground when the scaffold gave way and he fell. He reports that he landed on his feet. He did not strike his head and did not lose consciousness. He is complaining of pain in his lower back and his left foot. His vital signs include BP 130/80 mm Hg, HR 89 beats/minute, RR 16 breaths/minute, and pulse oximetry is 100% on room air. His Glasgow coma scale (GCS) is 15 and neurologic examination is normal.

292. Based on the radiographs of his left foot shown in the figures, which of the following statements is true?

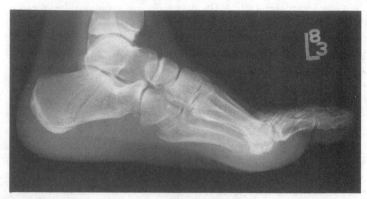

(Reproduced with permission from Tarek Hanna, MD.)

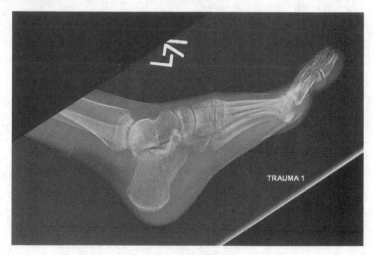

(Reproduced with permission from Tarek Hanna, MD.)

a. This injury is the second most commonly fractured tarsal bone
b. 10% of these injuries are associated with compression fractures of the lumbar spine
c. 90% of these injuries are bilateral
d. The mechanism of injury is usually secondary to rotational force at the subtalar joint
e. These fractures require operative repair to avoid gait defects

293. The patient is also complaining of lumbar back pain. A CT scan of his spine is performed and a representative image is shown in the figure. What is the most likely diagnosis based on this image?

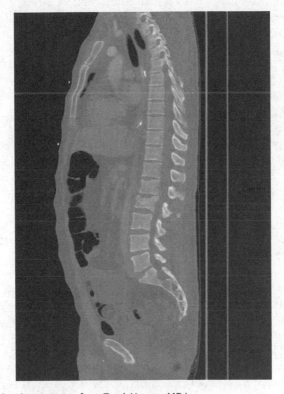

(Reproduced with permission from Tarek Hanna, MD.)

a. Lumbar transverse process fracture
b. Lumbar spinous process fracture
c. Lumbar wedge fracture
d. Lumbar burst fracture
e. Lumbar subluxation

294. A 39-year-old woman is brought to the ED by emergency medical services (EMS) on a backboard and cervical collar after being involved in a motor vehicle collision (MVC). The primary survey is unremarkable. However, the secondary survey reveals a deformity of the right arm involving the upper arm and elbow. Which of the following injury associations is paired correctly?

a. Olecranon fracture and median nerve injury
b. Posterior elbow dislocation and ulnar and brachial artery injury
c. Anterior elbow dislocation and brachial artery injury
d. Supracondylar fracture and radial nerve and median nerve injury
e. Humeral shaft fracture and axillary nerve injury

295. A 34-year-old man presents to the ED after an MVC and is diagnosed with a tibial plateau fracture. You are concerned that he may develop compartment syndrome. Which of the following is considered the earliest sign of compartment syndrome?

a. Pallor
b. Pulselessness
c. Paralysis
d. Pain disproportionate to injury or exam findings
e. Paresthesia

296. A 31-year-old man is riding his mountain bicycle down a steep hill when he hits a rock in the path and is thrown off the bicycle. In the ED, the individual complains only of left arm pain. Your primary survey is unremarkable and vital signs are within normal limits. After administering analgesic medication, you send the patient for a radiograph of his arm. Which of the following injuries is consistent with this patient's radiograph as seen in the figure?

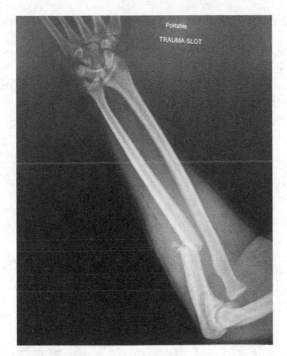

(Reproduced with permission from Adam J. Rosh, MD.)

a. Monteggia fracture
b. Galeazzi fracture
c. Nightstick fracture
d. Colles' fracture
e. Smith fracture

297. A 32-year-old dental hygienist presents to the ED with a painful lesion at the distal aspect of her right index finger. She reports a low-grade fever and malaise over the last week and subsequently developed pain and burning of the digit. In the past few days, she has noted erythema, edema, and the development of small grouped vesicles on an erythematous base as depicted in the figure. Which of the following is the most appropriate next step in management?

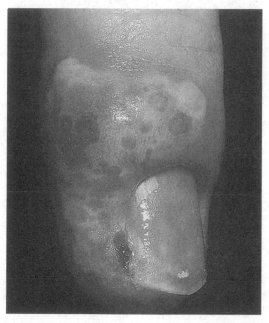

(Reproduced, with permission, from Wolff K, Johnson RA, Suurmond R. Fitzpatrick's Color Atlas & Synopsis of Clinical Dermatology. 5th ed. New York, NY: McGraw Hill; 2005. Figure 25-27.)

a. Perform an incision and drainage to facilitate healing and avoid bacterial suprainfection
b. Buddy tape the index finger to the middle finger
c. Prescribe an oral antiviral agent, such as acyclovir
d. Do not apply a dressing and keep the wounds open to air so that they dry out
e. Prescribe a prophylactic oral and topical antibiotic

298. A 26-year-old, restrained driver is brought in by EMS after a low-to-moderate speed MVC where he was at a stop sign and struck from behind. He was immobilized on a long spine board and a cervical collar was placed. He is hemodynamically stable and his primary survey is intact. He complains of pain in his left arm and the back of his neck. On secondary survey, there are no neurologic deficits noted. The CT C-spine was negative for fracture or dislocation. The patient continues to complain of pain upon palpation of the cervical spine. What is the next step in the management of this patient?

a. Remove the cervical collar and clinically clear his cervical spine
b. Instruct the patient to wear the hard cervical collar until his pain resolves
c. Place him in a soft cervical collar and discharge with outpatient follow-up
d. Admit him for emergent magnetic resonance imaging (MRI) of the cervical spine
e. Consult neurosurgery

The following scenario applies to questions 299 and 300.

A 24-year-old woman presents to the ED after accidentally slamming her finger in the car door 2 hours prior to arrival. There is no obvious deformity and she appears to have full range of motion of her ungual fingers. You notice blood collecting under her fingernail. The nail edges are intact.

299. What is the most appropriate next step in the management of this patient?

a. Apply a cold compress
b. Consult the hand surgery service
c. Order an X-ray of her hand
d. Perform a digital nerve block
e. Splint the patient's finger and refer for outpatient hand referral

300. What is the appropriate management of her subungual hematoma?

a. Apply a pressure dressing
b. Buddy tape the finger
c. Remove the nail from the nail bed
d. Scalpel insertion under the nail edge
e. Trephination of the nail

301. A 2-year-old child presents to the ED with right elbow pain. She reportedly "threw a tantrum" at naptime. Her father attempted to pick her up out of the crib by the arm with her feet dangling. She later refused to use her right arm and whimpers when anyone tries to move it passively. On examination, there is no deformity, joint swelling, erythema, or neurovascular compromise. The arm is held in slight flexion, pronated and abducted. A radiograph of her elbow is shown in the figure. What is the most appropriate next step?

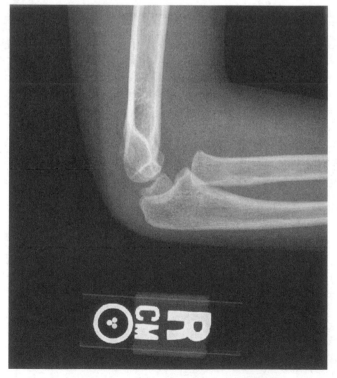

(Reproduced with permission from Tarek Hanna, MD.)

a. Attempt to flex and supinate the forearm with slight pressure held at the radial head
b. Apply traction to the wrist while pronating the arm and extending the elbow
c. Consult orthopedics
d. Apply an arm sling and refer for outpatient orthopedic referral
e. Order X-rays of the contralateral elbow for comparison

The following scenario applies to questions 302 and 303.

An 8-month-old infant is brought to the ED by her mother after she reportedly rolled off of the couch. The mother left the infant on the couch unattended for a few minutes. The mother heard a thud and then her daughter was heard crying. She ran back into the room to find the baby lying on the floor and crying. The mother immediately picked up the infant and brought her to the ED for evaluation. On physical examination, the vital signs include a BP of 76/50 mm Hg, HR of 140 beats/minute, RR of 26 breaths/minute, temperature of 36.8°F, and pulse oximetry of 98% on room air. The infant is well nourished. She is moving all four extremities spontaneously. There is soft tissue swelling in the region of the left lower leg. A radiograph is obtained and shown in the figure.

302. Based on the clinical scenario and radiograph, what is the most likely diagnosis?

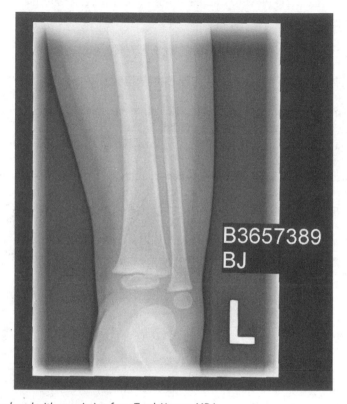

(Reproduced with permission from Tarek Hanna, MD.)

a. Greenstick fracture
b. Spiral fracture of the tibia
c. Normal radiograph showing open physis
d. Salter Harris IV fracture
e. Salter Harris V fracture

303. You inform the mother of the radiograph results and ask a few additional questions. The mother reports that the infant is able to sit unassisted; however, she does not pull to stand up or walk. What is the most appropriate management plan for this patient?

a. Place a left lower extremity splint with follow-up in the orthopedic clinic
b. Since the infant is nonambulatory, place an elastic wrap on the left lower extremity with follow-up in the orthopedic clinic
c. Consult orthopedics for fracture management
d. Obtain a skeletal survey, consult ophthalmology, and admit the child to the hospital
e. Obtain comparison radiographs of the right leg and arrange for 24-hour follow-up with her pediatrician

304. A 40-year-old man presents to the ED complaining of severe right hip pain that is present at rest and worse with movement. He reports that over-the-counter analgesics provide minimal relief and that the pain has become unbearable. A radiograph of his pelvis is shown in the figure. Which of the following is the most likely underlying cause of his hip pain?

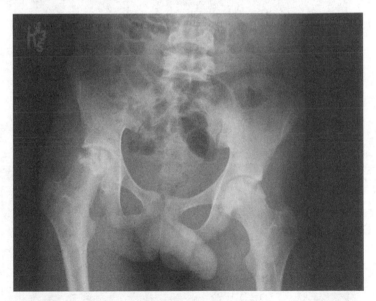

(Reproduced with permission from Tarek Hanna, MD.)

a. Sickle cell disease
b. Osteosarcoma
c. Hypertension
d. Prostate cancer
e. Gout

305. A 43-year-old warehouse worker is helping to stock large refrigerator boxes onto the forklift. One of the boxes starts to fall off the shelf and he tries to catch it before it falls. In doing so, his hand is hyperextended at the wrist and he experiences immediate wrist pain. In the ED, you note limitation of the normal motion of the wrist with palpable fullness on the volar aspect. The patient also complains of numbness and tingling in the distribution of the median nerve. Radiographs of the wrist are obtained and shown in the figure. What is the most likely diagnosis?

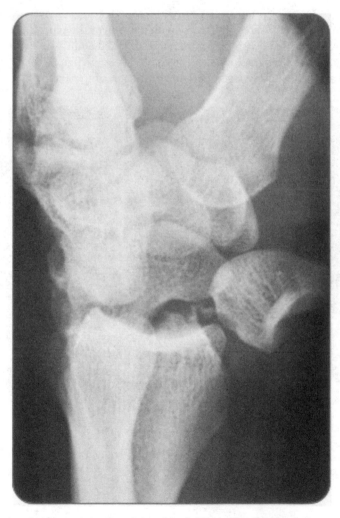

(Reproduced with permission from Adam J. Rosh, MD, and Rosh Review.)

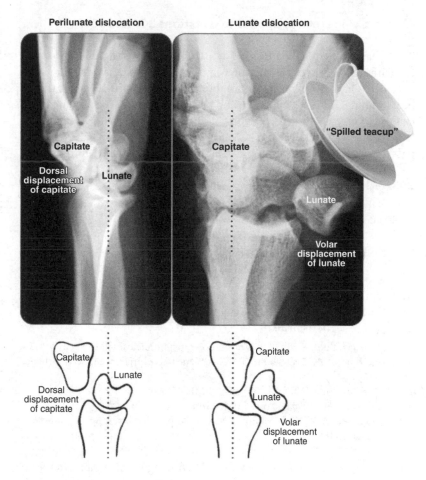

a. Lunate dislocation
b. Perilunate dislocation
c. Scapholunate dislocation
d. Capitate dislocation
e. Scaphoid fracture

The following scenario applies to questions 306 and 307.

A 24-year-old man with a history of asthma and IV drug use presents to ED with right knee pain since yesterday. He denies trauma or similar prior episodes. On arrival, vitals are notable for temperature 100.8°F, HR 101 beats/minute, BP 125/70 mm Hg, and pulse oximetry 97% on room air. On examination, you see an uncomfortable appearing male with an erythematous, swollen, and tender right knee. He endorses significant pain with both passive and active range of motion. Radiographs are negative for fracture.

306. What is the most likely diagnosis?

a. Reactive arthritis
b. Pseudogout
c. Gout
d. Septic arthritis
e. Rheumatoid arthritis

307. An arthrocentesis is performed. Gram stain and culture are pending. Which of the following synovial fluid results is most consistent with a diagnosis of septic arthritis?

a. Clear yellow fluid; WBC 10,000/mm^3; polymorphonuclear (PMN) cells 15%
b. Turbid fluid; WBC 50,000 mm^3; PMN 60%; negative birefringent needle-shaped crystals
c. Clear yellow fluid; WBC 20,000/ mm^3; PMN 25%
d. Cloudy fluid; WBC 90,000 mm^3; PMN 90%
e. Turbid fluid; WBC 50,000 mm^3; PMN 60%; positive birefringent rhomboid-shaped crystals

308. A 35-year-old man presents to ED with right ankle pain after a fall while running. Patient states he rolled his ankle on uneven ground and was unable to ambulate after the fall. The following radiographs were obtained. What is the diagnosis and management?

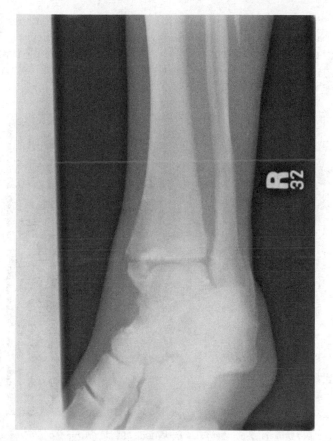

(Northwestern University, Feinberg School of Medicine, Department of Emergency Medicine.)

a. Monteggia fracture; splint and discharge with orthopedic follow-up
b. Maisonneuve fracture; orthopedic consult for surgical fixation
c. Bimalleolar fracture; orthopedic consult for surgical fixation
d. Galeazzi fracture; splint and discharge with orthopedic follow-up
e. Talar fracture; splint and discharge with orthopedic follow-up

309. A 48-year-old man presents to ED with left foot pain after falling off of a ladder. He estimates the ladder was 12 feet high. Primary survey is intact; however, secondary survey is notable for swelling and ecchymosis of the middle of his left foot. Radiograph is obtained as below. What is the diagnosis?

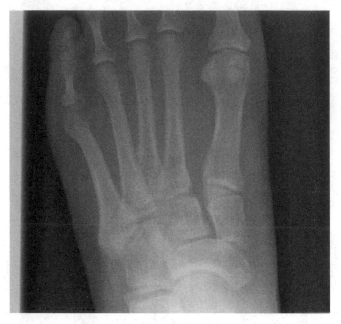

(Northwestern University, Feinberg School of Medicine, Department of Emergency Medicine.)

a. Jones fracture
b. Pseudo-Jones fracture
c. Navicular fracture
d. Stress fracture
e. Lisfranc injury

310. An 18-year-old woman presents to ED with severe left knee pain after tripping over a hurdle at a track meet. On examination, patient is unable to actively extend her knee. Radiograph is obtained as below. What is the diagnosis and management?

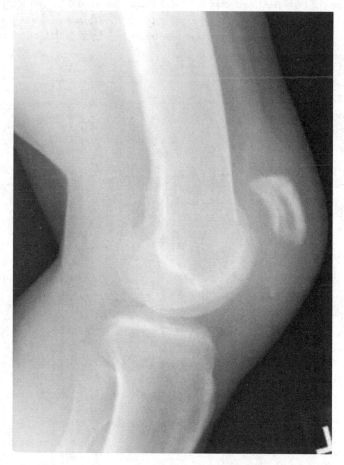

(Northwestern University, Feinberg School of Medicine, Department of Emergency Medicine.)

a. Patellar tendon rupture; knee immobilizer and orthopedic follow-up
b. Patellar fracture; knee immobilizer and orthopedic follow-up
c. Tibial plateau fracture; obtain CT and consult orthopedics
d. Quadriceps tendon rupture; knee immobilizer and orthopedic outpatient follow-up
e. ACL tear; knee immobilizer and orthopedic outpatient follow-up

311. A 55-year-old male is the restrained front-seat passenger in an MVC. On arrival to ED, primary survey is intact. Secondary survey is notable for a right leg that is slightly flexed at the hip, shortened, adducted, and internally rotated. Exam is also notable for loss of sensation of the posterior leg and foot, loss of dorsiflexion and plantar flexion, and loss of deep tendon reflex (DTR) at the ankle. Patient has palpable posterior tibial and dorsalis pedis pulses. Patient's exam is concerning for injury to which of the following?

a. Femoral nerve injury
b. Femoral artery injury
c. Sciatic nerve injury
d. Obturator nerve injury
e. Saphenous nerve injury

Musculoskeletal Injuries

Answers

279. The answer is d. The **scaphoid** is the **most common carpal bone injured in** a **FOOSH** injury. On examination, patients will exhibit tenderness at the **anatomic snuffbox** (ie, the space between the extensor pollicis longus and the extensor pollicis brevis) and pain referred to the anatomic snuffbox with longitudinal compression (ie, axial loading) of the thumb.

A triquetral **(a)** dorsal chip injury is the second most common carpal bone fracture and occurs with a FOOSH or direct blow to the dorsum of the hand. Lunate fracture **(b)** is the third most common carpal fracture. The capitate **(c)** is the largest carpal bone and comprises 5% to 15% of all carpal fractures. The pisiform **(e)** is the only carpal bone with one articulation (with the triquetrum). Anatomically, it is important because the deep branch of the ulnar nerve and artery pass in close proximity to the radial surface of the bone. It is an uncommon fracture.

280. The answer is b. Up to 15% of scaphoid fractures are not detected on initial X-rays. As the necrotic bone at the fracture site is resorbed, the fracture line often becomes apparent on radiographs 10 to 14 days after injury. In patients with snuffbox tenderness and negative initial radiographs, a **thumb spica splint** should be applied until films can be repeated 10 to 14 days postinjury. The application of the splint is especially important, because of the scaphoid's high risk for avascular necrosis (**AVN**) due to its distal to proximal blood supply. The blood supply to the scaphoid normally penetrates the cortex at the distal aspect of the bone. Therefore, there is **no direct blood supply to the proximal portion of the bone**, which predisposes this fragment to AVN and delayed union. The more proximal the scaphoid fracture, the greater the likelihood of developing **AVN**.

Placing an elastic wrap **(a)** will not provide adequate immobilization and will lead to increased complications if a fracture is present. Ice packs and ibuprofen **(c)** are recommended, but immobilization is also required. Even a CT scan **(d)** may not pick up the fracture immediately after injury. However, if there is snuffbox tenderness after 14 days and the radiograph remains negative, a CT scan is warranted. A short arm cast (e) is not the appropriate immobilization device for a suspected scaphoid fracture and the follow-up interval is too soon.

281. The answer is a. Pseudogout is the most common cause of acute **monoarticular arthritis** in the **elderly**. It affects women and men equally, primarily after their sixth decade of life. It is caused by the deposition of **calcium pyrophosphate crystals**. The **knee** is the most commonly involved joint, followed by the wrist and ankle. The synovial fluid **reveals rhomboid-shaped crystals** that are weakly **positive birefringent** under polarized light. Treatment is generally supportive with nonsteroidal antiinflammatory drugs (NSAIDs).

Gout **(b)** occurs commonly in middle-aged men and elderly adults. Uric acid crystals usually deposit in the lower extremities, particularly the great toe (podagra). Evaluation of synovial fluid reveals needle-shaped crystals that exhibit negative birefringence under polarized light. Septic arthritis **(c)** is a medical emergency that most commonly affects the knee in adults. Joint fluid generally reveals greater than 50,000 WBC/mm³ (mostly neutrophils). Rheumatoid arthritis **(d)** is an autoimmune disease that is characterized by a symmetric, progressive polyarthritis. Unlike osteoarthritis **(e)**, rheumatoid arthritis has systemic manifestations.

282. The answer is a. The cruciate ligaments are the two internal bands extending from the tibia to the femur, one anteriorly and the other posteriorly. They control anteroposterior and rotary stability of the knee and prevent hyperextension. The **ACL is the most frequently injured ligament in the knee.** It has a rich blood supply that accounts for the high incidence of **hemarthrosis** when the ligament is injured. A history that includes a **pop** or **snap** at the time of injury (eg, during a sudden turn in direction while playing sports) suggests a rupture of the ACL until proven otherwise, particularly when associated with the rapid development of a knee effusion.

The PCL **(b)** is significantly stronger than the ACL and collateral ligaments. Therefore, injury to it is rare and is usually associated with severe knee injuries. The MCL **(c)** and LCL **(d)** are often injured with excessive valgus (knee forced medially relative to leg) and varus (knee forced laterally relative to leg) forces, respectively. The patellar ligament **(e)** runs from the patella to the tibial tuberosity and functions to help extend the leg at the knee. The patellar ligament is commonly injured from a fall onto a partially flexed knee.

283. The answer is e. The patient has an **Achilles tendon rupture**. The individual gives a history of a sudden excruciating pain and having heard or felt a **pop** or **snap**. This entity is most common in **sedentary, middle-aged men**, or in episodic athletes (ie, "weekend warriors"). Other risk factors include fluoroquinolone antibiotic use (now a Black Box Warning), steroid injections, and chronic inflammatory conditions. The diagnosis can be made with the **Thompson test**. The patient is placed in the prone position. With normal function, squeezing the calf produces plantar flexion of the foot. With a complete tear of the Achilles tendon, plantar flexion will not occur. If doubt remains, MRI or ultrasound can be used to confirm the diagnosis. Treatment includes splinting the affected leg and discharging the patient with crutches. Orthopedic follow-up is required for repair.

Homans sign (**a**) is traditionally used to help diagnose a deep vein thrombosis (DVT). It is considered positive when passive dorsiflexion of the ankle elicits sharp pain in the calf. However, this sign is neither sensitive nor specific for DVT. The Lachman test (**b**) is used to detect an injury of the ACL. The McMurray test (**c**) is used to detect an injury to the meniscus of the knee. A ballotable patella (**d**) signifies a significant knee effusion.

284. The answer is c. This patient has **an anterior shoulder dislocation**. The glenohumeral joint is the most commonly dislocated joint in the body, mainly because of the lack of bony stability and its wide range of motion. Anterior dislocations account for 95% to 97% of cases and are most commonly seen in younger, athletic male patients and geriatric female patients. The mechanism of injury is usually an indirect force that involves an abduction plus extension plus external rotation. Directly, it may occur due to a posterior blow that forces the humeral head out of the glenoid rim anteriorly. Radiographs obtained must include an axillary view to determine positioning of the humeral head. Patients usually present in severe pain, holding the affected arm with the contralateral hand in slight abduction. The lateral acromial process is prominent giving the shoulder a full or **squared-off appearance**. Patients typically cannot internally rotate their shoulder. **Axillary nerve injuries** can occur in up to 54% of anterior dislocations; however, these are neuropraxic in nature and tend to resolve on their own. **Following the C5/C6 dermatome distribution, patients have a loss of sensation over the lateral aspect of the deltoid with decreased muscle contraction with abduction.** After proper muscle relaxation with conscious sedation or intraarticular injection, closed reduction may be attempted using a variety of methods. After reduction, it is imperative to repeat a neurovascular examination and obtain confirmatory radiographs.

Acromioclavicular joint sprains (**a**) occur primarily in men and account for 25% of all dislocations. However, the mechanism of injury primarily involves a fall or direct blow to the adducted arm causing a downward and medial thrust to the scapula. Posterior dislocations (**b and e**) are rare owing to the scapular angle on the thoracic ribs. They are seen, however, in convulsive seizures where the large internal rotator muscles overpower the weaker external rotators and cause the dislocation. Median nerve injuries (**d**) mainly involve weakness in the first three finger flexors. Ulnar nerve injuries (**e**) mainly involve weakness in the interossei muscles of the hand and paresthesia along the fifth digit.

285. The answer is b. The radiograph confirms an **anterior dislocation** of the left shoulder. Patients typically present in severe pain with the dislocated arm held in slight abduction and external rotation by the opposite extremity. The patient leans away from the injured side and cannot adduct or internally rotate the shoulder without severe pain. Associated fractures may occur in up to 50% of anterior dislocations. The most common of these is a **compression fracture of the humeral head**, known as a **Hill-Sachs deformity**.

Fracture of the anterior glenoid rim, or Bankart fracture (**a**), is also associated with anterior dislocations but is present in approximately 5% of cases. Choices (**c, d, and e**) are not commonly associated with anterior shoulder dislocations.

286. The answer is e. This patient most likely sustained a **closed-fist injury**, which has high infection rates and evidence of poor wound healing. Wounds sustained by punches to the jaw and human bites, also known as "fight bites," are classically over the **metacarpal joints**. Penetration deep into the joint space and infection are common given the positioning of the hand during the injury, human oral flora, and delay in seeking treatment. Infected wounds are **polymicrobial** and specifically include *Eikenella corrodens*, a facultative anaerobic gram-negative rod harbored in human dental plaque. It acts synergistically with aerobic organisms to increase the morbidity of these injuries. The joint spaces must be examined under full range of motion to detect any tendon lacerations or presence of foreign bodies. Hand radiographs should also be obtained to examine for any bony involvement. **IV antibiotics** and **admission** are the appropriate disposition. The antibiotics of choice are **directed at Staph sp, Strep sp, and gram-negative organisms** (typically ampicillin/sulbactam IV or amoxicillin/clavulanic acid (PO)) with broader coverage in the immunocompromised patient. The wounds should be left open with a sterile dressing, splinted in the position of function (hand-holding-glass position) and elevated. Human bites have resulted in the transmission of hepatitis B, hepatitis C, syphilis, and herpes. Although human immunodeficiency virus (HIV) is present in human saliva, it is in relatively small amounts and considered a low risk for transmission. Appropriate antivirals and testing should be considered in these patients.

You should never suture these lacerations **(a and b)**. Wound irrigation and tetanus prophylaxis **(c and d)** are warranted in conjunction with IV antibiotics.

287. The answer is e. A **boxer fracture is a fracture of the neck of the fifth metacarpal**. It is one of the most common fractures of the hand and usually occurs from a direct impact to the hand (eg, a punch with a closed fist).

Colles' fracture **(a)** is the most common wrist fracture seen in adults. It is a transverse fracture of the distal radial metaphysis, which is dorsally displaced and angulated. It usually occurs from a FOOSH. A Smith fracture **(b)** is a transverse fracture of the metaphysis of the distal radius, with associated volar displacement and angulation (the opposite of a Colles' fracture). The mechanism of injury is usually secondary to a direct blow or fall onto the dorsum of the hand. A scaphoid fracture **(c)** is the most common fracture of the carpal bones. It is typically seen in young adults secondary to a FOOSH. A Galeazzi fracture **(d)** involves a fracture at the junction of the middle and distal thirds of the radius, with an associated dislocation of the distal radioulnar joint (DRUJ).

288. The answer is d. The patient's clinical presentation is consistent with a **posterior shoulder dislocation**. Posterior dislocations are rare and account for only 2% of all glenohumeral dislocations. Posterior dislocations are traditionally associated with **seizures, lightening injuries**, and **electrocution injuries**. However, the most common dislocation seen in postseizure patients is an anterior dislocation. Classically, the patient holds the dislocated **arm across the chest in adduction and internal rotation**. Abduction is limited and external rotation is blocked. Radiographs may reveal a **"light bulb" sign**, which is the light bulb appearance when the humeral head is profiled in internal rotation. Posterior shoulder dislocations are frequently missed due to failure to suspect the injury and/or inadequate or misinterpreted plain films. There is often no obvious deformity and the shoulder may appear normal on anteroposterior (AP) or Grashey views. It is important to maintain a high index of suspicion and obtain the scapular Y and axillary views to confirm the diagnosis.

Although any type of injury can occur with a seizure (**a, b, c, and e**), the patient's clinical presentation is consistent with a posterior shoulder dislocation.

289. The answer is b. Dexamethasone and other **systemic steroids** are used in the treatment of gout in patients who cannot tolerate NSAIDs. **NSAIDs** are **contraindicated** in patients with comorbidities, such as peptic ulcer disease, GI bleeding, renal insufficiency, hepatic dysfunction, or are on warfarin.

Indomethacin (**a**), naproxen (**c**), and ketorolac (**e**) are all NSAIDs and would be contraindicated in this patient with renal insufficiency. Colchicine can be used in patients with renal insufficiency but is less commonly prescribed due to a narrow therapeutic window and risk of toxicity. Colchicine should be started within 36 hours of the onset of symptoms and is associated with side effects including vomiting and diarrhea. Intraarticular steroids such as triamcinolone acetonide, can be used for the treatment of gout. Topical steroid ointment (**d**) is not shown to be of benefit in the treatment of patients with gout.

290. The answer is c. The best way to **preserve an amputated part** is to rinse it with normal saline to remove gross contamination, wrap it in sterile gauze moistened with saline or lactated ringers, and place it in a sterile, watertight container. Then store this container in ice water.

Povidone-iodine (**a and d**) is a strong antiseptic solution that is used commonly in the hospital setting, particularly in the operating room to create a sterile field. However, it is thought to be injurious to fibroblasts and may limit wound healing. The amputated part should not be placed directly on ice or in ice water (**b**) because this may also damage the tissue. Reimplantation (**e**) of the thumb should be performed by a plastic surgeon in the operating room. The risk of tissue death increases the longer the severed part is not properly stored.

291. The answer is e. The patient sustained a **high-pressure injection injury** of his finger. This is a **surgical emergency**. These injuries may involve **extensive tissue loss** and are associated with **high infection rates**.

Most of these injuries involve grease, paint, or other industrial toxins. Paint generates a large, early inflammatory response, resulting in a high percentage of amputations. Within several hours after the digit has been injected, the extremity becomes painful and swollen. Initially, there may be anesthesia and even vascular insufficiency of the extremity. In the late stages, marked breakdown of the skin occurs, resulting in ulcers and draining sinuses. If the material injected into the extremity is radiopaque, it is possible to determine its degree of spread. Management involves **splinting** and **elevating** the extremity, administration of **antibiotics, tetanus prophylaxis** as indicated, **analgesia,** and immediate **hand surgery consultation.**

The patient requires admission, emergent orthopedic evaluation, and there is no indication for advanced imaging **(a, b, c, and d).**

292. The answer is b. This individual sustained a **calcaneal fracture** of the left foot. Ten percent of calcaneal fractures are associated with **compression fractures of the lumbar spine.** Therefore, it is important to examine the patient's entire spine. Calcaneal fractures are usually caused by an **axial load** such as a fall from a height with the patient landing on his or her feet. The examination reveals swelling, tenderness, and ecchymosis of the hindfoot and the inability to bear weight on the fracture.

The calcaneus is the most commonly fractured tarsal bone **(a).** The talus is the second most commonly injured tarsal bone. Calcaneal fractures are usually caused by compression injuries **(d),** not rotational injuries. Ten percent of calcaneal fractures are bilateral **(c).** Treatment varies depending on the extent of injury. In general, nondisplaced or minor extraarticular fractures only require supportive care with immobilization in a posterior splint and follow-up with an orthopedic surgeon **(e).** The management of intraarticular or displaced calcaneal fractures remains controversial regarding nonoperative versus immediate surgical reduction.

293. The answer is d. The CT image presented earlier demonstrates a **burst fracture of L2.** These fractures are commonly seen when a direct **axial load** is transmitted through the spine, in this case landing on the feet from a 15-foot fall. Burst fractures are unstable and require a thorough neurological examination and prompt neurosurgical consultation, as bone fragments and the disc may be retropulsed into the spinal cord. This type of injury is often seen in **conjunction with calcaneal fractures.** All patients with calcaneal fractures require dedicated imaging of their spine. **It is critical to distinguish burst fractures from simple compression fractures.**

While compression fractures only involve the anterior aspect of the vertebral body, burst fractures also have compression of the posterior vertebral body.

Solitary transverse process fractures (a) are stable and most often related to blunt trauma. Spinous process fractures (b), historically known as clay-shoveler fractures, occur most often from deceleration injuries and direct trauma and are noted to be stable. Simple wedge fractures (c) occur with longitudinal forces below the C2 level and can be differentiated from compression burst fractures by the absence of a vertical fracture of the vertebral body and less than 40% loss of height. Subluxation injuries (e) in the lumbar spine can be due to seatbelt injury (specifically lap-belt only) and can be associated with fractures of the vertebral bodies. These injuries can be quite devastating as they result in complete transection of the spinal cord.

294. The answer is c. Anterior elbow dislocations, although uncommon, have a much higher incidence of **vascular injury** than posterior dislocations. It is important to evaluate for an associated **brachial artery injury**.

Olecranon fractures (a) are associated with injury to the ulnar nerve not the median nerve. Individuals may experience paresthesias and numbness in the ulnar nerve distribution or weakness of the interossei muscles. Posterior elbow dislocations are associated with injuries to the ulnar and median nerves. They are not associated with brachial artery injuries (b). Supracondylar fractures (d), common in young individuals, are associated with injuries to the brachial artery and median nerve as the distal humeral fragment is displaced posteriorly, thus displacing the sharp fracture fragments anteriorly. Supracondylar fractures are not associated with injury to the radial nerve. Humeral shaft fractures (e) most commonly occur from a direct blow to the mid-upper arm. The fracture usually involves the middle third of the humeral shaft. The most common associated injury is damage to the radial nerve that causes wrist drop and loss of sensation in the first dorsal web space. Humeral shaft fractures are not associated with injury to the axillary nerve.

295. The answer is d. Pain disproportionate to injury or exam findings is the earliest sign of compartment syndrome. Compartment syndrome is defined as increased pressure within a closed space, ultimately compromising circulation and therefore function of tissues within the space. The end result is necrosis and damage to tissues. Up to 10% of tibial plateau fractures develop compartment syndrome. Compartment syndrome can occur in the setting of fractures (typically of long bones), vascular injury, crush injuries, circumferential burns, or iatrogenic etiologies (eg, surgical complications, IV infiltration). The earliest signs of compartment syndrome are **pain out of proportion to exam and pain on passive flexion of the muscle in the affected area. Compartment syndrome is a surgical emergency and requires orthopedic or surgical consult for fasciotomy.**

Pallor, pulselessness, paralysis, and paresthesia are all incorrect as they are late findings of compartment syndrome **(a, b, c, and e)**. The presence of a pulse does not rule out compartment syndrome.

296. The answer is a. The **Monteggia fracture** is a fracture of the **proximal one-third of the ulnar shaft** combined with a **radial head dislocation**. This injury commonly occurs from either a direct blow to the posterior aspect of the ulna or a FOOSH with the forearm in forced pronation. This fracture is associated with an **injury to the radial nerve**. It is always important to look for an associated fracture or dislocation when one is noted in a forearm bone. This diagnosis requires an orthopedic consult as the majority require surgical repair to provide stability to the elbow.

The Galeazzi fracture **(b)** is a fracture of the distal radial shaft associated with a distal radioulnar dislocation at the DRUJ. This fracture is often confused with Monteggia fracture. A way to remember the difference is to recall that Monteggia ends in an "a" and in this fracture, the ulna (also ends in "a") is fractured. A nightstick fracture **(c)** is an isolated fracture of the shaft of the ulna. This injury can occur after a direct blow to the ulna and usually occurs when an individual raises his or her forearm up to protect their face from a blow. A Colles' fracture **(d)** is a transverse fracture of the metaphysis of the distal radius with dorsal displacement of the distal fragment. The median nerve is at risk for injury in a Colles' fracture. A Smith fracture **(e)** is a transverse fracture of the distal radial metaphysis with volar displacement of the distal fragment. The median nerve is at risk for injury in the Smith fracture.

297. The answer is c. The patient has **herpetic whitlow**, a viral infection of the distal finger. This condition can be treated with **oral antiviral agents** such as acyclovir. It is caused by the **herpes simplex virus type I or II**. This condition typically occurs in health care providers with exposure to oral secretions, parents of children with primary oral infections, and in patients with coexistent herpes infections. There is generally a prodrome period of fever and malaise. Subsequently, there is localized burning, itching, and pain that precede the development of the classic clear herpetic vesicles. Typically, only one finger is involved. The diagnosis is usually made clinically, but, if doubt remains or if the presentation is atypical, it can be confirmed with a Tzanck smear or viral culture.

When managing this condition, it is important to note that surgical drainage is contraindicated (a) as this can result in secondary infection and delayed healing. It would be appropriate to splint the digit for comfort but you do not want to buddy tape it to the neighboring digit (b) because the tape wound be painful and cause additional damage to the skin underlying the vesicles. This practice would also increase the likelihood of spread to the adjacent digit. It would be inappropriate to leave the vesicles uncovered (d). A dry dressing should be placed over the vesicles to prevent transmission. Antibiotics (e) are not indicated unless there is evidence of bacterial superinfection.

298. The answer is c. Although CT-cervical spine imaging is negative, the patient **continues to have midline tenderness on examination** and therefore should be **discharged in a soft c-collar**. These patients should follow-up within 2 weeks and may require a routine MRI to evaluate for ligamentous injury. Occult ligamentous injuries can be missed on CT and plain radiographs, so patients with persistent midline tenderness require immobilization. The National Emergency X-Radiography Utilization Study **(NEXUS) Criteria** is a clinical decision rule to help determine which patients require imaging. Patients do not require C-spine imaging if all of the NEXUS criteria are met (see table).

NEXUS Criteria
Absence of posterior midline cervical tenderness
Normal level of conscious
No evidence of intoxication
No abnormal neurologic findings
No painful or distracting injuries

Because this patient has persistent midline cervical pain, his C-spine cannot be safely cleared clinically (a). This patient does not have any neurologic symptoms to necessitate an emergent MRI (d). Patients should never remain in the hard cervical collar as it is uncomfortable and can cause pressure sores to the occiput (b). The patient may need to see neurosurgery in follow-up but there is no indication for ED consultation (e).

299. The answer is c. The patient presents with a **subungual hematoma, a collection of blood underneath the nail** that usually results from trauma. The diagnosis is made by visual examination of the nail. If there is concern of injury to the underlying bone, **X-ray** imaging should be performed to **rule out associated fracture**.

While a cold compress (**a**) and digital nerve block (**d**) would assist with pain, it is more important to rule out underlying fracture. Hand surgery consultation (**b**) would be premature and unnecessary without further assessing for underlying fracture. If a distal phalanx tuft fracture is detected on X-ray, then splinting would be indicated (**e**).

300. The answer is e. An uncomplicated, painful subungual hematoma that does not involve disruption of nail edge should be **drained via trephination**. Trephination is performed using electrocautery or by twisting an 18 G needle through the nail. Once the trephination is performed, the blood that had collected under the nail will drain, alleviating pain and pressure. Multiple trephinations are sometimes needed.

Some experts suggest that painless hematomas may be left alone and do not require drainage Trephination and drainage is normally performed to alleviate pain and discomfort for the patient. If the nail edges are disrupted or the hematoma involves greater than 50% of the nail bed, the entire nail should be removed (**c**) to evaluate for nail bed laceration. Nail bed lacerations require repair with suturing since optimal initial management of the damaged nail bed decreases the likelihood of chronic painful nail plate deformity. Scalpel insertion under the nail edge (**d**) is the appropriate method to drain a paronychia. A pressure dressing (**a**) would cause increased pain and is not indicated. Buddy taping the finger (**b**) is not indicated.

301. The answer is a. The patient presents with **nursemaid's elbow,** or **radial head subluxation** due to immaturity of the annular ligament. This injury is most commonly seen in toddlers as the annular ligament strengthens over time. If there are no signs of joint effusion, the examiner can **flex and supinate the forearm with slight pressure held** on the radial head in an attempt to reduce the subluxation. The radial head should be palpated and during the maneuver, a click noted by the examiner has been shown to have a positive predictive value of over 90%. The child should begin to use the arm within minutes of the reduction, and immobilization is not needed for a first-time occurrence.

Pronation and extension of the forearm (**b**) is an incorrect method of reduction. An orthopedic consult (**c**) would be unnecessary for a nursemaid's elbow injury. A sling (**d**) for immobilization is not required. Reduction of a nursemaid's elbow is both diagnostic and therapeutic. X-ray images pre- and postreduction are not necessary unless there are signs of joint effusion, bruising, or deformity. In pediatrics, contralateral imaging is sometimes performed when there is diagnostic uncertainty between injury and normal anatomic variation, but there is no role for contralateral comparison (**e**) in this injury.

302. The answer is b. A **spiral fracture of the distal tibia** is known by the eponym **Toddler's fracture**. It is a fracture **commonly seen in ambulatory children aged 1 to 3 years**. The mechanism of injury usually involves a trivial fall or a twisting mechanism on a planted foot. Spiral fractures seen in nonambulatory children are highly suspicious for nonaccidental trauma (child abuse).

Greenstick fractures (**a**) are seen in children because the bones are soft and can bend resulting in incomplete fractures. X-rays demonstrate a "bow" fracture in which the bone becomes curved in its longitudinal axis. The outer cortex of the bone remains intact. The radiograph pictured demonstrates a fracture (**c**) and is not within normal limits. The Salter Harris classification is used to describe fractures involving the epiphyseal plate (physis) or growth plate. A Salter Harris I fracture is a fracture through the growth plate or physis. Diagnosis of this fracture is made clinically as the radiographs are negative. A Salter Harris II fracture involves the metaphysis and physis. A Salter Harris III fracture involves the physis and epiphysis. A Salter Harris IV fracture (**d**) involves the physis, metaphysic, and epiphysis. A Salter Harris V fracture (**e**) is a crush injury to physis. This fracture appears as decreased space between the epiphysis and diaphysis on radiograph.

303. The answer is d. Spiral fractures in children who are nonambulatory are highly suspicious for child abuse (nonaccidental trauma). In a child with suspected child abuse, a skeletal survey must be obtained to look for other occult fractures, both acute and subacute. Victims of suspected child abuse should also be evaluated by ophthalmology for retinal hemorrhages from shaking injuries. This child should be admitted to ensure safety and completion of the necessary medical and social evaluation. Additionally, the proper forms for suspected abuse need to be filed with Child

Protective Services. Social work should be consulted. The management of the toddler's fracture is a long leg cast for several weeks.

If child abuse is not suspected, a long leg lower extremity splint with orthopedic follow-up (a) is appropriate management. Compression wrapping does not provide adequate stabilization of this fracture and the appropriate management includes splinting even in the nonambulatory infant (b). For a nondisplaced spiral tibial fracture, orthopedic consultation from the ED (c) is not required but close follow-up with orthopedics is necessary. There is no indication for comparison radiographs in this case (e). With some bony injuries, comparison X-rays can be helpful to distinguish between acute injury versus congenital anatomic variance. However, in this case, it is unnecessary. If child abuse was not suspected and this was an isolated injury, analgesics and close follow-up with orthopedics (not the pediatrician) would be appropriate (e).

304. The answer is a. This X-ray demonstrates AVN of the **femoral head** with collapse of the femoral head. AVN is a known complication of **sickle cell disease**. AVN is the result of cellular death of bone components due to interruption of the blood supply. The anemia and vaso-occlusive crisis of sickle cell disease contribute to the interruption of the blood supply. The bone structures collapse, resulting in bone destruction, pain, and loss of joint function. Other risk factors for AVN include trauma (including femoral neck fracture) disrupting blood supply via the round ligament, hip dislocation (risk increases proportionally to duration), collagen vascular disease, Cushing's disease or chronic systemic steroid use, alcohol abuse, among other causes including idiopathic.

Osteosarcoma (b), hypertension (c), prostate cancer (d), and gout (e) have not been causally related to AVN of the hip.

305. The answer is a. The patient has a **lunate dislocation** as shown on the lateral radiograph of the wrist with volarly displaced lunate in the "**spilled teacup**" appearance. **Lunate dislocations** are usually caused by a **hyperextension** injury or a FOOSH. The **median nerve** runs through the carpal tunnel between the flexor carpi radialis and the palmaris longus. It provides sensation to the palmar aspect of the radial three and one-half fingers as well as the dorsal of the tips of the index and middle fingers and the radial half of the ring finger. The **median nerve may be compressed** in the carpal tunnel by the lunate, and the patient may display signs of **acute carpal tunnel syndrome**.

Perilunate dislocations (**b**) are the most common wrist dislocations and can also be associated with carpal tunnel syndrome. However, they have a different radiographic appearance.

Scapholunate dislocation (**c**) is sometimes defined on radiograph by the "Terry Thomas" or "David Letterman" sign, where there is a gap (>3 mm) in the space between the scaphoid and lunate (similar to a gap in the front teeth of these two people). Capitate dislocations (**d**) are rare. Scaphoid fractures (**e**) do not cause compression of the median nerve.

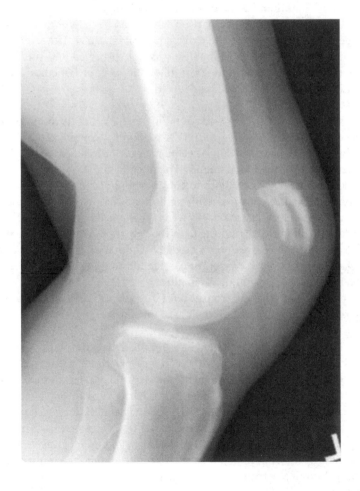

306. The answer is d. Septic arthritis is a bacterial infection of the joint space and its synovial fluid. It is an acute emergency and typically caused by either the hematogenous spread of bacteria to the joint capsule or by direct inoculation from recent arthrocentesis or joint surgery. In this case, the patient's history of IV drug abuse makes hematogenous spread more likely. Over 80% of cases are monoarticular and the most common joint affected is the knee. Patients classically present as above—with a painful, erythematous, warm joint and **endorse pain with both passive and active range of motion**. Risk factors for nongonococcal septic arthritis are history of IV drug use (as this patient), prosthetic joint, diabetes, immunocompromised states, the elderly, and those with indwelling catheters. Management includes analgesia, antibiotics, and investigation for primary source of infection if hematogenous spread is suspected. Orthopedics consultation is helpful to determine need for operative debridement or hardware removal if applicable.

Reactive arthritis **(a)** is a rare seronegative human leukocyte antigen B27 (HLA-B27) associated spondyloarthropathy secondary to a precipitating infection. It occurs most commonly in males under the age of 40 and typically affects large joints. It is classically characterized by a triad of urethritis, conjunctivitis (or uveitis), and arthritis ("can't see, can't pee, can't climb a tree"). Pseudogout **(b)** is a metabolic arthropathy caused by deposition of calcium pyrophosphate dihydrate crystals in the connective tissue. Patients typically present with pain, erythema, and warmth of the affected joint (similar to gout). Diagnosis is confirmed by arthrocentesis showing positively birefringent rhomboid crystals, and treatment may include NSAIDs, colchicine, or glucocorticoids. Gout **(c)** is another acute monoarticular arthropathy that presents similarly to pseudogout as mentioned above. It is distinguished by negatively birefringent needle-shaped monosodium urate crystals on arthrocentesis. Treatment is similar to pseudogout and may include NSAIDs, colchicine, or glucocorticoids. Rheumatoid arthritis **(e)** is a progressive systemic inflammatory polyarthritis. It more commonly affects women, and patients typically present with symmetric severe joint pain. While NSAIDs may be helpful in improving pain in acute flares, they do NOT prevent joint destruction. Importantly, many patients are on diseases modifying antirheumatic drugs (DMARDs) or biologics. While these medications do prevent disease progression, they also cause immunosuppression and increase susceptibility to underlying infection.

307. The answer is d. In septic arthritis, the fluid is typically cloudy or opaque in color and has a thin/watery viscosity. **Synovial WBC more than 50,000/ mm³ with synovial PMN 90% or more is most consistent with a diagnosis of septic arthritis.**

Answers **(a)** and **(c)** are incorrect because they are representative of normal synovial fluid, which has a thick viscosity, WBC less than 25,000 mm³, and PMN less than 30%. Answer **(b)** is incorrect as this is more representative of the crystal-induced arthropathy gout, with negative birefringent needle-shaped crystals. Answer **(e)** is also incorrect as this is representative of pseudogout.

308. The answer is B. Maisonneuve fracture. A Maisonneuve fracture is a **proximal spiral fracture of the fibula** that is **associated with a fracture of the medial malleolus or rupture of the deep deltoid ligament.** The typical mechanism of injury is ankle **eversion.** Many patients will only complain of ankle pain; therefore, it is critical to examine the entire leg as this will reveal **tenderness over the proximal fibula.** If tenderness over the proximal fibula is present, dedicated tibia-fibula radiographs should be obtained to make the diagnosis as below. Management in the ED involves analgesia and orthopedic consultation to plan for surgical repair.

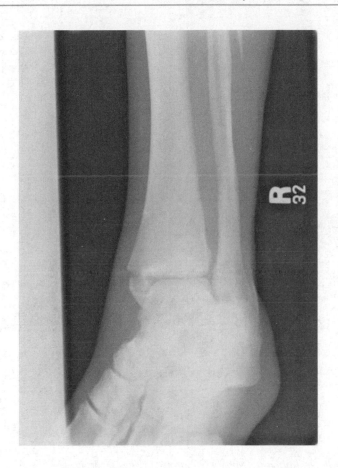

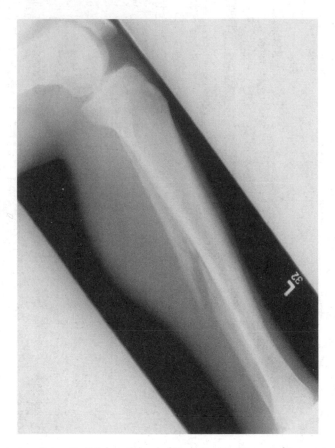

(Northwestern University, Feinberg School of Medicine, Department of Emergency Medicine.)

A Monteggia fracture (**a**) is a proximal ulnar fracture with radial head dislocation. A bimalleolar fracture (**c**) is a fracture of both the medial and lateral malleolus. A Galeazzi fracture (**d**) a fracture of the distal third of the radius with associated radioulnar joint dislocation. The talus (**e**) is the second most commonly fractured tarsal bone; however it is uncommon, accounting for only 3% to 6% of all foot fractures.

309. The answer is e. Lisfranc injury is a disruption of the tarsal-meta-tarsal (TMT) joint with or without an associated fracture. This is a **"can't miss" diagnosis** given that the Lisfranc ligament is a major stabilizer of the TMT joint, and injury or disruption to this ligament can cause mid-foot instability. Physical exam will typically demonstrate ecchymosis of the midfoot with swelling and pain at the TMT joint. Patients typically cannot bear weight, as in the case above. When a Lisfranc injury is suspected or confirmed, be sure to conduct a thorough neurovascular exam because the dorsal pedis artery crosses at the base of the first and second metatarsals, making it susceptible to potential injury.

A Jones fracture **(a)** refers to a fracture of the base of the fifth meta-tarsal. A pseudo-Jones **(b)** is a fracture of the base of the fifth metatarsal involving the lateral tuberosity. The navicular bone **(c)** is the most com-monly fracture midfoot bone and is important to diagnosis due to high risks of AVN. Stress fractures **(d)** typically occur secondary to repetitive low-intensity trauma where the rate of bone damage exceeds the rate of bone repair. This patient's injury is acute.

310. The answer is a. In a patient who is unable to actively extend the knee after an injury, suspect either a **patellar tendon rupture**, patella fracture, or quadriceps tendon rupture. The patellar tendon connects the patella to the tibia. While uncommon, patellar tendon rupture typically occurs in younger athletes. If ruptured, patient's will often have a high-riding patella (ie, patella alta) as seen in the radiograph. In contrast, the quadriceps ten-don connects the quadriceps muscle to the patella and when ruptured, results in a low-riding patella (ie, patella baja) on plain film.

Patellar fractures **(b)** are rare and typically occur with direct impact injuries (ie, high-energy dashboard injuries) or extensor mechanism injury. Patients will often have a palpable patellar defect with significant hemarthrosis, and are unable to perform a straight leg raise. Tibial plateau fractures **(c)** are fractures of the proximal aspect of the tibia. They have a bimodal distribution—typically occurring due to high-energy mechanisms in the young and low-energy mechanisms in the elderly. Patients will refuse to bear weight on the affected leg. Quadriceps tendon rupture **(d)** is more commonly seen in older patients with chronic illnesses or repeated steroid injections. Similar to patellar tendon rupture, disruption of the quadri-ceps tendon causes inability to extend the knee. The ACL **(e)** is the most commonly injured knee ligament and typically occurs due to noncontact athletic injuries. Patients often describe a "popping" sensation at the time of injury with subsequent knee swelling. Physical exam maneuvers may aid in diagnosis—including the Lachman test and anterior drawer test.

311. The answer is d. This patient's clinical presentation is concerning for a **posterior hip dislocation with associated sciatic nerve injury.** Posterior hip dislocations account for 90% of all hip dislocations and often occur due to "dashboard injuries" in MVCs (ie, posterior force transmitted to a flexed hip while patient is seated in vehicle). Around 10% of posterior hip dislocations are associated with sciatic nerve injury—which may present as above with a loss of sensation of the posterior leg and foot, loss or difficulty with plantar and dorsiflexion, and loss of DTR at the ankle. Reduction under conscious sedation should take place within 6 hours to decrease risk of AVN. Injury to the femoral nerve **(a)** is typically associated with anterior hip dislocations and presents as loss of sensation over the thigh, weakness of the quadriceps muscle, and loss of DTR at the knee. While injury to the femoral artery **(b)** is a complication of hip dislocations, this patient is vascularly intact. The obturator nerve **(d)** supplies sensation and innervation to muscles of the medial thigh. The saphenous nerve **(e)** arises from the femoral nerve and provides sensation to the anteromedial leg.

Recommended Readings

Bossart PJ. Chapter 83. Hip and femur injuries. In: Adams JA, Barton ED, Collings JL, et al, eds. *Emergency Medicine: Clinical Essentials.* 2nd ed. Philadelphia, PA: Saunders, 2013.

Castillo J. Chapter 85. Foot and ankle injuries. In: Adams JA, Barton ED, Collings JL, et al, eds. *Emergency Medicine: Clinical Essentials.* 2nd ed. Philadelphia, PA: Saunders, 2013.

Cydulka RK. Accuracy of Ottawa ankle rules to exclude fractures of the ankle and midfoot. *Ann Emerg Med.* 2004;43(5):675-676.

Gibbs M, Sara N. Chapter 89. Hand and wrist injuries. In: Adams JA, Barton ED, Collings JL, et al, eds. *Emergency Medicine: Clinical Essentials.* 2nd ed. Philadelphia, PA: Saunders, 2013.

Hopkins C. Chapter 84. Knee and lower leg injuries. In: Adams JA, Barton ED, Collings JL, et al. *Emergency Medicine: Clinical Essentials.* 2nd ed. Philadelphia, PA: Saunders, 2013.

Kaji AH, Newton EJ, Hockberger RS. Chapter 43. Spinal injuries. In: Marx JA, Hockberger RS, Walls RM, et al, eds. *Rosen's Emergency Medicine: Concepts and Clinical Practice*. 8th ed, Philadelphia, PA: Elsevier Saunders, 2018.

Knoop KJ, Stack LB, Storrow AB. *Atlas of Emergency Medicine*. New York, NY: McGraw-Hill, 2002: 305.

Sherman SC. *Simon's Emergency Orthopedics*. 8th ed. McGraw Hill Professional, China, 2019.

Stiell IG, Clement CM, McKnight RD, et al. The Canadian C-spine rule versus the NEXUS low-risk criteria in patients with trauma. *N Engl J Med*. 2003;349:2510-2518.

Tintinalli JE, Stapczynski J, Ma O, et al. eds. *Tintinalli's Emergency Medicine: A Comprehensive Study Guide*. 9th ed. New York, NY: McGraw-Hill, 2019.

Walls R, Hockberger R, Gausche-Hill M. *Rosen's Emergency Medicine—Concepts and Clinical Practice E-book*. Elsevier Health Sciences, 2017.

Wolff K, Johnson RA, Suurmond R. *Fitzpatrick's Color Atlas & Synopsis of Clinical Dermatology*. 5th ed. New York, NY: McGraw-Hill, 2005. Figures 25-27.

Headache, Weakness, and Dizziness

Jonah Gunalda, MD

Questions

The following scenario applies to questions 312 and 313.

A 21-year-old college student is brought to the emergency department (ED) by her roommate. The roommate states that earlier in the day the patient complained of a severe headache, stiff neck, and photophobia. On their way to the ED, the roommate states that she was confused. Her vital signs are blood pressure (BP) 110/80 mm Hg, heart rate (HR) 110 beats/minutes, respiration rate (RR) 16 breaths/minute, and temperature 102°F.

312. Which of the following is the most appropriate management of this patient?

a. Start empiric antibiotics and order a noncontrast head computed tomography (CT) before performing lumbar puncture (LP)
b. Order a noncontrast head CT and start antibiotics once CT is read by radiology
c. Give acetaminophen and IV fluid hydration and perform an LP
d. Perform an LP and select antibiotics based on the cerebral spinal fluid (CSF) results
e. Order a noncontrast head CT, perform an LP, then start antibiotics

313. The Gram stain of the patient's CSF reveals gram-negative diplococci. Which of the following is true regarding postexposure chemoprophylaxis?

a. Postexposure prophylaxis of the roommate is not warranted
b. The roommate should be given intravenous (IV) vancomycin
c. The roommate should have nasal swab for culture to determine need for chemoprophylaxis
d. The roommate should be given PO rifampin
e. The nurse, radiology technician, and registrar need chemoprophylaxis

314. A 29-year-old obese woman presents to the ED complaining of a generalized headache over the last 2 months. She has seen many doctors for it, but has yet to get a correct diagnosis. She describes the headache as moderate in intensity and worse with eye movement. Occasionally, it awakens her from sleep and is worse when tying her shoes. She is scared because her vision gets blurry for a few minutes every day. Her only medication is acetaminophen and an oral contraceptive. Her BP is 140/75 mm Hg, HR is 75 beats/minute, RR is 16 breaths/minute, and temperature is 98.9°F. On physical examination, you appreciate papilledema. Which of the following is the most appropriate next step in management?

a. Consult neurosurgery
b. Administer ceftriaxone 2 g IV then perform an LP to rule out meningitis
c. Order a magnetic resonance imaging (MRI) to look for carotid artery dissection
d. Prescribe her a triptan for her migraine headaches
e. Perform a CT scan, and if negative, perform an LP to measure the opening pressure

315. A 67-year-old woman presents to the ED complaining of a 2-day history of malaise, subjective fever, chills, diffuse headache, and right-sided jaw pain. She also notes diminished vision in her right eye. Her symptoms are minimally relieved with acetaminophen. She denies any sick contacts. The patient's BP is 130/75 mm Hg, HR is 95 beats/minute, RR is 16 breaths/minute, oral temperature is 100.6°F, and oxygen saturation is 99% on room air. She is tender on the right side of her scalp. You initiate empirical treatment. Which of the following tests will confirm your diagnosis?

a. Influenza assay
b. Rapid strep test
c. Erythrocyte sedimentation rate (ESR)
d. Complete blood count (CBC)
e. Temporal artery biopsy

316. A 25-year-old stockbroker presents to the ED complaining of 6 weeks of daily headaches. Her headaches are band-like in distribution and are not associated with nausea, vomiting, visual phenomena, or neurologic symptoms. Normally, they respond to acetaminophen, but they have increased in frequency in the past week as she stopped taking a medication that had been prescribed to prevent them. What type of headache is the patient likely experiencing?

a. Migraine headache
b. Cluster-type headache
c. Trigeminal neuralgia
d. Postherpetic neuralgia
e. Tension headache

317. A 22-year-old woman presents to the ED complaining of headache. She states that while at home, she experienced a headache that was associated with blurry vision in both eyes and a shimmering line in her vision. She subsequently lost her vision and felt uncoordinated, followed by increased pain at the base of her skull. Upon arrival in the ED, her vision returned to normal. A head CT scan and an LP are both negative. She now complains of a persistent, severe, pulsatile headache. She has had two similar episodes in the past year with the headache refractory to over-the-counter medications. Which of the following is likely to relieve her symptoms?

a. Diazepam
b. High-flow oxygen
c. Sumatriptan
d. Acetaminophen
e. LP with removal of 15 mL of CSF

318. A 25-year-old man presents to the ED complaining of headache for 2 days. He describes the pain as pulsatile and occipital. The patient had an LP 3 days earlier and was diagnosed with viral meningitis. Noncontrast head CT at that time was normal. He improved shortly thereafter with defervescence of his fever and resolution of his constitutional and nuchal symptoms. He states that his new headache is different than his previous in that it is exacerbated by standing or sitting upright and is relieved by lying down. It is not associated with photophobia or neck stiffness. The headache is not relieved by over-the-counter pain medications. He is afebrile and well-appearing. Which of the following is definitive therapy for this patient's headache?

a. One L bolus of IV normal saline
b. Treatment with standard pharmacologic agents for migraine
c. Treatment with meclizine
d. Consultation with anesthesia for a blood patch
e. Repeat LP to improve symptoms

319. A 57-year-old man with a past medical history of hypertension and migraines presents to the ED complaining of a headache that started 2 days ago. He states the headache began suddenly with peak intensity while he was defecating. The pain is continuous particularly in the occipital region and is associated with mild nuchal rigidity and mild photophobia. He denies having a recent fever. A noncontrast head CT is obtained and is normal. Which of the following is the most appropriate next step in management?

a. Provide IV metoclopramide and ketorolac
b. Perform an LP
c. Begin empiric treatment with IV antibiotics
d. Administer IV mannitol
e. Order CT angiography

The following scenario applies to questions 320 and 321.

A 21-year-old woman presents to the ED for a throbbing left-sided headache that began 4 hours prior to arrival and is associated with nausea, vomiting, and photophobia. She has a family history of migraine headaches. She states that she has had headaches like this in the past and they usually resolve after she sleeps in a cool, dark, quiet room. You order IV medications and after they are given, the nurse informs you that the patient may be having a stroke. She is grimacing, her tongue is protruding, and her head is turned to the left. You reassure the nurse that this is likely a medication side effect.

320. Which of the following medications is likely to have caused the patient's symptoms?

a. Morphine sulfate
b. Acetaminophen
c. Metoclopramide
d. Caffeine
e. Sumatriptan

321. What drug is commonly used to treat this medication side effect?

a. Dantrolene
b. Diphenhydramine
c. Droperidol
d. Glucagon
e. Haloperidol

322. A 55-year-old woman with a past medical history of diabetes presents to the ED with fever, headache, vision complaints, and right-sided weakness. She was treated for otitis media 2 weeks ago with amoxicillin. You obtain the CT scan seen in the figure. What is the most likely diagnosis?

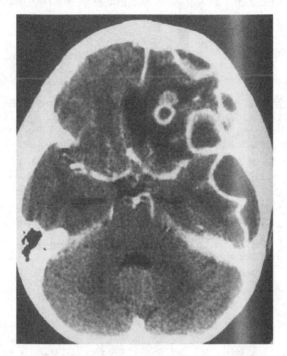

(Reproduced with permission from Schwartz DT, Reisdorff EJ. Emergency Radiology. New York, NY: McGraw Hill, 2000:430.)

a. Central nervous system (CNS) toxoplasmosis
b. Subdural hygroma
c. Glioblastoma multiforme
d. Brain abscess
e. Subarachnoid hemorrhage (SAH)

323. A 68-year-old man presents to the ED complaining of a daily head-ache for almost a month. He describes the headache as being dull, difficult to localize, most intense in the morning, and abating in the early afternoon. He also noticed progressive weakness of his right upper and lower extremity. Which of the following is most likely responsible for this patient's symptoms?

a. Intracranial neoplasm
b. Cluster headache
c. Tension-type headache
d. Idiopathic intracranial hypertension (IIH)
e. Waking or morning migraine

The following scenario applies to questions 324 and 325.

A 75-year-old man presents to the ED with a depressed level of conscious-ness. His wife is at the bedside and states he was stacking heavy boxes when he complained of a sudden intense headache. He subsequently sat down on the couch and progressively lost consciousness. She states that he had a headache the previous week. He had gone to visit his primary care physi-cian who sent him to have a CT scan of the brain, which was normal. Over the course of the past week, he complained of intermittent pulsating head-aches for which he took sumatriptan. In the ED, you intubate the patient and obtain the noncontrast head CT seen in the figure.

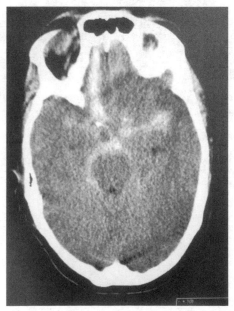

(Reproduced with permission from Adam J. Rosh, MD.)

324. What is the most likely diagnosis?

a. Meningoencephalitis
b. SAH
c. Normal-pressure hydrocephalus
d. Epidural hematoma
e. Subdural hematoma (SDH)

325. The patient takes warfarin for atrial fibrillation. Which of the following should be administered at this time?

a. Oral vitamin K via nasogastric tube
b. IV vitamin K
c. IV protamine sulfate
d. Crossmatched red blood cells (RBCs)
e. IV pantoprazole

326. A 43-year-old homeless man presents to the ED with fever and nuchal rigidity. His mental status is depressed, but his neurologic examination is otherwise nonfocal. Noncontrast head CT is normal. You obtain an LP for diagnostic purposes and initiate empiric antibiotic treatment for bacterial meningitis. The result of the CSF analysis is complete after 1 hour. The protein and glucose are within normal range, but the WBC count consists of 220 mononuclear cells. The Gram stain is negative. The patient was recently declared purified protein derivative (PPD) negative and had a normal chest X-ray. In addition to the treatment already initiated, what is the next most appropriate step in this patient's management?

a. Empiric treatment with isoniazid
b. Empiric treatment with acyclovir
c. Empiric treatment with antifungals
d. Antibiotic coverage for *Bartonella* sp
e. Addition of steroids to the antibiotic regimen

327. During a busy shift in the ED, you evaluate five patients whom you believe all require an LP to evaluate for meningitis. Of the following patients, who can undergo LP without a CT scan?

a. A 22-year-old man with fever and headache who had a witnessed seizure
b. A 49-year-old woman with acquired immunodeficiency syndrome (AIDS)
c. A 74-year-old man with new right lower extremity motor weakness
d. A 19-year-old man with a fever who is lethargic and disoriented
e. A 51-year-old woman who is febrile and complains of neck stiffness

328. A 53-year-old man presents to your ED stating he has an excruciating right-sided headache since leaving a movie theater 1 hour ago. He states that the headache is unilateral, severe, and associated with nausea and vomiting. His vision is blurry and notes seeing halos around objects. He denies trauma or a history of headaches in the past. Physical examination reveals right conjunctival injection and a mid-sized pupil that reacts only marginally. Which examination is likely to yield the correct diagnosis?

a. Measurement of intraocular pressure
b. Funduscopic examination
c. Fluorescein examination
d. LP with cell count
e. CT scan of the brain

329. A 35-year-old man presents to the ED complaining of a headache over the previous 4 weeks. He was assaulted with a baseball bat 4 weeks ago and was admitted to the hospital for observation in the setting of a small traumatic SDH. Repeat noncontrast CT scan of the head 2 weeks ago was normal with resolution of the hematoma. He states he has headaches several times each day. They last from 5 minutes to several hours. They are sometimes band-like; other times they are localized to the site where he was struck. They can be pulsating or constant and are associated with sensitivity to sound. A head CT scan this visit is normal. Which of the following is the most likely diagnosis?

a. Postconcussive syndrome
b. Posttraumatic hydrocephalus
c. Subdural hygroma
d. Cluster headache
e. Posttraumatic stress disorder (PTSD)

330. A 35-year-old woman presents to the ED complaining of headache and blurry vision. She has had daily headaches for 3 months associated with blurry vision. She is afebrile and has a normal neurologic and fundoscopic examination. She has not menstruated for 5 months and is not taking oral contraceptive pills (OCPs). She also complains of galactorrhea. Noncontrast head CT is normal. An LP is performed and reveals a normal opening pressure. Which of the following is the most appropriate next step in managing the patient's headaches?

a. Head CT with IV contrast
b. Treatment with bromocriptine
c. CSF analysis for xanthochromia and RBCs
d. MRI brain
e. Repeat LP with removal of 15 mL CSF

331. A 56-year-old man presents to the ED complaining of intermittent light-headedness and nausea throughout the day. He believes it started after eating leftover shrimp salad. On further questioning, he reports that the room is spinning around him. The symptoms are triggered by turning his head to the right. He denies hearing loss, tinnitus, or other associated symptoms. His BP is 137/85 mm Hg, HR is 67 beats/minute, RR is 14 breaths/minute, and temperature is 98.5°F. You can reproduce his symptoms by turning his head to the right. Which of the following is the most likely diagnosis?

a. Benign positional vertigo (BPV)
b. Food poisoning
c. Meniere disease
d. Labyrinthitis
e. Transient ischemic attack (TIA)

332. A 29-year-old woman presents to the ED complaining of double vision for 3 days. She states that she has been feeling very tired lately, particularly at the end of the day, when even her eyelids feel heavy. She feels better in the morning and after lunch when she is able to rest for an hour. Her BP is 132/75 mm Hg, HR is 70 beats/minute, RR is 12 breaths/minute, and temperature is 98.4°F. On examination, you find ptosis and proximal muscle weakness. What is the most appropriate diagnostic test to perform?

a. Edrophonium test
b. Serologic testing for antibodies to acetylcholine receptors (AChR)
c. CT scan of the head
d. Electrolyte panel
e. LP

The following scenario applies to questions 333 and 334.

A 40-year-old woman is brought to the ED by the paramedics complaining of bilateral foot weakness and numbness that started a few hours ago and is progressively worsening. She denies similar episodes in the past. On review of systems, she describes having abdominal cramps with nausea, vomiting, and diarrhea 2 weeks ago that resolved after 2 to 3 days. Her BP is 124/67 mm Hg, HR is 68 beats/minute, RR is 12 breaths/minute, and temperature is 98.8°F. On examination, you elicit 2/5 strength, decreased sensation, and loss of deep tendon reflexes in the lower extremities below the hips.

333. Which of the following is the most likely diagnosis?
a. Hypokalemic periodic paralysis
b. Guillain-Barré syndrome (GBS)
c. Peripheral neuropathy
d. Tetanus
e. Brain abscess

334. What life-threatening complication is associated with this disease process?
a. Permanent paralysis
b. Thrombocytopenia
c. Respiratory failure
d. Cardiogenic shock
e. Renal failure

335. A 58-year-old man presents to the ED complaining of generalized weakness for the last 2 days. He states that a few days ago he had abdominal cramps, vomiting, and diarrhea when his whole family got sick after a picnic. These symptoms resolved a day and a half ago, but he has not been eating well and now feels weak all over. He has a history of hypertension for which he takes hydrochlorothiazide (HCTZ). His primary physician recently increased his dose. His BP is 144/87 mm Hg, HR is 89 beats/minute, RR is 12 breaths/minute, and temperature is 98.7°F. The physical examination reveals hyporeflexia. His electrocardiogram (ECG) is shown in the figure. Which of the following is the most likely diagnosis?

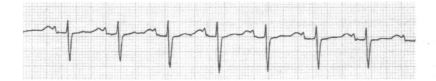

a. Hypernatremia
b. Hyponatremia
c. Hyperkalemia
d. Hypokalemia
e. Hypercalcemia

336. A 55-year-old man with hypertension, insulin-dependent diabetes mellitus, and end-stage renal disease on hemodialysis presents with severe generalized weakness and fatigue. He has no focal neurologic deficits, but is ill-appearing on examination. His ECG shows hyperacute T waves and a widened QRS complex. He then goes into cardiac arrest with pulseless electrical activity. In addition to CPR and epinephrine, which of the following medications should be given at this time?

a. Magnesium sulfate
b. Amiodarone
c. Procainamide
d. Furosemide
e. Calcium gluconate

The following scenario applies to questions 337 and 338.

A 35-year-old woman presents to the ED complaining of left arm weakness and right facial pain for 1 day. She denies any past medical history. On review of systems, she reports pain and decreased vision in her left eye approximately 4 months ago that has since resolved. She attributed it to being stressed and tired and did not see a physician at the time. Her BP is 126/75 mm Hg, HR is 76 beats/minute, RR is 12 breaths/minute, and temperature is 98.8°F. Her physical examination is unremarkable except for 4/5 strength in the left upper extremity.

337. Which of the following is the most likely diagnosis?

a. Myasthenia gravis
b. Multiple sclerosis (MS)
c. Vertebrobasilar artery occlusion
d. Encephalitis
e. GBS

338. Which of the following is the most appropriate initial diagnostic test?

a. Edrophonium test
b. Angiogram of the carotid arteries
c. LP and CSF analysis
d. Head CT
e. MRI of the brain

339. A 58-year-old woman is brought to the ED by paramedics complaining of worsening left arm and leg weakness. She reports a history of hypertension, diabetes, and tobacco use. She denies any past surgeries or other medical problems. Her BP is 165/83 mm Hg, HR is 110 beats/minute, RR is 18 breaths/minute, temperature is 98.4°F, and oxygen saturation is 98% on room air. Her capillary glucose is 147 mg/dL. On examination, the patient's speech is slurred and you notice a left-sided facial droop. Her left arm and leg strength is 2/5 and there is decreased sensation. The patient's head CT is normal. It has been 2.5 hours since the onset of symptoms. Which of the following is the most appropriate next step in management?

a. Admission for observation
b. Administer nitroprusside followed by thrombolytics
c. Administer heparin
d. Administer thrombolytic therapy
e. Administer aspirin

340. A 63-year-old woman is brought to the ED by EMS. She is accompanied by her husband. She developed right arm weakness that started 90 minutes ago. She has a history of hypertension and a long history of smoking cigarettes. She has no surgical history. The patient's BP is 215/118 mm Hg, HR is 97 beats/minute, RR is 14 breaths/minute, and temperature is 99.3°F. On examination, the patient is anxious and mildly aphasic. She has 2/5 motor strength and diminished sensation in the right upper extremity. An emergent head CT scan is normal. It has now been 2 hours since the onset of symptoms. Which of the following is the most appropriate next step in management?

a. Administer labetalol
b. Administer fibrinolytic therapy
c. Administer aspirin followed by fibrinolytic therapy
d. Administer phenytoin followed by fibrinolytic therapy
e. Administer mannitol followed by fibrinolytic therapy

341. An 82-year-old right-handed woman is brought to the ED by her daughter. According to her daughter, the patient has not been able to walk after waking up from a nap 30 minutes ago. She has a history of hypertension and diabetes. Her BP is 179/76 mm Hg, HR is 91 beats/minute, RR is 14 breaths/minute, and temperature is 98.9°F. On examination, you elicit neurologic deficits and emergently bring her to the CT scanner. The radiologist calls to report concern for a left middle cerebral artery stroke. Which of the following deficits are most consistent with this diagnosis?

a. Right-sided sensorimotor deficit in the arm greater than the leg, as well as aphasia
b. Left-sided sensorimotor deficit in the arm greater than the leg, as well as aphasia
c. Right-sided sensorimotor deficit in the leg greater than the arm, slowed response to questions, and impaired judgment
d. Right-sided sensorimotor deficit and left-sided facial droop
e. Isolated right leg motor deficit

342. A 67-year-old man is brought to the ED by his wife who is concerned that her husband's "face looks different." He has reportedly been nauseated, vomiting, and unsteady on his feet since the previous day. He also has been having blurred vision and difficulty swallowing. He also feels like the room is tilting from side to side. The patient's past medical history is notable for obesity and hypertension. His BP is 187/89 mm Hg, HR is 86 beats/minute, RR is 13 breaths/minute and temperature is 99.3°F. On examination, you find a right facial droop, diplopia, vertical nystagmus, and severe ataxia. Which of the following is the most likely diagnosis?

a. Lacunar infarct
b. BPV
c. Labyrinthitis
d. Posterior cerebral artery occlusion
e. Vertebrobasilar artery occlusion

343. A 57-year-old man presents to the ED with generalized weakness, body aches, abdominal discomfort, and nausea for 2 days. On review of systems, he also admits to recent polydipsia, polyuria, and an unintentional 10-lb weight loss. His medical history includes hypertension for which he takes no medications. He has a 20-pack-year smoking history. The vital signs are remarkable for mild tachycardia and hypertension. Laboratory results reveal a serum sodium 131 mEq/L, potassium 3.5 mEq/L, chloride 101 mEq/L, bicarbonate 22 mEq/L, blood urea nitrogen (BUN) 15 mg/dL, creatinine 1.1 mg/dL, glucose 125 mg/dL, and serum calcium level of 12.6 mEq/L. Which of the following is the most appropriate next step in management?

a. Administer calcitonin
b. Start normal saline IV bolus
c. Administer furosemide
d. Obtain chest radiograph
e. Obtain ECG

The following scenario applies to questions 344 and 345.

A 46-year-old woman presents to the ED with left-sided arm and leg weakness for 30 minutes. She has no medical problems except for chronic neck pain after a motor vehicle collision 5 years ago. On examination, she has right eye miosis, partial ptosis, and 3/5 strength in her left upper and lower extremities.

344. Which of the following describes the patient's ocular findings?
a. Oculomotor nerve palsy
b. Bell's palsy
c. Horner's syndrome
d. Kehr's sign
e. Nikolsky's sign

345. On further questioning, the patient states that earlier in the day she saw a chiropractor for her neck pain. After the session, she developed severe right-sided neck pain. About an hour later, she noticed difficulty using the left side of her body. Which of the following is the most likely diagnosis?
a. Internal carotid artery (ICA) dissection
b. Cavernous sinus syndrome
c. MS
d. Transverse myelitis
e. Spinous process fracture of a cervical vertebra

346. A 64-year-old man presents to the ED complaining of an episode of vertigo he experienced while exercising in the gym. He states that he has been having similar episodes with exercise for a week. His routine consists of running on a treadmill, lifting weights, and doing leg presses. The vertigo usually occurs mid-routine when he is lifting weights and resolves with cessation of exercise. He also noticed unusual left arm pain during these episodes. He has hypertension for which he takes antihypertensive medication and had a myocardial infarction 6 years ago. He decreased his smoking from one pack/day to five cigarettes/day over the last 6 years. His BP in the right arm is 148/80 mm Hg and in the left arm it is 129/74 mm Hg. Which of the following is the most likely diagnosis?

a. Superior vena cava syndrome
b. Aortic dissection
c. Subclavian steal syndrome
d. Angina pectoris
e. Vestibular neuronitis

347. A 36-year-old woman presents to the ED complaining of worsening weakness over the past few weeks. Initially, she attributed this to being overworked, but for the last few days she has been having difficulty getting out of her chair and walking up the steps to her fourth-floor apartment. She has no prior medical history and takes no medications. Her vital signs are unremarkable. On examination, she has 5/5 strength in her bilateral upper and lower extremities distally but 3/5 strength proximally. Sensory examination and reflexes are normal. You also notice a red confluent macular rash on her eyelids. Which of the following is the most likely diagnosis?

a. Myasthenia gravis
b. MS
c. Dermatomyositis
d. Rhabdomyolysis
e. Disseminated gonococcal infection

348. A 31-year-old woman presents to your ED with a headache. The headache started soon after she gave birth to her son 3 weeks ago. Her pregnancy and peripartum course were unremarkable and she is back on OCPs. The headache is aching, constant, slowly worsening, and severe. She denies changes to her vision, fevers, and chills. She reports that her left leg has become clumsy and weak. She has not fallen. What test would be most likely to provide you the diagnosis?

a. Serum AChR antibodies
b. LP with fluid analysis
c. CT venography of the head
d. Carotid angiography
e. Electroencephalogram (EEG)

349. A mother brings her 2-month-old son into the ED with poor feeding. Mom is concerned that he has seemed progressively lethargic for the past 1 week. He was previously healthy, was born by spontaneous vaginal delivery, and takes no medications. He is making a normal amount of wet diapers, but has not had a bowel movement since early the previous day. His physical examination reveals a floppy baby with drooping eyelids. A point-of-care glucose is normal and his CBC and comprehensive metabolic panel (CMP) are unremarkable. Head CT scan and LP are normal. His mom reports that he has also had a cough, which his grandfather has been treating with honey. What clinical condition is most consistent with this presentation?

a. Myasthenia gravis
b. Hypokalemic paralysis
c. Lambert-Eaton myasthenic syndrome (LEMS)
d. Todd paralysis
e. Infantile botulism

Headache, Weakness, and Dizziness

Answers

312. The answer is a. This patient presents with symptoms consistent with **meningitis**. **Antibiotics** are administered **empirically** as diagnostic workup proceeds. The best choice in this patient is **ceftriaxone**, which has good CNS penetration. In order to avoid transtentorial herniation in this patient with a **neurologic abnormality (confusion)**, a **noncontrast head CT** should be performed **before LP**. It is controversial whether or not a head CT needs to be performed before all LPs. However, if papilledema or a neurologic abnormality is present, head CT is mandatory.

It is not prudent to wait for official radiology results from a head CT before giving antibiotics (**b**). This will only delay treatment of a potentially fatal disease. Although this patient can benefit from acetaminophen and hydration (**c**), starting antibiotics empirically is more important. In addition, this patient requires a head CT before LP. As previously stated, antibiotics should be started early in management and not be delayed while waiting for results (**d and e**).

313. The answer is d. This patient's Gram stain is concerning for *Neisseria meningitidis*. Household close contacts (ie, roommate) or those exposed directly to the patient's oral secretions (ie, physician performing intubation) should receive postexposure chemoprophylaxis with antibiotics effective against *N. meningitidis* (rifampin, ciprofloxacin, or ceftriaxone).

Contacts exposed to other causes of meningitis (**a**) such as *Streptococcus pneumonia* or *Haemophilus influenzae* do not benefit from prophylaxis. Vancomycin (**b**) is not an antibiotic of choice against *N. meningitidis* in this scenario. Prophylaxis is most effective when administered within 24 hours (**c**) and should not be delayed for cultures. Although a frequent cause of anxiety, most normal health care workers (**e**) do not warrant treatment unless they are exposed to large droplet respiratory secretions.

314. The answer is e. The patient most likely has **IIH**, formerly pseudotumor cerebri, a neurologic disease seen primarily in **young obese women** of **childbearing age**. Clinically, patients complain of a generalized headache of gradual onset and moderate severity. It may worsen with eye movements or with the Valsalva maneuver. Visual complaints are common and may occur several times a day and can become permanent in 10% of patients. Patients typically have **papilledema** and visual field defects on physical examination. Diagnosis is made by a normal neuroimaging scan (ie, head CT scan) and an elevated intracranial pressure (ICP) (>25 mm Hg) measured by the opening pressure obtained from a lateral decubitus LP. This is also therapeutic as the aim is to preserve vision.

   This patient does not require immediate surgery (**a**) but may require a ventricular shunt in the future if she exhibits impending vision loss. Neurosurgery consultation can wait until after the diagnosis is made. Two grams of ceftriaxone (**b**) is therapy for meningitis, which this patient does not have. She is afebrile with no other constitutional or meningeal symptoms or signs. A carotid artery dissection (**c**) presents classically with the triad of unilateral headache, ipsilateral partial Horner's syndrome, and contralateral hemispheric findings, such as aphasia, visual disturbances, or hemiparesis. This patient does not exhibit any of these findings. Migraines (**d**) tend to be unilateral and pulsating and associated with nausea, vomiting, photophobia, phonophobia, blurred vision, and light-headedness. Patients should not exhibit papilledema.

315. The answer is e. This patient's clinical picture is consistent with **temporal arteritis (TA)**. Patients are usually **middle-aged** (age > 50) **women** who present with malaise, fevers, and headache. A complete physical examination would have revealed **temporal artery tenderness** to palpation. This patient also complains of symptoms consistent with **polymyalgia rheumatica**, a general achiness that may become confused with influenza. Temporal or giant-cell arteritis is a granulomatous inflammation that involves the large- and medium-sized arteries of the body, commonly the carotid artery and its branches. Symptoms are produced as a result of ischemia to the organs fed by the branches of the artery. Visual loss in one eye, transient diplopia, and jaw claudication are common symptoms when the branches of the internal and external carotid are affected. A **temporal artery biopsy** is the diagnostic test of choice and will confirm the diagnosis. However, it is important to note that TA is segmental in nature and false negatives do occur. Treatment up until the time of biopsy should include high-dose

glucocorticoids, namely, prednisone or methylprednisolone. This does not alter biopsy results and may prevent progression of the disease. Hospitalization is warranted in patients with severe debilitation or impending visual loss and may require high-dose steroids.

Symptoms of influenza (**a**) closely mimic those of polymyalgia rheumatica, were it not for the specific eye and jaw symptoms. Patients with streptococcal pharyngitis (**b**) may present with profound general malaise; however, they are typically more febrile and have a history of sick contacts and dry cough. Tonsillar exudates and anterior cervical adenopathy might be evident upon physical examination. An ESR between 50 and 100 mm/h (**c**) is a good initial test to further the suspicion of TA; however, it is not the diagnostic test of choice. An elevated C-reactive protein may also be present. A CBC (**d**) may indicate anemia, which results from the arterial inflammation that furthers the breakdown of RBCs. However, this and an elevated WBC count are nonspecific findings.

316. The answer is e. Tension headaches often occur **daily**, and classically cause bilateral occipital pain that is described as a **band tightening** around the head. In general, people experience a constant, dull pain that is not throbbing and without the ancillary features associated with migraines (eg, visual phenomena, aura, neurologic complaints, nausea, or vomiting). There is often secondary contraction of the neck and scalp musculature. First-line treatment includes **NSAIDs** and **acetaminophen**. If the headaches occur frequently enough to cause dysfunction in daily activities, patients may benefit from preventive therapy, such as amitriptyline, desipramine, or propranolol.

Migraine headaches (**a**) classically begin with visual phenomena or another aura and are pulsatile, unilateral, associated with nausea, vomiting, photophobia, and phonophobia. They may also have associated neurologic phenomena. Cluster headaches (**b**) are more common in men and are unilateral, boring, and may be associated with neurologic phenomena or autonomic activation. They are short lived and generally recur daily at the same time for days or weeks before the patient has remission of their symptoms. Trigeminal neuralgia (**c**) is thought to result from microvascular compression of the trigeminal nerve roots. It presents as shooting facial pain, in the distribution of the fifth cranial nerve (CN), particularly the second and third nerve roots. In fewer than 5% of cases, it involves the first division of the trigeminal nerve and patients will present complaining of headache. Treatment includes carbamazepine or other antiepileptic drugs.

Postherpetic neuralgia (d) is pain that continues after an eruption of herpes zoster. It is often described as a burning or stabbing pain that is constant in the dermatome originally affected by the zoster outbreak. In 50% of patients, it subsides after 6 months. In some patients, it lasts for years. Treatment is with gabapentin, phenytoin, or amitriptyline.

317. The answer is c. The patient is experiencing a **migraine** variant known as a **basilar migraine**. Its onset is similar to other migraines in that it can begin with scotomata or aura. The visual symptoms are often bilateral and followed by a brief period of cortical blindness. Symptoms related to the basilar circulation then predominate, including incoordination, dysarthria, vertigo, and numbness and tingling in the arms or legs. These symptoms generally last 10 to 30 minutes then resolve. Occasionally, transient coma or quadriplegia can develop but persist for only several hours. The resulting headache is **occipital and pulsating**. The symptoms may mimic a vertebro-basilar ischemic event. Treatment with first-line agents for migraine (most commonly a sumatriptan) is recommended. Threshold should be low to seek neurologic consultation and possible MRI/MRA (magnetic resonance angiography) unless the diagnosis is certain.

Diazepam (a) is useful for treating cervical muscle spasm and torticollis. It is unlikely to relieve the pain associated with a migraine although it may be useful for associated scalp and trapezius spasm. High-flow oxygen (b) is beneficial to migraine patients but is not the mainstay of treatment. Acetaminophen (d) is a useful first-line treatment with NSAIDs for migraine and tension-type headaches. Therapeutic removal of CSF (e) is indicated in cases of IIH.

318. The answer is d. The patient has a **post-LP headache**. The headache is thought to be caused by the removal of CSF during LP with a continued leakage of CSF. The headache is **positional** and many patients will experience relief of pain after being placed in the Trendelenburg position. A **blood patch** is placed by injecting an aliquot of the patient's blood in a sterile fashion just external to the dura mater at the same interspace where the LP occurred. The majority of patients have relief of symptoms with this procedure. Prevention of the post-LP headache includes using a 22-gauge or smaller needle, removing as little fluid as possible, and facing the bevel up when the patient is in the lateral position.

Administering IV fluids (a) is thought to increase intravascular volume and CSF production, thereby reducing symptoms. While IV fluid should be administered to this individual, it is not definitive treatment. Standard migraine treatments **(b)** are often ineffective in treating the post-LP headache. The headache often responds well to caffeine-based therapy. Meclizine **(c)** is a medication used to treat peripheral vertigo and is ineffective in the treatment of the post-LP headache. Repeat LP **(e)** is unlikely to yield new diagnostic information and is likely to exacerbate the headache.

319. The answer is b. The patient presents with a clinical history that is consistent with a **SAH**. Brain CT without contrast is the procedure of choice for diagnosing SAH and should be done in any individual with a new onset of a severe or persistent headache. It has a sensitivity of 95% for detecting SAH. **If the CT is negative, an LP should be performed.** A yellow supernatant liquid (xanthochromia), obtained by centrifuging a bloody CSF sample, can help distinguish SAH from a traumatic tap. If the diagnosis is still in question, angiography may be required.

Administration of metoclopramide and ketorolac **(a)** is useful in managing pain as a result of a migraine. Because of their antiplatelet activity, ketorolac and other NSAIDs are contraindicated in patients who may be actively bleeding. Treatment of meningitis **(c)** with IV antibiotics should not be delayed if the diagnosis is suspected. However, the patient's clinical history is inconsistent with this diagnosis. Infusion of IV mannitol **(d)** lowers ICP acutely via osmotic diuresis. It is indicated in patients displaying symptoms of increased ICP or when impending herniation is suspected. Angiography **(e)** is the gold standard for diagnosis of a cerebral aneurysm, but LP should be performed to confirm the presence of intracranial bleeding before contrast-based imaging.

320. The answer is c. Dystonic reactions may occur with the use of dopamine-blocking agents. Medications classically associated with dystonic reactions are typical antipsychotics (eg, haloperidol) but can also occur with the antiemetics used to treat migraines (eg, **metoclopramide**). Common dystonic reactions include oculogyric crises (eyes deviating in different directions), torticollis, tongue protrusion, facial grimacing, and difficulty speaking.

Morphine sulfate **(a)** has the principal side effect of respiratory depression. This effect and the drug's analgesic properties are reversed by naloxone. Localized reactions including erythema, swelling, and pruritus are common after intramuscular or subcutaneous injection. Anaphylaxis has been described but is rare. Acetaminophen **(b)** has the principal side effect of hepatotoxicity. In patients using it chronically without following dose-based guidelines, liver damage is possible. Caffeine (**d**) is a methylxanthine. Side effects include palpitations, anxiety, tremulousness, and dry mouth. Sumatriptan (**e**) has side effects related to the cardiovascular system. They include hypertension and coronary artery vasospasm. Several cases of myocardial infarctions have been observed after its use.

321. The answer is b. **Dystonic reactions** are generally not life threatening and respond almost immediately to administration of **diphenhydramine** given intravenously or intramuscularly. Other frequently used medication options include benzodiazepines and other anticholinergic medications (eg, benztropine).

While dantrolene (**a**) can function as a muscle relaxant, its side effect profile limits its use to more life-threatening conditions (eg, neuroleptic malignant syndrome, malignant hyperthermia). Droperidol (**c**) and haloperidol (**e**) are both first-generation antipsychotic medications and are potential causes of dystonia or other extrapyramidal symptoms. Glucagon (**d**) does not have a known role in the management of dystonia.

322. The answer is d. **Brain abscesses** are uncommon and the incidence has decreased over the past several years as a result of better antibiotic treatment of the remote infections that cause them. **Today, the majority of brain abscesses in developed countries are the result of contiguous spread from otitis media, mastoiditis, paranasal sinusitis, or meningitis.** They can also occur after trauma, classically after a basilar skull fracture. Presentation is often nonspecific, with almost half presenting with headache alone. Focal weakness, fevers, and nausea are other common presenting complaints. Antibiotic choice should be guided by suspected source and ability to penetrate the CNS. In general, MRI is more sensitive at detecting CNS infection than CT. With contrast CT, the walls of the abscess enhance and there is a central necrotic area of lower density (ring enhancing). On this CT with IV contrast, there are multiple ring-enhancing lesions with surrounding edema in the left frontal lobe. The large extraaxial collections with enhancing margins represent emphysemas. There is also midline shift secondary to mass effect of the abscesses.

CNS toxoplasmosis (**a**) is uncommon in the developed world outside of advanced human immunodeficiency virus (HIV) or other immunocompromised states. Patients often present with altered mental status, neurologic deficits, or seizures. On contrast-enhanced CT, there are often multiple, small, ring-enhancing lesions. Subdural hygromas **(b)** are fluid-filled subdural pockets containing xanthochromic fluid. They are often the result of trauma and present with signs and symptoms of increased ICP or with neurologic deficits. They are thought to result from tears in the arachnoid with fluid accumulation. Glioblastoma multiforme **(c)** is the most common and most aggressive of the primary brain tumors. On CT scans, glioblastomas usually appear as irregularly shaped hypodense lesions with a peripheral ring-like zone of contrast enhancement and a penumbra of cerebral edema. Spontaneous SAHs **(e)** present as severe headaches associated with nausea, vomiting, nuchal rigidity, and can have neurologic deficits associated with them. It appears on noncontrast CT as hyperdense fluid that may fill the cisterns and subarachnoid space.

323. The answer is a. Headaches caused by a mass lesion, such as an **intracranial neoplasm**, are classically described as **worse in the morning**, associated with **nausea and vomiting**, and **positional**. Rarely do patients present with focal neurologic symptoms. When they do, imaging is a necessary adjunct before leaving the ED. If a mass lesion is part of the differential diagnosis, LP should be deferred until neuroimaging has been performed because of the risk of herniation.

Cluster headaches **(b)** are rare, generally occur in male patients, last less than 2 hours, and present as unilateral eye or temporal pain. There is often unilateral tearing, swelling, or nasal congestion. In contrast to the migraine patient, patients with cluster headaches are typically restless. Cluster headaches respond to ergots, triptans, and often high-flow oxygen. Tension-type **(c)** headaches are bilateral, not pulsating, not worsened by exertion, and should not be associated with nausea or vomiting. They generally respond to NSAIDs or acetaminophen. Headaches associated with IIH **(d)** are exacerbated by changes in position (eg, squatting), are often frontotemporal, and may be associated with disturbances of gait and incontinence. They are difficult to control. Migraines **(e)** are generally unilateral, pulsating, associated with phonophobia or photophobia, nausea, and vomiting. They are slow in onset and generally last 4 to 72 hours. There is considerable heterogeneity in their presentation. Most patients with chronic migraines can describe their headache syndrome and are able to differentiate between their normal migraine and another headache. Change in the character, intensity, location, or duration of a migraine should prompt suspicion of another cause.

324. The answer is b. The CT scan depicts a **subarachnoid hemorrhage**. This patient may have had a sentinel bleed (a small SAH) the previous week as described by his wife. Noncontrast CT misses a small percentage of SAHs and therefore, in cases of high suspicion, an LP must be obtained to exclude the diagnosis.

Irritation of the meninges or inflammation of the brain **(a)** may not appear at all on noncontrast CT of the brain. If contrast is used, meningeal or cerebral enhancement may be apparent, but diagnosis of these conditions is not based on imaging. High clinical suspicion must be present for either condition, and LP with CSF analysis confirms the diagnosis. Hydrocephalus **(c)** appears as dilated ventricles on CT scan. If all of the ventricles are patent and dilated, it is termed communicating hydrocephalus. If part of the ventricular system is collapsed and the others dilated, an obstructive cause of hydrocephalus is present. Epidural hematomas **(d)** are the result of brisk arterial bleeds into the space between the dura and the calvarium. They are classically caused by trauma and are associated with a "lucid period" during which level of consciousness is normal before neurologic deterioration. On noncontrast CT, they appear as hyperdense intracranial collections of blood that are biconvex in shape. SDHs **(e)** are intracranial blood collections that result from tearing of the bridging veins between the dura and the brain. Risk factors for SDH include advanced age and chronic alcohol use. Both conditions are associated with decreased brain volume and provide stretch on these delicate veins. On noncontrast CT, SDHs appear as crescent-shaped collections of hyperdense blood.

325. The answer is b. In the setting of life-threatening bleeding as in this case, patient's taking warfarin should be given **vitamin K 10 mg IV**. Warfarin is a vitamin K antagonist and inhibits clotting factors II, VII, IX, and X along with plasma proteins C and S. IV vitamin K is preferred to oral vitamin K in life-threatening bleeding [eg, intracerebral hemorrhage, exsanguinating gastrointestinal (GI) hemorrhage].

Oral vitamin K **(a)** is recommended for non-life-threatening bleeding in patients taking warfarin, or those with a supratherapeutic international normalization ratio (INR) level. Protamine sulfate **(c)** is the antidote for bleeding from heparin. Crossmatched RBCs **(d)** has no mortality benefit in life-threatening intracerebral hemorrhage. IV pantoprazole **(e)** or other proton pump inhibitors may be given to patients experiencing GI bleeding, but these agents have no role in the management of life-threatening intracerebral hemorrhage.

326. The answer is b. The CSF analysis in this patient is consistent with a **viral or atypical cause of meningitis**. Although patients may have a mononuclear predominance and still have bacterial meningitis, viral causes should be considered. CSF should be sent for polymerase chain reaction (PCR) analysis and empiric treatment with **acyclovir** initiated for **herpes encephalitis**. The mortality of meningoencephalitis caused by herpes simplex virus (HSV) is exceptionally high if untreated.

Tuberculosis (TB) meningitis **(a)** should be considered in this homeless patient. Other risk factors for TB include an immunocompromised state and living in an endemic region. However, the patient is PPD negative with a normal chest X-ray, making this possibility less likely. In an immunocompromised patient, PPD may be less reliable so a CSF acid-fast stain and mycobacterial culture should still be sent. Fungal causes **(c)** of CNS pathology are also a diagnostic consideration but are less likely than viral causes. In this patient, fungal cultures are recommended in addition to CSF cryptococcal antigen. *Bartonella* sp **(d)** and other rare causes of meningitis are not considered until other first- and second-tier analyses are conducted. When given simultaneously with (or before, but not after) the first dose of antibiotics, corticosteroids **(e)** reduce the incidence of sensorineural hearing loss associated with bacterial meningitis in children. Steroids also decrease the risk of an unfavorable outcome in adults with bacterial meningitis.

327. The answer is e. Indications for brain CT scanning before LP include—patients who are **immunocompromised**, patients with **known CNS disease** (eg, tumor, stroke), patients who presented with a new-onset **seizure** or who had a seizure within 1 week of presentation, patients with **abnormal level of consciousness**, patients with a known **malignancy**, patients more than 60 years old, patients with **focal findings on neurologic examination**, and patients with **papilledema** seen on physical examination with clinical suspicion of elevated ICP.

All of the patients in this scenario **(a, b, c, and d)** fit one of these contraindications except for the 51-year-old woman with fever and neck stiffness.

328. The answer is a. The patient presents with **acute angle closure glaucoma** that results from obstruction of aqueous outflow of the anterior chamber of the eye with a resulting **rise in intraocular pressure**. It is the result of a shallow anterior chamber or a chamber distorted by the development of a cataract. Classically, it occurs when a patient leaves a prolonged dimly lit environment (eg, movie theater). When the iris becomes mid-dilated, it maximally obstructs the trabecular meshwork occluding aqueous humor flow. Intraocular pressures may rise from normal (10-21 mm Hg) to levels as high as 50 to 100 mm Hg. **Visual acuity is usually decreased** in the affected eye as a result of corneal edema. Treatment is aimed at lowering intraocular pressure with acetazolamide, ophthalmic β-blockers, prosta-glandin analogues, and pilocarpine to induce miosis. Patients may present complaining of headache, nausea, and vomiting but will often endorse that the symptoms began with acute eye pain. Ophthalmologic consultation and follow-up are indicated.

Funduscopic examination (**b**) is occasionally abnormal in acute glau-coma, but papilledema rarely develops acutely. Corneal examination with fluorescein (**c**) is used to diagnose corneal abrasions or other corneal pathology (eg, ulcers, keratitis). The cornea may appear normal or "steamy" in the setting of acute glaucoma as the edges accumulate edema from the increase pressure of the anterior chamber. The cornea normally should not take up fluorescein. LP (**d**) is used to diagnose intracranial pathology. The acute unilateral pain of glaucoma may make the clinician consider an SAH, but glaucoma should always be considered. CT scan of the brain (**e**) should be normal in patients diagnosed with glaucoma.

329. The answer is a. Thirty to 90% of patients complain of headache while recovering from head trauma. **Postconcussive headaches** are nota-ble for their **variability** in frequency, location, and associated symptoms. They are often exacerbated by physical activity or changes in position and may be clinically difficult to distinguish from other headache syndromes. In patients with preexisting migraines, increased frequency of their nor-mal migraine syndrome is often noted. Most patients have resolution of their headaches after 4 weeks. In 20% of patients, their postconcussive headache persists for longer than a year. Headache may be one feature of a larger postconcussive syndrome, including nervous system instability. This may include fragmentation of sleep, emotional lability, inability to tolerate crowds, restlessness, inability to concentrate, and anxiety.

Posttraumatic hydrocephalus (**b**) is a rare complication of minor head trauma. It presents with signs and symptoms of increased ICP, includ-ing headache, gait instability, dizziness, nausea, and vomiting. It is often transient and may appear as a mild dilatation of the ventricles. Subdural hygromas (**c**) can occur in the weeks following a trauma or may appear as incidental findings. They occasionally increase in size causing symptoms because of mass effect. Cluster headaches (**d**) happen daily at the same time for days or weeks. They are unilateral, short, and boring in quality. The autonomic instability of posttraumatic nervous instability overlaps considerably with PTSD (**e**), which has led some researchers to postulate that they share a similar mechanism.

330. The answer is d. The patient presents with symptoms consistent with a **prolactin-secreting pituitary adenoma**. The appropriate imaging modality to diagnose a pituitary adenoma is with high-resolution **MRI** with thin cuts through the sella. Women often present with amenorrhea, infertility, and galactorrhea. Men will present with decreased libido. In both cases, extension beyond the sella may present with visual field defects or other mass-related symptoms.

Noncontrast and contrast-enhanced CTs (**a**) are not particularly sensitive for these lesions. Bromocriptine (**b**) or other centrally acting dopamine agonists are used to treat pituitary macro- and microadenomas. The presence of RBCs or xanthochromia in the CSF (**c**) is diagnostic for an SAH. The clinical presentation is inconsistent with SAH. Removing CSF is treatment for IIH (**e**).

331. The answer is a. BPV is a transient **positional** vertigo associated with nystagmus. The problem occurs secondary to the creation and movement of canaliths (free-moving densities) in the semicircular canals of the inner ear with a particular head movement. Neurologic deficits are absent in BPV. Note that horizontal, vertical, or rotary **nystagmus** can occur in BPV. It is important to pay special attention to a patient with vertical nystagmus or nystagmus that changes directions or is not fatigable because it may be associated with a brainstem or cerebellum lesion (eg, stroke). BPV is treated with the **Epley maneuver** (a series of head and body turns that reposition the canalith), antiemetics, and antihistamines. Key differences between peripheral and central vertigo are seen in the table below.

Food poisoning (**b**) does not cause vertigo. If associated with vomiting and diarrhea, this can lead to dehydration and light-headedness, but not vertiginous symptoms. Meniere disease (**c**) is an inner ear disease of unclear etiology. It presents with recurrent attacks of vertigo and tinnitus, with deafness of the involved ear between attacks. Labyrinthitis (**d**) presents with hearing loss and sudden, brief positional vertigo attacks. TIA (**e**) of the vertebrobasilar system can present with vertigo, but is an unlikely diagnosis in this case of recurrent positional vertiginous symptoms.

	Peripheral Vertigo	**Central Vertigo**
Pathophysiology	Disorder of vestibular nerve (CN VIII)	Disorder of brainstem or cerebellum
Severity	Intense	Less intense
Onset	Sudden	Slow
Pattern	Intermittent	Constant
Nausea and vomiting	Usually present	Usually absent
Exacerbated by position	Most of the time	Less of the time
Hearing abnormalities	May be present	Usually absent
Focal neurologic deficits	Usually absent	Usually present
Fatigability of symptoms	Yes	No
Nystagmus	Horizontal, rotary	Vertical, nonextinguishing, or direction changing

332. The answer is a. These signs and symptoms are concerning for **myasthenia gravis**, an autoimmune condition in which **AChR** block acetylcholine binding and prevent normal neuromuscular conduction. The disease typically affects young women and older men, and presents with **generalized weakness worsening with repetitive muscle use** that is usually **relieved with rest**. Ptosis and diplopia are usually present. The **edrophonium test** is used to help diagnose myasthenia gravis. It involves administering edrophonium, a short-acting anticholinesterase, which prevents acetylcholine breakdown at the neuromuscular junction. With the increased acetylcholine levels at the neuromuscular junction, the patient experiences a subjective and objective improvement of symptoms by preventing rapid breakdown of acetylcholine at the neuromuscular junction.

Serologic testing **(b)** for antibodies to AChRs is often not immediately available, but is useful when positive and should be obtained in the workup of this patient. A negative test does not exclude the disorder. The electromyogram is diagnostic. You may consider a CT scan **(c)** to evaluate the patient for possible mass lesion or aneurysm that is causing her ptosis and diplopia. However, the clinical scenario is more consistent with myasthenia gravis. An electrolyte panel **(d)** will likely be normal. If the edrophonium test is normal, an LP **(e)** should be considered.

333. The answer is b. The patient has a **progressive ascending peripheral neuropathy**, also known as **GBS**. GBS is an autoimmune-mediated acute peripheral nerve demyelination disorder. Patients can usually recall a preceding viral illness (classically *Campylobacter* gastroenteritis). Subsequently, patients **develop ascending motor weakness** (that starts in the stocking-glove distribution and progresses proximally) and a loss of **deep tendon reflexes.** The patient may have concurrent or preceding sensory abnormalities (eg, paresthesia, neuropathic pain), but they are not necessarily present in GBS.

Hypokalemic periodic paralysis **(a)** is part of the heterogeneous group of muscle diseases known as periodic paralyses and is characterized by episodes of flaccid muscle weakness occurring at irregular intervals. Most of the conditions are hereditary and are more episodic than periodic. Peripheral neuropathy **(c)**, a common complication of longstanding diabetes, causes paresthesia in the distal lower extremities and not acute paralysis. Tetanus **(d)** caused by the *Clostridium tetani* toxin manifests as muscular rigidity preventing release of inhibitory neurotransmitters. Lockjaw is a common complaint in generalized tetanus. A brain abscess **(e)** typically presents with fever, headache, and focal neurologic findings, and is usually caused by an associated trauma, surgery, or infectious spread from another site.

334. The answer is c. The progressive paralysis in GBS is characterized by its **rapid ascending** nature. As the weakness ascends, it can cause **respiratory failure** due to paralysis of the diaphragm and accessory respiratory muscles. This is the primary life threat from GBS. Patients need to be monitored (with serial pulmonary function tests and other clinical examinations to evaluate for respiratory adequacy) and provided with ventilatory support as necessary.

GBS is a transient, not permanent **(a)**, condition. All other answer choices **(b, d, and e)** are not complications of this syndrome.

335. The answer is d. This patient presents with **hypokalemia**, secondary to increased potassium losses through vomiting and diarrhea as well as reduced oral intake. HCTZ is a potassium-wasting diuretic medication that can also cause hypokalemia. Potassium deficiency results in hyperpolarization of the cell membrane and leads to **muscle weakness, hyporeflexia, intestinal ileus, and respiratory paralysis.** Characteristic ECG findings include flattened T waves, U waves, and prolonged QT and PR intervals.

Hypernatremia **(a)** and hyponatremia **(b)** mainly affect the CNS, resulting in headache, anorexia, lethargy, and confusion. In more severe cases, hyponatremia causes seizures, coma, and respiratory arrest, whereas patients with profound hypernatremia develop ataxia, tremulousness, and spasms. Hyperkalemia **(c)** can lead to cardiac dysrhythmias and typically exhibits distinctive ECG findings, including peaked T waves, prolonged QT and PR intervals, and widened QRS complex that can progress to a sine wave pattern. Signs of hypercalcemia (**e**) include bony and abdominal pain, renal stones, and altered mental status (remembered by: "bones, stones, groans, and psychiatric overtones"). In addition, cardiac effects include bradycardia, heart blocks, and shortened QT interval on ECG.

336. The answer is e. **Hyperkalemia** may cause severe muscle weakness and fatigue. In any patient presenting with a chief complaint of generalized weakness, it is important to consider checking electrolytes so as not to miss severe hyperkalemia. Hyperkalemia is also a reversible cause of pulseless electrical activity and should be considered in any patient who presents with or develops cardiac arrest. ECG findings of hyperkalemia include hyperacute T waves, flattened or absent P waves, prolonged PR interval, QRS prolongation, conduction abnormalities (eg, slow atrial fibrillation), and sinusoidal morphology. Emergent management includes cardiac membrane stabilization with **calcium gluconate** (or calcium chloride through a central venous catheter), potassium shifting medications (eg, insulin with dextrose, nebulized albuterol), and potassium elimination (eg, furosemide, dialysis). Magnesium sulfate (**a**) is used to treat torsades de pointes, which is a form of polymorphic ventricular tachycardia resulting from a prolonged QT interval. Amiodarone (**b**) is an antiarrhythmic medication recommended for the use of ventricular tachycardia. Procainamide (**c**) may be used for stable ventricular tachycardia or for tachydysrhythmias associated with Wolff-Parkinson-White syndrome. Furosemide (**d**) is used to treat hyperkalemia, but its effects are delayed and it does nothing to stabilize the cardiac membranes.

337. The answer is b. Consider **MS** as a potential diagnosis in presentations of various neurologic symptoms that are difficult to explain by a single CNS lesion, particularly those occurring in a woman in her third decade of life. MS is a **multifocal demyelinating CNS disease** that in 30% of cases initially presents with **optic neuritis** (ie, unilateral eye pain and decreased visual acuity). Myasthenia gravis (**a**) commonly presents with muscle weakness that is exacerbated by activity, sleeplessness, or alcohol intake, and is relieved by rest. The most frequent initial symptoms include ptosis, diplopia, and blurred vision. Vertebrobasilar insufficiency (VBI) (**c**) presents with cerebellar and brainstem symptoms, such as vertigo, dysphagia, and diplopia, none of which are present in this patient. Encephalitis (**d**) is an infection of brain parenchyma and presents with altered mental status that may be associated with focal neurologic deficits. Patients might present with behavioral and personality changes, seizures, headache, photophobia, and generalized symptoms of fever, nausea, and vomiting. GBS (**e**) is the most common polyneuropathy. It is described as an ascending paralysis that is often preceded by a viral syndrome. Classically, it is associated with the loss of deep tendon reflexes.

338. The answer is e. The **demyelinating lesions** of MS are often well demonstrated on **MRI** of the brain, but cannot be well visualized on CT scan (**d**).

The edrophonium test (**a**) is used as an adjunct in the diagnosis of myasthenia gravis. A carotid artery angiogram (**b**) is useful when evaluating the carotid arteries for trauma, dissection, or thrombus. CSF analysis (**c**) can help aid you in the diagnosis of MS, which often shows oligoclonal bands and elevated protein. However, MRI is the initial test of choice.

339. The answer is d. The patient is a candidate for **fibrinolytic therapy**. She is having an **acute ischemic stroke** (in the distribution of the middle cerebral artery), has no contraindications to the thrombolytic therapy, and is being evaluated within the 4.5-hour therapeutic window from the onset of symptoms. The head CT may initially appear normal and starts to show the extent of injury within 6 to 12 hours after the onset of symptoms.

Exclusion criteria for the use of thrombolytics include the following:

- Intracranial hemorrhage on noncontrast head CT (absolute)
- Minor or rapidly improving stroke symptoms
- Clinical suspicion for SAH
- Active internal bleeding within last 21 days
- Known bleeding diathesis
- Within 3 months of serious head trauma, stroke, or intracranial or spinal surgery
- Within 14 days of major surgery or serious trauma
- Recent arterial puncture at noncompressible site
- LP within 7 days
- History of intracranial hemorrhage, A-V malformation
- Witnessed seizure at stroke onset
- Recent myocardial infarction
- Systolic BP greater than 185 mm Hg or diastolic BP greater than 110 mm Hg

Current guidelines (a) recommend that thrombolytics be administered within 3 to 4.5 hours of the patient's symptom onset (depending on which guidelines are referenced). Any patient whose symptoms are present upon waking up from sleep is excluded because it cannot be certain when the symptoms began. The general consensus in the neurology literature is to *not* treat hypertension in patients with acute ischemic stroke unless they are candidates for thrombolysis and their BP is greater than 185 mm Hg systolic or 100 mm Hg diastolic (b). Labetalol is often recommended over nitroprusside. Labetalol preserves normal cerebral autoregulation whereas nitroprusside, a vasodilator, may divert blood from the injured tissue, and cause increased ischemia. Heparin therapy (c) has not been shown to reduce stroke-related mortality or disability in the setting of acute stroke. If the patient is not a candidate for thrombolytics, aspirin (e) should be given in the setting of acute ischemic stroke. Maintenance therapy with daily aspirin or another antiplatelet agent has been shown to help reduce stroke recurrence after a TIA.

340. The answer is a. This patient's BP of 215/118 mm Hg needs to be lowered to **185/110 mm Hg** to make her a more optimal candidate for thrombolytic therapy. **Labetalol** is an appropriate choice in this case. Other agents to consider include nitroprusside in combination with labetalol, and nicardipine.

Fibrinolytic administration (b) at this level of hypertension carries a risk of intracranial bleed, and untreated hypertension above 185/110 is a contraindication to fibrinolysis. Daily aspirin (c) has been shown to reduce the incidence of strokes. However, aspirin should not be administered within 24 hours of fibrinolytic use because it increases the risk of post-thrombolytic bleed. Antiseizure prophylaxis with phenytoin (d) is not indicated in ischemic strokes, although a small percentage of stroke patients will seize within the first 24 hours. Hyperventilation and mannitol (e) are sometimes used for temporary, emergent management of increased ICP owing to cerebral edema in an ischemic stroke, which peaks at 72 to 96 hours. There is no role for mannitol in acute stroke in a patient without signs of elevated ICP.

341. The answer is a. The **middle cerebral artery** is the most common site of intracranial cerebral artery thrombosis. Clinical findings can include **contralateral hemiplegia, hemianesthesia, and homonymous hemianopsia.** The **upper-extremity** deficit is usually more severe than the lower-extremity deficit. **Aphasia** occurs if the dominant hemisphere is involved. Gaze preference is in the direction of the lesion.

The symptoms of MCA infarct are contralateral, not ipsilateral **(b)**. Choice **(c)** describes the deficits associated with anterior cerebral artery (ACA) infarction are greater deficits in lower extremity and include altered mentation because of frontal lobe involvement. Crossed deficits such as contralateral motor and ipsilateral CN findings **(d)** occur in brainstem strokes, which are supplied by the posterior circulation. Pure motor **(e)** or sensory loss occurs in lacunar infarcts, which involve small penetrating arteries.

342. The answer is e. Do not get confused with the multiple signs and symptoms in this case! They involve three distinct areas of the brain—the brainstem (facial droop, dysphagia, vertigo, and vertical nystagmus), cerebellum (ataxia, vertigo, and vertical nystagmus), and visual cortex (diplopia). All of these anatomical areas are supplied by the **posterior circulation**, specifically the **vertebrobasilar artery**. A mnemonic to help remember the presentation of a vertebrobasilar stroke is the "**3 Ds**"—**dizziness (vertigo)**, **dysphagia**, and **diplopia**. Cerebellar nerve and CN deficits are observed on both sides of the body.

Lacunar infarcts **(a)** are small infarcts that are usually caused by a hypertensive vasculopathy, but may occur in diabetics and can affect both the anterior and posterior cerebral vessels. Lacunar strokes involve penetrating cerebral arterial vessels lying deep in the gray matter (internal capsule) or brainstem. BPV **(b)** is a transient positional vertigo associated with nystagmus. Neurologic deficits are absent in BPV. Note that horizontal, vertical, or rotary nystagmus can occur in BPV; however, vertical nystagmus is always worrisome as it may indicate a brainstem or cerebellum lesion. Labyrinthitis **(c)**, an infection of the labyrinth, presents with hearing loss and sudden brief positional vertigo attacks and does not involve other neurologic deficits. The posterior cerebral artery **(d)** delivers blood supply to the occipital cortex and upper midbrain. Clinical findings include contralateral homonymous hemianopsia, hemiparesis, hemisensory loss, memory loss, and ipsilateral CN III palsy, that is pupil sparing.

343. The answer is b. This common presentation of **hypercalcemia** is initially managed with **aggressive isotonic saline IV hydration** to restore volume status. Hypercalcemia impairs renal concentrating ability, and patients typically present with **polyuria**, **polydipsia**, and **dehydration** and may develop **kidney stones**. Increased calcium levels also cause generalized weakness, bone pain, neurologic symptoms (ataxia and/or altered mental status), GI dysfunction (abdominal pain, nausea, vomiting, and/or anorexia), and ECG abnormalities (shortened QT interval). A handy mnemonic for symptoms of hypercalcemia is "bones, stones, groans, and psychiatric overtones."

Calcitonin (a) decreases calcium levels by reducing bony osteoclast activity and intestinal calcium absorption. It does not produce an immediate effect and is generally not started in the ED. Loop diuretics such as furosemide (c) increase renal elimination of calcium but worsen volume depletion. Patients need to be hydrated first. Obtaining a chest radiograph (d) is a good idea while the patient is getting IV hydration. This patient has a significant smoking history and recent weight loss, which should raise your suspicion of a neoplastic lung process causing hypercalcemia. Malignancy is an important cause of hypercalcemia; others include endocrine abnormalities (hyperparathyroidism, hyperthyroidism, pheochromocytoma, and/or adrenal insufficiency), granulomatous disease (sarcoidosis and/or TB), drugs (thiazides and/or lithium), and immobilization. The patent should have an ECG (e), which may show a shortened QT interval. Very high calcium levels may cause heart block. However, you should not delay treatment to obtain the ECG.

344. The answer is c. Unilateral findings of ptosis, miosis, and anhidrosis are seen in **Horner's syndrome** that results from **interrupted sympathetic nerve supply to the eye**.

Palsy of the oculomotor nerve (CN III) (a) results in a "down and out" eye because of the dysfunction of the extraocular muscles innervated by the oculomotor nerve. In addition, the pupil appears mydriatic as a result of the loss of function of the ciliary parasympathetic nerves. Ptosis is common because the oculomotor nerve innervates the levator palpebrae. Bell's palsy (b) involves unilateral facial paralysis as a result of peripheral involvement of the facial nerve (CN VII). In patients with a central facial nerve lesion, the forehead is spared. Kehr's sign (d) refers to left shoulder pain associated with splenic pathology. Nikolsky's sign (e) is sloughing of the outer epidermal layer with rubbing of the skin seen in dermatologic diseases, such as pemphigus vulgaris and scalded skin syndrome.

345. The answer is a. This patient has an **ICA dissection** secondary to chiropractic neck manipulation. ICA dissection can occur spontaneously or in minor neck trauma and should be considered in a **young patient with acute stroke**. ICA dissection should also be suspected in patients with **neck**

pain and Horner's syndrome because of the disruption of ipsilateral ocu-losympathetic fibers. In this scenario, it presents with ipsilateral Horner's syndrome and contralateral ischemic motor deficits. Other causes of acute Horner's syndrome include tumors (eg, Pancoast tumor), stroke, herpes zoster infection, and trauma.

Cavernous sinus syndrome **(b)** presents with headache, ipsilateral eye findings, and sensory loss in the distribution of the ophthalmic branch of the trigeminal nerve (V1). Eye findings include proptosis, chemosis, Horner's syndrome, and ophthalmoplegia caused by the involvement of CNs III, IV, and VI. It does not cause decreased strength in the extremities. MS **(c)** is an inflammatory demyelinating CNS disease, resulting in various neurologic abnormalities, such as optic neuritis, transverse myelitis, and paresthesias. Transverse myelitis **(d)** is a pathologic inflammation of the spinal cord (often postviral or autoimmune) that results in sensory loss and paresis. An isolated spinous process fracture **(e)** typically occurs in the setting of trauma and is considered a stable vertebral fracture. It does not result in motor weakness.

346. The answer is c. This patient presents with **VBI** causing vertigo and **claudication** (atypical arm pain with exercise). These symptoms are consistent with **subclavian steal syndrome**. This phenomenon occurs in patients with subclavian artery occlusion or stenosis proximal to the ver-tebral artery branch, which causes retrograde blood flow in the vertebral artery with ipsilateral arm exercise. Collateral arteries arising from the sub-clavian artery distal to the obstruction deliver blood to the arm. During arm exercise, these vessels dilate and siphon blood from the head, neck, and shoulder to increase perfusion of ischemic arm muscles. This results in temporary reversal of blood flow in the vertebral artery leading to VBI and symptoms of vertigo, dizziness, syncope, dysarthria, and diplopia. Arm pain is a result of muscle ischemia.

Superior vena cava syndrome **(a)** is caused by an obstruction of the superior vena cava typically caused by the compression of a tumor. The most common complaints include edema and venous distention of the face and upper extremities. Facial plethora and telangiectasias are also commonly noted. Aortic dissection **(b)** can cause a difference in BP in the extremities. In general, patients complain of tearing chest pain that radiates into their back. If suspicion is high for aortic dissection, a CT scan with contrast or echocardiography should be performed to rule out the diagnosis. Angina pectoris **(d)** refers to myocardial ischemia caused by insufficient coronary blood flow to meet myocardial oxygen demand. It typically presents with symptoms of chest discomfort relieved with rest or nitroglycerin. Patients might complain of arm pain or radiation of pain to the arms, but the presentation does not involve neurologic deficits. Vestibular neuronitis (**e**) refers to acute self-limiting dysfunction of the peripheral vestibular system that causes vertigo.

347. The answer is c. This patient presents with **symmetric proximal muscle weakness** and characteristic **heliotrope rash** of **dermatomyositis**. It is an idiopathic inflammatory myopathy with associated dermatitis. The characteristic of the disease is progressive symmetric proximal muscle weakness with possible dysphagia, symmetric heliotrope rash in the periorbital region or neck, elevated creatinine kinase, and abnormal electromyogram and muscle biopsy. There is also an associated risk of malignancy.

Myasthenia gravis (**a**) is an autoimmune disorder of the neuromuscular junction in which anti-AChR antibodies compete with acetylcholine at the nicotinic postsynaptic receptors. The disease causes characteristic progressive reduction in muscle strength with repeated muscle use. Bulbar muscles are most commonly involved, and patients report worsening of symptoms at night and improvement with rest or in the morning. MS (**b**) is an inflammatory demyelinating CNS disease, resulting in various neurologic abnormalities, such as optic neuritis, transverse myelitis, and paresthesias. Rhabdomyolysis (**d**) refers to muscle fiber breakdown because of a variety of etiologies, such as trauma, burns, ischemia, seizures, excessive muscular activities, sepsis, and myopathies. Its complications include hyperkalemia, metabolic acidosis, and acute renal failure. Disseminated gonococcal infection (**e**) is a systemic disease secondary to the presence of *Neisseria gonorrhoeae* in the bloodstream. In the early bacteremic phase, patients present with fevers, migratory polyarthritis, and rash. This evolves from disseminated erythematous macules into hemorrhagic pustular lesions. Serious complications may include meningitis, osteomyelitis, and endocarditis.

348. The answer is c. This patient has historical features concerning for a **dural venous sinus thrombosis (DVST)**. This should be suspected in any patient with a hypercoagulable state (eg, postpartum, OCP use), headache, and neurologic deficit. Any type of headache description could be associated with DVST, but it is classically progressively worsening, and initially nonspecific (leading to many being missed on initial presentation). The venous obstruction from the thrombus leads to decreased blood flow, and potentially focal neurologic findings (eg, arm or leg weakness or vision changes).

The diagnosis is made with **contrast-enhanced venography** (either CT or MR). Occasionally, the sinus thrombus can be seen on noncontrast head CT. These are treated with anticoagulation, and very rarely thrombolysis.

Myasthenia gravis (**a**) could be diagnosed with serum AChR antibodies. This would typically present as weakness that worsens throughout the day, without persistent focal findings or headache. LP (**b**) and fluid analysis could diagnose idiopathic IIH or meningitis, but should not be performed in a patient with a neurologic deficit before normal head imaging. Carotid angiography (**d**) can be used to help diagnose carotid dissection. This presentation could conceivably be consistent with dissection, but DVST is much more congruent. EEG (**e**) can identify seizures. It is unlikely that this patient's symptoms are related to seizure.

349. The answer is e. Infantile botulism is a life-threatening condition in an infant. It is caused by the ingestion of *Clostridium botulinum* spores that subsequently reproduce in the gut and release their toxin (which prevents the release of acetylcholine at the neuromuscular junction). It is classically associated with the **consumption of honey** (or spoiled canned goods in adults). Symptoms are varied and can range from subtle bulbar weakness (drooping lids and/or abnormal swallowing) to lethargy and poor feeding to respiratory depression or apnea. Stool assays can provide the diagnosis and treatment is with botulinum immunoglobulin and supportive care (potentially intubation and mechanical ventilation). The initial differential diagnosis must include hypoglycemia, sepsis, and trauma (including nonaccidental trauma), which were evaluated by the provider in this question.

Myasthenia gravis (**a**) causes progressive bulbar and proximal weakness as the patient becomes fatigued. These symptoms wax and wane over time, improve with rest, and are not overall progressive. Hypokalemic paralysis (**b**) is a genetic disorder in which blood potassium levels are abnormally low. It manifests with intermittent attacks of muscle weakness and improves with potassium repletion. LEMS (**c**) is an autoimmune neuromuscular disorder with antibodies directed against the presynaptic portion of the neuromuscular junction. These patients are often older adults, and the syndrome is often paraneoplastic. The classic description would be subtle weakness in the proximal muscles that improves with repeated stimulation. Todd's paralysis (**d**) is a postictal hemiparesis. Possibly due to neurologic fatigue or substrate depletion, this is a transient phenomenon in patients who have recently suffered a seizure. It is a common stroke mimic.

Recommended Readings

Edlow JA. Diagnosing patients with acute-onset persistent dizziness. *Ann Emerg Med.* 2018;71:625-631.

Friedman BW. Managing migraine. *Ann Emerg Med.* 2017;69(2)202-207.

Godwin SA, Cherkas DS, Panagos PD, et al. Clinical policy: Critical issues in the evaluation and management of adult patients presenting to the emergency department with acute headache. *Ann Emerg Med.* 2019;74:e41-e74.

Goldman B, Johns P. Chapter 170. Vertigo. In. Tintinalli JE, Ma O, Yealy DM, et al, eds. *Tintinalli's Emergency Medicine: A Comprehensive Study Guide.* 9th ed. New York, NY: McGraw-Hill, 2020.

Koyfman A, Long B. Chapter 165. Headache. In: Tintinalli JE, Ma O, Yealy DM, et al, eds. *Tintinalli's Emergency Medicine: A Comprehensive Study Guide.* 9th ed. New York, NY: McGraw-Hill, 2020.

Pediatrics

Nicholas A. Kuehnel, MD

Questions

350. A 6-month-old girl is brought to the emergency department (ED) because of persistent crying for the past 6 hours. Her teenage father informs you that she has been inconsolable since waking from her nap. No recent illness, trauma, fever, or other complaints are reported. On physical examination, the patient is alert, awake, and crying. You note swelling, deformity, and tenderness of the left tibia. When inquired about this finding, the caretaker responds, "Her leg got stuck between the rails of her crib." You obtain the radiograph as seen in the following figure. Which of the following is the next best step in management?

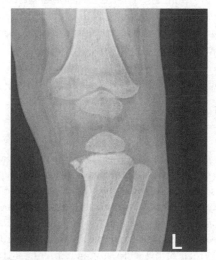

(Reproduced with permission from Ethan S. Wiener, MD.)

a. Genetic workup for osteogenesis imperfecta and other bone abnormalities
b. Orthopedic consultation for closed reduction
c. Serum electrolytes including calcium and phosphate
d. Perform skeletal survey and contact Child Protective Services
e. Placement of posterior splint and discharge home with orthopedic follow-up

351. A 4-year-old boy is brought to the ED by his concerned mother after she noticed lesions under his nose and around his mouth. The patient is otherwise well with no change in behavior, fever, or vomiting reported. On physical examination, you note a well-nourished, well-developed child in no acute distress with multiple small round, honey-colored crusted lesions with slightly erythematous centers. What is the predominant organism involved?

a. Group B Streptococcus
b. *Staphylococcus aureus*
c. *Streptococcus pyogenes*
d. *Streptococcus pneumoniae*
e. *Salmonella*

352. A 3-year-old boy with a history of sickle cell disease presents to the ED after he developed a low-grade fever, runny nose, and an erythematous discoloration of both cheeks. His vital signs are heart rate (HR) of 110 beats/minute, respiratory rate (RR) of 24 breaths/minute, and pulse oximetry of 98% on room air. The patient looks well and is in no acute distress. You note a macular lesion on both cheeks. The rash is not pruritic and there is no associated cellulitis or suppuration. What is the most serious complication to consider in this patient?

a. Osteomyelitis
b. Viral encephalitis
c. Pneumonia
d. Aplastic anemia
e. Meningitis

353. A 9-month-old boy is brought to the ED with a 2-day history of fever, vomiting, and fussiness. The patient has had multiple episodes of emesis that follow intense periods of fussiness after which the patient seems to relax and go to sleep. He has had normal stooling. In between these episodes, he has slightly decreased energy but otherwise seems well. Oral intake is decreased and urine output has been decreased since the day of symptom onset. Which of the following statements is true regarding this condition?

a. The majority of patients present with vomiting, colicky abdominal pain, and currant jelly stools
b. Air enema is the therapeutic intervention of choice
c. Plain films of the abdomen usually confirm the diagnosis
d. Surgical intervention is often indicated
e. Most of these have a "lead point" as the underlying pathologic cause

354. A 7-year-old girl with sickle cell disease and a previous history of admissions for acute painful crises presents with a 1-day history of fever and cough. She is tachypnic on presentation with a temperature of 102°F. Auscultation of the chest reveals rales on the right. A chest radiograph confirms the diagnosis of pneumonia. After initial treatment with antibiotics and intravenous (IV) fluids, patients with this condition are most at risk of developing which complication?

a. Acute chest syndrome
b. Sepsis
c. Empyema
d. Stroke
e. Congestive heart failure

355. A previously well 21-month-old girl presents with 7 days of fever and rash. She had been seen by her primary care physician (PCP) during this episode and diagnosed with a "viral illness." On further questioning, the mother indicates that the patient has had red eyes, but no discharge. She has had no vomiting, diarrhea, cough, congestion, or complaints of pain. She has, however, seemed very irritable and fussy throughout the last few days and cannot seem to get comfortable. On examination, the patient is highly irritable and only intermittently consolable. Vital signs reveal blood pressure (BP) 100/60 mm Hg, HR 170 beats/minute, RR 22 breaths/minute, and temperature 101°F rectally. Her conjunctivae are mildly injected with no purulent discharge. The oropharynx is clear though she has dry and cracked lips. There are two anterior cervical nodes measuring 2.5 cm each. The heart is tachycardic without a murmur. The lungs are clear, and abdomen is soft and nontender with no hepatosplenomegaly. The skin reveals a diffuse, blanching, erythematous, and macular rash. The extremities have no swelling or tenderness. Laboratory evaluation reveals white blood cell (WBC) 13,500/μL, Hgb 9.5 mg/dL, platelets 870/μL, C-reactive protein (CRP) 8.9, erythrocyte sedimentation rate (ESR) 85, and normal electrolytes; liver function tests reveal aspartate aminotransferase (AST) 110 U/L and alanine aminotransferase (ALT) 88 U/L. Which of the following is the most appropriate next step in the management of this patient?

a. Consult cardiology for echocardiogram
b. Perform Epstein-Barr viral titers, strep test, antinuclear antibody, and bone marrow biopsy
c. Reassure the parents that the initial diagnosis was probably accurate
d. Administer IV antibiotics and perform lumbar puncture (LP)
e. Admit for administration of intravenous immunoglobulin (IVIG) and aspirin

356. An 8-day-old boy is brought to the ED by his mom who describes the newborn as breathing fast, feeding poorly, and appearing blue. He has no history of fever or vomiting. The patient was born full term at home to a G4P3 mother with an uncomplicated antenatal course. The mom had prenatal laboratory tests but is unaware of the results. On examination, the patient is lethargic with central and peripheral cyanosis. His BP is unobtainable in the extremities by automatic pressure meter. His HR is 180 beats/minute, RR is 70 breaths/minute, and rectal temperature is 95.4°F. The oxygen saturation on room air is 65%, which does not improve with administration of 100% oxygen by face mask. Auscultation reveals a harsh 3/6 systolic murmur with an active precordium. Lungs reveal diffuse, bilateral rales, and wheezes. Liver edge is palpated 3 to 4 cm below right costal margin. Which of the following is the most important next step in the management of this patient?

a. Intubation for administration of 100% oxygen
b. STAT portable chest radiograph and electrocardiogram (ECG)
c. Administration of IV antibiotics and full sepsis workup
d. Administration of prostaglandin bolus followed by continuous drip
e. Immediate surgical intervention and activation of extracorporeal membrane oxygenation (ECMO) team

357. A 27-day-old neonate presents to the ED with a complaint of a 2-day history of nonbilious vomiting. He has had no fever and no diarrhea. He has always been a "spitter," according to his mom, but this seems more excessive and forceful. The patient has had no wet diapers over the course of the previous 12 hours and is fussy in the examination room. There are no other complaints. The mother has just finished feeding the child formula as you walk into the room and you see the newborn have an episode of projectile vomiting. The examination reveals HR 180 beats/minute, RR 50 breaths/minute, temperature 99.8°F, and pulse oximetry of 95% on room air. The remainder of the examination is benign except for slightly prolonged capillary refill. You order the appropriate radiographic studies and consult the appropriate services. If you were to check a set of electrolytes in this patient, what would be the most likely result?

a. Na 137, K 3.7, Cl 112, HCO$_3$ 22, glucose 110
b. Na 137, K 3.1, Cl 89, HCO$_3$ 39, glucose 55
c. Na 145, K 6.2, Cl 122, HCO$_3$ 35, glucose 55
d. Na 145, K 3.1, Cl 89, HCO$_3$ 16, glucose 80
e. Na 122, K 6.2, Cl 122, HCO$_3$ 35, glucose 55

358. A 15-month-old girl is brought to the ED by emergency medical services (EMS) secondary to seizure activity noted at home. The patient is previously healthy child and her immunizations are up-to-date. She has had no cough, congestion, vomiting, diarrhea, or rash. This afternoon, the patient was being observed in the playroom when her eyes rolled back and she began having generalized tonic-clonic activity that lasted for approximately 2 minutes. When EMS arrived, the patient was in her mother's arms, tired but arousable, and in no apparent distress. On examination, BP is 95/50 mm Hg, HR is 155 beats/minute, RR 32 is breaths/minute, and temperature is 103.1°F. She has normal tympanic membranes, oropharyngeal exam reveals several tiny erythematous and vesicular appearing lesions in the posterior oropharynx, lungs and heart examinations are normal, and abdomen is soft and nontender. Skin examination is clear with brisk capillary refill. Over the course of your evaluation, the patient becomes increasingly inter active and playful. Which of the following is the most appropriate course of action for this patient?

a. Obtain complete blood count (CBC), blood culture, urinalysis, urine culture, and chest radiograph, and determine treatment on the basis of the results of these tests
b. Obtain blood and urine for culture, administer ceftriaxone, and discharge home
c. Reassure parents that this is a benign condition and that no further testing is indicated at this time
d. Obtain routine blood work and head computed tomographic (CT) scan and call for neurology consultation for first-time seizure
e. Obtain head CT scan and perform LP secondary to fever and seizure to rule out meningitis

359. A 13-year-old adolescent boy is brought to the ED by his mother for a complaint of right knee pain for 1 to 2 weeks. The only notable trauma that the patient can recall was jumping on a trampoline. On the morning of presentation, the patient complained of increased pain and was noted to be limping. He denies fever. No other trauma or recent illness was noted by the family. On examination, the patient is afebrile with normal vital signs. He has no previous medical problems and is noted to be overweight but is in otherwise good health. The lower extremity examination reveals no swelling or erythema over any of the joints. His knee has no focal tenderness or pain with range of motion, but the hip is noted to be painful with internal and external rotation. He has a normal neurosensory examination of the distal extremity. A radiograph is performed. Which of the following is the most likely diagnosis?

a. Legg-Calvé-Perthes disease
b. Slipped capital-femoral epiphysis (SCFE)
c. Septic arthritis
d. Osgood-Schlatter disease
e. Transient synovitis of the hip

360. A 3-week-old girl is brought to the ED by her parents after they noticed blood in her stool. The patient was born full term following an uncomplicated pregnancy and delivery. She has been feeding well (breast-feeding primarily) and active without fever, respiratory problems, or fussiness. She has had several episodes of nonforceful, nonbilious emesis after feeds with multiple wet diapers each day. She normally has several soft and seedy stools. In the last day, the parents noticed streaks of blood in her stool and on the day of presentation she had grossly bloody stool. The patient does not seem to be in any distress or discomfort. On examination, HR is 155 beats/minute, RR is 44 breaths/minute, and temperature is 98.9°F. The patient is awake, active, and in no apparent distress. Her abdomen is soft and nontender with normal bowel sounds and no masses. Examination of her anus does not reveal a fissure. Which of the following is the most likely diagnosis?

a. Acute gastroenteritis
b. Milk protein colitis
c. *Clostridium difficile* colitis
d. Intestinal malrotation
e. Necrotizing enterocolitis

361. A 9-day-old boy is brought to the ED for fever and fussiness. He was born full term. However, the delivery was complicated by premature rupture of membranes (PROM) and the mother had a fever for which she was treated with antibiotics before delivery. The baby did well in the nursery, and has been at home and feeding without any difficulties until the day of presentation when he became fussier, less interested in feeding, and his parents noted an axillary temperature of 101.5°F. On presentation, his HR is 160 beats/minute, RR is 48 breaths/minute, temperature is 102.4°F, and pulse oximetry of 97% on room air. His anterior fontanelle is open and flat, conjunctivae are clear, neck is supple without masses. His heart, lung, and abdominal examinations are normal. The skin shows tiny (1-3 mm) pustules with a surrounding rim of erythema on the patient's trunk. No vesicular lesions are noted. Which of the following is the most likely organism responsible for this patient's condition?

a. *Escherichia coli*
b. *Listeria monocytogenes*
c. Group B Streptococcus
d. *S. aureus*
e. Herpes simplex virus (HSV)

362. A 5-month-old previously healthy girl presents to the ED with a 5-day history of constipation and decreased feeding. The patient is a full-term product of an uncomplicated antenatal course and delivery. She also had recent nasal congestion and cough that resolved with administration of tea prepared by a family friend. The mother denies any recent fever or vomiting. On examination, HR is 165 beats/minute, RR is 22 breaths/minute, and temperature is 99.9°F. The BP was not obtained. The patient has a weak cry, is notably flaccid, and ill-appearing. You note that patient is drooling. Her pupils are poorly responsive and she is not tracking to light or faces. Which of the following is the most likely cause of this condition?

a. Type I spinal muscular atrophy
b. Brain tumor
c. Infant botulism
d. Meningitis
e. Organophosphate poisoning

363. A 6-month-old boy is brought to the ED after being found apneic and cyanotic at home. The patient's mother called 911 and began cardio-pulmonary resuscitation (CPR). The patient responded within seconds to minutes. On arrival at the ED, he was noted to be awake and responsive, but slightly mottled with mild respiratory distress. Within minutes of arrival, the patient becomes apneic suddenly, cyanotic, and bradycardic. Which of the following is the most important initial response?

a. Administer epinephrine
b. Provide oxygen via nonrebreather facemask
c. Jaw thrust, chin lift, and bag-valve-mask ventilation
d. Endotracheal intubation
e. Chest compressions

364. A 4-year-old boy is brought to the ED by his parents who state that he is having difficulty breathing. The patient has a 1-week history of fever, congestion, and cough. Over the last 2 days, he has appeared tired with intermittent vomiting and persistently increased RR despite administration of acetaminophen. On presentation, his vital signs are BP 75/40 mm Hg, HR 185 beats/minute, RR 50 breaths/minute, temperature 100.5°F, and pulse oximetry of 88% on room air. He is ill-appearing and listless. He has diffuse rales noted on auscultation, pulses are weak and thready, and his liver is palpable 3 to 4 cm below the right costal margin. After several attempts at a peripheral IV, the patient becomes increasingly somnolent. Which of the following is the most appropriate method of obtaining access in this patient?

a. Internal jugular central line
b. Femoral vein central line
c. Saphenous vein cutdown
d. Large bore IV in antecubital fossa
e. Tibial intraosseous (IO) line

365. A 3-year-old girl is brought to the ED with acute onset of respira-tory distress. She recently immigrated to the United States. Her initial vitals include BP of 110/60 mm Hg, HR of 115 beats/minute, RR of 28 breaths/minute, and oxygen saturation of 88% on room air. She is also febrile to 103.5°F. She is anxious, ill-appearing, sitting forward in her mother's lap, and drooling. Her mother reports sore throat that began 2 days ago and that she was going to see her pediatrician this week for her initial vaccinations. Given this patient's history and presentation, which of the following should be of particular concern?

a. Epiglottitis
b. Retropharyngeal abscess
c. Epstein-Barr virus (EBV) pharyngitis
d. Ludwig's angina
e. Peritonsillar abscess

366. A 5-month-old boy formerly born at 34 weeks gestation, is brought to the ED by his mother who reports difficulty breathing over the past 2 days. He has no other past medical history and has received the full course of vaccines at both his 2- and 4-month visits. The child has had rhinorrhea and cough. Upon physical examination, the patient has a HR 160 beats/minute, RR 70 breaths/minute, temperature 101.1°F, and pulse oximetry of 87% on room air. He has copious nasal discharge, audible wheezing with diffuse rhonchi, and rales upon chest auscultation. He also has intercostal retractions and nasal flaring. Given this patient's history and physical examination, which of the following is the most likely etiology of his symptoms?

a. Foreign body aspiration
b. Asthma
c. Pneumococcal pneumonia
d. Acute bronchiolitis
e. Parvovirus B19

367. A 4-year-old girl is brought to the ED after falling from a tree. She hit her head on the ground and has significant temporal swelling on the left side. In transit to the hospital by her parents, the patient had multiple episodes of emesis. On arrival to the ED, the patient is confused and agitated and then becomes acutely unresponsive and apneic. You make the decision to intubate the patient. Which of the following is the most appropriate endotracheal tube (ETT) to use in this intubation?

a. 4.0 uncuffed ETT
b. 4.5 cuffed ETT
c. 5.0 cuffed ETT
d. 5.5 uncuffed ETT
e. 4.5 uncuffed ETT

368. A 2-year-old boy is brought to the ED shortly after a choking episode. His parents noted he had been playing with coins just before the episode. There is no history of fever or runny nose in the past few days. The parents tried to feed him after the episode, but he has been unwilling to take anything orally. On examination, the patient is calm with stable vital signs and a pulse oximetry of 98% on room air. He spits saliva in a cup every couple of minutes, but is otherwise in no apparent distress. His oropharynx is unremarkable and lungs are clear. His radiograph is seen in the figure. Which of the following most likely accounts for the patient's symptoms?

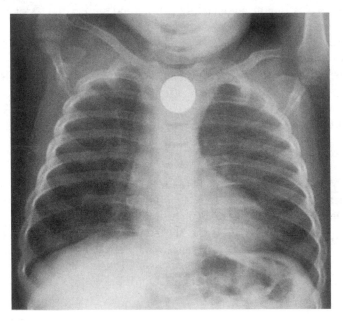

(Reproduced with permission from Adam J. Rosh, MD.)

a. Foreign body aspiration
b. Bronchospasm
c. Foreign body ingestion
d. Epiglottitis
e. Allergic reaction

369. A 2-year-old girl is brought into the ED with 2 days of fever and runny nose. On the day of presentation, she developed a dry, harsh, and "barking" cough. Her HR is 123 beats/minute, RR is 25 breaths/minute, temperature is 103.3°F, and pulse oximetry of 98% on room air. On evaluation you note an alert, responsive but somewhat anxious female, in moderate respiratory distress. Auscultation reveals stridor with clear and equal air entry bilaterally without rales or wheezing. You also note subcostal and intercostal retractions at rest. The remainder of her examination is unremarkable. After receiving a single treatment of racemic epinephrine, she feels better and her breathing improves. Which of the following is the most appropriate next step in management?

a. Chest radiograph
b. CBC and blood culture
c. Lateral soft tissue radiograph of the neck
d. Broad-spectrum antibiotics IV antibiotics
e. One-time dose of oral dexamethasone

370. A 3-month-old boy is brought into the ED by his mother with a chief complaint of "not eating" over the past 24 hours. The patient has been doing well without any prior medical problems until the day of presentation when the mother noted sweating and irritability, particularly with feeding. In the ED, the patient attempts to feed but within minutes stops and begins to cry. Vital signs include HR of 240 beats/minute, RR of 50 breaths/minute, temperature of 98.2°F, and pulse oximetry of 98% on room air. On physical examination, the patient is pale and clammy to touch. Breath sounds are clear on auscultation. Pulses are normal and symmetric in all extremities. An ECG is seen in the figure. Which of the following is the most appropriate next step in management?

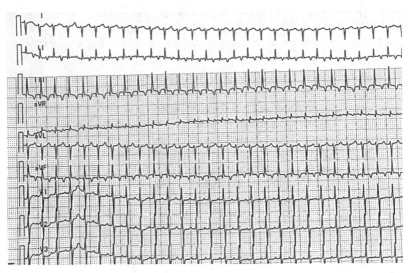

(Reproduced, with permission, from Shah BR, Lucchesi M. Atlas of Pediatric Emergency Medicine. New York, NY: McGraw Hill; 2006: Figure 5-10.)

a. Synchronized cardioversion at 0.5 J/kg
b. Verapamil 0.1 mg/kg bolus
c. Defibrillation at 2 J/kg
d. Adenosine at 0.1 mg/kg followed by 0.2 mg/kg if first dose is ineffective
e. Ice slurry bag to infant's face

371. A 4-year-old uncircumcised boy is brought to the ED by his caretaker for an 8-hour history of swelling and redness of the penis. The caretaker states that she retracted the foreskin over the penis to clean it and could not move it back afterward. The patient's vital signs are within normal limits. On examination, he is crying and becomes irritable whenever you try to examine the genital area. The glans is edematous and erythematous. The testicular examination shows bilateral descended testicles with a normal cremasteric reflex. Which of the following is the most appropriate next step in management?

a. Manual reduction of the foreskin over the glans
b. Dorsal slit incision or circumcision
c. Topical lidocaine
d. Catheterization to prevent obstruction and urinary retention
e. Topical steroids to reduce the swelling

372. A 10-week-old girl is brought to the ED after 5 hours of abdominal distension and vomiting greenish-colored emesis. The infant has been previously healthy and was born full term. On the day of presentation, she has been unable to hold any fluids down without vomiting. Her vital signs include HR of 185 beats/minute, RR of 65 breaths/minute, and temperature of 100.8°F. Abdominal examination reveals a diffusely tender abdomen that is tympanitic to percussion. Which of the following is the definitive study of choice?

a. Upper GI series
b. Abdominal ultrasound
c. Findings on physical examination
d. CBC, electrolytes, and urine analysis
e. Serum lactate

373. A 5-year-old boy who fell from the monkey bars and landed on his left elbow is brought into the ED for evaluation. The patient has no significant medical history. On physical examination, you note the patient is holding his left arm in an adducted position. There is obvious swelling around the elbow with decreased range of motion secondary to pain. He complains of hand numbness, but the motor and vascular examination is normal. The radiograph shown in the figure shows posterior displacement of the capitellum with evidence of a dark shadow posterior to the distal humerus. Which of the following is the most serious complication associated with this injury?

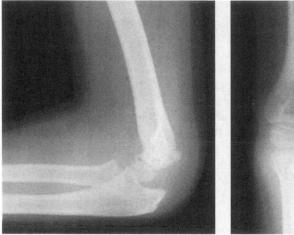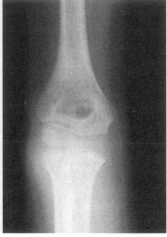

(Reproduced, with permission, from Simon RR, Sherman SC, Koenigsknecht SJ. Emergency Orthopedics: The Extremities. 5th ed. New York, NY: McGraw Hill; 2007: Figure 6-18.)

a. Transection of the brachial artery
b. Malunion of distal humerus
c. Motor deficit from injury to the ulnar nerve
d. Chronic arthritis of the elbow
e. Chronic deformity of the hands and fingers caused by contractures

374. A 7-year-old boy presents to the ED 1 hour after slipping and landing on his right outstretched hand. He was evaluated and splinted by emergency medical technicians (EMTs) and brought to the ED. On examination, you note a deformity of his right wrist. There are no neurovascular deficits. A radiograph of the wrist is shown in the figure. Which of the following is true regarding physeal fractures in children?

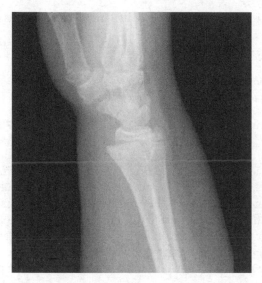

(Reproduced, with permission, from Shah BR, Lucchesi M. Atlas of Pediatric Emergency Medicine. New York, NY: McGraw Hill; 2006: Figure 19-3.)

a. Salter-Harris type IV is defined as a crush injury of the growth plate.
b. The most common type of fracture is the Salter-Harris type II.
c. This patient's radiographic findings are consistent with Salter-Harris type V.
d. Fractures through the physis, metaphysis, and epiphysis are classified as Salter-Harris type III.
e. The worst prognosis is seen with Salter-Harris type I fractures.

The following scenario applies to questions 375 and 376.

A 9-year-old boy with a history of sickle cell anemia is brought into the ED after sudden onset of left-sided hemiplegia. The mother states that her son had rhinorrhea and nasal congestion for the past 2 days, but has otherwise been in a good state of health.

375. What is the best diagnostic modality to evaluate for possible cerebro-vascular accident (CVA)?

a. Cerebral angiography
b. LP
c. Magnetic resonance imaging and angiogram (MRI/MRA) of the head and neck
d. Noncontrast computerized tomography (CT) scan of the head
e. Positron emission tomography (PET) scan

376. What treatment should be initiated immediately in this patient?

a. Oral aspirin 3 to 5 mg/kg
b. Exchange transfusion
c. IV alteplase
d. IV unfractionated heparin
e. Subcutaneous low molecular weight heparin

The following scenario applies to questions 377 and 378.

A 3-year-old boy presents to the ED with his adoptive mother for a new rash. He was adopted 2 weeks ago from Thailand and his vaccination history is unknown. He has had a fever for the past 3 days and a mild cough and rhinorrhea for the past 2 days. The rash started behind his ears the previous night and in the morning of the day of presentation it spread further to his neck and chest. On examination, he is ill-appearing, awake, alert, and crying. A maculopapular rash is present on his head, neck, and upper trunk. You also note scleral injection bilaterally. There are no lesions in his mouth.

377. Which of the following is the most likely causal organism?

a. Roseola
b. Measles
c. Erythema infectiosum
d. Rubella
e. Varicella

378. The mother has also been taking care of her 10-month-old niece for the past week while the infant's parents are out of town. The infant is afebrile and has not exhibited any similar symptoms. Which of the following is the most appropriate management of the 10-month-old niece?

a. Supportive care
b. Measles vaccine administration
c. Measles immunoglobulin (IG) administration
d. Hospitalization with respiratory isolation
e. Obtain measles IgM level

379. A 6-week-old full-term boy presents with concern for yellowing of the eyes. His mother reports that he has been feeding well and acting normally. The child has been solely breastfed since birth and had normal urine output and stool output but noted lightening stool color from seedy yellow to pale, yellow/gray in appearance. Birth history reveals an uncomplicated normal spontaneous vaginal delivery without vacuum assist. Hepatitis B immunization and Vitamin K injection were given at birth. Newborn screen and patient's transcutaneous bilirubin level at birth discharge were normal. No recent travel or animal exposures. Vital signs on presentation show temperature 98.9°F, BP 96/44 mm Hg, HR 164 beats/minute, RR 32 breaths/minute, and pulse oximetry 99%. Patient is calm with scleral icterus bilaterally and mild jaundice to face and chest. Heart sounds are normal and lungs clear. Abdomen soft and nontender with liver edge 1 cm below the costal margin. Capillary refill is brisk. No bruising noted on skin exam. Initial labs are notable for elevated total bilirubin level of 14.1, and direct bilirubin 9.2, with elevation in transaminases with AST 85 and ALT 101. CBC shows a slightly low hemoglobin of 10.4, but otherwise normal. What is the next best step in management?

a. Obtain a right upper quadrant ultrasound to evaluate the biliary tree
b. Discharge home with recommendation to switch to formula feed
c. Consult Pediatric Infectious Diseases to evaluate for infectious hepatitis
d. Consult Pediatric Gastroenterology to evaluate for inherited disorder of biliary metabolism
e. Consult Pediatric Hematology to evaluate for autoimmune hemolytic anemia

The following scenario applies to questions 380 and 381.

380. An 18-month-old girl presents with 2 days of fever and fussiness. Her mother states that she had 2 days of upper respiratory symptoms prior to the fever starting. Additionally, her mother noticed her pulling at her left ear. She has been drinking well and eating normally with normal urine output and stool output. Patient's mother has been giving acetaminophen for fevers every 4 hours. Patient's immunizations are up to date. Past medical history significant for 3 previous episodes of otitis media, last treated 3 months prior. She has an allergy to penicillin. Vital signs on presentation show temperature 102.1°F, BP 101/62 mm Hg, HR 174 beats/minute, RR 36 breaths/minute, and oxygen saturation 99%. HEENT (head, eyes, ears, nose, and throat) exam shows mild rhinorrhea with moist mucus membranes. No conjunctivitis. Right ear exam shows a normal external canal, with a slightly erythematous, nonbulging, tympanic membrane. Left ear exam shows a normal external canal, with an erythematous and bulging, tympanic membrane with purulent middle ear effusion. Which of the following is the best therapy for this child?

a. Ibuprofen
b. Amoxicillin
c. Ibuprofen and a prescription for amoxicillin to be given in 48 hours if no improvement
d. Ibuprofen and cefdinir
e. Referral to pediatric otolaryngologist for tympanostomy tubes

381. Three days after initiating the recommended therapy, the above patient re-presents to the ED with concern for bloody stools. Mother reports that the patient seemed to be overall improving when she had a large stool in her diaper that was "very red" colored. Mother denies abdominal pain or vomiting. No new rashes noted. Vital signs on presentation show temperature 99.0°F, BP 98/64 mm Hg, HR 144 beats/minute, RR 24 breaths/minute, and oxygen saturation 99%. Abdomen is soft, nontender, nondistended. No hepatosplenomegaly. No rashes noted on skin exam. What is the next best step in management for this patient?

a. Hemoccult stool to determine presence or absence of blood
b. Ultrasound abdomen to evaluate for intussusception
c. Discontinue antibiotic due to allergic reaction
d. Plan films of the abdomen to evaluate for small bowel obstruction
e. Collect stool culture to evaluate for infectious colitis

382. A 10-year-old boy from Wisconsin presents to the ED with complaint of left ankle and foot pain after completion of his youth basketball game earlier today. Patient rates pain as a 3/10 at rest and 6/10 with activity. He does not remember any specific injury, but states that it hurt "really bad" every time he tried to jump to rebound the ball. He has experienced this pain before, but never this bad. At presentation, vital signs show temperature 98.5°F, BP 102/60 mm Hg, HR 104 beats/minute, RR 18 breaths/minute, and oxygen saturation 100%. Skin exam is normal without rash. There is no joint swelling. Left lower extremity shows 5/5 strength with flexion and extension at each joint, plantar flexion with squeezing of calf muscles, no point tenderness, erythema, or swelling of ankle, though pain with heel squeeze. Remainder of examination is normal. This patient's condition is most consistent with which of the following:

a. Sprain of the anterior talofibular ligament
b. Apophysitis of the calcaneal epiphysis
c. Salter-Harris fracture of the fibular head
d. Achilles tendon rupture
e. Lyme disease arthritis of left ankle

383. Parents of a 7-month-old child present with their daughter for concern for new abnormal eye movements. She is an otherwise healthy child, with normal development, who started having eye movements several days prior. Over the last week, the movements have become more frequent and are now occurring several times daily. They describe the eye movements as "erratic rapid zig-zag movements in all directions." There has been no known trauma or bruising. No family history of seizures. No recent travel. Family does own a dog, a tarantula, and a coral snake. At presentation, vital signs show temperature 100.2°F, BP 98/56 mm Hg, HR 154 beats/minute, RR 24 breaths/minute, and oxygen saturation 98%. HEENT exam shows flat anterior fontanelle, pupils equally reactive with red reflex present bilaterally, normal scalp exam, and normal tympanic membranes bilaterally without hemotympanum. Skin exam is normal without bruising or obvious puncture wounds. Abdomen is soft, with no hepatosplenomegaly and normal movement of all extremities with 2+ deep tendon reflexes in bilateral upper extremities and lower extremities. What is the most concerning cause of patient's eye movements?

a. Toxin envenomation from coral snake bite
b. Increased intracranial pressure due to subarachnoid hemorrhage from traumatic head injury
c. New onset seizure disorder
d. Opsoclonus-myoclonus syndrome due to neuroblastoma
e. Retinoblastoma

384. A 15-year-old adolescent boy presents with new onset headache. Patient states that the headache started during his second period class. He describes initially having difficulty seeing the words on his paper due to white spot being in the center of his vision. This has since resolved but he now describes an 8/10 headache located in bilateral frontal regions, and describes lights as very bright and sounds as very loud. He does play football, but has not had a headache, dizziness, or nausea after playing. Vital signs on presentation show temperature 97.9°F, BP 112/66 mm Hg, HR 68 beats/minute, RR 14 breaths/minute, and oxygen saturation 99%. HEENT exam is overall normal with equally reactive pupils and normal tympanic membrane exam. Photophobia and phonophobia are present. What is the best next step in the care of this patient?

a. Administer 100% oxygen via nonrebreather
b. Oral acetaminophen
c. IV morphine
d. IV antibiotics followed by LP
e. IV prochlorperazine, ketorolac, diphenhydramine, and 20 mL/kg normal saline bolus

Pediatrics

Answers

350. The answer is d. This is a case where **nonaccidental trauma (NAT)** should be considered. This is a classic example of a **"bucket handle" fracture.** Metaphyseal corner fractures, known as bucket handle fractures, are considered **pathognomonic for abuse** and are caused by rapid shearing forces or twisting motion. Spiral fractures in a nonambulating child, fractures of the posterior ribs, sternum, scapula, or spinous processes may be the only presentation of child abuse; multiple fractures in various stages of healing are also highly indicative of abuse. Any type of trauma that does not fit the mechanism should raise suspicion and alert the physician of the possibility of abuse. In this case, the fracture pattern mandates further workup for NAT. According to the American Academy of Pediatrics (AAP), the **skeletal survey** is the initial test of choice for all children less than 2 years of age with concern for possible abuse. Additional workup may be indicated based on the age and presentation of the child. In this case, a head CT scan and ophthalmology consultation should also be strongly considered. All states have mandatory reporting of child abuse. It is also mandatory to contact the local **Child Protective Services** to further investigate the situation.

Osteogenesis imperfecta (**a**) is a rare genetic condition caused by mutations of the type I procollagen gene. Children may present with fractures in the setting of little or no trauma. Classic blue sclerae may be present. This type of injury should not be simply splinted and discharged home (**e**). A simple posterior long leg splint may be adequate treatment for this fracture at this time but not for the overall disposition. Orthopedic surgery (**b**) should be included early in the intervention, but their expertise is not necessarily critical in the immediate treatment algorithm. Electrolyte abnormalities (**c**) that may be responsible for pathological fractures in children are exceedingly rare when compared to child abuse and should only be considered once NAT is excluded or in the presence of other abnormalities in the physical examination.

351. The answer is c. This is a case of **impetigo.** It is a superficial skin infection most commonly caused by *S. pyogenes* (group A β-hemolytic

Streptococcus). When large pustules are observed (>1 cm), the term used to describe this condition is bullous impetigo, which is more strongly associated with *S. aureus*. The typical presentation of impetigo includes **honey-crusted lesions on erythematous skin**. These tend to be pruritic and easily spread by the patient. Although possible, systemic infection is uncommon so patients typically are well appearing. Treatment includes either oral or topical antibiotic therapy. Topical therapy with mupirocin is very effective and is usually first-line treatment, unless widespread infection, in which case cephalexin can be considered. Hand washing is also critical to limit the spread of infection to other family members. Treatment of the skin lesions does not prevent the development of nephritis.

Group B Streptococcus (a) does not generally cause impetigo. It is a well-known cause of severe perinatal infection, such as pneumonia and meningitis. *S. aureus* (b) is commonly associated with impetigo whose appearance is circular, scaly, and ring-like lesions. This etiology is usually combined with Streptococcus. *S. aureus* is the sole isolate in 10% of cases; therefore, it is important to treat for both organisms. *S. pneumoniae* (d) is a well-known pathogen involved in many types of infection such as osteomyelitis, pneumonia, meningitis, pericarditis, peritonitis, and cellulitis; however, it does not usually cause impetigo. *Salmonella* (e) is known to cause infectious diarrhea, meningitis, and osteomyelitis, particularly in sickle cell patients.

352. The answer is d. This is a case of **erythema infectiosum** or Fifth disease, which is caused by **parvovirus B19**. It is characterized by an eruption that presents initially as an erythematous malar blush (**slapped cheek appearance**) followed by an erythematous maculopapular eruption on the extensor surfaces of extremities that evolves into a reticulated, lacy, mottled appearance. Fever and other symptoms may be present but are uncommon. In patients with chronic hemolytic anemia (eg, sickle cell disease), **aplastic anemia** is a serious complication. Pregnant women should avoid exposure to this virus, because it may cause fetal hydrops in 10% of cases.

Sickle cell patients can develop osteomyelitis (a); however, the described clinical presentation is not consistent with this diagnosis. Patients with osteomyelitis caused by *Salmonella* species are generally those with sickle cell disease. However, the most common organism that causes osteomyelitis in patients with sickle cell disease is *S. aureus* (similar to the general population). Encephalitis (b) is an inflammation of the brain parenchyma and is not commonly caused by parvovirus. Common etiologic agents of encephalitis include herpes simplex, herpes zoster, varicella zoster, West Nile virus, and toxoplasmosis. Pneumonia (c) is a common diagnosis in patients of all ages. In children, the most common causative agents of pneumonia are viral. The most commonly found bacterial agent is *S. pneumoniae*. Meningitis (e) is an infection of the meninges that surround the brain that is caused by viral and bacterial entities. The most common bacterial agents vary with age. *E. coli*, group B Streptococcus, and *L. monocytogenes* are seen in very young infants. *S. pneumoniae, Neisseria meningitides*, and *Haemophilus influenzae* are seen in older children.

353. The answer is b. This is a classic story and presentation for **intussusception** in which a part of intestine telescopes inside of another resulting in ischemia that can lead to infarction of bowel. This is a **true gastrointestinal (GI) emergency**. The most common type of intussusception is ileo-colic and most commonly idiopathic in etiology. Ileo-ileal and colo-colonic intussusceptions are possible though rare in comparison. The most common age group is 3 to 12 months with greater than 80% occurring within the first 2 years of life. **Air enema is both diagnostic and therapeutic** and has been widely adopted as the intervention of choice for these patients.

Although the classic triad consists of colicky abdominal pain, vomiting, and currant jelly stools, fewer than 20% of patients will present with all of these findings (a). Plain films cannot typically confirm or refute the presence of intussusception, though air present in the cecum indicates no ileocolic intussusception (c). Radiographs are important, however, to exclude the presence of free air before attempting an enema reduction. From a diagnostic perspective, ultrasound has been employed and demonstrated to have very high sensitivity for intussusception. Although surgical consultation (d) is warranted before reduction for cases of perforation identified with the air enema or unsuccessful reductions, relatively few patients ultimately require surgical correction. There is a lead point in a small minority of patients in the classic age range (e). The incidence of pathologic lead points increases as the age of the patient increases beyond the classic age group. Lead points can be hypertrophied Peyer's patches, a Meckel's diverticulum, a polyp, or a tumor.

354. The answer is a. Acute chest syndrome by definition is the presence of a new infiltrate on chest X-ray plus one of the following: fever more than 38.5°C, chest pain, hypoxia, or increased work of breathing.

This is **one of the most serious and life-threatening complications of sickle cell disease.** One must be very cautious with IV fluid hydration because overaggressive fluid administration can lead to pulmonary edema in patients who have pneumonia or previously suffered from acute chest syndrome. Administration of IV antibiotics, transfusions for anemia, and oxygen are the mainstays of therapy.

Disseminated infection leading to sepsis **(b)** and empyema **(c)** are complications of bacterial pneumonia in general. Patients with sickle cell disease have an inherent preponderance to infection by encapsulated bacteria due to auto-splenectomy, but these are not specific complications of fluid and antibiotic administration. Stroke **(d)** is another complication of sickle cell disease but it is not caused by fluid resuscitation. Likewise, patients with long-standing anemia are at risk for congestive heart failure **(e)** and, indeed, many patients with sickle cell disease have an enlarged heart. However, this is a chronic complication and not one specifically associated with treatment of pneumonia and acute chest syndrome.

355. The answer is e. This is a patient with **Kawasaki disease (KD).** This entity is defined by **fever lasting for a minimum of 5 days** and *four of the following five criteria*:

- Cervical lymphadenopathy of greater than 1.5 cm
- Dry, cracked lips or other oral mucous membrane involvement (strawberry tongue)
- Truncal, nonvesicular rash
- Nonpurulent conjunctivitis
- Swollen or edematous hands and feet

KD is a systemic **inflammatory vasculitis** of unknown etiology. The characteristic constellation of symptoms, which this patient meets, requires immediate action to prevent complications of the disease. Another common finding, and one that many practitioners use to help in the diagnosis of "atypical" cases, is intense irritability of the child. The most serious sequelae involve **coronary artery aneurysms.** These occur in approximately 20% to 25% of untreated patients. This number is reduced to 2% to 4%, if treatment with **IVIG** occurs within the first 10 days of symptom onset. Additional treatment with **high-dose aspirin** is recommended both for its antiplatelet and antiinflammatory effects.

Although this patient will require a cardiology consultation and echo-cardiogram **(a)**, it is not the next step in management because it is critical to not delay treatment. The absence of coronary artery aneurysms should not dissuade you from initiation of treatment and their presence does not, in the short-term, alter therapy. There are no laboratory values that contribute to making the diagnosis, although there are some characteristic findings. If the patient clinically meets diagnostic criteria, no additional labs are needed; however, if full criteria are not met, labs can be acquired to aid in diagnosis of incomplete KD. Typically, these patients have elevated serum markers of inflammation, ESR, and CRP, and can have elevated transaminases, as is present in this case. Hypoalbuminemia may also be present. The other classic finding is a thrombocytosis, which typically does not present itself until at least a week into the disease and can reach over 1 million/mm^3 in some cases. Additional laboratory tests (b) are not required except in cases where the diagnosis is truly in question. Therefore, reassurance (c) and continued septic workup (d) are incorrect. Antibiotics have no role in the treatment of this condition.

356. The answer is d. The most important next step is administration of **prostaglandin bolus followed by a drip**. This patient is in severe cardiac failure due to **impending closure of his ductus arteriosus**. The patient is presenting in a classic time frame, which usually ranges from **7 to 10 days**. **Ductal-dependent congenital heart lesions** that present in this manner typically include transposition of the great arteries, truncus arteriosus, total anomalous pulmonary venous return, left heart hypoplasia, and aortic coarctation. The most important next step is administration of a medication that will assist the ductus to remain open while preparing for surgical intervention.

Oxygen (a) is a stimulant to close the ductus (as is appropriate in normal neonates) and should not be administered; it can be used for a brief period of time as a diagnostic tool as it can help differentiate the location of the lesion. In lesions with right-to-left mixing, the saturations will not improve. In pulmonary conditions causing this presentation or in cardiac conditions without right-to-left shunting, the saturations will improve. There should be a low threshold for intubation as prostaglandin administration can cause apnea. The other choices, chest radiograph and ECG (b), would need to be done; however, the patient requires immediate intervention with prostaglandin. The next step is not to place the patient on ECMO (e). Antibiotics would likely be administered to this patient early on because sepsis should be considered as this is a home birth, the patient is hypothermic, and this intervention is critical for early goal-directed therapy (c).

Still, the presentation is classic for closure of the ductus arteriosus and recognition of this condition is critical.

357. The answer is b. This patient has **pyloric stenosis** and will exhibit a **hypochloremic, hypokalemic metabolic alkalosis. Hypoglycemia** is common in newborns of this age who experience poor intake of calories and who have very poor glycemic reserves. The low chloride and high bicarbonate are the result of hydrochloric acid loss from stomach with repeated episodes of vomiting leading to an alkalemia. As a result, the patient will physiologically try to balance ions and trade intracellular H^+ for extracellular K^+, thus lowering the serum potassium. Pyloric stenosis typically presents between 3 and 6 weeks of life. It is most common in first-born male patients. In the majority of cases, a palpable mass will not be felt in the epigastric region, though it can sometimes be felt in the operating room (OR) under anesthesia.

Answer **(a)** is incorrect because these values are physiologically normal. Answers **(c)** and **(e)** are incorrect because both the potassium and the chloride are elevated and this is not consistent with pyloric stenosis. Answer **(d)** is incorrect because the bicarbonate is low. Low bicarbonate can be a very late finding in pyloric stenosis and is a sign of severe physiologic disturbance secondary to hypovolemia, resulting in a patient progressive to a hypovolemic shock-like state.

358. The answer is c. This patient had a **simple febrile seizure.** Approximately, 2% to 5% of children will experience a febrile seizure during their lifetimes. Febrile seizures occur between the **ages of** 3 months and 5 years, are associated with fever, and are categorized as either simple or complex. Simple febrile seizures are **generalized** and last **less than 15 minutes** typically at the start of an illness. Complex febrile seizures are prolonged, recur within 24 hours, or are focal. The approach to a patient with a febrile seizure is, for all intents and purposes, identical to that of the same patient who has not had a seizure, so long as the seizure has stopped by the time you are evaluating the patient. If the seizure continues, treat as you would any other seizure with indicated medications (ie., benzodiazepines) with attention to the primary survey and correction of hypoglycemia when present. Once the patient is stable, and the seizure has abated, potential sources of the fever should be identified. This patient, having a temperature of 103°F and lesions consistent with Coxsackie virus infection on the posterior pharynx, does not need any testing. In approximately half of all children with simple, febrile seizures, the source is viral. In well-appearing children meeting the criteria for a simple febrile seizure, minimal testing is necessary.

In the presence of an otherwise normal examination, other diagnostic tests (**a and b**) are not indicated. CBC and blood cultures in otherwise well-appearing, fully immunized children of this age are no longer indicated to evaluate for occult bacteremia. Neither a head CT scan nor a neurology consultation (**d**) is warranted for a first-time febrile seizure. An LP to rule out meningitis (**e**) is not indicated in this patient who has regained normal mental status, appears well, and has no neurologic deficit.

359. The answer is b. This is a case of a patient with an **SCFE**. SCFE is a condition of the femur where the femoral head slips or shears off from the neck of the femur through the physis. It is more common in **boys** than in girls, typically in **early or mid-adolescence** and is more common in African-American children than in Caucasian children. Its cause is unknown. SCFE can present either with a complaint of tightness that progresses to more significant pain, a limp or, more dramatically, with extreme pain and inability to bear weight. It is not uncommon for a child to present with a complaint of knee pain after minimal trauma. A careful examination will often better localize the origin of the pain to the hip. It is usually unilateral, though it can be bilateral in upward of a quarter of the cases. The diagnosis is made on radiograph. It is classically described as the "ice cream falling off of the cone" appearance. Treatment includes admission and surgical correction.

Legg-Calvé-Perthes (**a**), also known as avascular necrosis of the femoral head, typically affects younger children aged 2 to 6 years and is uncommon in African American as compared with Caucasian children. Septic arthritis (**c**) is typically characterized by fever, intense pain, inability to bear weight, and large effusions with elevated inflammatory markers. Osgood-Schlatter (**d**) disease is the most common cause of knee pain in this age group. It is caused by the patellar tendon avulsing on its insertion at the tibial tuberosity. It is characterized by localized tenderness and treatment is conservative. Transient synovitis (**e**) of the hip is typically a postinfectious condition of young, toddler-aged children. It would be unlikely to occur in a 13-year-old.

360. The answer is b. This is a case of **milk protein colitis**, a common cause of rectal bleeding in this age group. Some neonates have sensitivity to cow's milk protein (which is fundamentally different from human milk proteins) that leads to an allergic antibody response causing a true colitis and bloody stools. Approximately, a third of these patients will have a similar reaction to soy milk proteins. The resulting symptoms are dramatic but generally without other consequence except in cases where the exposure is long-standing and bleeding is ongoing. This can lead to malnourishment, anemia, and poor growth. Milk protein colitis is more frequently seen in bottle-fed infants but can be seen in exclusively breast-fed infants where the proteins are thought to transfer from the mother's milk into the infant, which results in the same symptoms as if the patient were drinking milk directly. Treatment is **elimination of offending agent from the diet**, which typically results in total resolution of symptoms. Most patients will grow out of their sensitivity by 2 years of age and milk products can be reintroduced at that time.

Acute gastroenteritis (**a**) typically presents with multiple episodes of vomiting and diarrhea. It can occur with or without fever. *C. difficile* colitis (**c**) does cause bloody stool, but it generally follows an antibiotic exposure or is associated with other risk factors. It would be highly unusual in an otherwise healthy 3-week-old without risk factors. Both intestinal malrotation (**d**) and necrotizing enterocolitis (**e**) are GI and surgical emergencies that can be associated with blood in stool but occur in ill-appearing infants.

361. The answer is c. This is a case of **neonatal sepsis**, an invasive bacterial infection occurring during the first 90 days of life. The most common causes of newborn sepsis are **group B β-hemolytic Streptococcus (GBS) and *E. coli*.** Approximately, a third of women are carriers of GBS in their vagina and exposure is through the birth canal. There is **increased risk with PROM** that is thought to result in ascending infection. Increased colony counts result in increased risk for neonatal sepsis and thus the tendency to screen pregnant women and to treat at the time of delivery for either screen-positive women or women with fever or PROM. Any neonate younger than 4 weeks with fever higher than 100.3°F requires a full workup to search for the source of infection. This workup includes a CBC, blood culture, urinalysis and urine culture, and an LP for cell counts and culture. One should consider sending the cerebrospinal fluid (CSF) for HSV culture and polymerase chain reaction, particularly if there are any maternal risk factors, suspicious skin lesions, or in any infant who is very ill. Empiric antiviral therapy should also be administered in such cases pending test results, as there is sufficient evidence now that neonates with HSV meningitis may not have typical herpetic skin lesions. In this case, the lesions on this patient's trunk are most consistent with a benign newborn rash called erythema toxicum neonatorum and are unrelated to the fever.

The other organisms listed are all known causes of neonatal sepsis. *E. coli* (a) incidence is similar to GBS and is the most common of the enteric pathogens that cause this condition. It is the most common cause of urinary tract infections (UTIs) in infants, which can lead to bacteremia as well. *Listeria* (b) is a commonly cited source of infection in neonatal sepsis but with much lower incidence. Exposure is primarily from unprocessed meats and unpasteurized produce. *S. aureus* (d) is an unlikely pathogen in an immunocompetent patient of this age. HSV (e) is an important pathogen to consider in neonatal sepsis. Obtaining the maternal history is important to help diagnose this condition, though many patients who ultimately are diagnosed with neonatal HSV have no known maternal history of vaginal herpes.

362. The answer is c. This is a classic case of **infant botulism** characterized by **generalized weakness, pupillary unresponsiveness, and hypoventilation**. Patients often present with an initial complaint of **constipation**. They are noted to have a particularly **weak cry**. The condition is caused by release of the botulinum toxin from *Clostridium botulinum*. The toxin prevents release of acetylcholine from the neuromuscular junction. Older children present with complaints of diplopia, dysarthria, and dysphagia. Young infants are particularly susceptible from ingestion of honey, which can harbor *C. botulinum* spores. The pH in infant stomachs does not digest the spores. **Honey is not recommended for any infant younger than 1 year**.

This is not a case of spinal muscular atrophy (ie, Werdnig-Hoffmann disease) (a), which is an autosomal recessive disorder characterized by muscle weakness that can affect every aspect of eating, breathing, and moving and will often be apparent from very early on—even before the age of this child. Brain tumors (b) can cause some of these symptoms but would not typically present with generalized weakness and poorly responsive pupils. This child does not show particular signs of increased intracranial pressure like vomiting or persistent irritability. Similarly, this patient is not showing signs of meningitis (d). She is afebrile and is not irritable. Organophosphate poisoning (e) causes increased muscarinic and nicotinic tone from the inhibition of acetylcholinesterase. The symptoms may be similar to this patient with drooling and weakness. In addition, diarrhea, autonomic dysfunction, and CNS disturbances are common. This condition is unlikely in a nonmobile infant and exposures are uncommon in this setting.

363. The answer is c. This patient has become apneic and requires assisted ventilation. The correct approach is to do a **jaw thrust and chin lift** in order to provide optimal airway positioning and **begin bag-valve-mask ventilation**. This is the most important skill to learn in pediatric resuscitation. In many cases, providing oxygenation and ventilation appropriately is all that is needed to resolve the bradycardia and circulatory issues. **The most common cause of arrest in children is respiratory arrest.** This is a classic case of respiratory arrest causing cyanosis and subsequent bradycardia.

Epinephrine (**a**) is certainly in the algorithm for bradycardia, but the first step in resuscitation is always addressing the airway. Oxygen should be administered to this patient and a nonrebreather face mask (**b**) can provide high oxygen delivery. However, the patient is not actively breathing, so this method is ineffective. Endotracheal intubation (**d**) may be necessary to establish a definitive airway in this patient. However, it will take time to set up and perform. The simplest and quickest intervention is jaw-thrust or chin-lift with bag-valve-mask ventilation. Chest compressions (**e**) are soon to follow in this patient's resuscitation if ventilation is not effective alone, but the initial intervention is attention to airway and breathing.

364. The answer is e. This patient is in shock. Attempts at peripheral IV access are acceptable, but should be limited to two attempts within 60 seconds and then **IO insertion should be attempted**. IO lines can be performed quickly and reliably. The preferred sites for insertion are the **proximal tibia**, followed by the distal tibia and distal femur. In the emergent situation, most medications can be administered through the IO line and onset of action is similar to venous administration.

Internal jugular central line (**a**), femoral vein central line (**b**), and saphenous cutdown (**c**) are all very good methods of establishing IV access in many critically ill adults and some pediatric patients but require both greater skill and time. IO access is proven to be quick and reliable in the pediatric population and should be utilized when peripheral access is difficult to obtain in an unstable patient. A large-bore IV in the antecubital fossa (**d**) is also a good method of vascular access, but peripheral access was not obtained in this individual.

365. The answer is a. Epiglottitis is a life-threatening inflammatory condition of the epiglottis, aryepiglottic, and paraglottic folds. The etiology is usually infectious, with *H. influenzae* type b (Hib) as the classic and most common etiology before the introduction of the Hib vaccination. Most cases now appear in adults and nonimmunized children. Epiglottitis is most commonly seen as secondary infections following viral illnesses (the most notorious was primary varicella before the widespread use of that vaccine). Signs and symptoms include a **prodromal period** of 1 to 2 days with high fever, dysphagia, pooling of secretions, and dyspnea. Patients usually sit in an erect or "tripod" position, leaning forward with neck extended to provide the maximum diameter of the airway. Lateral radiographs of the neck may show the classic thumbprint sign of an enlarged, inflamed epiglottis, although a CT scan of the neck may delineate the condition further. However, CT scans are typically difficult to obtain because of the fact that patients are not stable enough to leave the ED and need continuous monitoring in case of airway compromise. The classic approach to a patient with suspected epiglottitis is to leave them in their caretaker's arms, try to avoid agitating them, and call immediately for ENT (ear, nose, and throat) and anesthesia assistance in the ED. Direct laryngoscopy in the ED is contraindicated because it may induce laryngospasm. These patients require direct visualization, often only in the OR, with the appropriate surgical service prepared to place a surgical airway emergently. The lone emergency physician should have multiple airway adjuvants ready when intubating these patients. The patient should be sedated but paralytic medications should be avoided during the intubation procedure. IV antibiotics and steroids are indicated to help treat the infection and decrease swelling.

Retropharyngeal abscesses (**b**) may present somewhat similarly but not typically in the same level of extremis as this patient, and is typically in children under 4 years of age. The classic physical examination finding is an inability to extend the neck because this stretches the inflamed prevertebral soft tissue area. Retropharyngeal abscess should be suspected when there is a widened prevertebral soft tissue stripe on the lateral neck film. EBV pharyngitis (**c**) may present with erythema or exudate of the tonsils, dysphagia, fever, and cough. In addition, patients may be very uncomfortable and moderately ill appearing, but will typically not present with airway compromise and hypoxia. In addition, clinical mononucleosis is usually a condition of older children and adolescents. Ludwig's angina (**d**) is an infection of the submandibular space. Peritonsillar abscess (**e**) is often a secondary infection of strep throat and will present with trismus, difficulty swallowing, and fever typically over 4 years of age.

366. The answer is d. Bronchiolitis is a common cause of respiratory distress in infants, especially younger than 6 months, and the most common virus associated with bronchiolitis is **respiratory syncytial virus (RSV)**. Diagnosis is made clinically on the basis of the constellation of symptoms. Patients at risk of increased disease severity are those who have chronic lung disease (especially ex-preemies), complex congenital heart disease, or an immunocompromised state. These patients are eligible for receiving palivizumab, an injectable antibody that confers passive immunity and can reduce the likelihood of severe lower respiratory tract disease caused by RSV in susceptible individuals. RSV bronchiolitis presents similarly to other viral illnesses including rhinovirus, parainfluenza virus, coronavirus, echovirus, and Coxsackie virus. The clinical condition of bronchiolitis is caused by RSV in approximately 70% of cases, especially during the peak months of November to April. The diagnosis is confirmed by a rapid antigen test of a nasal aspirate, but this is typically only useful in patients whose diagnosis is unclear or in whom management may be different based on concomitant conditions. Management is largely supportive with IV hydration and high-flow oxygen to improve minute volume. Respiratory precautions are necessary to limit transmission.

Foreign body aspiration (**a**) can happen in infants of this age and, if undetected initially, can cause similar symptoms. Often, a radiograph will show an ingested object or stridor may be present. It is believed that bronchiolitis is a precursor to asthma (**b**) and that infants who develop bronchiolitis are more likely to develop asthma as they get older, though the diagnosis of asthma does not apply to someone with their first wheezing episode at this age. Pneumococcal pneumonia (**c**) is the predominant cause of bacterial pneumonia in this age group, although the incidence has declined with the consistent administration of Prevnar (pneumococcal conjugate vaccine). This patient would have received two doses of the vaccine by this age, if his immunizations are up-to-date. Pneumococcus can result as a secondary infection as well but this clinical scenario is classic for bronchiolitis. Parvovirus B19 (**e**) is the etiologic agent of Fifth disease. Fifth disease is a mild illness that occurs most commonly in children. The child typically has a fever associated with a "slapped-cheek" appearance to the face and a lacy red rash on the trunk and limbs.

367. The answer is b. Cuffed tubes are preferable for providing a better seal without an increased risk for endothelial damage from overinflation of the balloon. Cuffed ETTs also allow better ventilation in patients with poor lung compliance. It is important not to blow the balloon up to a pressure greater than 20 cm H_2O with this complication in mind. There are two acceptable methods for choosing the appropriate cuffed ETT size. One relies on the length-based resuscitation tape that should be available and utilized in the resuscitation of all small children. The other utilizes a formula that has been endorsed by the American Heart Association for calculation of the appropriate tube size for a cuffed tube is ETT size (mm of internal diameter of tube) = **(age in years/4) + 3.5.** The calculation in this patient would yield a size of 4.5 mm for a cuffed tube.

To calculate the size of an uncuffed ETT, the calculation is as follows: size (in mm) = (age in years/4) + 4. That would yield an ETT size of 5.0 mm for an uncuffed tube. This is not one of the choices. All other answer choices **(a, c, d, and e)** are incorrect.

368. The answer is c. Foreign body ingestion and aspiration are common in this age group with peak occurrence between 6 months and 4 years. In this patient, the position of the coin on the anterior-posterior chest film aids with the diagnosis. When the coin is in the esophagus, it is seen head-on in the anteroposterior (AP) projection. When it is localized in the trachea, it is seen in the sagittal plane because the cartilaginous tracheal rings in children are incomplete and remain open posteriorly, causing the coin to sit sagittal or sideways. After assessing the patient's airway and breathing, it is important to assess characteristics of the foreign body ingested. Ingested foreign bodies usually get obstructed in three common locations—thoracic inlet (60%-80%), at the gastroesophageal junction (10%-20%), and at the aortic arch (5%-20%). A good way to remember this is by their level in the spine—C4-C6, T8, and T4, respectively. Once they pass the pylorus, most foreign bodies pass through the remainder of the GI tract. Objects larger than 2 × 5 cm, sharp objects (eg, needles, tacks), or disc/button batteries should be considered for emergent removal if pre-pylorus.

Although foreign body aspiration **(a)** is a possibility, the position of the coin in the radiograph and the absence of respiratory symptoms make this diagnosis unlikely. If there is a suspicion for an aspirated foreign body, the patient should undergo bronchoscopy. Bronchospasm **(b)** occurs as a reaction to aspirated foreign bodies and should always be considered in patients presenting with cough or respiratory symptoms. Patients with epiglottitis **(d)** classically present with drooling and assume a "tripod position" to assist their breathing and will often show evidence of respiratory distress. Allergic reaction (e) is unlikely given the absence of dermatologic or respiratory symptoms.

369. The answer is e. This is a case of **laryngotracheitis** or **croup**. It is the most common cause of stridor and upper respiratory obstruction in children 6 months to 3 years old. It usually begins with constitutional symptoms and subsequently patients develop the characteristic **"seal-like" cough** described as barky. The etiology is most commonly the parainfluenza virus. Diagnosis is usually clinical. Treatment includes steroids which help decrease laryngeal edema. Dexamethasone is the most commonly used steroid, with onset of within 6 hours. For severe croup (marked stridor at rest, respiratory distress leading to agitation of child), nebulized racemic epinephrine is administered due to its quick onset to decrease bronchospasm and mucosal edema. After administration of racemic epinephrine, patients should be observed for at least 2 hours to assure that the disease does not progress, which was previously thought to be due to rebound from the medication. Some home-based treatments, such as taking a child outdoors to breathe cool air or into the bathroom to breathe the steam produced when running hot water in the shower both seem to aid in symptomatic relief, but have not been supported by evidence-based studies.

Radiographs of the chest (a) to evaluate for pneumonia and the soft tissues of the neck (c) are not indicated in patients presenting with classic findings for croup. CBC and blood culture (b) are of no utility in a patient with this classic viral illness. Antibiotics (d) are not effective in patients with a viral illness.

370. The answer is e. The ECG shows a narrow complex tachycardia at 240 beats/minute with no variability and absent P waves. This is diagnostic of **supraventricular tachycardia (SVT)**. SVT is the most common pathologic arrhythmia of childhood. It is sometimes confused with sinus tachycardia, which presents at a rate of less than 225 beats/minute in infants and less than 150 beats/minute in older children and adults. This finding, coupled with variability with respirations and evidence of normal P waves, will prove to be useful in differentiating sinus tachycardia from SVT. This dysrhythmia is typically well tolerated in young children and infants. SVT will often present with a history of **pallor, poor feeding, tachypnea, and lethargy, or irritability**. Older children will describe palpitations, light-headedness, and shortness of breath. Signs of congestive heart failure or shock may be present. SVT can occur in children with no structural lesions and is associated with fever, infection, or sympathomimetic drugs (ie, cold medicine or bronchodilators), but is most often idiopathic. Stability is the most important factor in managing patients with SVT. Stable patients usually have normal mental status and only mild symptoms. Unstable patients typically present in congestive heart failure or shock. First-line intervention should be **vagal maneuvers**, increasing parasympathetic response to induce conversion to normal sinus rhythm. In infants and young children, an **ice slurry in a bag**, placed over the child's face and holding in place for 20 seconds is most effective. Care must be taken to not cover the nose and the mouth. In older children, maneuvers such as blowing through a straw while sitting up followed immediately by lowering the head and raising the leg to increase venous return has also been shown to be effective.

In cases where vagal maneuvers fail, adenosine (**d**) is safe and effective and has a short half-life. It is the first-line IV therapy in patients with stable SVT, but should be used only after vagal maneuvers have been attempted and failed. It must be administered rapidly through a large-bore IV in a vein as close to the heart as possible (antecubital is classic and generally adequate) and followed by a 10- to 20-mL normal saline bolus using the double stopcock method to flush it quickly. Adenosine will block conduction at the atrioventricular (AV) node leading to a brief period of asystole, which can be very disconcerting to those receiving or administering the medication. Synchronized cardioversion (**a**) is the treatment for any unstable patient or when other treatment options failed. Sedation should be provided prior to any cardioversion. Verapamil (**b**) should be avoided in infants because it can cause potentially lethal hypotension. Defibrillation (**c**) is the treatment for patients in ventricular fibrillation or pulseless ventricular tachycardia.

371. The answer is a. Paraphimosis is a true urological emergency. It occurs when the foreskin of an uncircumcised male is retracted beyond the glans and not returned to its normal position. Ensuing congestion and edema make it difficult for it to be retracted back to its normal position. **Manual reduction** is the first-line treatment for paraphimosis after appropriate analgesia is provided. Manual reduction is performed by placing your thumbs over the glans as you attempt to gently pull the engorged foreskin tissue back over the head of the penis. Ice can be applied to the penis to help decrease swelling. In addition, a dorsal penile nerve block can be used for analgesia making it easier to perform a manual reduction.

Dorsal slit (**b**) should be considered after the initial attempts at manual reduction have failed and typically in consultation with a urologist. Topical lidocaine (**c**) is not described for treatment of this condition. Topical steroids (**e**) can be considered in the treatment of phimosis, not paraphimosis. Catheterization (**d**) is rarely indicated as most paraphimoses are retractable in the ED and urinary retention is uncommon.

372. The answer is a. The patient's clinical presentation is very concerning for **malrotation with midgut volvulus**. Malrotation occurs when there is an inappropriate fixation of the intestines at the ligament of Treitz during fetal life. Signs and symptoms of malrotation may be nonspecific and include **bilious vomiting and abdominal distension**. Most cases present in the first year of life. The most catastrophic presentation of malrotation occurs when the abnormally fixed mesentery twists around itself and the superior mesenteric artery. This rotation can lead to bowel infarction, shock, sepsis, and death, all of which can occur within a few hours. The definitive diagnostic study of choice is an **upper GI series**. Contrast in the gut will fail to demonstrate the classic "C-loop" of the four parts of the duodenum and instead show the "corkscrew" appearance classic of this condition.

Ultrasound (**b**) is not the imaging modality of choice for malrotation. It is commonly used to diagnose pyloric stenosis. Some physicians begin the workup with a plain film of the abdomen (**c**) looking for air-fluid levels, dilated loops, or pneumatosis coli that can be seen in patients with severe distention. The classic plain film finding is that of the "double bubble." However, plain films are less sensitive and specific than an upper GI series and could not be used as a definitive diagnostic study. CBC, electrolytes, and urine analysis (**d**) will not provide sufficient information to rule this disease out but may show electrolyte abnormalities, dehydration, leukocytosis, and elevated specific gravity. Serum lactate (**e**) rises late in the disease process and is an indicator of ischemia.

373. The answer is e. The patient's presentation and radiographic findings are consistent with a **supracondylar fracture**. Supracondylar fractures are the most common type of elbow fracture in children and important to recognize early because of the **risk of injury to the arteries and nerves**

that pass through this area. Patients typically present with pain, swelling, and decreased range of motion with the arm held in adduction. Most fractures occur after a fall on an outstretched hand with the distal humerus displacing posteriorly. Posterior fractures are classified in three categories. Type I fractures show only an increased anterior fat pad sign and evidence of a posterior fat pad that is always pathologic, although not specific for this condition. Type II fractures have an obvious nondisplaced fracture. Type III show posterior displacement of the capitulum and have no cortical contact between the fracture fragments. Types II and III require operative reduction and fixation. The most serious complication of supracondylar fractures is **Volkmann ischemic contracture**. This occurs when high pressure builds up in the forearm compartments leading to a compartment syndrome. It can also be caused by kinking of the brachial artery with subsequent ischemia if not repaired. If the condition is not addressed, there is potential for permanent damage to nerves and muscles of the forearm leading to contractures. Patients who develop pain upon passive extension of the fingers, forearm tenderness, or refuse to open the hand have a very high risk of developing this condition.

Ulnar nerve injury (c) is rare in supracondylar fractures. The most commonly injured nerve is the anterior interosseous nerve. Brachial artery transection (a) is uncommon and generally results in a pulse deficit on examination. Malunion (b) and arthritis (d) are far less common and less serious sequelae than contractures.

374. The answer is b. The physis, or growth plate, is a common site of fractures in pediatric patients. The most widely used system of classification for these fractures is the Salter-Harris classification. In this system, there are five classifications of injuries. In general, the higher the Salter-Harris classification, the worse the prognosis and the higher the chance for growth arrest. This X-ray reveals a **Salter-Harris type II** fracture that involves the physis and metaphysis. Salter-Harris II is the **most common type**, accounting for approximately 75% of fractures involving the growth plate. Salter-Harris I occurs when the fracture involves the growth plate. There may be no radiographic evidence of these fractures. This injury should be suspected in any patient who is tender around the physis of a bone in the absence of obvious radiographic fracture. Treatment for this injury includes early immobilization and referral. Prognosis is usually good. Salter-Harris III occurs when a fracture breaks through the growth plate and into the epiphysis. Salter-Harris IV involves the metaphysis, physis, and epiphysis.

Salter-Harris V is a crush injury to the growth plate and has a high potential for growth arrest (Figure).

	Salter-Harris Fracture Classification	
	Type	**Characteristics**
	I	**S - Slipped** Epiphyseal slip, separation through the physis (growth plate) Excellent prognosis, managed nonoperatively
	II	**A - Above growth plate** Fracture through a portion of the physis (growth plate) that extends through the metaphysis Excellent prognosis, managed nonoperatively
	III	**L - Lower than growth plate** Fracture through a portion of the physis (growth plate) that extends through the epiphysis and into the joint Often unstable
	IV	**T - Through the growth plate** Fracture across the metaphysis, physis (growth plate), and epiphysis Prone to limb length discrepancies
	V	**ER - ERasure of growth plate** Crush injury to the physis (growth plate) Prone to limb length discrepancies

(Reproduced with permission from Adam J. Rosh, MD, and Rosh Review.)

All other answer choices (**a, c, d, and e**) are incorrect based on this information.

375. The answer is c. The optimal study of choice when assessing for a possible acute stroke in children is **MRI/MRA of the head and neck with diffusion weight imaging**, as it is more sensitive for early ischemia. The most common risk factor for arterial ischemic strokes is an arteriopathy, which is any disease process that affects arteries. Arteriopathies include nontraumatic dissection, vasculitis, moyamoya, postvaricella arteriopathy/vasculitis, transient cerebral arteriopathy, primary vascular disorder, and sickle cell disease. A **recent minor infection** [ie, viral upper respiratory infection (URI)] is a positive predictor of arteriopathies. This has been thought to be due to infection promoting systemic procoagulant effects and local inflammation leading to vascular injury, both of which contribute to thrombosis. Arterial ischemic strokes most frequently affect males, 5 to 9 years of age, and involve the middle cerebral artery, which results in the most common presentation of **hemiplegia.**

Cerebral angiography (**a**) should be pursued in any spontaneous intracerebral hemorrhage in young patients. LP (**b**) is useful in the diagnosis of stroke mimics, such as meningitis, acute subarachnoid hemorrhage, or idiopathic intracranial hypertension, but is not the diagnostic study of choice for acute ischemic stroke. CT (**d**) may be falsely negative in up to 12.5% and is not sensitive for early ischemia. Also, though it does not pertain to the mentioned vignette, CT is not sensitive for ischemia that involves the posterior circulation of the brain and MRI/MRA should be used if suspecting stroke in this region. PET scans (**e**) are not very useful in diagnosing acute ischemia as it is a test for brain function; the radionuclide tracer accumulates in areas with more blood flow and glucose consumption function, indicating areas of higher levels of activity. This is not very helpful in the acute setting but can be used in identifying subacute or chronic areas of ischemia as there will be less radionuclide uptake in these regions.

376. The answer is b. Patients with sickle cell disease in whom a stroke is suspected, **exchange transfusion** should be started immediately to treat the acute stroke. The exchange transfusion should not be delayed until confirmation of stroke is made through MRI or any further imaging. A partial run of exchange transfusion is adequate in order to obtain confirmatory imaging as long as a hemoglobin level of 10 is reached; studies have shown that the blood viscosity at this hemoglobin level prevents further clumping of sickled red blood cells, thus decreasing the likelihood of new or further stroke development.

Aspirin 3 to 5 mg/kg (**a**) may be started if antithrombotic or thrombolytic medication is not used and there is no contraindication to its use (ie, intracranial hemorrhage). IV alteplase (**c**) is not approved for use in children by the Food and Drug Administration (FDA) as safety data in the pediatric population is lacking. It may be considered in an adolescent who otherwise meet criteria for use in adults, but should be utilized after emergent consultation with a neurologist who has expertise in acute stroke management. Current recommendations are the use of low molecular weight heparin (e) or unfractionated heparin (d) for up to 1 week after an ischemic stroke. Anticoagulation rather than antiplatelet therapy is recommended for those patients with strokes whose etiology is confirmed to be either due to a cardioembolic source or extracranial dissection. This differs from those with sickle cell disease in which etiology of stroke development is due to the clumping together of the sickled red blood cells, leading to obstruction within the blood vessel.

377. The correct answer is b. The **measles virus** causes a highly contagious airborne disease that infects approximately 20 million annually, mainly in the developing countries of Asia and Africa. Measles classically presents with the **"three C's" of cough, coryza, and conjunctivitis.** This is usually accompanied with a **maculopapular rash that starts on the head and then spreads to the trunk and extremities.** The patient will likely have a fever for 4 to 7 days prior to the rash onset. **Koplik's spots** (tiny white spots surrounded by a red ring present on the buccal mucosa) are pathognomonic but present for less than a day and therefore may not be found on examination.

Roseola (a) is caused by human herpesvirus 6 (HHV-6) and begins with sudden onset of high fever. The fever will subside after a few days followed by a rose-colored maculopapular rash on the trunk that spreads to the legs and neck once the child is afebrile. The rash resolves within 1 to 2 days. Patients with roseola are well-appearing. Erythema infectiosum (c), also known as "Fifth's disease," is a childhood exanthem caused by Parvovirus B19. It usually starts with cold-like symptoms (ie, cough and/or rhinorrhea) and a low-grade fever, followed shortly by the development of a rash. Infected patients are generally well-appearing. The associated rash is most prominent on the face and the patient appears to be flushed with reddish cheeks (slapped cheeks). The rash can also present on the upper arms and torso. This rash can last from a few days up to a couple weeks. The patient is not contagious until the rash develops. Rubella virus (d) presents with a fever and rash that starts on the head and spreads to the trunk and limbs and is also accompanied by posterior cervical lymphadenopathy (which the patient described in this question does not display). Rubella infections also do not typically have associated cough, coryza, and conjunctivitis as seen with measles infections. Varicella (e) is a childhood exanthem caused by the varicella-zoster virus. It usually starts with nonspecific constitutional symptoms, such as a low-grade fever and malaise for 1 to 2 days, which then proceeds to an extremely pruritic, vesicular rash. When inspecting the rash, it is characteristic to find lesions in multiple stages.

378. The correct answer is c. For infants **less than 1 year** of age or those who have a contraindication to receiving the measles vaccine, **measles IG** should be administered within 72 hours.

Children older than 1 year of age who are not immunized against measles should receive the vaccine **(b)** within 72 hours of exposure provided there is no contraindication (ie, immunocompromised state, previous reaction to the vaccine). Supportive care **(a)** and respiratory isolation **(d)** are appropriate for individuals with active disease, but not indicated for exposure. Obtaining a serum IgM level **(e)** is not an element of postexposure prophylaxis and therefore not required for nonimmunized individuals with recent measles exposure.

379. The correct answer is a. This infant is resenting with high concern for symptoms and laboratory findings of biliary atresia. **Biliary atresia** is a condition that occurs due to abnormal development of the biliary system. Without a proper biliary system for bile to be excreted from the liver, it builds up within the liver tissue leading to secondary cirrhosis and eventually liver failure. Clinical signs often include jaundice and a history of **"clay colored stool."** Laboratory findings will be consistent with a primary cholestatic process and varying degrees of transaminitis depending on how early the disease is caught. **A right upper quadrant ultrasound** is needed to evaluate the liver and for abnormalities of the biliary system.

Gastroenterology consult **(d)** is prudent for medical management and evaluation of alternative causes of hepatitis; however, rare inherited disorders of bile excretion and metabolism less commonly cause elevated transaminases. Consultation with an infectious disease specialist **(c)** can be considered if concern for primary hepatitis or TORCH (toxoplasmosis, rubella, cytomegalovirus, herpes simplex) infection from birth, though the patient in this scenario had no concerning birth history, fevers, or known exposures. Hemolysis can be a source of elevated bilirubin and AST. However, the elevation in bilirubin would be indirect or unconjugated which is opposite of the direct hyperbilirubinemia that this patient has. Therefore, consultation with hematology is not indicated **(e)**. Breast milk jaundice **(b)** is a cause of hyperbilirubinemia directly related to breast milk's effect on bilirubin metabolism; however this would cause an indirect hyperbilirubinemia.

380. The correct answer is (d). This is a case of a **viral URI** with associated **acute otitis media (AOM)**. Treatment for otitis media evolved significantly over the last several years. According to the 2013 AAP, in children **aged 6 months to 23 months**, pain control and antibiotic therapy is recommended for AOM. **First-line therapy** recommended for AOM is high-dose **amoxicillin**, 40 to 50 mg/kg to be taken twice daily (80-90 mg/kg total). **Cefdinir** is a third-generation cephalosporin which is a recommended therapy as second line or in patients with penicillin allergies.

Although penicillin is first line, this child is allergic to penicillin, thus options **(b)** and **(c)** are incorrect, and an alternate therapy is needed. Answer **(c)** could be considered if the child were over 23 months. In children older than 2 years of age (for whom secondary complications are less likely), the recommended treatment is analgesics (topical, oral, or a combination of both) with a 48- to 72-hour period of observation for improvement or persistence of symptoms. This will avoid unnecessary antibiotics in many children. Answer **(a)** is incorrect as pain control alone is not a recommended therapy option at this age. Answer **(e)** could be considered in a patient who had more frequent ear infections; however, this patient has only had three previous infections in their life, and would still require antibiotic therapy.

381. The correct answer is a. The patient in this vignette is overall well appearing and improving from their previous AOM. Additionally, the only new symptom that this patient is experiencing is **red stool.** First step in management to develop your differential is to determine whether this patient's red stool is due to blood (hematochezia) or another cause. **Cefdinir** is known to cause red or orange colored, hemoccult negative stools as a side effect of the medication.

Red stool from cefdinir is not an allergic reaction, and the antibiotic can be continued **(c)**. Intussusception **(b)** should be considered and evaluated for with ultrasound in this age group, if there is acute, intermittent abdominal pain with new bloody stools (classically described as currant jelly stools); however, this patient's hemoccult would be negative, thus necessitating no further evaluation. With no abdominal pain, distention, or bilious emesis, a small bowel obstruction is unlikely **(d)**. Infectious colitis **(e)** is unlikely in the absence of fever, diarrhea, and hemoccult positive stools.

382. The correct answer is b. Patient described in this vignette has calcaneal apophysitis, commonly known as **Sever's disease. Apophysitis** is a common condition in children occurring at **ages of rapid growth.**

Calcaneal apophysitis can occur bilaterally in up to 60% of patients and is due to repetitive microtrauma from Achilles tendon contraction and tension on the calcaneal epiphysis. Mechanism is similar to the apophysitis of the tibial tuberosity seen in Osgood-Schlatter disease. History consistent with a subacute injury, worse with jumping, and examination with pain with heel squeeze is most consistent with Sever's disease.

Sprain of the anterior talofibular ligament (**a**) is the most commonly affected ligament involved in sprain of the ankle, but would most often present with an acute injury involving inversion of the ankle while plantar flexed and have point tenderness at insertion point on talus bone. Salter-Harris fracture (**c**) is unlikely as well given lack of point tenderness, swelling, or point tenderness over the fibular head. Achilles tendon rupture (**d**) is an emergent condition requiring splinting or surgical repair depending on severity; however, one would not expect plantar flexion with squeezing of the calf if the tendon were completely ruptured, and strength with plantar flexion would be significantly limited. Lastly, given that the patient is from Wisconsin, a Lyme endemic area, (**e**) there is no history of known tick bite or rash, fever with malaise, or true arthritis of the ankle joint. Lyme arthritis typically presents during the third stage of illness weeks after infection and most commonly involves large joints such as the knee.

383. The correct answer is d. The erratic eye movement described in the vignette is consistent with **opsoclonus-myoclonus syndrome**. Of the listed choices, the only option that is known to be associated with this syndrome is **neuroblastoma**. Opsoclonus-myoclonus is a condition that describes eye movements that are involuntary, arrhythmic, and multidirectional saccades with horizontal, vertical, and torsional components. Neuroblastoma presents with opsoclonus-myoclonus as a paraneoplastic condition in a small percent of patients; however in 50% of patients with this eye movement disorder, it is associated with neuroblastoma. Diagnosis can be confirmed through urinary tests for **urine metanephrines** [homovanillic acid (HVA) and vanillylmandelic acid (VMA)] and imaging to identify location of the primary tumor.

A seizure disorder (**c**) can be considered; however, most common cause of seizures at this age is febrile seizures, and no fever, or generalized tonic-clonic like movements were reported, along with absence of a post ictal period. Retinoblastoma (**e**) is the most common intraocular cancer of children; however, abnormal eye movements are not typically associated with this disease, rather, leukocoria, where the pupil appears white when light is shined on it, different from the typical "red reflex" or red coloration of the pupil when viewed through an ophthalmoscope. Abnormal, "dancing" eye movements are associated with scorpion stings; however, coral snake envenomation (a) carries a neurotoxin which more commonly presents with weakness and eventually respiratory failure due to diaphragm paralysis. Lastly, though NAT (b) must remain on your differential as the story is often unknown to care giver or undisclosed, there is no history suggestive of increased intracranial pressure such as vomiting, lethargy, or inability for up-gaze, along with exam showing no bruising on skin exam and no bulging anterior fontanelle or hematomas.

384. The correct answer is e. The patient in this vignette is presenting with acute onset headache associated with **phonophobia and photophobia**, preceded by visual changes consistent with **aura**. This combination of findings is most consistent with new onset **migrainous headache**. In status migrainosus, IV therapy is recommended. A "cocktail" or combination therapy has shown to be more effective than any single agent. Diphenhydramine is used in combination with the prochlorperazine to decrease its extrapyramidal side effects, such as akathisia, as this can be uncomforting to the patient.

Mild migraine headaches can be treatment with oral therapies (b). Administration of 100% oxygen therapy (a) is the treatment of cluster headache. This patient's headache description is more consistent with a migraine. There are no indications for antibiotic therapy and LP (d) in this afebrile patient with a normal neurologic exam. Opiate pain medications (c) should not be used in the treatment of migraine headaches.

Recommended Readings

Brousseau DC, Duffy SJ, Anderson AC, Linakis JG. Treatment of pediatric migraine headaches: a randomized, double-blind trial of prochlorperazine versus ketorolac. *Annals Emer Med.* 2004;43:256-262.

Centers for Disease Control and Prevention, Measles Vaccinations. Available at: http://www.cdc.gov/measles/hcp/. Accessed February 5, 2018.

Gershel J, Crain E. *Clinical Manual of Emergency Pediatrics.* 6th ed. Cambridge University Press, 2018.

Leung S, Bulloch B, Young C, et al. Effectiveness of standardized combination therapy for migraine treatment in the pediatric emergency department. *Headache.* 2013;53:491-497.

Lieberthal AS, Carroll AE, Chonmaitree T, et al. Clinical practice guideline: the diagnosis and management of acute otitis media. *Pediatrics.* 2013;131:e964-999.

Morgan L. Evaluation and management of the child with suspected acute stroke. *Clin Pediatr Emerg Med.* 2015;16(1):29-36.

Nadkarni V, Berg R, Berg M, et al. Chapter 8. Pediatric resuscitation. In: Walls R, Hockberger R, Gausche-Hill M, eds. *Rosen's Emergency Medicine: Concepts and Clinical Practice.* 9th ed. Philadelphia, PA: Elsevier, 2017.

Shah B, Mahajan P, Amodio J, et al. *Atlas of Pediatric Emergency Medicine.* 3rd ed. McGraw Hill, 2019.

Shaw K, Bachur R. *Fleisher and Ludwig's Textbook of Pediatric Emergency Medicine.* 7th ed. Wolters Kluwer, 2015.

Weiss SL, Peters MJ, Alhazzani W, et al. Executive summary: surviving sepsis campaign international guidelines for the management of septic shock and sepsis-associated organ dysfunction in children. *Pediatr Crit Care Med.* 2020;21(2):e52-e106.

Vaginal Bleeding

Dana Resop, MD

Questions

The following scenario applies to questions 385 to 387.

A 24-year-old woman with a history of depression presents with vaginal bleeding and lower abdominal pain. Her last menstrual period (LMP) was 3 weeks ago. Vital signs include blood pressure (BP) 96/60 mm Hg, heart rate (HR) 110 beats/minute, and temperature 98.6°C. Exam shows lower abdominal tenderness in the left lower quadrant.

385. What is the most important laboratory test in determining your differential diagnosis?

a. Complete blood count (CBC)
b. Blood type
c. Urine pregnancy test
d. Creatinine level
e. Thyroid-stimulating hormone (TSH)

386. The patient's HR improves with 1-L intravenous (IV) crystalloid and her pain improves with 50 μg fentanyl intravenously. She has a positive urine pregnancy test and quantitative β-human chorionic gonadotropin (β-hCG) is 300 mIU/mL. Her hemoglobin is 11 g/dL, blood type is AB+ (Rh positive), creatinine is 0.7 mg/dL, and TSH 1.3 U/mL. Pelvic exam shows left adnexal tenderness but no swelling. Trace blood is noted in the vaginal vault. Cervical os is closed. What is the next step in managing this patient?

a. Magnetic resonance imaging (MRI) of the abdomen
b. Type and cross 2 units packed red blood cells (PBRCs) and infuse
c. Inject $Rh_0(D)$ immunoglobulin
d. Pelvic ultrasound
e. Coagulation panel

387. Pelvic ultrasound shows a small fluid collection within the endometrial cavity, but no other contents. There is a moderate amount of free fluid in the abdomen. No masses are identified on ultrasound. What is an appropriate disposition plan for this patient?

a. Consult gynecology for surgery
b. Admit to general surgery for serial hematocrits and abdominal exams
c. Discharge home with plan for repeat β-hCG and pelvic ultrasound in 2 to 3 days
d. Discharge home with plan to see OB (Obstetrics) in a week
e. Give methotrexate for inevitable miscarriage

The following scenario applies to questions 388 and 389.

A 28-year-old G4P3 woman at 36 weeks gestational age presents with sudden onset, severe abdominal pain associated with vaginal bleeding after she was involved in a motor vehicle collision (MVC). She denies associated uterine contractions. She reports loss of fetal movements shortly after the onset of pain. All three of her previous children were born via cesarean section. Her vitals are significant for a BP of 70/40 mm Hg and an HR of 140 beats/minute.

388. Which of the following is the most likely diagnosis?

a. Uterine rupture
b. Premature labor
c. Placenta accreta
d. Placenta previa
e. Ruptured ovarian cyst

389. What is the most appropriate next step in her management?

a. Establish IV access and begin fluid resuscitation
b. Check fetal heart tones with bedside ultrasound
c. Perform a speculum examination
d. Administer intramuscular morphine
e. Administer IV tocolytics

390. A 24-year-old G2P0010 woman in her second trimester of pregnancy presents to the emergency department (ED) with vaginal spotting for the past 1 day. She denies any abdominal pain and is otherwise in her usual state of health. Her vital signs are BP of 120/65 mm Hg, HR of 76 beats/minute, respiratory rate (RR) of 16 breaths/minute, and temperature of 98.9°F. Which of the following is the most likely cause of this patient's symptoms?

a. Ectopic pregnancy
b. Placenta previa
c. Abruptio placentae
d. Uterine rupture
e. Ovarian torsion

391. A 24-year-old G3P1112 woman presents to the ED with vaginal bleeding and passage of blood clots after having a home delivery approximately 2 hours prior to arrival. She was in labor for more than 12 hours. Her vital signs include a BP of 110/70 mm Hg, HR of 120 beats/minute, RR of 14 breaths/minute, and oxygen saturation of 99% on room air. She is afebrile and in mild distress. Pelvic examination is significant for a large and boggy uterus; no tears are seen on vaginal exam. What is the most likely diagnosis?

a. Genital tract trauma
b. Endometritis
c. Uterine atony
d. Ectopic pregnancy
e. Uterine inversion

392. A 40-year-old G1P0101 woman presents to the ED with suprapubic pain and general malaise for the last 3 days. Her past medical history is significant for an emergency cesarean section 2 weeks ago without any other gynecologic history. Her vital signs include BP of 100/60 mm Hg, HR of 115 beats/minute, and temperature of 101°F. Her abdomen is soft with significant suprapubic tenderness to light palpation, but no rebound or guarding. Pelvic examination reveals a scant amount of dark red vaginal blood and yellow discharge. What is the most likely diagnosis?

a. Uterine atony
b. Retained products of conception
c. Uterine inversion
d. Endometritis
e. Ovarian torsion

393. A 30-year-old G2P2 woman with a history of *Chlamydia* presents to the ED with acute onset of severe lower abdominal pain associated with vaginal bleeding that began 2 hours prior to arrival. She denies any prior medical history but does report having a tubal ligation after the birth of her second child. Her vitals are significant for a BP of 90/60 mm Hg and HR of 120 beats/minute. On physical examination, her cervical os is closed and she has right adnexal tenderness with blood in the posterior vaginal vault. Given this patient's history and physical examination, which of the following is the most likely diagnosis?

a. Heterotopic pregnancy
b. Pelvic inflammatory disease (PID)
c. Placenta previa
d. Ectopic pregnancy
e. Abruptio placentae

394. A 17-year-old woman presents to the ED with nausea and vomiting and vaginal spotting. Her LMP was 9 weeks ago and has had "morning sickness" over the past several weeks. For the past 1 week, her nausea and vomiting has been so severe that she is unable to tolerate more than a few sips of water or juice. Her vitals include BP of 190/100 mm Hg, HR of 110 beats/minute, and temperature of 99°F. Her uterine fundus is palpable at the umbilicus. Urine pregnancy test is positive and the following sonographic image is obtained. What is the most likely diagnosis?

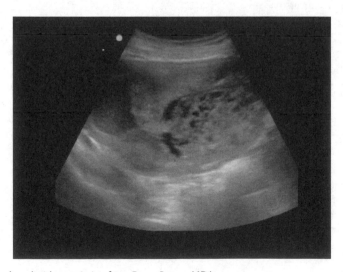

(Reproduced with permission from Dana Resop, MD.)

a. Ectopic pregnancy
b. Hydatidiform mole
c. Ovarian torsion
d. Abruptio placentae
e. Intrauterine twin pregnancy

395. A 25-year-old G1P0 woman presents to the ED with vaginal bleeding. She had a positive home pregnancy test, however has yet to be evaluated by a physician. She does not know her LMP. She denies a history of trauma or any other associated symptoms. She reports using two absorbent pads per hour and denies passing fetal tissue. On physical examination, her cervical os is open.

Which of the following is the most appropriate diagnosis?

a. Threatened abortion
b. Complete abortion
c. Inevitable abortion
d. Incomplete abortion
e. Missed abortion

Questions 396 and 397 refer to the following scenario:

396. A 38-year-old G2P1001 woman presents to the ED complaining of vaginal bleeding that started earlier in the day. She has used two pads over the last 12 hours. She describes mild lower abdominal pain. Her BP is 105/75 mm Hg, HR is 78 beats/minute, and temperature is 98.9°F. Pelvic examination reveals clotted blood in the vaginal vault with a closed cervical os. Transvaginal ultrasound documents an intrauterine pregnancy (IUP) with fetal HR of 120 beats/minute. Which of the following is the correct diagnosis?

a. Threatened abortion
b. Complete abortion
c. Inevitable abortion
d. Incomplete abortion
e. Missed abortion

397. The patient's last pregnancy was 10 years ago. She and her partner have been trying to conceive for the last 6 months. She asks if today's events indicate anything about her ability to become and stay pregnant. Which of the following is the most appropriate response?

a. Miscarriage is very rare; if she miscarries it means she likely cannot have a baby
b. There is good evidence that bed rest prevents miscarriage
c. Finding a live fetus on ultrasound increases likelihood of successful pregnancy
d. If she has a stressful job, it is dangerous for her pregnancy
e. She should see a fertility specialist because she is of advanced maternal age

398. A 28-year-old woman presents to the ED with heavy menstrual flow for the last 2 days with passage of quarter-sized blood clots. She reports using approximately two pads every hour. The patient states that she has occasional heavy intermenstrual bleeding in the past and has been treated with oral contraceptives. She reports feeling light-headed, however denies syncope, palpitations, chest pain, abdominal pain, or weakness. Her initial vital signs include a BP of 135/70 mm Hg, HR of 96 beats/minute, RR of 14 breaths/minute, and oxygen saturation of 99% on room air. The patient is obese and has a pronounced hairline. Which of the following conditions is most consistent with this patient's history and physical examination?

a. IUP
b. Polycystic ovarian syndrome (PCOS)
c. Ectopic pregnancy
d. Follicular cyst rupture
e. Corpus luteum cyst rupture

399. A 22-year-old woman presents to the ED with diffuse pelvic pain and vaginal bleeding. She has a history of dysmenorrhea. She also reports pain with defecation and dyspareunia. She has felt this way before, but that the pain has now worsened and is intolerable. Her abdomen is soft with normal bowel sounds. There is no rebound, guarding, or costovertebral tenderness. Her pelvic examination is significant for blood in the posterior vaginal vault, a closed os, and no palpable masses or cervical motion tenderness. Which of the following is the most likely diagnosis?

a. Ureteral colic
b. Pregnancy
c. Ruptured ectopic pregnancy
d. Endometriosis
e. Appendicitis

400. A 22-year-old woman presents to the ED with vaginal bleeding that began earlier in the day. Her LMP was 2.5 weeks ago and she denies any history of irregular or notably heavy menstrual bleeding. Her vital signs are within normal limits. A pelvic examination is performed. Her cervical os is closed and small clots are noted in the posterior vaginal vault. She denies adnexal and cervical motion tenderness. She has mild abdominal cramps but no localizing pain. Her pregnancy test is negative. What is the most likely diagnosis?

a. Threatened abortion
b. Normal menstruation
c. Ectopic pregnancy
d. Abnormal uterine bleeding
e. PID

401. A 28-year-old G2P0010 woman presents to the ED complaining of vaginal spotting. She had a positive home pregnancy test 2 weeks ago. Pelvic examination is performed and reveals blood in the vaginal vault and a closed internal os. Transvaginal ultrasound confirms an IUP with a gestational age of 11 weeks. Her BP is 130/75 mm Hg, HR is 82 beats/minute, RR is 16 breaths/minute, and temperature is 99.1°F. Laboratory results reveal a white blood cell count (WBC) 10,500/μL, hematocrit 40%, platelets 225/μL and blood type B-negative. Which of the following is the most appropriate intervention prior to discharge from the ED?

a. Administer 50 μg of anti-D immune globulin
b. Administer 2 g of IV magnesium sulfate
c. Administer IV penicillin G
d. Administer oral ferrous sulfate
e. Administer 1 unit of PRBCs

402. A 6-year-old girl presents to the ED with her mother who is concerned that the child is being sexually abused. The mother noted a small amount of malodorous blood in the child's underwear on the day of presentation. The patient denies complaints, including history of abuse. Your external physical examination is unremarkable. Which of the following statements is true?

a. A pelvic examination should never be performed in the ED on a pediatric patient
b. The patient should be transferred to a certified sexual assault center for evidence collection
c. The most likely cause of her symptoms is a vaginal foreign body
d. The patient should be evaluated for an underlying bleeding disorder
e. The mother should be reassured that no specific intervention is required

403. A 70-year-old woman presents to the ED after noticing small amounts of vaginal spotting in her underwear over the last several weeks. She is sexually active. Pelvic examination reveals a smooth, shiny, and friable vaginal epithelium with introital stenosis. There is no vaginal discharge, cervical motion tenderness, cervical bleeding, or adnexal tenderness. What is the most likely diagnosis?

a. PID
b. Cervicitis
c. Atrophic vaginitis
d. Endometrial cancer
e. Urinary tract infection

The following scenario applies to questions 404 and 405.

A 28-year old G1P0 woman presents to the ED complaining of sudden onset of severe abdominal pain and vaginal bleeding. She is 32 weeks pregnant. Her BP is 180/60 mm Hg and HR is 98 beats/minute. She is in distress secondary to pain. Her uterus is firm and tender to palpation.

404. What is the most likely diagnosis?

a. Placental abruption
b. Placenta previa
c. Eclampsia
d. Hyperemesis gravidarum
e. Ectopic pregnancy

405. What is the most common risk factor for the development of this condition?

a. Hypertension
b. Cocaine use
c. Tobacco use
d. Multiparity
e. Abdominal trauma

406. A 63-year-old woman presents with 2 weeks of vaginal bleeding that became worse today. She is changing her menstrual pads every 6 hours. She is not on hormone therapy. Vital signs show an HR of 80 beats/minute and BP of 125/73 mm Hg. She is afebrile. Abdominal exam reveals soft abdomen and no tenderness. Labs are normal with a hemoglobin of 14 g/dL. Pelvic exam reveals trace blood in vagina, closed os, and no lesions on external or internal visual exam. What is the most appropriate disposition plan?

a. Consult gynecology for emergent evaluation
b. Admit patient to gynecology for endometrial biopsy
c. Admit patient to medicine for serial hemoglobin/hematocrits and abdominal exams
d. Discharge home with repeat CBC in 2 weeks
e. Discharge home with follow-up with gynecology within 1 to 2 weeks

407. A 32-year-old G2P2002 woman presents with heavy, irregular vaginal bleeding. This has been attributed to fibroids and she has required transfusions in the past. She has no history of easy bruising or bleeding otherwise. She reports passing golf-ball sized clots for 3 days and feeling lightheaded. Her vital signs and labs are normal with the exception of her hemoglobin is 6 g/dL. Her pregnancy test is negative. In addition to transfusion and arranging follow-up with gynecology, what treatment might you consider to help temporize her bleeding?

a. Pelvic packing
b. Bakri uterine balloon catheter
c. Copper intrauterine device (IUD)
d. Oral progestin
e. Desmopressin

Vaginal Bleeding

Answers

385. The answer is c. A **urine or** serum β-hCG should be one of the first ancillary tests ordered in **any female of reproductive age**, especially in those presenting with vaginal bleeding or abdominal pain regardless of their sexual, contraceptive, and menstrual history. Recent period does not rule out pregnancy; up to 15% of patients with ectopic pregnancy report no missed menses. Urine tests are rapid and reliable, but follow-up serum quantitative β-hCG may be warranted if the urine test is positive. A patient with vaginal bleeding or abdominal pain who has a positive pregnancy test needs to have the status of her pregnancy determined and **ectopic pregnancy excluded**. Diagnosis of pregnancy may also distinguish between an emergent cause of vaginal bleeding (eg, ectopic pregnancy) versus a non-emergent cause (eg, pathologic cervical lesion).

A CBC **(a)** may be helpful in distinguishing such conditions as immune thrombocytopenia and to evaluate for anemia. Although a blood type **(b)** may be necessary in a patient with severe vaginal bleeding and hemodynamic instability, this patient is currently stable. A blood type is also indicated if the patient is found to be pregnant in order to determine her Rh status. Creatinine **(d)** evaluates for kidney function and although this number is helpful, it does not drive the evaluation in this clinical case. Similarly, abnormal TSH levels **(e)** may indicate a cause for abnormal uterine bleeding, but does not cause focal abdominal pain. Remember the most important initial step in evaluating a woman of reproductive age presenting with abdominal pain or vaginal bleeding is to **determine pregnancy status.**

386. The answer is d. Ultrasound of the pelvis is the first-line imaging modality for acute gynecologic complaints in both pregnant and non-pregnant patients. Radiology ultrasound can evaluate for pregnancy, ovarian or uterus pathology, ovarian torsion, and pelvic free fluid. Radiology or point-of-care ultrasound demonstrating free fluid in the abdomen may indicate hemorrhage from possible ruptured ectopic and direct care in an unstable pregnant patient.

MRI of the abdomen without contrast (a) may be ordered for pregnant patients with abdominal pain concerning for diagnoses such as appendicitis and pelvic vein thrombosis in order to avoid ionizing radiation during pregnancy, but is not appropriate as primary imaging modality in a possibly unstable patient. Gadolinium is pregnancy class C as it may be teratogenic and should be avoided in pregnancy. Vital signs of mild tachycardia and borderline hypotension could be hemorrhagic shock, but with improvement of vital signs with minimal interventions provided here and without history to indicate life-threatening hemorrhage, empiric transfusion of blood (b) is not indicated. If the clinician is suspicious of potential hemorrhage, blood can be typed and crossed with units to hold at the blood bank if needed. Rh immunoglobulin is not indicated in this Rh-positive patient (c). Rh-negative women diagnosed with ectopic pregnancy, miscarriage, or any vaginal bleeding should receive this injection within 72 hours of onset of bleeding to prevent alloimmunization. A coagulation panel (e) may be considered in the outpatient setting to determine if recurrent abnormal uterine bleeding is induced by conditions such as von Willebrand disease, but this test is not helpful in the setting of acute bleeding in a patient in the ED.

387. The answer is a. Gynecology should be emergently consulted for diagnosis of ruptured ectopic pregnancy. This patient has **free fluid in her abdomen**, which is blood from a ruptured ectopic and a **surgical emergency** until proven otherwise. Although a small amount of free fluid in the pelvis may be physiologic, a moderate to large amount in the setting of no identified IUP is concerning for ectopic. Next steps should include gynecology consultation for admission and surgery as well as continuing any needed resuscitation. Patients with symptoms of ectopic pregnancy but no evidence of rupture may have admission to gynecology for exploratory surgery or serial exams. Serial β-hCG levels with repeat ultrasound (c) and outpatient follow-up (d) is appropriate for stable patients who have normal vital signs and no indications of ruptured ectopic. This patient's pain and ultrasound findings both indicate that is not the case. Mean β-hCG are actually lower in ectopic pregnancies than in normal pregnancies which could contribute to the low count seen in this case. Similarly, methotrexate (e) is not appropriate treatment for ruptured ectopic pregnancy. General surgery (b) will generally defer management of ectopic pregnancy to gynecology in most practice settings.

388. The answer is a. Uterine rupture is a rare and often catastrophic complication of pregnancy that manifests variably with abdominal pain, loss of uterine contractions (when rupture occurs during labor), vaginal bleeding, and maternal hemorrhagic shock, but may only be initially evident by signs of fetal distress. The **most important risk factor is previous cesarean section**. Other risk factors include congenital uterine anomalies, multiparity, previous uterine instrumentation, and abdominal trauma (such as the case in this scenario). This is an **obstetric emergency** that necessitates emergent surgical intervention (cesarean section) for stabilization of both mother and child.

Premature labor **(b)** is not likely to present with hemodynamic instability and loss of uterine contractions. Placenta accreta **(c)** occurs when the placenta abnormally implants into the uterus and invades deep into the uterine wall. This is a potentially life-threatening cause of maternal hemorrhage that usually manifests as painless vaginal bleeding following delivery. Placenta previa **(d)** occurs when the placenta partially or completely overlies the cervical os and usually presents with painless vaginal bleeding in the second trimester of pregnancy. Ruptured ovarian cysts **(e)** are possible in pregnant patients. Although ruptured cysts are often painful, they are not likely to lead to this degree of hemodynamic instability. The other more life-threatening causes should be higher up on the differential diagnosis.

389. The answer is a. The patient is **hemodynamically unstable** and likely developing hemorrhagic shock, therefore **large-bore IV access** should be established and she requires immediate **fluid resuscitation** with crystalloid and likely will ultimately require transfusion of blood products. Consideration of patient positioning (elevating the patient with pillows 15 degrees onto the left lateral decubitus position) may also improve BP as it will prevent the uterus from compressing the inferior vena cava. In this case, strict spinal precautions should be considered when manipulating the patient.

Fetal survival is dependent on maternal survival. Therefore, the initial care should always be directed at the mother. It will be important to check the status of the fetus by assessing fetal heart tones ultrasound **(b)**, however this should not take precedence. Ultimately a full physical examination, including a speculum examination **(c)** will be necessary; however, the primary goal at this point is resuscitation of the mother. Although intramuscular morphine **(d)** will address the patient's pain, intramuscular injections are difficult to titrate to pain and BP and may in fact be harmful to the patient at this point by further dropping her BP. Small, carefully titrated doses of a short-acting opiate such as fentanyl may be used to treat patient's discomfort while monitoring for worsening hypotension. The patient is not in labor nor is she experiencing uterine contractions; IV tocolytics (e) are of no benefit in this scenario.

390. The answer is b. Placenta previa, a condition where the placenta partially or completely overlies the internal cervical os, is the most probable etiology for this patient's second-trimester **painless, vaginal bleeding**. This bleeding is rarely severe and the physical examination is usually unremarkable except for a gravid uterus. It is important to note, however, that **bimanual and speculum pelvic examinations should not be done until after placenta previa can be ruled out on ultrasound**. Transvaginal ultrasound can be done because of the wide angle of the probe and low probability of penetrating the cervical os. Vaginal examination may then be performed, but cervical manipulation may worsen separation of placental margin, requiring surgical intervention to control bleeding.

It is important to emphasize on the importance of the patient's presentation regarding painful or painless vaginal bleeding. Pain can help differentiate the diagnosis of vaginal bleeding in pregnancy. Abruptio placentae (c) and uterine rupture (d) tend to be painful causes of vaginal bleeding and ovarian torsion (e) is usually painful and may cause bleeding. Ectopic pregnancy (a) is usually more painful after it ruptures but may present as painless vaginal bleeding in the first trimester prior to rupture.

391. The answer is c. Postpartum bleeding is **loss of more than 500 mL of blood following delivery** and classified as **early** (within 24-48 hours) or **late** (up to 1-2 weeks postpartum). Causes of early postpartum bleeding include **uterine atony** (the most common cause), genital tract trauma, retained products of conception, and uterine inversion. Late bleeding episodes may be caused by endometritis or retained products of conception. Uterine atony is common after **prolonged labor**. Physical examination will reveal a **large and boggy uterus** and blood in the vaginal vault. Treatment consists of bimanual massage and IV oxytocin to stimulate uterine contractions. Ergot alkaloids may be given in refractory cases. Evaluation for retained products of conception should be considered if these treatments are not effective.

Genital tract trauma (a) is a possible cause of early postpartum bleeding, but this patient's physical examination is more consistent with uterine atony. As explained, endometritis (b) is a late cause of postpartum hemorrhage and manifests as fever, abdominal pain, and foul-smelling lochia with a tender, swollen uterus on examination. Ectopic pregnancy (d) is extremely unlikely given this patient's history of just giving birth. Uterine inversion (e) occurs during delivery and is generally due to overaggressive traction on the umbilical cord during delivery of the placenta. This causes severe pain and is also unlikely given the patient's physical examination.

392. The answer is d. Postpartum bleeding is classified as **early** (within 24-48 hours) or **late** (up to 1-2 weeks postpartum). Causes of early postpartum bleeding include uterine atony, genital tract trauma, retained products of conception, and uterine inversion. Late bleeding episodes may be caused by **endometritis** or retained products of conception. Patients with endometritis most often present with **fever, vaginal discharge, general malaise, and vaginal bleeding.** Upon pelvic examination, the uterus will be soft and tender to the touch. The majority of infections are caused by normal vaginal flora, such as anaerobes, enterococci, and streptococci. Patients generally should be admitted and those who do not respond to initial antibiotic therapy may warrant broader-spectrum coverage and further evaluation for pelvic abscess or pelvic thrombophlebitis.

Uterine atony (a) and uterine inversion (c) are earlier causes of postpartum bleeding. Although retained products of conception (b) is a possibility in this patient and may predispose to infection, her presentation is acutely concerning for infection given her fever and significant abdominal tenderness. Ovarian torsion (e) generally presents with sudden onset, unilateral pelvic pain and the physical examination will often reveal an enlarged, tender ovary. This patient's clinical picture is more consistent with an infectious etiology.

393. The answer is d. This patient has two risk factors for **ectopic pregnancy** including **tubal ligation** and **previous sexually transmitted infection (STI).** Tubal ligation increases the likelihood of having an ectopic pregnancy by providing an outlet for improper implantation of an embryo into the fallopian tube or somewhere outside of the uterus. Chlamydia and other STIs also increase the likelihood of ectopic pregnancy due to tubal scarring. As always, **determining the patient's** β-hCG **status is crucial in the beginning stages of her workup.** In a normal pregnancy, the β-hCG doubles every 48 to 72 hours, but usually increases at a slower rate in ectopic pregnancy. In a stable patient, a transvaginal ultrasound may be warranted to determine the size and location of the ectopic and any associated free fluid indicating associated rupture. β-hCG levels dictate whether a transvaginal (>1500 mIU/mL) or transabdominal (>6500 mIU/mL) approach is expected to visualize the pregnancy, but should not determine if an ultrasound should be performed. However, this patient is hemodynamically compromised and has most likely ruptured. Surgical intervention is warranted in these cases. Patients with ectopic pregnancies may also present with back or flank pain, syncope, or peritonitis. Other risk factors include previous ectopic pregnancy, IUD use, previous PID, infertility, in vitro fertilization (IVF), tobacco use, and recent elective abortion.

Heterotopic pregnancy (**a**) occurs when there are concurrent intrauterine and extrauterine pregnancies. The incidence of heterotopic pregnancy is increasing in prevalence, but still clinically rare, occurring in approximately 1/4000 pregnancies. However, it is common in women on fertility treatments, and should be considered even if ultrasound confirms an IUP in this group. PID (**b**) often presents with gradual pelvic pain and vaginal discharge with other systemic signs of an infectious etiology, such as fever and chills. Placenta previa (**c**) occurs when the placenta partially or completely overlies the cervical os and usually presents with painless vaginal bleeding in the second trimester of pregnancy. Abruptio placentae (**e**) occurs when the placenta separates from the uterine lining and also presents in the second or third trimester of pregnancy. Placental abruption classically presents with painful vaginal bleeding.

394. The answer is b. Molar pregnancy (hydatidiform mole) is associated with severe nausea and vomiting (hyperemesis gravidarum), uterine size larger than expected for dates, hypertension, and intermittent vaginal bleeding or passage of grape-like contents. Risk factors include a previous history of molar pregnancy, and very young or advanced maternal ages. Typical laboratory findings include anemia and a β-hCG higher than expected. Pelvic ultrasound classically shows intrauterine echogenic material, sometimes with discrete fluid collections (grape-like clusters), as shown in the figure. Treatment includes dilation and curettage (D&C) with future monitoring and evaluation for the development of **choriocarcinoma**.

There is no evidence of ectopic pregnancy (**a**) on the ultrasound image shown. Ovarian torsion (**c**) presents with sudden onset, unilateral pelvic pain, and may be associated with nausea and vomiting. There is no evidence of torsion on the image provided. Abruptio placentae (**d**) presents as sudden onset abdominal pain with associated vaginal bleeding in the second or third trimester of pregnancy. This is unlikely given the early stage of this pregnancy. There is no evidence of intrauterine twin pregnancy (**e**) on the ultrasound image shown.

395. The answer is c. She has an **inevitable abortion,** which occurs in the **first trimester** and manifests as **vaginal bleeding** with an **open internal cervical os without passage of fetal products.** Determining whether the internal os is open can be difficult and is often confused with the normally distended external os. In patients who have significant bleeding or signs of infection in setting of inevitable abortion, gynecology consultation for D&C with full evacuation of the pregnancy is warranted. Outpatient management may include pharmacologic treatment or D&C, if miscarriage does not progress. The woman is at risk for Rh isoimmunization if she is Rh-negative, therefore a type and screen should be obtained. First-trimester vaginal bleeding occurs in approximately 40% of pregnancies with approximately half eventually resulting in spontaneous miscarriage.

Types of Spontaneous Abortions			
Abortion Classification	Characteristics	Cervical Os	Passage of Fetal Tissue
Threatened	Abdominal pain or bleeding in the first 20 weeks of gestation	Closed	None
Inevitable	Abdominal pain or bleeding in the first 20 weeks of gestation	Open	None
Incomplete	Abdominal pain or bleeding in the first 20 weeks of gestation	Open	Yes (Some products of conception remain in uterus)
Complete	Abdominal pain or bleeding in the first 20 weeks of gestation	Closed	Complete passage of fetal parts and placenta and contracted uterus
Septic	Infection of uterus during miscarriage, fever and chills. Usually due to *Staphylococcus aureus*	Open with purulent cervical discharge and uterine tenderness	None or may be incomplete

(Reproduced with permission from Adam J. Rosh, MD, and Rosh Review.)

A threatened abortion **(a)** is defined as any vaginal bleeding with a closed os and no passage of fetal tissue during the first 20 weeks of gestation. A complete abortion **(b)** is the passage of all fetal products and products of conception with a now closed os. An incomplete abortion **(d)** is the partial passage of fetal products or products of conception but with an open cervical os and some products remaining. A missed abortion **(e)** occurs when a nonviable fetus remains in the uterus with a closed os.

396. The answer is a. In a **threatened abortion**, the patient has vaginal bleeding in the first 20 weeks of gestation, with a closed internal cervical os. The risk of miscarriage is approximately 35% to 50% depending on the patient population and severity of symptoms.

A complete abortion **(b)** means all fetus and products of conception have passed and the os is now closed. Inevitable abortions **(c)** have an open internal cervical os but no passage of fetal products. An incomplete abortion (**d**) is the partial passage of fetal products or products of conception but with an open cervical os and some products remaining. A missed abortion (**e**) occurs when a nonviable fetus remains in the uterus with a closed os.

397. The answer is c. Patients who have **viable fetus on ultrasound are less likely to miscarry (3% to 6% miscarriage rate).** Although half of patients experiencing early pregnancy vaginal bleeding ultimately miscarry, this is much less common in those with viable fetus on ultrasound. As described in the previous question, **miscarriage is very common, occurring in up to one-third of pregnancies in the 35 to 40-year-old age group and around 15% to 20% in younger patients.** Despite it being common, **miscarriage can be quite stressful for patients and families** and is **an opportunity for clinicians to acknowledge this stressful event and provide additional education.**

Although bed rest is often recommended (**b**), there is no evidence that moderate daily activities increase risk of miscarriage. Most miscarriages are due to chromosomal abnormalities or uterine malformation, so patients should be reassured that their activity (**b**) and stress level (**d**) or other events are unlikely to be the cause of any miscarriage. This patient currently has a successful pregnancy and does not need to see a fertility specialist at this time, but should follow closely with her outpatient provider and discuss her next steps if she has more than one consecutive miscarriage.

398. The answer is b. This patient exhibits signs of **hyperandrogenism** and **anovulation** as evidenced by her history of **irregular, heavy menstrual periods** (previously termed metromenorrhagia), and being treated with oral contraceptives. Her physical examination is consistent with hirsutism, which is a result of increased serum testosterone. Many of these patients are also obese. For these reasons, **PCOS** is the most probable cause of this patient's symptoms.

Intrauterine and ectopic pregnancy (**a and c**) should always be ruled out with a β-hCG, however are unlikely to lead to this constellation of signs and symptoms. Follicular cysts (**d**) are very common and usually occur within the first 2 weeks of the menstrual cycle. Pain is secondary to stretching of the capsule and cyst rupture. Follicular cysts usually resolve within 1 to 3 months and do not result in bleeding. Corpus luteum cysts (**e**) occur in the last 2 weeks of the menstrual cycle and are less common. Bleeding into the capsule may occur, but these cysts usually regress at the end of the menstrual cycle. In general, cysts are usually asymptomatic unless they are complicated by rupture, torsion, or hemorrhage. Ultrasound is the preferred mode of imaging.

399. The answer is d. Endometriosis is defined by the presence of endometrial glands and tissue outside the lining of the uterus. This tissue may be present on the ovaries, fallopian tubes, bladder, rectum, appendix, or other GI tissue. There are many different hypotheses as to how this ectopic tissue forms, the most commonly accepted being "retrograde menstruation." Pain most commonly occurs before or at the beginning of menses. Other symptoms include dyspareunia and pain with defecation. Clinical suspicions can only be confirmed with direct visualization under diagnostic **laparoscopy. Treatment includes analgesia for acute episodes and hormonal therapy to suppress the normal menstrual cycle.** Surgical intervention is taken for those cases that are truly refractory to these treatments.

Ureteral colic (**a**) is unlikely given the lack of lateralizing flank or abdominal pain or urinary complaints. Pregnancy (**b**) including ectopic pregnancy (**c**) should be ruled out with a quick and easy β-hCG; however, both are less likely in this scenario given the history of recurrent, cyclical exacerbations. The probability of appendicitis (**e**) is low given that this patient's abdominal examination is unremarkable.

400. The answer is b. The patient is likely experiencing **normal menstruation.** It is important to remember that sometimes patients come to the ED with benign or normal conditions in which education and reassurance are the treatments of choice.

In this case, it is true that her menstrual flow is early; however, a one-time occurrence does not make the diagnosis of abnormal uterine bleeding (**d**) or endometriosis. Given her negative β-hCG, an ectopic pregnancy (**c**) or threatened abortion (**a**) can be ruled out. PID (**e**) presents with fever, abdominal pain, purulent vaginal discharge, and a positive STI history, not otherwise asymptomatic vaginal bleeding.

401. The answer is a. Rh isoimmunization occurs when an Rh-negative female is exposed to Rh-positive fetal blood during pregnancy, miscarriage, or delivery. Initial exposure leads to primary sensitization with production of immunoglobulin-M antibodies placing the current and future pregnancies at risk. Patients with threatened abortions, who have Rh-negative blood, are at increased risk for Rh isoimmunization and therefore should receive **anti-D immune globulin.** A **50-μg** dose is used prior to 12 weeks gestational age and a **300-μg** dose thereafter (the 300 μg can be given at less than 12 weeks gestational age if the 50-μg dose is unavailable).

Eclampsia is a syndrome of hypertension, proteinuria, generalized edema, and seizures that usually occurs after the second trimester in pregnancy and is treated with IV magnesium sulfate **(b)**. There is no indication for treatment with antibiotics **(c)**. Ferrous sulfate **(d)** is used as a supplement to help treat anemia, however this patient is not anemic. This patient does not require a blood transfusion **(e)**.

402. The answer is c. Although sexual abuse is possible, a **vaginal foreign body** is a much **more common** cause of vaginal bleeding in this population. This often is due to a small object, such as a bead, piece of cloth or toilet tissue in the vaginal vault. This manifests as small amounts of malodorous vaginal spotting. This patient requires further work-up to exclude a vaginal foreign body, which would need to be removed.

Although pelvic examination may be difficult in the pediatric population **(a)**, it is an essential part of the physical examination. This may require sedation to adequately visualize the vaginal vault. If there are any signs of genital trauma, it is important to describe the examination carefully in the medical record. Transfer to a certified sexual assault center **(b)** should be considered if there is any concern for sexual abuse, even if examination shows no trauma or abnormality. Remember that obtaining a history from a 6-year-old may be unreliable and you should maintain a level of clinical suspicion. Abnormally heavy vaginal bleeding may be a presenting symptom of von Willebrand factor (VWF) deficiency **(d)**, however is unlikely in a child of this age. Vaginal bleeding is abnormal in a 6-year-old **(e)** and therefore requires further investigation.

403. The answer is c. Up to 40% of postmenopausal women will develop **atrophic vaginitis,** a condition that may cause **vaginal dryness, spotting, itching, dyspareunia,** as well as urinary frequency, urgency, and incontinence. Patients with confirmed atrophic vaginitis may be started on estrogen replacement and treated symptomatically with local moisturizers and lubricants.

Although the patient is sexually active, the history and physical examination are less consistent with PID **(a)** and cervicitis **(b)**. Many postmenopausal patients who develop vaginal bleeding are concerned that they have developed endometrial cancer **(d)** and should be referred for outpatient evaluation. However, given the constellation of signs and symptoms this is less likely; outpatient endometrial ultrasound evaluation could be considered. Urinary tract infection (**e**) is less likely based on the information provided.

404. The answer is a. The patient is experiencing **placental abruption**, which occurs when the placenta prematurely separates from the uterus during the second or third trimester of pregnancy. Placental abruption is characterized by **sudden onset abdominal pain and vaginal bleeding**. The condition is **life-threatening** to both the mother and the fetus.

Placenta previa (**b**) occurs when the placenta partially or completely overlies the cervical os leading to painless vaginal bleeding in the second or third trimester. Eclampsia (**c**) is a syndrome of hypertension, proteinuria, generalized edema, and seizures that usually occurs after the second trimester. Hyperemesis gravidarum (**d**) is a syndrome of severe nausea and vomiting associated with weight loss and electrolyte disturbances. Ectopic pregnancy (**e**) can manifest as abdominal pain and vaginal bleeding, however presents in the first trimester.

405. The answer is a. Hypertension is the most common risk factor for the development of placental abruption.

Other risk factors for placental abruption include cocaine use (**b**), tobacco use (**c**), multiparity (**d**), abdominal trauma (**e**), chronic alcohol abuse, advanced maternal age, and history of previous placental abruption. None of these are the most common.

406. The answer is e. All patients with postmenopausal bleeding without clear explanation should have referral for **outpatient ultrasound and gynecology for endometrial biopsy to evaluate for endometrial hyperplasia**.

Although this patient's story is concerning for possible malignancy as cause of bleeding, admission for endometrial biopsy (**b**) is not indicated in this otherwise comfortable patient with normal hemoglobin and stable vitals. Similarly, she does not need admission for serial monitoring by exam or labs (**c**). She has no abdominal or pelvic pain to indicate vascular issue or infection, so does not need emergent imaging or emergent gynecologic evaluation (**a**). Repeat labs in 2 weeks (**d**) is a reasonable additional step, but the definitive test for endometrial malignancy is biopsy regardless her serial labs or clinical symptoms.

407. The answer is d. Vaginal bleeding in nonpregnant patients may be treated with hormonal treatments in a patient without contraindications. Monophasic oral contraceptive pills containing low-doses of estrogen and progesterone treatments such as 10 mg medroxyprogesterone acetate can be used to treat abnormal uterine bleeding. Contraindications to hormone treatments include history of thromboembolism (eg, pulmonary embolism or deep vein thrombosis), liver disease, and breast cancer. Estrogens are additionally contraindicated in women over 35 who smoke or have vascular disease. Nonsteroidal anti-inflammatory drugs (NSAIDs) can also temporize bleeding.

Copper IUDs **(c)** do not decrease bleeding, but hormone IUDs that release progestin improve some patients' heavy bleeding and have fewer contraindications than oral hormone treatments, so are a referral option, but not usually available in the emergency setting. Although life-threatening exsanguination from the uterus seen in the postpartum period may be treated with pelvic packing **(a)** or a uterine balloon tamponade **(b)**, these are not used in the patient with abnormal uterine bleeding from fibroids or ovulatory dysfunction.

Vaginal bleeding in nonpregnant patients is generally divided into structural versus nonstructural etiologies. This patient has had leiomyomas, or fibroids, identified as her cause of abnormal uterine bleeding. **Structural causes of abnormal uterine bleeding**, represented in the mnemonic "**PALM**" include polyps, adenomyosis, leiomyoma, malignancy (including hyperplasia). **Nonstructural causes of abnormal uterine bleeding** are named in the mnemonic "**COEIN**" ("coin") naming coagulopathy, ovulatory dysfunction, endometrial, iatrogenic and not-yet-classified etiologies. Patients with patterns concerning for abnormal menstrual bleeding need outpatient follow-up to evaluate for these etiologies, but, if otherwise healthy, most can use NSAIDs and hormone therapies to temporize heavy bleeding until follow-up can occur.

Recommended Readings

Borhart J. Chapter 31. Vaginal bleeding. In: Walls RM, Hockberger RS, Gausche-Hill M, et al, eds. *Rosen's Emergency Medicine: Concepts and Clinical Practice.* 9th ed. Philadelphia, PA: Elsevier, 2018.

Hang BS. Chapter 100. Abnormal uterine bleeding. In: Tintinalli JE, Ma O, Yealy DM, et al, eds. *Tintinalli's Emergency Medicine: A Comprehensive Study Guide.* 9th ed. New York, NY: McGraw-Hill, 2020.

Heaton HA. Chapter 98. Ectopic pregnancy and emergencies in the first 20 weeks of pregnancy. In: Tintinalli JE, Ma O, Yealy DM, et al, eds. *Tintinalli's Emergency Medicine: A Comprehensive Study Guide.* 9th ed. New York, NY: McGraw-Hill, 2020.

Robertson J, Long B, Koyfman A. Emergency medicine myths: ectopic pregnancy evaluation, risk factors, and presentation. *Clin Rev Emerg Med.* 2017;53(6):819-828.

Salhi BA, Nagrani S. Chapter 178. Acute complications of pregnancy. In: Walls RM, Hockberger RS, Gausche-Hill M, et al, eds. *Rosen's Emergency Medicine: Concepts and Clinical Practice.* 9th ed. Philadelphia, PA: Elsevier, 2018.

Vasquez V, Desai S. Chapter 181. Labor and delivery and their complications. In: Walls RM, Hockberger RS, Gausche-Hill M, et al, eds. *Rosen's Emergency Medicine: Concepts and Clinical Practice.* 9th ed. Philadelphia, PA: Elsevier, 2018.

Young JS. Chapter 100. Emergencies after 20 weeks of pregnancy and the postpartum period. In: Tintinalli JE, Ma O, Yealy DM, et al, eds. *Tintinalli's Emergency Medicine: A Comprehensive Study Guide.* 9th ed. New York, NY: McGraw-Hill, 2020.

Ultrasound in Emergency Medicine

Dana Resop, MD, and Jessica Schmidt, MD, MPH

Questions

408. A 35-year-old woman presents to the emergency department (ED) via emergency medical services (EMS) after being involved in an automobile collision. She was the restrained front seat passenger in a car struck on the front passenger door with significant cabin intrusion. She required prolonged extraction from the vehicle. Two large-bore IVs were established with 2 L of normal saline (NS) infused during extrication and transport. She is confused, amnestic to the event, and complains of pain in her left forearm and abdomen. Her vital signs upon arrival to ED are blood pressure (BP) 80/65 mm Hg, heart rate (HR) 140 beats/minute, respiratory rate (RR) 35 breaths/minute, temperature 97.9°F, and oxygen saturation 100% on a nonrebreather (NRB) mask. She is diaphoretic. Her abdomen is nondistended, soft, and tender to palpation along the left upper and lower quadrants. She has a 4-cm laceration to her left forearm with active oozing

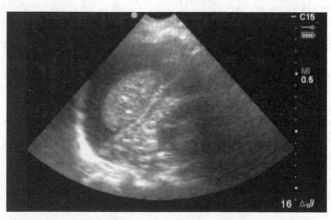

(Reproduced with permission from Mark Favot, MD, RDMS, RDCS.)

of blood but no other extremities injuries are noted. She is neurovascularly intact. A third liter of NS is started, type O–negative blood is ordered, and the type and crossmatch is sent to the laboratory. Chest and pelvis radiographs are negative for acute injury. You obtain a focused assessment by sonography for trauma (FAST) examination, shown in the following figure. What is the next best step in the management of the patient?

a. Continue intravenous (IV) fluids and obtain a computed tomographic (CT) scan of her head
b. Continue IV fluids and obtain a CT scan of her abdomen and pelvis
c. Wait for the hemoglobin result and if low, administer two units of packed red blood cells (PRBCs)
d. Transport the patient to the operating room (OR) for emergent therapeutic laparotomy
e. Perform a tube thoracostomy on the left hemithorax by placing a 36 F chest tube in the fifth intercostal space in the midaxillary line

409. A 16-year-old girl presents to the ED complaining of severe, sudden-onset, sharp pain located in the right lower quadrant (RLQ) of the abdomen that started 1 hour before presentation. She had a single episode of nonbloody emesis. She denies diarrhea, vaginal bleeding, vaginal discharge, urinary frequency, or dysuria. The patient denies any sexual activity in her past. She is G0P0 and her last normal menstrual period (LMP) was 3 weeks ago. Her BP is 130/75 mm Hg, HR is 115 beats/minute, RR is 18 breaths/minute, temperature is 99.3°F, and oxygen saturation is 100% on room air. She appears very uncomfortable and is holding her RLQ. Her abdomen is tender in the RLQ with voluntary guarding. Rovsing's, psoas, and obturator signs are all negative. Pelvic examination shows right adnexal tenderness. There is no adnexal mass, cervical motion tenderness, or discharge noted. Urine pregnancy test is negative. Which of the following statements regarding the ultrasound findings in ovarian torsion is correct?

a. Ovarian torsion cannot be ruled out by ultrasonography alone
b. Venous and arterial blood flow detected with Doppler sonography of the ovary rules out ovarian torsion
c. Free fluid in the pouch of Douglas rules out ovarian torsion
d. A unilateral, edematous, and enlarged ovary rules out ovarian torsion
e. Presence of an adnexal mass measuring 5 cm in largest diameter rules out ovarian torsion

410. A 23-year-old woman presents to the ED with intermittent abdominal discomfort located in the left lower quadrant (LLQ) for the past 3 days. She denies vomiting, diarrhea, dysuria, vaginal bleeding, or vaginal discharge. The patient states she is sexually active with one partner and her LMP was 2 weeks ago. Her BP is 115/70 mm Hg, HR is 75 beats/minute, RR is 15 breaths/minute, temperature is 98.6°F, and oxygen saturation is 100% on room air. Physical examination is unremarkable. Urine pregnancy test is positive. Bedside transvaginal pelvic ultrasound is obtained as seen in the figure. Which of the following is the earliest ultrasound finding confirming intrauterine pregnancy (IUP)?

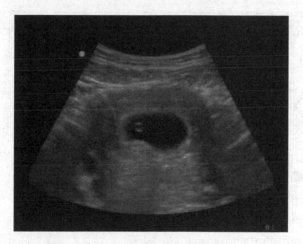

(Reproduced with permission from Jessica Schmidt, MD, MPH)

a. Gestational sac with visualized endometrial stripe
b. Gestational sac containing yolk sack and embryonic pole with visualized endometrial stripe
c. Blighted ovum with visualized endometrial stripe
d. Intradecidual sign with visualized endometrial stripe
e. Gestational sac containing yolk sac with visualized endometrial stripe

411. EMS was dispatched to the scene of an unconscious 38-year-old man with labored breathing. Paramedics intubate the patient on scene, place two large-bore IVs, and begin an NS bolus. On arrival, his BP is 70/30 mm Hg, HR is 140 beats/minute, temperature is 98.9°F, and oxygen saturation is 100% on an NRB mask. He is diaphoretic, moving all four extremities spontaneously, but he is not following commands. He has distended jugular veins and a midline trachea. A single stab wound is noted just below the xiphoid process. No abdominal distension is appreciated. Your FAST examination is shown in the following ultrasound image. What is the next best step in the patient's management?

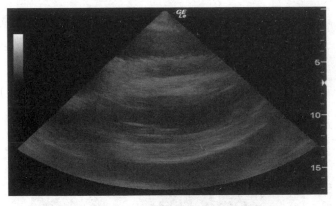

(Reproduced with permission from Mark Favot, MD, RDMS, RDCS.)

a. ED resuscitative thoracotomy
b. Immediate transfer to the OR for emergent laparotomy and pelvic binding
c. Immediate transfer to OR for emergent thoracotomy
d. STAT CT scan of the abdomen and pelvis to evaluate for hollow viscus injury
e. Perform a STAT bedside pericardiocentesis.

412. A 42-year-old woman presents to the ED complaining of right upper quadrant (RUQ) abdominal pain, nausea, and vomiting that started 5 hours before presentation. The pain is sharp and radiates to her right flank and back. The pain is constant but waxes and wanes in intensity. She reports sharp pains in her RUQ after eating meals for the past year. Her BP is 145/75 mm Hg, HR is 110 beats/minute, RR is 16 breaths/minute, temperature is 100.3°F, and oxygen saturation is 100% on room air. Her abdomen is nondistended and tender to palpation in the RUQ. When the patient tries to inhale during deep palpation of the RUQ, she pauses because of extreme pain. You perform a bedside ultrasound scan and see the following figure. Her gallbladder wall thickness is measured at 7 mm. Which of the following ultrasound findings does *not* indicate the diagnosis of acute cholecystitis in this patient?

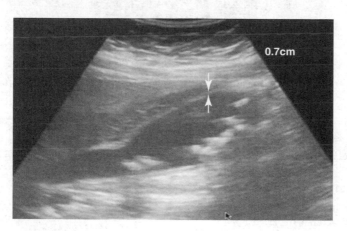

a. Cholelithiasis
b. Sonographic Murphy sign
c. Dilated common bile duct (CBD)
d. Gallbladder wall thickening
e. Pericholecystic fluid

413. A 63-year-old dentist presents with acute onset flashes and loss of vision in the right eye. He has worn glasses since he was a young child, but otherwise has no medical issues. His exam shows no afferent pupillary defect, equal pupils bilaterally, and normal extraocular eye movements. He reports seeing flashes of light occasionally in the right eye when he moves his eyes from side to side and feels like he cannot see well to his right side. Vision is 20/20 bilaterally with glasses. You perform an ultrasound and see the image shown below:

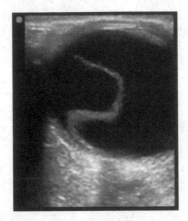

(Reproduced with permission from Dana Resop, MD.)

What is the most likely diagnosis?

a. Retinal detachment
b. Intracranial hypertension
c. Lens dislocation
d. Vitreous hemorrhage
e. Ischemic stroke

The following scenario applies to questions 414 to 416.

A 70-year-old man presents to the ED complaining of dull, aching pain in his left back and flank that began 1 day before presentation while watching TV. The pain is constant and does not radiate. He denies history of trauma or heavy lifting, and nothing seems to make the pain worse or better. His BP is 170/95 mm Hg, HR is 88 beats/minute, RR is 17 breaths/minute, temperature is 97.6°F, and oxygen saturation is 100% on room air. His physical examination and laboratory studies are unremarkable.

414. A bedside ultrasound is obtained as seen in the figure with the transverse and sagittal views of the aorta. Which of the following is the most sensitive way to measure the diameter of an abdominal aortic aneurysm?

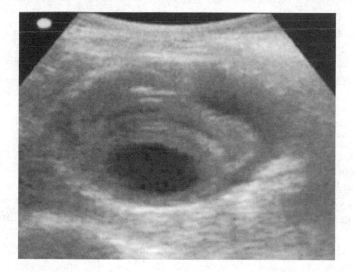

a. While viewing the aorta in a sagittal plane, measure anterior to posterior diameter from inner wall to inner wall
b. While viewing the aorta in a transverse plane, measure anterior to posterior diameter from inner wall to inner wall
c. While viewing the aorta in a transverse plane, measure anterior to posterior diameter from outer wall to outer wall
d. While viewing the aorta in a sagittal plane, measure the anterior posterior diameter from outer wall to outer wall
e. While viewing the aorta in a transverse plane, measure anterior to posterior diameter from outer wall to inner wall

415. After you perform the ultrasound examination and make the appropriate measurements of the abdominal aorta, you present the patient to your attending physician who asks you to expand your differential diagnosis. Which of the following diagnoses can be accurately identified using point-of-care ultrasound?

a. Retroperitoneal hemorrhage
b. Ureterolithiasis
c. Mesenteric ischemia
d. Acute pancreatitis
e. Cauda equina syndrome

416. After you finish discussing the patient, your attending physician leaves to examine the patient and you plan to return the ultrasound machine to its original location in the ED. Which of the following statements is true regarding cleansing procedures for an external ultrasound transducer?

a. All external transducers should be fully sterilized between each use
b. Ultrasound gel is bactericidal
c. If the sonographer wears gloves while performing an examination, it is not necessary to clean the ultrasound transducer between uses
d. The combination of soap and warm water is a safe and effective means to clean external ultrasound transducers
e. Alcohol-based products are safe to use to clean the ultrasound transducer

417. A 55-year-old woman was brought to ED after being struck by an automobile on her left side while she was crossing an intersection. She was found lying supine in the street, alert, and oriented to person, place, and time. On arrival, the patient complains of pain in the left hip and pelvic region. Vital signs in the ED are BP 95/60 mm Hg, HR 135 beats/minute, RR 28 breaths/minute, temperature 97.5°F, and oxygen saturation 100% on an NRB mask. She is pale and diaphoretic, lung sounds are clear bilaterally, and her abdomen is soft and nondistended. Her pelvis appears stable, but exquisite pain is elicited with rocking of the pelvis. There is no leg length discrepancy and she is neurovascularly intact. There is ecchymosis on the perineum and blood at the urethral meatus. You perform a FAST examination as seen in the following figures. A pelvic radiograph shows a markedly widened view of the pubic symphysis. After pelvic binding is applied, what is the next best step in the management of this patient?

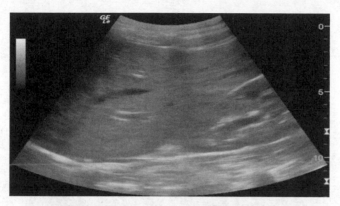

(Reproduced with permission from Mark Favot, MD, RDMS, RDCS.)

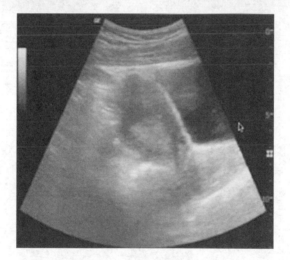

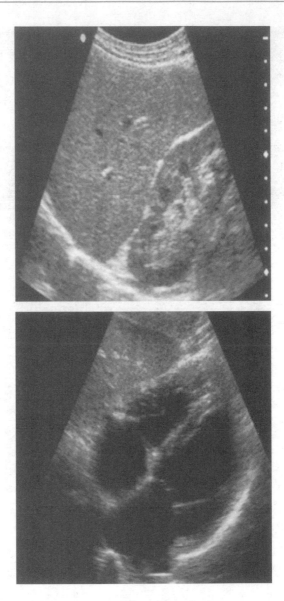

a. Retrograde cystourethrogram with contrast
b. Transport to the OR for emergent laparotomy
c. Transport to the interventional radiology suite for embolization
d. Foley catheter insertion to evaluate for hematuria
e. CT scan of the thorax with IV contrast

418. A 30-year-old man presents to the ED complaining of sudden onset, severe, stabbing pain in his left side and back radiating to his groin, which started 5 hours before presentation. The pain comes and goes, but never completely goes away. The patient denies hematuria, dysuria, fever, vomiting, changes in bowel habits, recent trauma, or heavy lifting. His BP is 155/80 mm Hg, HR is 105 beats/minute, RR is 18 breaths/minute, temperature is 99.5°F, and oxygen saturation is 100% on room air. He is in obvious pain and cannot seem to find a position of comfort after several repeated doses of analgesia. He has left-sided costovertebral angle tenderness. Laboratory results include blood urea nitrogen (BUN) 12 mg/dL and creatinine 0.7 mg/dL. Urinalysis shows 2+ blood and RBC 20 to 50/hpf. A bedside renal ultrasound is obtained as shown. Which of the following is the most appropriate next step in his management?

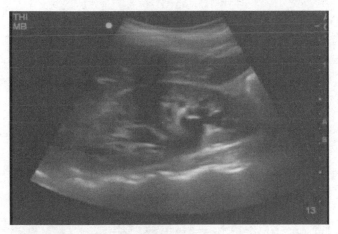

(Reproduced with permission from Leonard Bunting, MD, RDMS.)

a. Prescribe a nonsteroidal anti-inflammatory drug (NSAID), encourage increased oral fluid intake and discharge home with a urine strainer and outpatient urology follow-up
b. Administer 2 L of IV fluid, vancomycin and ceftriaxone, admit to the intensive care unit (ICU), and consult urology emergently
c. Obtain a kidney, ureter, bladder (KUB) study
d. Treat the patient with oral nitrofurantoin for 7 days as an outpatient
e. Treat the patient with IV fluids and analgesia and arrange for urology consultation in the ED

419. A 48-year-old man fell from the second story roof of his home and landed on his right side. EMS arrived at the scene, placed him in spinal precautions, and established an IV. On arrival to the ED, he complains of RUQ and right lateral chest pain that is worse with deep breathing. His BP is 130/80 mm Hg, HR is 110 beats/minute, RR is 25 breaths/minute, temperature is 98.9°F, and oxygen saturation is 95% on room air. He is taking rapid shallow breaths and holding his right hemithorax. His trachea is midline and he does not have jugular venous distention (JVD). He is tender to palpation down the right lateral chest wall. You do not palpate crepitus. His breath sounds are equal to auscultation. His abdomen is nondistended, but tender in the RUQ. IV access is established and you perform a FAST examination, as shown in the figure. What is the next best step in the management of this patient?

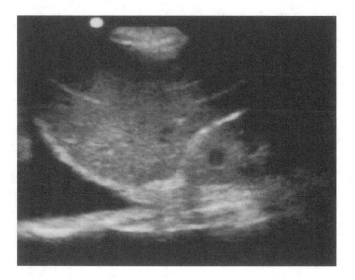

a. Chest tube thoracostomy
b. Rapid sequence intubation
c. CT scan of the thorax with IV contrast
d. CT scan of the abdomen and pelvis with IV contrast
e. Transport to the OR for emergent laparotomy

420. A 55-year-old man presents to the ED complaining of burning epigastric abdominal pain radiating to his back with associated vomiting and diarrhea. His BP is 180/90 mm Hg, HR is 100 beats/minute, RR is 20 breaths/minute, temperature is 98.9°F, and oxygen saturation is 100% on room air. His abdomen is soft and nondistended, but there is marked tenderness in the epigastrium. Abnormal laboratory results include aspartate aminotransferase (AST) 500 U/L, alanine aminotransferase (ALT) 600 U/L, alkaline phosphatase 450 U/L, amylase 1500 U/L, lipase 2000 U/L, and total bilirubin 3.0 mg/dL. You obtain a bedside ultrasound as shown in the figure. What does the ultrasound image demonstrate?

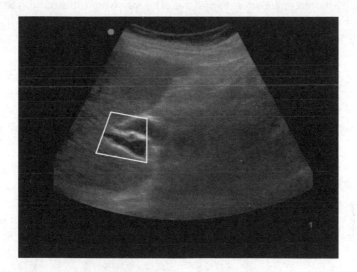

a. Free fluid in Morrison (hepatorenal) space
b. Abdominal aortic aneurysm
c. Portal vein thrombosis
d. A dilated extrahepatic bile duct
e. Mantle clock sign

421. A 25-year-old woman with a history of pelvic inflammatory disease (PID) presents to the ED with RLQ abdominal pain that has been sharp, constant, and nonradiating for the last 2 days. She reports vomiting and vaginal spotting. She denies fever, change in bowel habits, or vaginal discharge. Her LMP was 6 weeks ago and has been having unprotected sex with two partners. Her BP is 110/75 mm Hg, HR is 80 beats/minute, RR is 16 breaths/minute, temperature is 99.1°F, and oxygen saturation is 100% on room air. She is tender in the RLQ with no rebound or guarding. Her cervical os is closed and there is scant vaginal bleeding on speculum examination. She has right adnexal tenderness without cervical motion tenderness. Urine pregnancy test is positive. The following ultrasound image is obtained of the uterus. What finding is demonstrated in this image?

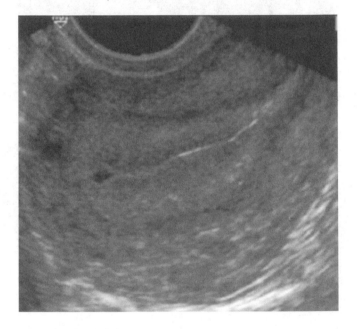

a. Gestational sac with yolk sac in the uterus
b. Gestational sac with yolk sac in the adnexa
c. Molar pregnancy
d. Intrauterine contraceptive device
e. Pseudogestational sac

422. A 30-year-old woman who is 8-weeks pregnant, presents to the ED with vomiting more than 10 times a day for the past 5 days. She reports vaginal spotting over the last day as well. Her BP is 135/75 mm Hg, HR is 100 beats/minute, RR is 18 breaths/minute, temperature is 97.9°F, and oxygen saturation is 100% on room air. Her mucous membranes are dry and her abdomen is nontender with a gravid uterus extending half way between the pubic symphysis and umbilicus. There is scant blood in the vaginal vault with a closed cervical os. Laboratory results reveal serum sodium 143 mEq/L, potassium 3.9 mEq/L, chloride 95 mEq/L, bicarbonate 19 mEq/L, BUN 15 mg/dL, creatinine 1 mg/dL, and glucose 105 mg/dL; urinalysis shows a specific gravity greater than 1.030 g/mL and 3+ ketones; and quantitative β-human chorionic gonadotropin (β-hCG) is 1,500,000 mIU/mL. Which of the following ultrasound findings confirms the suspected diagnosis?

a. Thick-walled unilocular anechoic cystic structure measuring 4 cm diameter on the ovary
b. Cluster of grapes in the uterine cavity
c. Hypoechoic stripe between the endometrium and chorionic membrane
d. Multiple thin-walled multilocular cystic masses on each ovary measuring approximately 6 cm in diameter
e. Hypoechoic solid spherical mass in the uterine wall

423. A 35-year-old man with a history of IV drug abuse (IVDA) presents to the ED with left anterior forearm pain and redness after injecting heroin 4 days ago. He denies fever, chills, and malaise. His BP is 140/70 mm Hg, HR is 85 beats/minute, RR is 16 breaths/minute, temperature is 99.2°F, and oxygen saturation is 100% on room air. There is an area of erythema on his proximal anterior forearm extending 5′5 cm. The area is warm and painful to touch, with a central area of induration, but no obvious fluctuance. The patient has full range of motion of his left elbow and wrist and is neurovascularly intact. Bedside soft tissue ultrasound is performed. Which of the following images is diagnostic for an underlying abscess?

a.

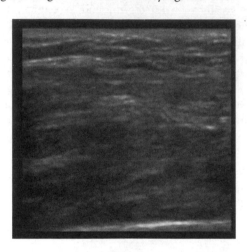

b.

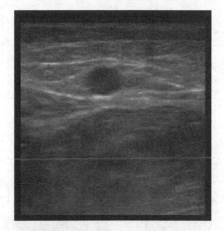

(Reproduced with permission from Dana Resop, MD.)

c.

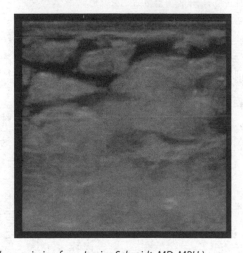

(Reproduced with permission from Jessica Schmidt, MD, MPH.)

d.

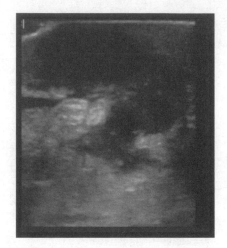

(Reproduced with permission from Dana Resop, MD.)

e.

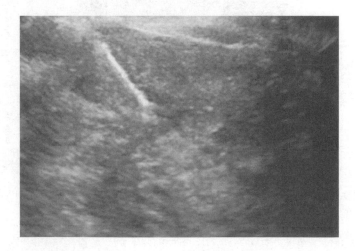

424. A 58-year-old-woman presents to the ED with the complaint of left-sided back pain, fever, vomiting, and fatigue. Her symptoms started 15 days ago with lower abdominal pain and dysuria, which has progressively worsened and moved to her left flank. The pain was initially consistent with her previous urinary tract infections (UTIs) and she tried home remedies before coming to the hospital. Four days ago, she was started on oral cipro-floxacin for pyelonephritis. She has been compliant with her medications, but she seems to be getting worse. Her history is significant for multiple UTIs and diabetes. Her BP is 150/85 mm Hg, HR is 110 beats/minute, RR is 18 breaths/minute, temperature is 101.5°F, and oxygen saturation is 100% on room air. She is nontoxic appearing, has mild left-sided costovertebral angle tenderness and left upper quadrant (LUQ) tenderness. Laboratory results reveal white blood cell (WBC) 15,000/µL, hematocrit 48%, platelets 250/µL, sodium 135 mEq/L, potassium 4.5 mEq/L, chloride 110 mEq/L, bicarbonate 23 mEq/L, BUN 20 mg/dL, creatinine 1.2 mg/dL, and glucose 250 mg/dL. Urinalysis shows 1+ leukocyte esterase, 1+ blood, 1+ bacteria, 5 to 10 RBC/hpf, and 5 to 10 WBC/hpf. A bedside left renal ultrasound is obtained as shown in the figure. Which of the following is most suggestive of renal abscess?

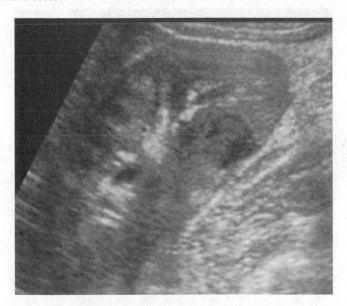

a. Solitary anechoic cystic structure with internal septations and areas of echogenic debris
b. Solitary anechoic smooth cystic structure with no internal echoes
c. Prominent echolucent renal pelvis and calyces
d. Multiple anechoic smooth cystic structures with no internal echoes
e. An irregular heterogeneous solid structure that is hyperechoic relative to sur-rounding parenchyma

The following scenario applies to questions 425 and 426.

A 35-year-old man presents to the ED complaining of left leg pain and swelling that started when he woke up this morning. He was aboard a transatlantic flight from England the previous day. There is no history of trauma, he has never experienced leg pain like this in the past, and currently has no chest pain or shortness of breath. His BP is 130/75 mm Hg, RR is 16 breaths/minute, HR is 75 beats/minute, temperature is 99.3°F, and oxygen saturation is 98% on room air. His left leg is larger in circumference when compared to his right. It is slightly red, warm to touch with soft compartments, symmetric pulses, and intact sensation. The left calf is tender to palpation and with dorsiflexion of the ankle. An ultrasound of his left lower extremity is performed as shown in the figure.

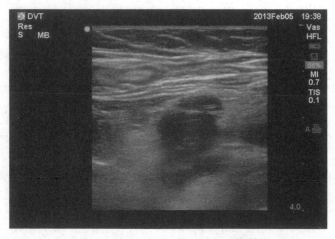

(Reproduced with permission from Leonard Bunting, MD, RDMS.)

425. Which of the following ultrasound findings is most consistent with an acute deep venous thrombosis (DVT)?

a. Noncompressible anechoic cystic structure in the popliteal fossa
b. Noncompressible anechoic femoral vein without internal echoes
c. Noncompressible spherical echogenic structure superficial to femoral artery
d. Noncompressible middle section of the great saphenous vein
e. Semi-compressible cystic structure with fluid dissecting into the soft tissue planes of the calf

426. The patient had the ultrasound examination performed as seen in the above image; however, you fail to recognize the image as representing an acute DVT because you were erroneously expecting to see echogenic material within the common femoral vein. Your error is discovered by the ED Ultrasound Director during a regularly scheduled Quality Assurance (QA) session. She immediately brings this to your attention. What is the most appropriate course of action?

a. Call the patient to inform him of the error and refer him to his primary care physician in the next 24 to 48 hours
b. Apologize to your ED Ultrasound Director for your error in interpretation
c. Apologize to your ED Ultrasound Director for your error in image acquisition
d. Call the patient to inform him of the error and request that he come to the ED immediately for further evaluation and treatment
e. Go home and practice lower extremity venous ultrasound on a friend

427. A 27-year-old man presents via ambulance after being involved in an automobile accident in which he was the restrained backseat passenger. The car was T-boned and stuck on the patient's rear passenger side door. There was significant cabin intrusion of the car, but he was able to climb out of the other side of the car and was ambulatory on scene. He is complaining of neck and right-sided chest pain that is sharp and worse with breathing. He has no other complaints. His BP is 135/70 mm Hg, HR is 110 beats/minute, RR is 20 breaths/minute, temperature is 98.2°F, and oxygen saturation is 100% on room air. His breath sounds are clear bilaterally. He has marked tenderness of the right lateral thorax with no crepitus or ecchymosis. His abdomen is soft, nondistended, and nontender. A supine AP chest radiograph is normal. You place the ultrasound on the patient's anterior chest wall and obtain the following images. Which of the following diagnoses does the ultrasound finding support?

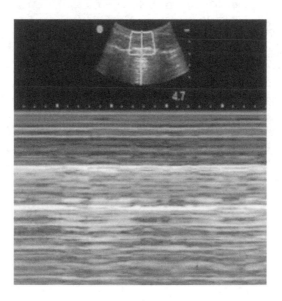

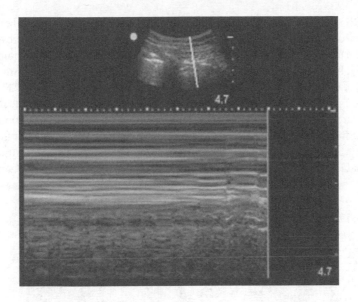

a. Pulmonary contusion
b. Aortic transection
c. Rib fracture
d. Pneumothorax
e. Hemothorax

428. A 45-year-old man presents to your ED after a fall sustained when he tripped on his rug and fell into his coffee table. He hit his left side on the edge of the table. He complains of pain in the left flank and pain in his left shoulder when he takes a deep breath. His vital signs include a BP of 140/75 mm Hg, HR of 95 beats/minute, RR of 16 breaths/minute, temperature of 98.9°F, and oxygen saturation of 100% on room air. The lungs are clear to auscultation bilaterally and the abdomen is tender in the LUQ. There is no rebound, guarding, or organomegaly. There is no ecchymosis noted in the left flank. You obtain a bedside FAST examination, shown in the following image. What is the next best step in the management of this patient?

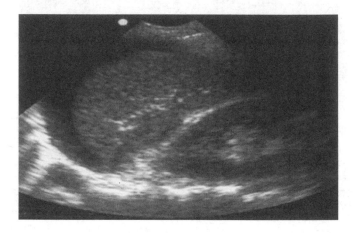

a. Transfuse two units of O-negative blood and start crossmatched blood once available
b. Perform CT scan of the abdomen and pelvis with IV contrast
c. Transfer to the OR for emergent laparotomy
d. Upright chest radiograph to rule out free air under the diaphragm
e. Prescribe ibuprofen for pain control and have him follow-up with his primary care physician in 5 days for a repeat abdominal examination

The following scenario applies to questions 429 and 430.

A 55-year-old man presents to your ED with acute onset of chest pain that radiates to the back and abdomen that began immediately following sexual intercourse. He denies dyspnea or light-headedness. The pain is severe and constant and 10/10 in intensity. Vitals signs include BP 192/109 mm Hg, HR 68 beats/minute, RR 16 breaths/minute, temperature 98.9°F, and oxygen saturation 96% on room air. He is in obvious distress secondary to pain. His neurologic and mental status examinations are normal. Pulses are equal in all four extremities, lung sounds are clear to auscultation, his heart has a regular rate and rhythm without murmurs, and his abdomen is soft and nontender. After ordering an upright chest radiograph, you perform a point-of-care cardiac ultrasound, which reveals the following figure.

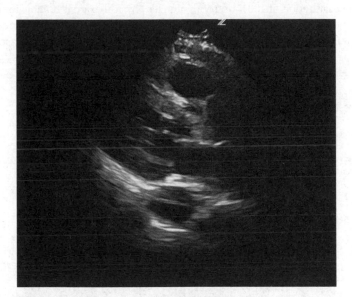

(Reproduced with permission from Mark Favot, MD, RDMS, RDCS.)

429. What finding does the ultrasound image demonstrate?

a. Pericardial effusion
b. Aneurysm of the thoracic aortic root
c. Thoracic aortic dissection
d. Normal cardiac anatomy
e. Right ventricular dilation

430. What is the next most appropriate step in the management of this patient?

a. Perform an emergency pericardiocentesis
b. Request a stat transesophageal echocardiogram (TEE)
c. Order a CT angiogram (CTA) of the thorax, abdomen, and pelvis
d. Admit the patient for a stress echocardiogram
e. Begin IV heparin therapy

The following scenario applies to questions 431 and 432.

A 40-year-old woman presents with 3 days of progressive RUQ abdominal pain worsen after eating fatty or spicy foods. She denies any fevers, vomiting, jaundice or changes in stool. Her vital signs are notable for a BP of 160/85 mm Hg, HR of 96 beats/minute, RR of 14 breaths/minute, temperature of 97.4°F, and oxygen saturation of 100% on room air. Her physical exam is notable for obesity and tenderness to palpation in the RUQ without any peritoneal findings. She was given 4 mg IV morphine with resolution of her pain. An ultrasound was performed and the following image was obtained.

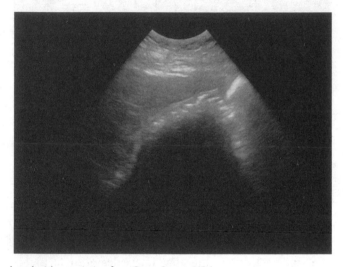

(Reproduced with permission from Dana Resop, MD.)

431. What is the next best step in management for this patient?

a. Start IV ceftriaxone and metronidazole
b. Obtain urinalysis to assess for hematuria
c. Discharge home with oral antibiotics
d. Arrange outpatient surgical follow-up
e. Consult general surgery for emergent operative intervention

432. One of your colleagues asks you to clarify what you are seeing on the ultrasound images. Which artifact is represented in the above image?

a. Posterior acoustic enhancement
b. Acoustic shadowing
c. Reverberation
d. Anisotropy
e. Refraction

433. A 59-year-old man presents with 12 hours of increased abdominal distention, nausea, and decreased flatus. His past medical history is significant for diabetes, hypertension, and hyperlipidemia. His surgical history is significant for appendectomy and tonsillectomy and adenoidectomy. Vital signs include a BP of 188/64 mm Hg, HR of 56 beats/minute, RR of 16 breaths/minute, temperature of 97.2°F, and oxygen saturation of 98% on room air. Laboratory values are significant for a 132 mEq/L, potassium 4.1 mEq/L, chloride 92 mEq/L, bicarbonate 18 mEq/L, BUN 16 mg/dL, creatinine 0.9 mg/dL, and glucose 244 mg/dL. Physical exam demonstrates diffuse tenderness to palpitation with abdominal distension and hyperacute bowel sounds. What ultrasound findings would increase your concern for bowel wall ischemia?

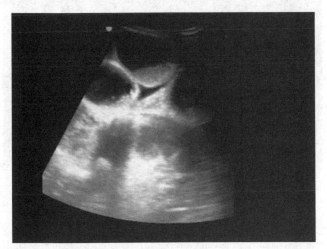

(Reproduced with permission from Dana Resop, MD.)

a. Dilated bowel loop greater than 2.5 cm
b. To and fro peristalsis
c. Bowel wall thickness less than 3 mm
d. Clear transition point in the RLQ
e. Extraluminal trace free fluid

434. A 29-year-old G2P1 woman presents to the ED with 2 days of painless vaginal bleeding. Her LMP was 5 weeks prior and she is not using contraception. She denies any abdominal pain or cramping, excessive vomiting, lightheadedness, syncope, passing clots, or heavy bleeding. Vitals signs include a BP of 124/80 mm Hg, HR of 68 beats/minute, RR of 14 breaths/minute, temperature of 98.1°F, and oxygen saturation of 99% on room air. Pelvic exam includes a closed os, scant blood in the vaginal vault, and no abnormal discharge, cervical motion tenderness, or adnexal tenderness. Laboratory results reveal hemoglobin 12.4 g/dL, quantitative β-hCG is 1400 mIU/mL, Rho positive, and urinalysis shows a specific gravity greater than 1.010 g/mL, 1+ blood, negative leukocyte esterase, and negative bacteria. You perform a bedside transvaginal ultrasound and see the following image. What is your next step in management?

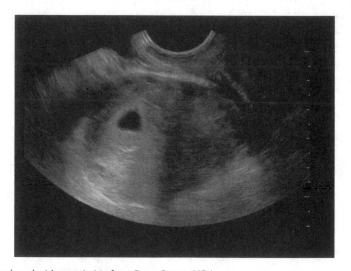

(Reproduced with permission from Dana Resop, MD.)

a. Arrange for repeat β-hCG in 48 to 72 hours
b. Start IV antibiotics for tuboovarian abscess
c. Prescribe prenatal vitamins and arrange OB (Obstetrics) follow-up in 2 weeks
d. Administer Rhogam
e. Consult GYN (Gynecology) for ruptured ectopic pregnancy

435. A 78-year-old man arrives by EMS for shortness of breath. He has a history of heart failure, atrial fibrillation, and chronic obstructive pulmonary disease (COPD). He has become progressively short of breath and notes a 20-pound weight gain in the last 10 days. He denies fevers, chest pain, notable cough, or sputum production. His vital signs include a BP of 180/90 mm Hg, HR of 110 beats/minute, RR of 23 breaths/minute, temperature of 97.9 F, and oxygen saturation of 78% on room air. He is placed on supplemental oxygen with improvement of saturation to 91%. A point-of-care ultrasound of his lungs is seen in figure below:

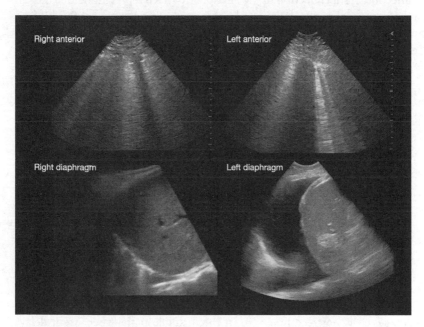

(Reproduced with permission from Dana Resop, MD.)

What is your diagnosis based on the patient presentation and ultrasound images?

a. COPD exacerbation
b. Fluid overload
c. Third-degree heart block
d. Pneumonia
e. Pneumothorax

Ultrasound in Emergency Medicine

Answers

408. The answer is d. The LUQ view of this FAST examination shows an **anechoic fluid collection in the perisplenic space** representing free fluid in the peritoneal cavity. In the **setting of trauma, free peritoneal fluid is presumed to be blood**. In the supine position, the hepatorenal (Morrison) space and the inferior liver tip are the most dependent portions of the peritoneal cavity making it the most sensitive region to find free fluid, even if the injury is not to a structure in the RUQ. When fluid is seen in the LUQ, it is most often seen between the spleen and left kidney, but is variably found along any area of the spleen (eg, near diaphragm or at inferior spleen tip). In female patients, fluid often collects between the anterior wall of the rectum and posterior wall of the uterus (the pouch of Douglas). A small amount of physiologic fluid may be normal, but should be taken in clinical context. In male patients, the pouch of Douglas equivalent is the rectovesical pouch, between the anterior wall of the rectum and posterior wall of the bladder, and is the most dependent location in the peritoneum when patients are in the upright position.

Obtaining a CT of head (**a**) is a good consideration with the mechanism of injury and depressed mental status. However, the more likely cause of the depressed mental status in this patient is profound shock. Taking the patient for a CT scan will delay definitive management in the OR. Although CT scan of the abdomen and pelvis (**b**) may provide diagnostic images, it is not recommended in the unstable patient because it delays definitive therapy. Abdominal exploration and hemorrhage control by the trauma surgeon are both diagnostic and therapeutic. Hemoglobin levels can be misleading in the early stages of hemorrhage (**c**). Initial hemoglobin studies will be near normal because the concentration of hemoglobin remains the same despite low blood volume. This patient has lost a significant volume of blood and laboratory studies should not delay the initiation of a blood transfusion in an unstable patient. Had the ultrasound image presented shown anechoic fluid cephalad to the diaphragm, then a hemothorax would be the likely source of bleeding and a chest tube (**e**) would need to be inserted.

409. The answer is a. The diagnosis of **ovarian torsion** can be difficult to rule out despite all imaging modalities available to the clinician. The **gold standard to ruling out ovarian torsion is laparoscopy** and should be reserved for patients with high clinical suspicion for torsion in the setting of negative imaging studies. However, patients with **normal-sized ovaries and without ovarian or adnexal masses** (measuring 3 to 4 cm in diameter) **are extremely unlikely to have ovarian torsion**.

An edematous and enlarged ovary (**d**) is the most common ultrasound finding in patients with ovarian torsion. Ovaries could also appear medialized or with peripherally displaced follicles and often have associated pelvic free fluid. Ovarian enlargement, in the case of torsion, results from venous and lymphatic congestion secondary to crimped vascular supply to and from the ovary. Venous and arterial flow detected with Doppler sonography of the ovary (**b**) does not rule out ovarian torsion. The ovary is a dual-blood-supply organ meaning that blood flow to one area of ovary does not mean that blood flow to other areas of the ovary is adequate. Free fluid in the pouch of Douglas (**c**) is a very nonspecific finding that can often be found in the case of ovarian torsion. Presence of a right adnexal mass measuring 5 cm in diameter (**e**) does not rule out ovarian torsion and may in fact increase a likelihood of torsion.

410. The answer is e. The ultrasound (see figure) reveals a **gestational sac** containing the **yolk sac**, characterized by a **ring-like echogenic structure located at the periphery of the gestational sac**. A **gestational sac surrounding a yolk sac confirms gestational product**. IUP can be confirmed if the endometrial stripe can be visualized with both the gestational and yolk sacs. The yolk sac can be detected by transvaginal ultrasound between 5 and 6 weeks and transabdominal ultrasound at 6 weeks.

An intrauterine gestational sac (**a**) is suggestive of an IUP; however, isolated fluid collections in the uterus are not uncommon with ectopic pregnancy. Isolated fluid collections in the uterus are called pseudo-gestational sacs and can be falsely reassuring of an IUP. An intrauterine gestational sac with yolk sac and embryonic pole (**b**) confirms an IUP, but it is not the earliest finding. An embryo can be detected on transvaginal ultrasound around 6 weeks and transabdominal ultrasound around 7 weeks. Blighted ovum (**c**) is consistent with embryonic demise. It is characterized by a gestational sac with a gestational age greater than 7 weeks and absence of embryonic product development inside. Intradecidual sign (**d**) is an embryo completely embedded within the endometrial decidua but does not displace the endometrial stripe. This finding is difficult to recognize and easily mimicked by small fluid collections in the uterus. Therefore, the intradecidual sign is not a reliable confirmation of IUP. The **double decidual sign** is another finding **diagnostic of an IUP**. It is characterized as a gestational sac surrounded by two echogenic layers of tissue. Although this is the earliest sign of an IUP, it is technically difficult to differentiate from small fluid collections within the uterus. Generally, it is accepted that the yolk sac within this intrauterine fluid collection is the first definitive sign of IUP. We recommend identification of a yolk sac within a gestational sac to confirm IUP.

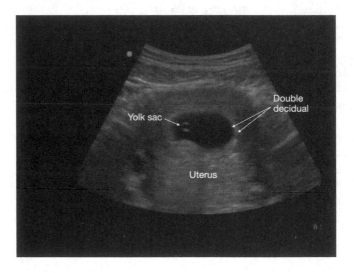

411. The answer is e. This patient has an **anechoic fluid** collection between the heart and pericardium consistent with **hemopericardium**. The patient's clinical presentation of hypotension, elevated jugular venous pressure, and hemopericardium is consistent with **pericardial tamponade**, which is a life-threatening condition. **Pericardiocentesis** should be attempted, in addition to fluid resuscitation, as a temporizing measure so the patient can be transferred to the OR for definitive repair of his injuries. The classic presentation of pericardial tamponade is associated with **Beck's**

triad—hypotension, JVD, and muffled or distant heart sounds. However, when the classic presentation is not appreciated clinically, ultrasound provides valuable information that can rapidly guide management.

There are multiple dynamic findings on ultrasound that suggest cardiac tamponade. The **earliest finding** is collapse of the right atrium (RA) during ventricular systole (atrial diastole, when the RA pressure is lowest). Then **collapse of the right ventricle (RV) during early diastole (when the intra-cavitary pressure inside the RV is lowest)**. During end ventricular diastole, both ventricles should be maximally dilated, but in tamponade, the RV will appear collapsed during passive filling in diastole, giving it the appearance of being "jumped on." Another **sonographic finding** that supports the diagnosis of **cardiac tamponade** is a **plethoric inferior vena cava**. Normally, the inferior vena cava transiently narrows during inspiration when blood is pulled into the thoracic cavity during inspiration. This occurs secondary to negative pressure in the thoracic cavity that is generated by respiration and creates a gradient for blood to flow across the diaphragm between the abdomen and thorax. In cardiac tamponade, the inferior vena cava will appear plethoric and have no respiratory variation as blood flow into the heart is blocked by the high intrapericardial pressure. However, if the patient's circulatory volume is low secondary to hemorrhage elsewhere, respiratory variation may still be present.

ED resuscitative thoracotomy (**a**) is not indicated in this case. The most widely accepted **indication for ED thoracotomy** is in a **penetrating trauma** patient with a **loss of vital signs in or near the ED**. Taking the patient to the OR for laparotomy (**b**) is not the best choice, because the patient has no evidence of hemoperitoneum. Transfer to the OR for thoracotomy (**c**) should occur after a temporizing pericardiocentesis is performed. If the tamponade is not immediately addressed, the patient is at risk of deteriorating into pulseless electrical activity. A CT scan (**d**) is not indicated because a diagnosis of pericardial tamponade was made by ultrasound.

412. The answer is c. This patient's RUQ ultrasound (Figure) reveals a **thickened gallbladder wall, pericholecystic fluid, cholelithiasis**, and a sonographic Murphy sign. Considering the history, physical examination findings, and bedside ultrasound images, **cholecystitis** is the most likely diagnosis. A dilated CBD is a finding that may be seen in association with choledocholithiasis or cholangitis, but the presence or absence of a dilated CBD is not required for diagnosis of cholecystitis.

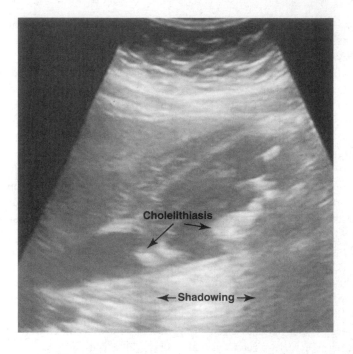

There are numerous ultrasound findings that suggest cholecystitis. However, no ultrasound finding alone is enough to make the diagnosis of cholecystitis and must be considered with the entire clinical picture. The combination of a sonographic Murphy sign and cholelithiasis **(a and b)** has a sensitivity of 91% and specificity of 66% for cholecystitis. The sonographic Murphy sign is considered more specific for cholecystitis than hand palpation because the gallbladder is compressed under direct visualization as the patient inhales. The presence of cholelithiasis does not mean cholecystitis, but their presence supports the diagnosis. At least 95% of patients found to have cholecystitis have gallstones present. Gallbladder wall thickening **(d)** is another finding suggestive of cholecystitis. Measurement of the anterior gallbladder wall should be less than 3 mm. A wall thickness of 3 to 5 mm is indeterminate particularly after a meal, as the postprandial gallbladder contracts giving a thickness up to 5 mm. A gallbladder wall greater than 5 mm is abnormal. However, congestive heart failure (CHF) and chronic liver disease and other systemic disorders are known to cause thickened gallbladder walls without the presence of cholecystitis. Pericholecystic fluid

(e) is a later finding of cholecystitis characterized by a collection of fluid around the gallbladder wall. Of all the ultrasound findings, pericholecystic fluid is the most specific finding for cholecystitis. However, similar to gallbladder wall thickening, CHF and chronic liver disease can lead to pericholecystic fluid without the presence of cholecystitis.

413. The answer is a. This ultrasound image shows a **retinal detachment**. Ultrasound of the eye can be advantageous in the ED as it **allows visualization of the posterior chamber (behind the iris) without dilating the eyes**. When evaluating the eye with ultrasound, minimize pressure exerted on the eye by the ultrasound probe. Proper technique consists of liberal application of ultrasound gel over the closed eyelid and the sonographer's hand stabilizing the probe by resting on the patient's forehead or nasal bridge. The ultrasound probe only requires contact with the gel to obtain adequate images of the globe and therefore does not need to rest on the closed eyelid itself.

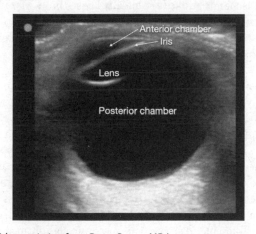

(Reproduced with permission from Dana Resop, MD.)

The vitreous material of a normal posterior chamber is anechoic (black). The retina is the layer of photoreceptor cells along the back of the eye and is very echogenic (bright white). **Retinal detachment is identified by a bright linear ribbon seen moving within the eye**. In the attached figure, the detached retina can be seen as the bright S-shaped ribbon that **tethers to the back of the eye at the optic nerve**. Urgent ophthalmology consultation is needed to salvage vision and protect from any further vision loss. As this patient has intact central vision with visual acuity of 20/20, his retinal detachment does not involve the macular and urgent surgery may save him from significant vision loss (and likely career as a dentist).

Patients can have self-limited bleeding into the posterior chamber, called a vitreous hemorrhage (**d**). This is seen on ultrasound as poorly organized hypoechoic, mobile material that does not adhere to the sides of the globe. This patient does not have hemorrhage seen on this image, although it can occur from traction from a retinal detachment. Lens dislocation (**c**) requires some trauma to face or eye to displace, so this is unlikely in this patient. The lens can be seen on ultrasound between the anterior and posterior chambers, but is not in the plane of view in the attached figure. The patient has no headache, and vision loss due to increased intracranial pressure (**b**) is unlikely to affect only one eye. Increased intracranial pressure may result in changes of the appearance of the optic disc and nerve sheath at the back of the eye, but ultrasound has not been validated for diagnosis. Ischemic stroke (**e**) typically causes binocular vision changes and should not be associated with "flashes," a phenomenon that occurs when the traction from the detached retinal torques and physically depolarizes photoreceptor cells.

414. The answer is c. In the case of an unstable patient, many clinicians may go directly to the **distal aorta** to evaluate for abdominal aortic aneurysm because it is the **most common location for aneurysmal development**. The distal aorta can usually be identified with the probe placed just superior to the umbilicus. In the stable patient, however, a systematic approach is used to evaluate the abdominal aorta for pathology. The abdominal aorta is broken into a proximal, middle, and distal segment. The proximal segment is defined by the aorta visualized just below the xiphoid process to the takeoff of the superior mesenteric artery. The middle segment is the area just distal to the superior mesenteric artery. The anatomic significance of the middle segment is any aneurysm within 1 to 2 cm of the superior mesenteric artery that is highly likely to include the renal arteries. The distal segment of the aorta is just proximal to the aortic bifurcation into the common iliac arteries. The anterior to posterior diameter of each segment is measured in the **transverse orientation** from **outer wall to outer wall**. The aorta tapers from proximal to distal with the upper limit of normal 2.5 cm in the proximal segment and 1.8 cm in the distal segment. The diagnosis of abdominal **aortic aneurysm** can be made when a measurement **greater than or equal to 3 cm** is recorded in any one of the three segments.

Measuring from inner wall to inner wall (**b**) or outer wall to inner wall (**e**) may miss mural thrombus that is present and lead to under measurement. Sagittal sections of the aorta can also be obtained to further evaluate the contour of the aorta and assess for luminal irregularities (ie, thrombus or intimal flap suggesting aortic dissection). However, caution should be used when measuring anterior to posterior diameter on sagittal sections (**a and d**) because of cylinder tangent effect. A longitudinal beam slice through the center of the vessel will show an accurate maximal diameter. However, caution should be used as an off-center slice of the sidewall of the vessel will give a falsely reduced AP diameter.

415. The answer is b. Of the listed diagnoses only **ureterolithiasis** (or the resulting hydronephrosis) can be reliably diagnosed using ultrasonography. A high-quality randomized-control trial published in *New England Journal of Medicine* demonstrated that point-of-care ultrasound was equivalent to radiology-performed comprehensive renal ultrasound and CT of the abdomen/pelvis in patients with suspected ureterolithiasis in terms of patient-oriented outcomes.

The alternative answer choices are all much better evaluated with CT or magnetic resonance imaging (MRI) than with ultrasound. The major branches of the aorta (**c**) can be seen sonographically, but obstructions to flow causing mesenteric ischemia will not be well seen. The pancreas (**d**) is located in the retroperitoneum (**a**) and is not easily visualized on ultrasound. Cauda equina syndrome (**e**) is a compression of the distal portion of the spinal cord. These structures are protected by the vertebral column and are not well-visualized on ultrasound because of the posterior acoustic shadowing caused by the bony structures.

416. The answer is d. It is important to clean all external ultrasound transducers between each use. **Warm soapy water** is a safe and effective means to do this, as the rubber matching layer of the ultrasound transducer will prevent any water or soap from reaching the piezoelectric crystals housed inside the transducer.

Only internal transducers (eg, endocavitary or endovaginal probes) require full sterilization in between each use (**a**). Ultrasound gel is neither bacteriostatic nor bactericidal (**b**). The sonographer should always sanitize his or her hands before and after an exam and wear gloves when performing an ultrasound examination; whether or not they are worn does not change the fact that the transducer should be cleaned after every use (**c**).

Many alcohol-based solutions are not safe to be used on ultrasound transducers as the alcohol can penetrate the rubber matching layer and destroy the piezoelectric crystals **(e)**; manufacturer's recommendations should guide selection of cleaning products.

417. The answer is c. This patient has a **negative FAST examination**. This patient's examination and radiograph are consistent with an **open book pelvis fracture**. Pelvic fractures have a high association with **retroperitoneal hemorrhage**. **Ultrasound is not sensitive or specific for evaluating the retroperitoneal space**. The optimal management choice is transport to interventional radiology for embolization of the bleeding retroperitoneal vessels from the pelvic fracture.

A CT scan of the thorax, **(e)** will not identify her most likely source of unstable vitals, vascular injury from an unstable pelvic fracture. CT of the abdomen and pelvis can help guide management; CT scan is very sensitive and specific for solid-organ injury, hollow viscous injury, and retroperitoneal injury. However, considering this patient's injuries and instability, CT scan is not the best answer. Emergent exploratory laparotomy **(b)** would allow for evaluation and treatment for occult peritoneal injuries and the pelvis can be packed in an effort to limit hemorrhage. However, the patient may still need vascular embolization for bleeding in the retroperitoneal tissues of the pelvis despite the surgeon's effort. Therefore, laparotomy delays definitive management of the bleeding. Evaluating for hematuria **(a and d)** is not priority at this time as the patient is not stable. There is already high suspicion for urogenital injury given her pelvic fracture and finding of blood at the urethral meatus. Once stabilized, the patient should undergo a retrograde cystourethrogram **(a)** to evaluate for severity of urogenital injury before Foley placement.

418. The answer is e. This patient's presentation, physical examination, and laboratory studies are classic for **ureterolithiasis**. The ultrasound findings of dilated anechoic renal calyces and a prominent anechoic renal pelvis are suggestive of moderate **hydronephrosis**. The gold standard for evaluation for ureterolithiasis is spiral CT scan of the abdomen and pelvis without IV contrast; however, this requires exposure to ionizing radiation. In patients with a high pretest probability for the disease (eg, this patient), ultrasound is an ideal first-line imaging modality. Identification of **moderate hydronephrosis** in a patient with suspected renal colic is an **indication for urology evaluation and possibly intervention** (eg, lithotripsy, ureteral stenting), if the patient fails conservative management. This patient has intractable pain, so requires urology evaluation in the ED setting instead of outpatient follow-up.

Patients with uncomplicated ureteral stones (ie, no evidence of infection), who have adequate pain control and are tolerating oral intake in the ED, can be discharged home with outpatient urology follow-up (a). Septic patients and those who have infected ureteral stones are at a high risk for significant morbidity and mortality and require prompt resuscitation and treatment with empiric antimicrobial medications. The patient in the question stem had no evidence of infection by history, physical examination, or urinalysis and thus does not require IV antibiotics and admission to the ICU (b). A KUB radiograph would offer no value in a patient with a very high pretest probability of nephrolithiasis who has moderate hydronephrosis seen on ultrasound (c). The patient has no evidence of a lower UTI and therefore treatment with nitrofurantoin is not appropriate (d).

419. The answer is a. This patient's FAST examination shows an **anechoic fluid collection above the right hemidiaphragm** as seen in the first figure below. In addition, there is loss of normal mirror artifact and continuation of the spinous shadow beyond the diaphragm. Mirror artifact around the diaphragm is a normal finding and, when absent, raises suspicion for underlying pathology. Mirror artifact occurs at the diaphragm because sound travels at a very different speed in soft tissue than it does in air. The dramatic difference in the speed of sound transmission between the liver and the lung lead to near 100% reflection of sound waves at the tissue-air interface of the diaphragm. The reflected sound waves then cross back through the liver where they are again reflected at various angles before some make it back to the ultrasound probe. The ultrasound machine assumes the signal has traveled in a straight line and incorrectly interprets these signals as if they had originated far beyond the diaphragm. Therefore, a liver-like image is projected superior to the diaphragm almost as if the diaphragm is a mirror of the true liver. Because of this interference, tissues deep to the diaphragm, such as the hyperechoic surface of the spine, are not visible superior to the diaphragm. Compare this to the second image, which is normal.

When there is a **hemothorax or pleural effusion present**, there is no reflection of sound at the diaphragm. Sound waves can travel through the fluid in the thorax and reflect off of the spinal column, allowing it to be seen superior to the diaphragm. In the setting of trauma, a fluid collection above the diaphragm is presumed to be a hemothorax. Chest tube thoracostomy is required to prevent further accumulation of blood from compromising respiratory status and monitor loss of blood. An immediate output of greater than 20 mL/kg of blood or continued bleeding of greater than 3 mL/kg/h is generally viewed as an indication for thoracotomy in the OR.

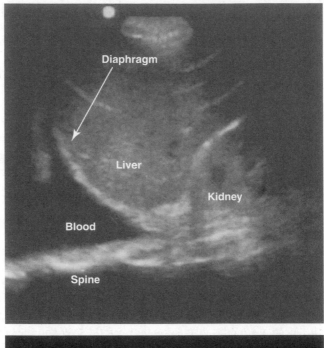

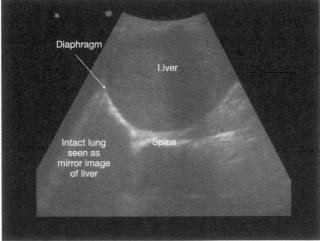

(Reproduced with permission from Dana Resop, MD.)

Rapid sequence intubation (**b**) is not indicated at this time. The patient is having difficulty breathing because of pain. However, his oxygen saturation is acceptable and his normal mental status suggests appropriate ventilation. Should the patient become hemodynamically unstable, develop hypercapnia, or hypoxia refractory to noninvasive oxygen supplementation, intubation would be indicated. A CT thorax, abdomen, and pelvis with IV contrast (**c and d**) should be considered after the hemothorax is addressed. Emergent laparotomy (**e**) is not indicated in this case, as the patient has no free fluid in the abdomen and the patient's vital signs are acceptable.

420. The answer is d. This patient's history and physical examination is nonspecific; however, the laboratory values suggest **biliary tract obstruction with pancreatitis**. The ultrasound image demonstrates a **dilated CBD**, which in this example is identified by using color flow Doppler to determine which structure within the portal triad (CBD, portal vein, and hepatic artery) does not demonstrate any color flow signals. This is the CBD. On ultrasound, the CBD is normally much smaller than the portal vein. When dilated, it becomes similar in size to the neighboring portal vein that gives the appearance of a "**double barrel shotgun**" or "**parallel channel**." Suspicion of biliary obstruction requires an evaluation of the CBD to assess for dilation. The CBD is most easily seen at the portal triad consisting of the portal vein, CBD, and hepatic artery. The main lobar fissure tracks to the gallbladder and is an excellent landmark for locating a contracted gallbladder. A CBD that appears similar in size to the portal vein highly suggests CBD obstruction. In most people, a **CBD width of less than 6 mm is considered normal**. However, instances exist where a CBD diameter greater than 6 mm is normal. The CBD dilates with age and after cholecystectomy. Postcholecystectomy patients have a normal CBD diameter up to 1 cm. Age can be accounted for by adding 1 mm for every decade older than age 60. For example, an 8-mm-diameter CBD in a patient aged 80 years is normal.

Fluid in Morrison space (**a**) can be seen in many conditions including abdominal trauma with solid organ injury leading to hemoperitoneum, a perforated hollow viscus, and ascites. While it is possible that the patient in question does have free fluid in the abdominal cavity, the ultrasound image presented did not demonstrate this. The vessel in the image is the portal vein, not the abdominal aorta (**b**). Portal vein thrombosis (**c**) requires the sonographer to use pulsed Doppler imaging (which was not done on this ultrasound examination). The mantle clock sign (**e**) is a term used to describe the appearance of the normal superior mesenteric artery in short axis as it overlies the abdominal aorta and is not shown in the image provided.

421. The answer is e. The acquired image shows an **endometrial stripe** with a **tiny pseudogestational sac** suggesting lack of an IUP. The patient's history, physical examination, and ultrasound are all suggestive of **ectopic pregnancy**.

There is no yolk sac visualized (**a**) in the image provided making the sac a pseudogestational sac rather than a gestational sac. The image provided is of the uterus and not the adnexa (**b**). A molar pregnancy is seen as an enlarged uterus containing a heterogeneous mass of complex anechoic, hypoechoic, and hyperechoic material (**c**). An intrauterine device can be seen sonographically, but it appears as a hyperechoic linear echo within the endometrium of the uterus (**d**).

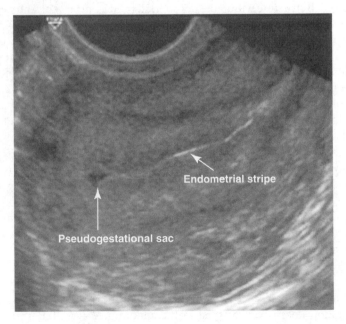

422. The answer is b. This patient presents with vaginal bleeding, uterine size too large for dates, and symptoms of hyperemesis gravidarum. Her metabolic panel and urinalysis are consistent with vomiting and dehydration. Her **quantitative β-hCG is extremely high**. The β-hCG in normal pregnancies usually levels off at 10 weeks around 100,000 mIU/mL. The most likely diagnosis in this case is a **molar pregnancy**. A molar pregnancy can be confirmed by direct visualization of the hydatidiform mole with pelvic ultrasound. The classic appearance of a **hydatidiform** is a **cluster of grapes** or **snowstorm appearance** in the intrauterine cavity.

A thick-walled unilocular anechoic cystic structure 4 cm in diameter on the ovary (**a**) is consistent with a corpus luteum cyst. The corpus luteum cyst is a thick-walled cyst greater than 2 cm in diameter and typically a benign finding in pregnancy. The corpus luteum cyst is usually unilateral. If the patient has multiple large multilocular anechoic cystic masses on each ovary (**d**), it is suggestive of theca lutein cyst. Theca lutein cysts are exacerbated corpus luteum and have an association with very high β-hCG levels. They are commonly seen in patients with gestational trophoblastic disease and with ovarian hyperstimulation from fertility medications. Both corpus luteum cyst and theca lutein cyst usually resolve spontaneously. A hyperechoic stripe between the endometrium and chorionic membrane (**c**) is consistent with a **subchorionic hemorrhage**. This can present with vaginal bleeding in the first trimester and can increase risk of miscarriage. This finding, however, does not explain a uterus too large for dates, hyperemesis, and elevated quantitative β-hCG. Hypoechoic solid spherical mass in the uterine wall (**e**) is consistent with uterine fibroids. Uterine fibroids can create problems with dysfunctional uterine bleeding and pelvic pain; however, they are generally considered a benign finding. They are often palpable and can mislead the examiner for a uterus too large for dates; however, they do not explain the hyperemesis and elevated β-hCG.

423. The answer is d. Subcutaneous abscesses have a variety of sonographic appearances. The abscess cavity itself can have a spherical or lobulated appearance. The **fluid content of an abscess is usually very dark** (hypoechoic) in appearance relative to surrounding soft tissue; however, in some cases the abscess cavity may be isoechoic to surrounding soft tissue.

The sonographic appearance of cellulitis (**c**) is primarily related to the presence of edema. Differentiating inflammatory edema from chronic dependent edema can be challenging. Classically, cellulitis is described as cobblestone-like and characterized by thickened and abnormally bright subcutaneous tissues traversed by a lattice of broad dark bands of edema. When there is posterior acoustic enhancement deep to an area of cobblestoning, one should be concerned for an underlying abscess. Normal soft tissue (**a**) ultrasound findings from superficial to deep are as follows: normal skin is typically thin and homogeneous with a bright layer of connective tissue separating the skin from the subcutaneous tissues. The subcutaneous tissues are primarily fat, appearing dark relative to surrounding soft tissue. Intertwined in the fat are bright layers of connective tissue breaking the fat layer into fat lobules. Mixed in the subcutaneous layer are **veins (b)**, which are thin-walled tubular structures that easily compress and are not pulsatile. Arteries are much thicker-walled tubular structures that are pulsatile. Nerve tissue is often described as honeycomb-like when viewed in cross-section. Between the subcutaneous tissue and muscle is the bright layer of fascia. Muscle appears relatively dark with a regular pattern of internal striations in long axis and speckled in appearance in short axis. Bone is characterized by a very bright outer cortex with clean acoustic shadowing in the far field. Retained foreign bodies **(e)** are an important potential source of soft tissue infection and often easily overlooked. Radiography works well for radiopaque objects such as metal, glass, and gravel. However, radiolucent matter such as wood, plastic, and organic compounds (eg, cactus spines or thorns) are frequently missed. If historical clues suggest a foreign body could be present, ultrasound is an excellent adjunct to radiography when evaluating for retained foreign bodies. Depending on the composition and size of the foreign body, variable degrees of acoustic shadowing are created. Gravel and wood cast an acoustic shadow similar to that of gallstones. Wood fragments (depending on size) cast a brightly echogenic anterior surface similar to bone. Foreign bodies retained for longer than 24 to 48 hours are frequently surrounded by an echolucent halo, resulting from reactive hyperemia, edema, abscess, or granulation tissue, which may be helpful in locating retained foreign bodies.

424. The answer is a. This patient's history is concerning for the development of **a renal abscess**. Ultrasound evaluation is an **excellent screening tool for renal or perinephric abscess** development, although the sensitivity of point-of-care ultrasound for abscess is unknown. The sonographic appearance of an abscess, regardless of the location, is variable in terms of the cavity shape and degree of internal echo. Classically, an abscess cavity appears as a spherical cystic structure. The purulent matter in the cavity is represented by **internal septations** and **echogenic debris,** either floating or collecting in dependent portions of the cavity. A renal abscess is contained within the renal cortex, while a perinephric abscess extends beyond the renal cortex into the perinephric fat.

Smooth cystic structures with no internal echoes **(b)** are consistent with renal cyst. Simple renal cysts are common and, when present in small numbers, they have little clinical significance. They are often exophytic and extend outward from one of the poles of the kidney. However, when the surface area of both kidneys is occupied by an abundance of renal cysts (d), the suspicion for polycystic kidney disease is high. Patients with polycystic kidney disease are prone to renal insufficiency and cerebral aneurysm. A prominent echolucent renal pelvis and calyces (c) is consistent with a mild to moderate hydronephrosis. Hydronephrosis indicates renal outflow obstruction, and with coexisting infection it requires emergent urology evaluation prompt antibiotic therapy and aggressive resuscitation and often admission to an ICU setting. However, the presence of hydronephrosis alone is not consistent with renal abscess. An irregular heterogeneous solid structure that is hyperechoic relative to surrounding parenchyma (e) is concerning for renal malignancy. The most common malignancy of the kidney is renal cell carcinoma, which carries a poor prognosis if not detected early. Any solid mass or cystic mass with internal septations requires further imaging with CT scan or MRI for further evaluation to help differentiate benign from malignant mass. Though a solid appearing mass could represent an abscess, it is more suggestive of renal malignancy.

425. The answer is b. Emergency ultrasound evaluation of the lower extremity for DVT requires sequential compression of the major deep veins starting with the common femoral vein at the junction of the saphenous vein and continuing distally to the trifurcation of the popliteal vein. The common femoral vein bifurcates into the femoral and deep femoral veins. The femoral vein travels through the obturator canal to the popliteal fossa where it becomes the popliteal vein. The popliteal vein further divides into the peroneal, anterior, and posterior vein known as the trifurcation. **Normal deep veins collapse under moderate pressure applied by the sonographer.** A study is **positive for DVT when the deep vein under interrogation does not collapse fully when pressure is applied to the skin with the ultrasound probe.** An artery is differentiated from the vein by its thicker wall and pulsatile nature. In the image provided, the thick-walled vessel (artery) is flattening with transducer pressure, while the thin- walled vessel (vein) adjacent to it is not collapsing under the same pressure because an acute intraluminal clot is present and preventing compression of the vein.

An anechoic cystic structure in the popliteal fossa (a) is consistent with a Baker cyst. A Baker cyst develops from a communication between the synovium of the knee and semimembranosus bursa. Chronic inflammation of the knee leads to increased synovial fluid production that tracks into the cyst causing cyst enlargement. The Baker cyst can be differentiated from a DVT on ultrasound by noting that the cyst has a spherical structure as opposed to the tubular shape of a vein. The cyst can enlarge and rupture leading to intense pain and swelling of the calf. The fluid of a ruptured Baker cyst tracks through the tissue planes of the calf. The volume loss of the cyst makes it somewhat compressible when pressure is applied to the cyst. A noncompressible spherical structure superficial to the femoral artery is consistent with a lymph node (c). Lymph nodes are differentiated from DVT by the spherical shape of the lymph node compared to the tubular structure of the vein. Lymph nodes also tend to lie superficial to the vasculature. The sonographer can also apply Doppler to the lymph node showing blood flow in and out of the node hilum as well as throughout the node itself. The great saphenous vein (d) is a superficial vein. Thrombosis of the saphenous vein is not associated with embolic disease. However, thrombosis of the proximal segment, near its confluence with the common femoral vein, is often treated as a DVT because of potential proximal propagation into the common femoral vein. Rarely, one will find a semicompressible cystic structure with surrounding fluid dissecting into the soft tissue planes of the adjacent calf muscles (e), which would be consistent with an abscess with surrounding cellulitis and not an acute DVT.

426. The answer is d. Error disclosure is an important principal of high-quality patient care. When one introduces point-of-care ultrasound to their practice of emergency medicine, it is very important that a robust QA and feedback process is in place in order to identify and disclose errors in interpretation. Not only do these errors need to be communicated to the performing physician, when the error has the potential to compromise patient care (ie, a missed acute DVT), they need to be **promptly communicated to the patient** so that corrective actions may take place. In the case of a missed acute DVT, this involves **bringing the patient back to the ED** so that treatment with anticoagulation can be initiated.

Referral to primary care (a) is an inappropriate plan for this patient with an acute DVT that was misdiagnosed in the ED and will lead to further delays in care. There was no error image acquisition and it is not necessary to apologize to the ED Ultrasound Director (a and b). While further practice (e) is probably a good idea, it is not the most appropriate next step in this clinical scenario.

427. The answer is d. This is an example of a **stratosphere sign or a barcode sign** with a **lung point** diagnostic of a **pneumothorax**. The "B" in B mode stands for brightness. B mode is the mode of ultrasonography used with routine imaging. When a sound wave returns to the transducer, it is converted to a grayscale pixel that corresponds to the amplitude or "loudness" of that reflected sound wave. The different shades of gray pixels represent the amount of reflected sound based on the acoustic impedance of the tissues scanned. From these pixels, an image is generated and displayed on the monitor for interpretation. With real-time (B-mode) imaging, the parietal and visceral pleura are visualized as an echogenic surface deep to the chest wall. During a normal respiratory cycle, the mobile visceral pleura slides over the fixed parietal pleura. The presence of a sliding lung sign virtually rules out a pneumothorax. **The absence of a sliding lung sign is highly sensitive for pneumothorax**. However, false positives can be caused by pulmonary contusions, bullous emphysema, or acute respiratory distress syndrome (ARDS).

The "M" in M mode stands for motion. When the machine is switched to M mode, a line will appear on the B-mode image that is simultaneously displayed. This line corresponds to a single piezoelectric channel that can be focused on an area of interest. In this case, the line is focused through the lung-chest wall interface. Once the line is focused on an area of interest, the channel is plotted in a graph with time on the horizontal axis and depth on the vertical axis. By plotting this single channel of ultrasound waves over time, the movement of tissue relative to the ultrasound probe can be interpreted. When scanning a normal thorax in M mode, the soft tissues of the chest wall generate a series of horizontal lines, while the aerated lung sliding deep to the chest wall gives a grainy appearance. This is called the *seashore sign*. If air gets between the visceral and parietal pleura, the movement of the visceral pleura is no longer appreciated. Instead of the grainy beach-like image, a series of horizontal lines is projected. These horizontal lines look like a continuation of the horizontal lines from the chest wall giving a **stratosphere or bar-code sign**. Once the stratosphere sign is appreciated, the probe is positioned posterolaterally in an effort to find where the visceral and parietal pleura contact. The site where the pneumothorax ends and normal lung starts is called the lung point. At the *lung point*, the screen will show stratosphere sign with brief periods of seashore sign as the visceral pleura slides into view with respiratory cycles. **Visualizing the lung point is 100% specific for the diagnosis of pneumothorax.**

Pulmonary contusion **(a)** is less likely with a normal chest radiograph and the presence of a stratosphere sign with lung point. If real-time imaging showed the loss of a sliding lung sign and a lung point was not shown, pulmonary contusion would be more likely. Aortic transection (**b**) is a rare, often rapidly fatal diagnosis that is typically the result of massive deceleration forces causing a shearing type of injury to the aorta at or near the ligamentum arteriosum. The image provided is not one of the aorta, and this diagnosis would be best made by CT in a stable patient. The patient may have rib fractures (**c**), but these are not responsible for the ultrasound findings seen in the question. A hemothorax (**e**) would be represented by an anechoic fluid collection in the dependent portions of the thorax.

428. The answer is b. The perisplenic view of this FAST examination shows an **anechoic stripe** in the **subphrenic space** representing **free fluid in the peritoneal cavity**. In the **setting of trauma**, free peritoneal fluid is presumed to be **blood**. Blood in the perisplenic region most commonly collects in the subphrenic space. Blood in the left subphrenic space irritates the diaphragm giving referred pain to the left shoulder. This is called Kehr's sign. Given the history, physical examination, and ultrasound findings, this patient likely has a **splenic rupture**. Many low- to moderate-grade liver and spleen injuries can be managed nonoperatively or with interventional radiology by embolizing bleeding vessels. Because this patient is **clinically stable**, further imaging with a **CT scan is the next best step** in management.

If the patient had been hemodynamically unstable, it would be appropriate to begin a blood transfusion (**a**) or transfer the patient to the OR (**c**) for emergent management. Solid organ injury does not lead to pneumoperitoneum, thus an upright chest radiograph would not be helpful (**d**). Further imaging and observation is required to ensure that the patient does not deteriorate. Discharging the patient home directly from the ED on ibuprofen (**e**) is inappropriate in the setting of an intraperitoneal bleed.

429. The answer is c. This is a parasternal long axis (PLAX) view of the heart demonstrating a **dissection flap** seen running from left to right (transversely) across the descending thoracic aorta, which is seen immediately posterior to the left atrium (LA). It is important when you acquire a PLAX image that you adjust your depth to include the descending thoracic aorta. This is consistent with a diagnosis of **thoracic aortic dissection**.

There is no anechoic fluid between the pericardium and the epicardium of the heart (**a**), and thus no pericardial effusion is seen. Patients who have pericardial effusion with an acute aortic dissection have an extremely high mortality as this means that the dissection flap has dissected retrograde through the pericardium which envelopes the first 1 cm of the aortic root at the sinuses of Valsalva. In this patient, the aortic root is normal in appearance and caliber (<4 cm in diameter) and thus the patient does not have a thoracic aortic aneurysm **(b)**. The RV is seen in the near field, anteriorly, and nothing about it suggests that it is dilated or failing in this view **(e)**. PLAX is not the best view to make this determination. In order to see RV failure, one would need to see video clips of the heart to evaluate the size and kinetics of the RV. And lastly, because there is pathology seen in the descending thoracic aorta, this is not a normal cardiac examination **(d)**.

430. The answer is c. This is a stable patient with a thoracic aortic dissection. The next step should involve **consulting the appropriate service**, which will require knowing the type of dissection that the patient has. A Stanford type A dissection involves the aortic root, ascending aorta, or aortic arch, whereas a Stanford type B dissection begins distal to the takeoff of the left subclavian artery. Of the choices provided, **CTA is the best imaging study to make this critical determination**.

Since the patient does not have a pericardial effusion with tamponade, a pericardiocentesis **(a)** should not be performed. Should this patient with an aortic dissection develop tamponade, a pericardiocentesis should only be performed if the patient has suffered or is like to imminently suffer a cardiac arrest, as violating the pericardium may precipitate the patients demise if a surgeon capable of performing the necessary operation is not present. A TEE **(b)** would be an appropriate test in an unstable patient or one with a contrast allergy. Admitting the patient to the hospital for a stress test **(d)** is a potentially dangerous action in a patient with an aortic dissection and should not be pursued. Anticoagulation with IV heparin **(e)** would be the appropriate treatment if the patient had an acute pulmonary embolism, but nothing about the image presented suggests that this is the case. Anticoagulation in this scenario may lead to patient demise.

431. The answer is d. The patient is suffering from symptomatic cholelithiasis as seen by the **multiple gallstones with acoustic shadowing**. Her pain was well-controlled with a single dose of IV analgesia and although she will require surgical consultation in the future, she does not necessitate immediate surgical intervention.

The patient does not have evidence of cholecystitis which would require antibiotics **(a)** or emergent surgery **(e)** given she lacks sonographic features of acute infection including a thickened gallbladder wall (>3 mm) or pericholecystic fluid. The presence of gallstones and a sonographic

Murphy's sign (pain with palpation of the RUQ with the ultrasound probe) is nonspecific and can be seen in cholelithiasis and cholecystitis. Obtaining a urinalysis to assess for hematuria (**b**) could be considered in evaluation of kidney stones; however, the above image represents a gallbladder and not a kidney. Sending the patient home with antibiotics (**c**) would be inappropriate given no clear infection has been identified.

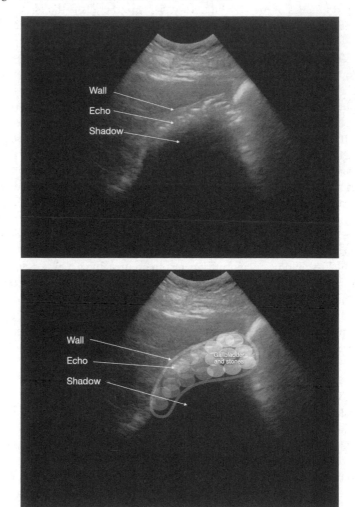

(Reproduced with permission from Dana Resop, MD.)

432. The answer is b. The image shows multiple layering gallstones which appear as hyperechoic round objects within the gallbladder lumen. These gallstones produce a **dark area distal to the stones**. This **artifact is created by a highly dense structure** (in this case, gallstones) which either reflect or absorb the sound waves creating a void behind them which is depicted as black. This is commonly referred to as the wall echo shadow (WES) sign.

Posterior acoustic enhancement **(a)** is created by increased "through transmission" of certain fluid-filled structures (eg, bladder, gallbladder) which creates increased echogenicity posterior to the fluid-filled structure. Reverberation artifact **(c)** occurs when the ultrasound beam bounces back and forth between two parallel reflective surfaces. Refraction **(e)** occurs when the ultrasound beam hits an object at a nonperpendicular angle and the two beams propagate at through tissue different speeds. Refraction can cause an object to appear at a slightly different location than it truly is, such as looking at an object under water. Finally, anisotropy **(d)** is seen in muscle or tendon fibers when sound waves hitting a reflective tissue plane at a nonperpendicular reflects the ultrasound beam away from the transducer, resulting in a hypoechoic appearance where in fact there should be echoes.

433. The answer is e. The small bowel can be characterized on ultrasound by hypoechoic lumen with finger-like projections, which are the plicae circularis. Ultrasound can be used to diagnose **small bowel obstruction** and include the presence of **fluid-filled loops of bowel greater than 2.5 cm** and **lack of forward peristalsis** (often referred to as the "washing machine" sign). Occasionally, the collapsed lumen distal to the obstruction may also be seen. Choices **(a, b, and d)** represent classic features of small bowel obstruction. Sonographic features concerning for **bowel ischemia** include bowel wall thickening greater than 4 mm **(c)** and **extraluminal free-fluid** luminal gas (hypoechoic areas with ring-down artifact) or absence of any peristalsis (observed for at least 5 minutes).

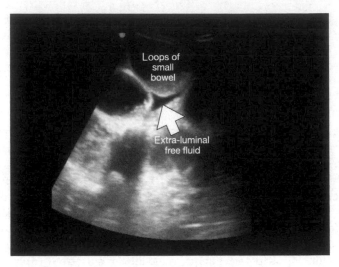

Loops of
small
bowel

Extra-luminal
free fluid

(Reproduced with permission from Dana Resop, MD.)

434. The answer is a. The patient is presenting with painless vaginal bleeding early in pregnancy with a low β-hCG. **The ultrasound does not definitely show an IUP, but instead shows an empty sac.** This could be an early gestational sac or a pseudogestational sac. When the β-hCG is less than the **discriminatory zone** of 1500 to 2000 mIU/mL, it may be too early to visualize an IUP on ultrasound, and a **repeat β-hCG should be arranged in the next 48 to 72 hours. An IUP should not be diagnosed unless a yolk sac is also visualized within the gestational sac.**

This patient does not have secondary signs of a ruptured ectopic pregnancy. These would include any mass-like structures, free fluid in the pelvic, significant pain, or abnormal vital signs. If any of these are present, or if there is strong clinical suspicion, Gynecology should be consulted for concern for possible ectopic pregnancy **(e)**. A low β-hCG does not rule out ectopic pregnancy; the entire clinical scenario should be considered. If this patient has a β-hCG greater than 2000 mIU/mL with no definitive IUP on ultrasound, this would also warrant an OB consult for concern for ectopic pregnancy given an IUP is expected to be seen and the sac could represent a pseudogestational sac. The patient does not require Rhogam **(d)** as she is Rh positive and is not a risk of isoimmunization. Additionally, she has no signs of infection or mass on ultrasound to suggest tubo-ovarian abscess **(b)** and so does not require antibiotics. Although all pregnant patients should be taking prenatal vitamins (**c**), she requires closer follow-up for a repeat β-hCG, making choice (**c**) not the most appropriate next step in management.

435. The answer is b. The ultrasound shows multiple **B-lines** in bilateral fields and pleural effusions at the bases of chest cavity, consistent with **fluid overload** and heart failure exacerbation. B-lines are artifacts seen on lung ultrasound and are bright echoes that extend from the pleural line at the top of the screen all the way to the base of the screen. These are contrasted to comet tails, which also start at pleural line, but do not continue to the bottom of the screen and are found in normal lung. A-lines are sonographic artifacts from normal, fully inflated lung. B-lines are sound artifacts from intact lung with thickening or edema of the tissue around the alveoli. **If more than three B-lines are seen in a field, they can indicate conditions such as fibrosis, infection, or fluid overload.** In this patient's images, there are multiple B-lines that have become confluent.

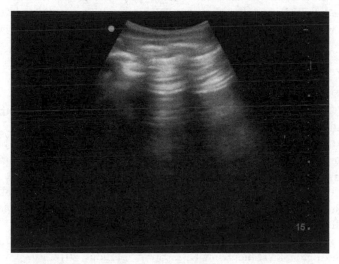

(Dana Resop, MD)

A thorough lung ultrasound exam may evaluate multiple rib spaces at both the anterior and posterior chest, but in this patient, the diagnosis is made quickly with only views of the superior lung fields. Anterior lung fields are typically evaluated at the third and fourth rib interspaces, along the midclavicular line, with a low-frequency probe. (In contrast, a high-frequency probe is often used to evaluate the same lung spaces for pneumothorax). **Pleural effusions** of anechoic fluid superior to the diaphragm in the lower lung fields are seen on this patient's ultrasound as well. The effusion on the patient's right is trace and is just a small black triangle located where the diaphragm meets the spine, but the left is larger and lung with atelectasis can be seen floating in the fluid.

Lung ultrasound can be helpful to rule out other pathologies in a patient with shortness of breath and respiratory failure. A COPD exacerbation **(a)** results in hyperinflation of the lungs and should have an ultrasound showing many A-lines, but no significant number of B-lines. Heart block **(c)** can cause profound bradycardia (<40 beats/minute) resulting in dyspnea and fluid overload, but this patient has an HR of 110 beats/minute. Pneumonia **(d)** can cause B-lines on ultrasound, but pneumonia is usually a focal process (B-lines found at only one lobe of one lung) and tends to occur in lower lungs, so in this patient with B-lines in bilateral upper lung fields, this is less likely. Pneumothorax **(e)** can be diagnosed on ultrasound by the lack of lung sliding, but this patient has B-lines at bilateral upper fields which rules out a pneumothorax at these locations.

Recommended Readings

Boyd JS, Rupp JD, Ferre RM. Emergency ultrasound. In: Knoop KJ, Stack LB, Storrow AB, Thurman R, eds. *The Atlas of Emergency Medicine.* 4th ed. New York, NY: McGraw-Hill. Available at: http:// accessmedicine.mhmedical.com.ezproxy.library.wisc.edu/content .aspx?bookid=1763&sectionid=125439068. Accessed May 17, 2020.

Butts C. Chapter 66. Ultrasound. In: Roberts JR, Thomsen C, et al, eds. *Roberts and Hedges' Clinical Procedures in Emergency Medicine and Acute Care.* Philadelphia, PA. Elsevier, 2019: 1434-1441.e1

Dawson M, Mallin M. *Lung: Introduction to Bedside Ultrasound.* Volume 1. Lexington, KY: Emergency Ultrasound Solutions, 2012.

Kimberly HH, Stone MB. Chapter e5, e49-366. Emergency ultrasound. In: Walls RM, Hockberger RS, Gausche-Hill M, et al. eds. *Rosen's Emergency Medicine: Concepts and Clinical Practice.* 9th ed. Philadelphia, PA: Elsevier, 2018.

Tolbert TN, Dickman E. Ultrasonography for small bowel obstruction. AEUS on Vimeo. Academy of Emergency Ultrasound: 2013. Available at: https://vimeo.com/69551555 Accessed June 15, 2020.

Environmental Exposures

Corlin Jewell, MD

Questions

436. A 58-year-old man presents to the emergency department (ED) with blister formation on both feet that he first noticed 2 days ago. He denies past medical history, medication use, or drug allergies. His social history is significant for alcohol dependence and he recently became homeless. He denies any sick contacts or recent travel. Upon physical examination, the lesions are fluid-filled. His feet are grossly cyanotic and tender to the touch. Pulses are present by Doppler. His foot is shown below. What is the most likely diagnosis?

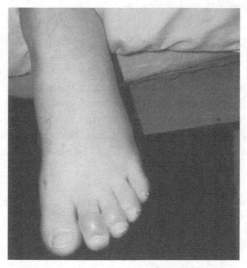

(Reproduced, with permission, from Knoop KJ, Stack LB, Storrow AB. Atlas of Emergency Medicine. New York, NY: McGraw Hill; 2002:517.)

a. Chilblains
b. Frostbite
c. Trench foot
d. Thermal burn
e. Herpes simplex infection

437. A 32-year-old otherwise healthy man develops dizziness, nausea, and confusion after running a race on a very humid day. Emergency medical services (EMS) are available on-site and the patient is given intravenous (IV) fluids. The patient appears off-balance when walking over to the stretcher and is generally confused. He is oriented to self and time but not place. He is warm and diaphoretic to touch, and it is difficult to obtain contact information from him. The patient is brought to the ED where he slowly begins to improve. He is admitted to the hospital for further management. Laboratory tests are drawn, which show multiple electrolyte abnormalities and elevated hepatic transaminases. Given his symptoms and laboratory findings, what is the most likely diagnosis?

a. Heat syncope
b. Heat edema
c. Rhabdomyolysis
d. Heat stroke
e. Heat exhaustion

438. A 42-year-old man presents to the ED after sustaining an electric shock while he was changing a wall outlet. The patient complains of pain in the finger that was shocked. Visual inspection reveals localized erythema at the tip of the distal phalanx, with good capillary refill. There are 2+ radial and ulnar pulses with full range of motion of all joints in the affected extremity. Chest auscultation reveals a regular rate and rhythm with a normal S_1 and S_2 along with clear breath sounds bilaterally. There are no other signs of trauma. What diagnostic test should be performed next in the complete evaluation of this patient?

a. Urinalysis
b. Basic metabolic panel
c. Chest radiograph
d. Electrocardiogram (ECG)
e. Arterial Doppler

439. An 18-year-old man presents to the ED with right leg pain and swelling after visiting a local beach in the United States. While swimming in the ocean, he felt a sharp sting on his right leg. Upon physical examination, there is no gross deformity of the right lower extremity. There are palpable dorsalis pedis and posterior tibial pulses. Tenderness is noted over the lateral calf with many punctate, erythematous lesions as seen in the figure. Which of the following should be applied to the skin first?

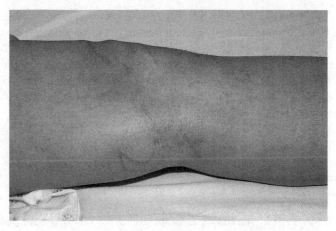

(Reproduced with permission from Corey Long, MD.)

a. Salt water
b. Cold freshwater
c. Vinegar
d. Urine
e. Capsaicin cream

440. A 49-year-old man presents to the ED with pain, erythema, and swelling to his left forearm after a chemical spill that he sustained while at work. He irrigated the area with water and applied a cold packet before arriving; however, the burning sensation in his arm has worsened. The patient works in a glass factory and reports exposure to a rust-removing agent. Which of the following tissue-saving treatments must be administered emergently?

a. Limb tourniquet
b. Topical calcium gluconate
c. Alkalinization of urine with IV sodium bicarbonate
d. Silver sulfadiazine ointment
e. Surgical debridement

441. A 23-year-old male construction worker is brought by ambulance to the ED with bilateral knee pain. He reports mixing cement the day before and kneeling in the process. The patient states that his jeans were soaked through most of the day, but he did not attempt to wash the cement off of them. Upon physical examination, you see marked tissue necrosis of both knees extending down to the bone in some places. Which chemical was this patient most likely exposed to?

a. Hydrocarbon
b. Phenol
c. Ammonia
d. Formic acid
e. Lime

442. A 40-year-old veterinary assistant presents to the ED with puncture wounds over her right hand. She reports being bitten by a cat 2 days ago while at work. On the day of presentation, she noticed redness and pain in that area. She denies fever, chills, nausea, vomiting, or other constitutional symptoms. Her vitals include a blood pressure (BP) of 125/75 mm Hg, heart rate (HR) of 90 beats/minute, respiratory rate (RR) of 14 breaths/minute, oral temperature of 99.7°F, and oxygen saturation of 99% on room air. Two puncture wounds are seen on the dorsum of her right hand with surrounding erythema and edema. The cat's immunizations are up-to-date. Which of the following combinations of potential pathogens and antibiotic choices are most appropriate?

a. *Staphylococcus aureus* and cephalexin
b. *Pasteurella multocida* and amoxicillin/clavulanic acid
c. *Streptococcus* and clindamycin
d. Methicillin-resistant *S. aureus* (MRSA) and vancomycin
e. *S. aureus* and bacitracin ointment

443. You are the physician staffing a clinic in the Rocky Mountains when a 29-year-old mountain-climber presents with nausea, vomiting, dizziness, anorexia, and mild ankle swelling. He recently flew in from Seattle to hike in the Rocky Mountains. He denies fever, cough, abdominal pain, rash, dyspnea, headache, and dysuria. He denies recent alcohol use. Which diuretic is the drug of choice for the treatment of this patient?

a. Furosemide
b. Hydrochlorothiazide
c. Bumetanide
d. Fosinopril
e. Acetazolamide

444. A 25-year-old scuba diver presents to the ED with multiple areas of periarticular joint pain and red pruritic skin. Vital signs include a BP of 110/65 mm Hg, HR of 88 beats/minute, RR of 14 breaths/minute, an oral temperature of 98°F, and oxygen saturation of 97% on room air. She has pain upon palpation of bilateral knees and ankles with full range of motion in these joints. There are no effusions, erythema, or crepitus noted over the knees or ankles. The erythema does not follow a specific dermatomal pattern and covers most of the lower extremities, torso, and back with areas of excoriation where patient reports scratching. There are no other lesions. Which of the following is the most likely diagnosis?

a. Sexually transmitted infection (STI)
b. Decompression sickness
c. Descent barotrauma
d. Ascent barotrauma
e. Nitrogen narcosis

445. A 19-year-old rookie Navy Seal presents to the ED following an episode of syncope upon ascent from a dive. The length and depth of the dive was within decompression regulation. He currently complains of feeling light-headed with a moderate frontal headache. Vital signs include a BP of 130/65 mm Hg, HR of 86 beats/minute, RR of 16 breaths/minute, and oxygen saturation of 93% on room air. He appears somewhat confused and is oriented only to person and place. He has no focal neurologic deficits. What underlying event is the likely cause for his symptoms?

a. Pulmonary embolism
b. Cardiac ischemia
c. Transient ischemic attack
d. Dysbaric air embolism
e. Nitrogen narcosis

446. A 23-year-old man presents to the ED after sustaining a bee sting. The pain is isolated to his left arm where the bee sting occurred. Upon physical examination, you see a single puncture wound with surrounding erythema and swelling. He denies respiratory distress and is phonating well. Chest auscultation reveals clear breath sounds bilaterally without wheezing. The oropharynx is patent without tongue or lip swelling or uvular displacement. Vital signs are within normal limits. Which of the following is the most appropriate next step in management?

a. Subcutaneous epinephrine 0.01 mL/kg
b. IV epinephrine 0.01 mL/kg
c. IV steroid administration
d. Observation
e. Oral antihistamine administration

447. A 31-year-old man presents to the ED with left calf pain, malaise, nausea, and myalgias since a recent trip to Arkansas. His vitals include a BP of 128/70 mm Hg, HR of 76 beats/minute, RR of 16 breaths/minute, oral temperature of 99°F, and oxygen saturation of 98% on room air. There are diffuse petechiae noted on his left lower extremity from the anterior distal tibia to the mid-thigh. Closer examination reveals a single small necrotic lesion at the level of the lateral mid-calf with surrounding edema as shown in the following figure. The patient's calf is tender to the touch and pain is worse with dorsiflexion. Which of the following is the most likely cause of his symptoms?

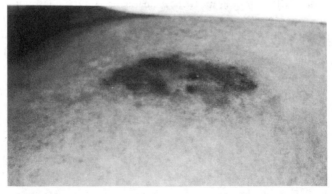

(Reproduced, with permission, from Knoop KJ, Stack LB, Storrow AB. Atlas of Emergency Medicine. New York, NY: McGraw Hill; 2002:531.)

a. Deep venous thrombosis (DVT)
b. Scorpion sting
c. Brown recluse spider bite
d. Black widow spider bite
e. Drug-induced thrombocytopenia

448. A 44-year-old woman was on a hiking trip through the Andes to see Machu Picchu. She develops a headache, anorexia, and light-headedness forcing her to descend and present to the ED. Her initial vital signs include a BP of 120/60 mm Hg, HR of 93 beats/minute, RR of 18 breaths/minute, and oxygen saturation of 96% on room air. She is placed on supplemental oxygen. Her lungs are clear to auscultation with no palpable crepitus of the chest wall and there is no peripheral edema noted. Physical examination is negative for ataxia or altered mental status. Her past medical history is negative for asthma, heart failure, chronic obstructive pulmonary disease (COPD), or tobacco use. She has an anaphylactic allergy to sulfonamide medications. Which of the following medications is indicated in this patient?

a. Acetazolamide
b. Dexamethasone
c. Nifedipine
d. Furosemide
e. Morphine

449. A 20-year-old man was brought in by EMS after he was found lying face down, unresponsive in a field by his friends. He regained consciousness after a few minutes, but is still confused in the ED. On examination, you notice the cutaneous lesion depicted in the figure. The patient denies any recent travel or sick contacts. He also denies any symptoms except for some generalized confusion. What other physical examination finding may help confirm this patient's diagnosis?

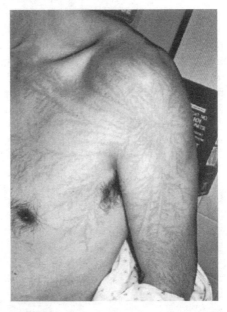

(Reproduced, with permission, from Tintinalli J, Kelen G, Stapczynski J. Emergency Medicine: A Comprehensive Study Guide. New York, NY: McGraw Hill; 2004:1238.)

a. Orthostatic vital signs
b. Otoscopic evaluation of tympanic membranes
c. Hemoptysis
d. Auscultation of systolic cardiac murmur
e. Palpating the cervical spine for tenderness

450. A 24-year-old man presents to the ED with diffuse body pain, pruritus, erythema, and dizziness after reportedly waking up covered in bugs after falling asleep while camping outside. His initial vital signs include a BP of 118/75 mm Hg, HR of 102 beats/minute, RR of 18 breaths/minute, and oxygen saturation of 98% on room air. What is the most appropriate next step?

a. Provide tetanus prophylaxis
b. Begin local wound care
c. Assess airway, breathing, and circulation
d. Start IV fluid administration
e. Give oral antihistamines

451. A 40-year-old homeless man is brought to the ED unresponsive after a snowstorm. EMS found him curled up on a bus stop bench covered only with a small blanket. His core temperature is 28°C. He is well-known to the hospital for multiple admissions for poorly treated schizophrenia. He has no other past medical history, does not take his medications, and has never used illicit drugs. His ECG is shown in the figure. Shortly after this is obtained and while his clothing is being removed, the patient's pulse can no longer be palpated. What is the most appropriate next step in treatment?

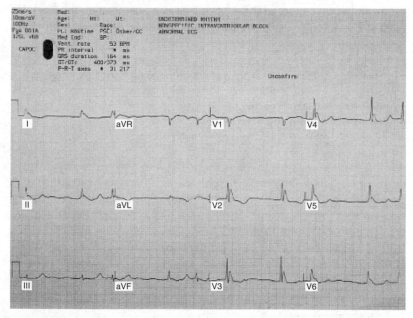

(Reproduced, with permission, from Knoop KJ, Stack LB, Storrow AB. Atlas of Emergency Medicine. New York, NY: McGraw Hill; 2002:516.)

a. Defibrillation
b. Cardiac pacing
c. Pronounce the patient deceased
d. Chest compressions and rewarming
e. Cardiopulmonary bypass

452. A 26-year-old man presents to the ED in severe pain with a Gila monster attached to his arm after he was bitten. He is the animal's main handler. He reports localized 10/10 pain. He denies weakness, nausea, or light-headedness. The animal attached itself 45 minutes ago. The animal is carefully removed from his arm by staff. What is the most appropriate next step?

a. Check for any remaining embedded teeth and begin wound care
b. Administer antivenin
c. Give tetanus prophylaxis
d. Administer broad-spectrum antibiotics
e. Apply suction device

453. An anxious college student presents to the ED at 2:00 am stating a bat woke him up from sleep. He heard something flying around his bedroom, and when he turned the lights on, he saw a bat fly into his closet. He is unsure of whether or not he was bitten. Which is the most appropriate management?

a. Provide reassurance and discharge home
b. Administer human rabies immune globulin and human diploid cell rabies vaccine
c. Administer oral ciprofloxacin
d. Admission for 24 hours of observation
e. Administer human diploid cell rabies vaccine

454. A 21-year-old man presents to the ED with a painful and itchy rash covering his hands and arms. The rash started 2 days ago with small pruritic vesicles and slowly progressed into variable sized bullae. The distribution includes the palms and a linear streaking pattern over both forearms. He denies fevers, chills, nausea, vomiting, or diarrhea. He recently started working for a lawn care company and has been clearing overgrown gardens. He does not wear gloves or long-sleeved shirts. His past medical history is negative for allergies, asthma, or previous rashes. Which of the following treatments is most recommended?

a. Oral systemic steroids
b. Oatmeal baths
c. Careful aspiration of the bullae
d. Hospital admission for further testing
e. Epinephrine 0.3 mg via intramuscular injection

455. A 40-year-old man from Connecticut presents to the ED with the inability to move both sides of his face. One week ago, he noted that the left side of his face began to droop. The following day, he began to notice a similar drooping of the right side of his face. He denies facial paresthesias, diplopia, focal extremity weakness, or headache. Physical examination shows bilateral cranial nerve VII palsy. He has intact cerebellar and extremity muscle strength bilaterally. What history would help guide further testing?

a. Bull's eye rash
b. Snake bite exposure
c. Family history of muscular dystrophy
d. Exposure to poison sumac
e. History of atherosclerosis

The following scenario applies to questions 456 and 457.

During the month of June, a 26-year-old man who lives in the northeastern United States presents with a worsening headache. He is an avid hunter and has recently returned from his nearby cabin after a week of hunting. He also has myalgias, fever, and a rash. The rash is nonblanching with small dark petechiae on his ankles, wrists, and hands. His headache is getting worse and is no longer responding to ibuprofen. On further history, he did notice ticks on the deer he was cleaning.

456. What further testing is necessary to initiate treatment?

a. Lumbar puncture
b. Skin biopsy
c. Start empiric treatment without further testing
d. Serology
e. Nasopharyngeal swab

457. What action can decrease the incidence of this disease?

a. DEET (N,N-Diethyl-meta-toluamide) repellant
b. Tiki torches
c. Washing of fruit and vegetables
d. Vaccination
e. Living on the west coast

458. A 25-year-old man is fishing off the coast of Florida when a large wave hits the boat and he falls overboard. He immediately emerges and is coughing up water. The boat returns to land and he is taken to the ED for further workup and treatment. By the time he arrives, he is asymptomatic and his lungs are clear to auscultation bilaterally. His arterial blood gas is normal. What is the most appropriate disposition?

a. Discharge home
b. Observation in the ED for approximately 2 hours, then discharge with antibiotics
c. Observation in the ED for at least 4 hours, then discharge without antibiotics
d. Admission is required due to salt water immersion
e. Admission is required due to fresh water immersion

459. A 26-year-old kite surfer was wading into the water to launch his kite. He was walking in murky salt water when he suddenly felt a sharp poke in his foot. He quickly lifted his foot and saw a stingray swim away. On examination, there is a small puncture wound on the dorsum of his foot without obvious debris present. The pain is sharp and burning and progressively increases. He is 45 minutes away from any help; however, there is a hotel nearby. What immediate treatment is most likely to improve his pain?

a. Pouring vinegar over the foot
b. Immersing the foot in hot water
c. Elevation and cold compresses on the affected limb
d. Urination on the foot
e. A half-cut onion applied to the wound

460. You are performing a ride-along with an EMS crew during a heavy thunderstorm and are dispatched to the scene of a lightning strike with multiple victims. Which victim should receive the most immediate attention?

a. Ambulatory adolescent boy complaining of hearing loss
b. Adult woman that appears in significant distress with obvious right arm deformity
c. Pregnant young woman complaining of abdominal pain
d. Pulseless middle-aged man who is not spontaneously breathing
e. Unconscious young adult woman with palpable pulse and rapid shallow breathing

461. A 19-year-old man is brought to the ED by his friends because he is acting unusual. The patient himself has a hard time describing the history and appears confused. He is flushed, but his skin is dry to the touch. His temperature is 100.6° F and his HR is 110 beats/minute. They deny any drug use, but the patient is unable to provide a urine sample. His friends state that they were hiking prior to the onset of symptoms and show you a picture on their phone of a plant that the patient ingested (see figure below). What plant did the patient most likely ingest?

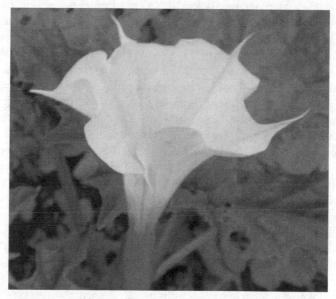

(Reproduced with permission from Adam J. Rosh, MD, and Rosh Review.)

a. Foxglove
b. Jimsonweed
c. Water hemlock
d. Coca (cocaine)
e. Monkshood

Environmental Exposures

Answers

436. The answer is b. Frostbite usually occurs when tissue temperature falls below 0°C (32°F). There are three phases to the freezing injury cascade. **Phase 1** (prefreeze, without actual ice formation) occurs when the tissue reaches a temperature below 10°C and includes initial skin cooling, increased blood viscosity, vasoconstriction, and microvascular leakage that causes localized edema formation. Patients typically lose cutaneous sensation in the tissue during this phase. **Phase 2** (freeze-thaw) occurs when extracellular crystal formation begins, thereby causing intracellular shrinkage, protein and lipid derangements, cell dehydration, and collapse of the cellular network. Finally, **phase 3** (vascular stasis and progressive ischemia) begins once the tissue is rewarmed and involves further coagulation, interstitial leakage, cytokine release, and cell death. This results in blister formation, cyanosis, and ultimately mummification of the tissue. The bullae formed may also have a hemorrhagic appearance, but not always. It is important to note that **wind and moisture** may increase the freezing rate. Management includes **rapid rewarming in a circulating water bath with water temperatures of 37°C to 39°C**. Tissue massage, which furthers tissue loss, should be avoided as should dry heat sources, such as a space heater. Rewarming is a painful procedure that requires parenteral analgesia. Patients may also have a degree of dehydration and benefit from warmed crystalloid administration.

Chilblains **(a)**, also known as pernio, is an abnormal vascular response to cold resulting in erythema, itching, and inflammation of the skin. Pernio is commonly seen in the homeless population as a result of chronic dry-cold exposure and mostly affects the face, hands, and pretibial areas, particularly in young women or those with autoimmune disorders Trench foot **(c)**, also known as immersion injury, is also common in the homeless population. This occurs when skin is exposed chronically to wet and cold environments; however, the ambient temperature is above freezing. It usually presents as a loss of sensation with pallor and mottled skin that is sodden and friable. Thermal burns **(d)** may present with bullae formation but do not elicit cyanosis and this patient's history is not consistent with thermal injury. Herpes **(e)** is also unlikely given the distribution, history provided, and lack of contacts with similar lesions.

437. The answer is d. The patient has **heat stroke**. Heat stroke lies at the severe end of a spectrum including heat exhaustion, heat cramps, and heat edema. Patients may have symptoms common to other heat-related illness, such as general malaise, fatigue, headache, diaphoresis, and nausea. However, they will also exhibit **neurological abnormalities**, including inappropriate behavior, confusion, ataxia, seizures, decerebrate/decorticate posturing, and coma which differentiate heat stroke from other forms of heat-related illness. Clinically, they may show signs of **dehydration** including dry mucus membranes, tachycardia, and orthostatic hypotension. Heat exhaustion and heat stroke cannot be delineated based on the presence of anhidrosis alone, as over half of patients with heat stroke still exhibit sweating. It is important to bring the patient to a cool location and start IV fluid replacement, typically 1 to 2 L initially of normal saline (NS) in the pre-hospital setting. Fluids should be continued at a rate which ensures good urine output following arrival to the hospital. Cold water immersion (CWI) therapy, in which the patient is immersed up to the neck in water just above the freezing point, is strongly recommended as the most rapid method of cooling. Cold and slightly salted oral rehydration can also be used initially if the patient is protecting their airway. **Hepatic transaminases** can be seen in cases of heat-related illness, with levels peaking 24 to 72 hours after the thermal insult. Other laboratory abnormalities can include hypernatremia, hypokalemia, elevated creatinine, and elevated creatine kinase (CK). The liver injury is secondary to centrilobular necrosis and is typically fully reversible. Both heat exhaustion and heat stroke are caused by dehydration and intravascular cell depletion, which can progress to cardiovascular shock, profound mental status changes, and increased temperature.

Heat syncope **(a)** results from the dilatation of cutaneous vessels to assist in the delivery of heat to the skin's surface. Blood distributes more to the periphery, thereby causing syncope with a quick return to normal mentation. Elderly patients and those who stand for long periods are especially prone to this. Heat edema **(b)** occurs in patients who are not acclimated to warmer temperatures and thereby develop swollen feet and ankles. This is not a central process and altered mental states do not occur. Rhabdomyolysis **(c)** may result in any case where there is muscle breakdown caused by dehydration, stress, or exogenous factors. The patient may have mild rhabdomyolysis; however, it alone does not explain his symptoms. Had this patient's mental status been intact, the correct answer would have been heat exhaustion (d), which will eventually lead to heat stroke if treatment is not initiated and thermoregulatory responses fail.

438. The answer is d. The patient sustained a **low-voltage (<1000 V) electrical injury** from the wall socket. All patients sustaining such an injury warrant an **ECG** and **cardiac monitoring** in the ED. In the United States, household wiring has 120 V of **alternating current** with a frequency (number of switches from positive to negative current) of 60 Hz. Alternating current causes continuous muscle contraction which can result in **tetany** pulling the victim into the current and can also cause **cardiac conduction abnormalities** resulting in ventricular fibrillation. Direct current usually just causes a single powerful muscle spasm often throwing the victim away from the current and therefore has an increased percentage of blunt trauma injury. The current is equal to the voltage over the resistance (Ohm's law). High-voltage injuries (>1000 V) typically only happen in industrial settings or those that have come into contact with power lines. This patient sustained a superficial thermal burn and most likely did not become part of the circuit as there are no clear entry or exit wounds which are seen in direct-contact injuries. Provided the ECG and telemetry are unremarkable, disposition of this patient should include localized wound care, close follow-up, and instructions to return if there are any worsening symptoms.

Although a urinalysis (a) to screen for myoglobin and a basic metabolic panel (b) to check renal function might be performed, it is not necessary given the nature of this patient's injury. A chest X-ray (c) and arterial Doppler (e) will not prove efficacious given the benign clinical examination.

439. The answer is a. This patient sustained an injury from a **venomous marine animal**. Marine species, such as sea urchins, stingrays, catfish, cone shells, and starfish inject venom via spines located on their body. In certain cases, these spines can shear off and remain embedded in the body. In this case, radiographs may be useful in delineating the calciferous material deposited in the skin for removal. Other marine species, such as jelly fish, fire coral, Portuguese man-o-war, and anemones, inject their venom through specialized harpoon-like structures called **nematocysts** which are discharged upon mechanical or chemical stimulation. This type of marine envenomation is much more prevalent and is the most likely cause for this patient's distress. The number of nematocysts on each tentacle can number in the thousands. These stinging cells can remain activated after several days of the animal being beached. The venom contains various peptides and enzymes that may cause progression of symptoms, including nausea, muscle cramps, dyspnea, angioedema, and anaphylaxis. The preferred initial treatment is to use a **salt water** rinse to remove any remaining tentacles. After this, hot freshwater immersion has been shown to be effective in treating pain from jellyfish stings. The patient should be given tetanus prophylaxis, analgesics, and antihistamines as needed. Dried nematocysts may be reactivated after water exposure so they should be physically removed with gloved fingers or forceps and NOT washed off.

In certain species, such as the box jellyfish found off the Australian coast, the area should be treated with vinegar (4%-6% acetic acid) **(c)**, which can deactivate the nematocyst. In other species, such as those commonly found in the United States, application of vinegar can actually stimulate the nematocysts. Cold freshwater **(b)** should be avoided as it can activate the nematocysts. Using urine **(d)** was a common myth, but has actually been shown to worsen symptoms. Capsaicin cream **(e)** should not be used in cases of jellyfish stings.

440. The answer is b. Chemical burns are a common occupational hazard and can be caused by a variety of solvents containing acidic or alkaline substances. Initially, it is important to remove any contaminated clothing and begin to irrigate the affected skin for at least 15 to 30 minutes with copious amounts of water. The next step is assessment of the affected area, size, and depth of the burn as some patients will need transfer to a burn center. This patient was chemically burned by a **rust-removing agent**, which commonly contains **hydrofluoric acid (HF)**. **Pain out of proportion to sustained injury** is usually seen in these cases. HF is a relatively weak acid; however, its extreme electronegativity makes it **very dangerous**. Fluoride avidly binds to available cations, including calcium and magnesium, thereby causing hypocalcemia and hypomagnesemia. **Profound hypocalcemia** has been demonstrated in HF exposure, especially with extensive burns. The free fluoride ions also inhibit Na/K ATPase and the Krebs cycle resulting in cellular destruction. The patient requires continuous ECG monitoring (given the risk of electrolyte abnormalities) and administration of exogenous cations, such as topical **calcium gluconate gel** applied every 15 to 30 minutes until pain begins to be relieved. This acts as a chelating agent to the fluoride ions. IV or intradermal calcium gluconate may also be used. Calcium chloride should be avoided as it can cause severe tissue necrosis upon extravasation. Blisters should be removed and debrided because they may contain fluoride ions.

Placing a tourniquet (a) upon the limb may cause ischemia and further cell death. Alkalinization of urine with sodium bicarbonate (c) would not be of benefit in this type of exposure. Silver sulfadiazine (d) may be applied later on for wound care, but data on its clinical utility has not shown a definite benefit. The extent of this injury at this time does not warrant surgical debridement (e); however, close wound monitoring should be performed to identify cases in which tissue necrosis progresses.

441. The answer is e. This patient was exposed to **lime**, which is present in **cement**. When water interacts with dry **cement**, calcium hydroxide is released, resulting in an increased pH of 10 to 13. Amateur cement workers, like the patient in the question, may not recognize the dangers of this substance and may stand or kneel in the substance for a prolonged period of time. **Alkali burns cause liquefaction necrosis**, resulting in quick dissolution of the involved tissues. Acid burns form a coagulation necrosis, which can serve to slow down the rate of further tissue penetration. The best treatment of lime exposure is **extensive irrigation** during initial contact. This patient will need further surgical debridement and wound care because of his exposure.

Hydrocarbons (a) are present mainly in gasoline and paint thinners. Phenols (b) are found in dyes, deodorants, disinfectants, and agriculture solvents, which causes cell denaturation upon contact. Ammonia (c) is present in many household cleaners, refrigeration units, and fertilizers. It acts differently depending on what form it is in. For example, ammonia may freeze skin on contact or affect breathing because of its vapors. Formic acid (d) is a caustic organic acid used in many industries. Treatment for exposure to all of these chemicals includes copious irrigation and observation for systemic side effects.

442. The answer is b. Cat bites involve small **puncture wounds** often extending down through skin into tendons and bones owing to the nature of the animals' sharp teeth. The reported incidence of infection from these bites varies wildly in the literature ranging from 16% to 80%, with many patients presenting only after an infection has incurred. It is important to note that **cat bites have a much higher infection rate compared to dog bites.** This is due to the typical puncture wound that inoculates bacteria deep into the tissues and subsequently becomes enclosed as the skin heals. *P. multocida* is a gram-negative, facultative anaerobic rod found in the oral cavity of the majority of healthy cats and may cause severe systemic infection, especially in immunocompromised individuals. *P. multocida* is primarily treated with **amoxicillin/clavulanic acid**. Patients need to be followed closely as these infections may seed deep into joints and other subcutaneous tissues requiring debridement. It is important to note that this bacterium is also carried on claws therefore scratches can also cause infection.

All other organisms (**a, c, d, and e**) are potential pathogens, though they are less likely in this scenario. The other antibiotic choices do not provide appropriate coverage for *P. multocida*. This bacterium is resistant to first-generation cephalosporins (**a**), vancomycin (**d**), and clindamycin (**c**). Topical antibiotics, such as bacitracin (**e**), would not be effective.

443. The answer is e. An avid **mountain-climber** who ascends rapidly and presents with new headache, nausea, and vomiting, should prompt you to diagnose **acute mountain sickness (AMS)**. Early on, symptoms may mimic an acute viral syndrome or alcohol hangover with nausea, vomiting, headache, and anorexia. However, these symptoms progress to include **peripheral edema, oliguria, retinal hemorrhages, and finally high-altitude pulmonary or cerebral edema if the patient continues to ascend**. Risk factors for AMS include, but are not limited to, rapid ascent, history of COPD, history of sickle-cell disease, obesity, cold exposure, heavy exertion, and sleeping at higher altitudes. In mild cases, further ascent should be halted for 12 to 36 hours to allow for acclimatization. For more severe symptoms or symptoms that do not improve with rest, the **initial treatment** is **immediate descent**. A descent of 1000 to 3000 feet reverses high-altitude sickness in most cases. Supplemental **oxygen** is indicated in all cases. **Carbonic anhydrase inhibitors, such as acetazolamide,** have been proven effective not only for treatment but also for prophylaxis. This works by reducing resorption of bicarbonate in kidneys, inducing a metabolic acidosis that stimulates respiration which increases Pao_2. Symptomatic treatment for vomiting and headache may also be indicated. Hyperbaric oxygen therapy is indicated in severe cases.

Other diuretics, such as furosemide (**a**) and bumetanide (**c**), are indicated in treatment of congestive heart failure. They do not alkalinize the urine and can induce hypotension and shock given their strong diuretic effect if the patient is already volume depleted. Hydrochlorothiazide (**b**) is a thiazide diuretic that is used for hypertension, not AMS. Fosinopril (**d**) is an angiotensin-converting enzyme (ACE) inhibitor and not a diuretic.

444. The answer is b. This patient is suffering from **decompression sickness**, more commonly known as **"the bends."** This term refers to a spectrum of states whereupon **bubbles of nitrogen** gas come out of solution and collect in the blood and tissues as pressure is decreased during ascent. To help illustrate, picture a bottle of soda being opened, allowing the bubbles to rapidly come out of the solution to the top. Clinically, the degree of collection is a result of the depth and length of the dive. Other risk factors include inherent fatigue, heavy exertion, dehydration, and flying after a dive. A patent foramen ovale may also prove to be dangerous in causing gas bubbles to embolize to the arterial system. Decompression sickness can progress from its initial musculoskeletal involvement to include the cardiovascular, respiratory, and central nervous system (CNS). **Divers should ascend in a slow, gradual manner to avoid to collection of nitrogen gas in these tissues.** IV fluid hydration and 100% supplemental oxygen should be administered immediately. Transport to the nearest **hyperbaric chamber** is the definitive therapy.

STI **(a)** can present in a somewhat similar fashion, particularly disseminated gonorrhea, however, less likely due to the acute onset of symptoms after diving. Descent barotrauma **(c)** is uncomfortable and includes sinus, ear, and skin squeeze. This can result in tympanic membrane damage and pain to palpation over the sinuses but has few long-term effects. Ascent barotrauma **(d)** involves similar symptoms in addition to pneumomediastinum and pneumothorax due to rapid expansion of the gas within the tissues, particularly if the patient was holding their breath during ascent. Nitrogen narcosis **(e)**, also known as "rapture of the deep," is a phenomenon in which prolonged dives produce a euphoric effect upon the diver because of the collection of nitrogen gas in the tissues. This may prove dangerous in the face of an emergency with a false sense of security and impaired motor skills.

445. The answer is d. This patient as a new diver ascended to the surface too quickly causing an **air embolism.** Nitrogen gas bubbles form and subsequently travel to the arterial system through the pulmonary veins into the cardiac chambers. **Arterial gas embolism** may also occur if the patient has a patent foramen ovale. **Symptoms** are usually **sudden and dramatic, usually occurring during or immediately after ascent.** Divers, who may have been thought to have drowned, actually passed out during ascent because of an underlying embolism. Treatment includes IV fluids, administration of 100% oxygen, and transfer to a center which can provide **hyperbaric oxygen therapy.** Air transport should be avoided.

Although cardiac ischemia (**b**) may occur because of this, it is not the precipitating event. Pulmonary embolism (**a**) in an otherwise healthy individual with no risk factors is low probability as the inciting event as history is more consistent with air embolism. Transient ischemic attacks (**c**) may present in a variety of ways, but given this clinical scenario, a serious diving-related cause must be investigated first. Nitrogen narcosis (**e**) occurs with breathing gasses at depths greater than 70 feet and this condition clears with resurfacing. Clinically, patients appear as if they are intoxicated with ethanol.

446. The answer is d. History taking should include prior bee stings, **as each successive sting increases the possibility of anaphylaxis given sensitization**. The ABCs must be initially addressed. Stings most commonly present with localized burning, erythema, and edema at the sting site lasting for about 24 hours. The patient is asymptomatic and only warrants **observation** at this time. Toxicity and anaphylaxis are typically evident soon after the sting and include vomiting, diarrhea, fever, and neurologic manifestations, such as seizures and altered mental status. The patient most likely sustained a sting from a honeybee or bumblebee given the single puncture wound. Bees possess retroserrate-barbed stingers, which are removed upon stinging, thereby eviscerating and killing the insect. Vespids, such as wasps, hornets, and yellow jackets, do not contain this mechanism and may sting many times. "Killer bees," as popularized by the film industry, contain the same amount of venom as other species. The difference is that they are more aggressive and prone to swarm and follow a victim for a longer distance.

The patient does not warrant epinephrine administration (**a and b**) in any form as there are no systemic signs of anaphylaxis. Steroids (**c**) and antihistamines (**e**) are usually given in patients with systemic signs. β_2-agonists (eg, albuterol) may also be given for respiratory symptoms.

447. The answer is c. The **necrotic lesion** in connection with travel to the **south-central United States** is classic for a **brown recluse spider bite**. The brown recluse spider can be distinguished by its **violin-shaped cephalothorax**. The initial bite is usually painless and within a few hours forms a small papule, which can progress to erythema and blistering over the next several hours. Initial lesions may appear target-shaped, as blood supply to the central area is diminished and the tissue becomes necrotic. The surrounding tissue becomes indurated and an eschar forms over the central lesion. This eschar falls off over the course of the first 1 to 2 weeks following envenomation leaving behind an ulcer which heals by secondary intention. Associated systemic symptoms include fever, chills, myalgias, hemolysis, petechiae, and eventually seizure, renal failure, and death. However, these are rare in the United States. Initial treatment includes addressing the ABCs, wound care, analgesia, and tetanus prophylaxis. Patients with laboratory abnormalities or systemic symptoms should be admitted. Antibiotics may become warranted if bacterial superinfection ensues.

Although associated with travel, a DVT (a) is less likely given the clinical scenario including the single necrotic lesion seen on the leg. Drug-induced thrombocytopenia (e) can also cause petechia, however is less likely given the information provided in the question. Scorpion stings (b) present differently with immediate localized pain and are followed by neurologic symptoms including salivation, muscle fasciculation, and blurred vision. The venom of a black widow spider (d) causes symptoms that can be mistaken for peritonitis due to painful muscle spasm and resultant abdominal rigidity. Spasms usually resolve spontaneously, but can progress to hypertension and cardiovascular failure in rare cases. Black widow spiders have a signature hourglass bright-red marking on the underside of the abdomen.

448. The answer is b. Dexamethasone is recommended because the patient has an allergy to sulfonamide medications. This patient is experiencing **AMS** with no signs of high-altitude pulmonary edema or high-altitude cerebral edema. The first-line treatment is **descent** and **oxygen supplementation**, which is already accomplished in this patient. Other treatment considerations include hyperbaric oxygen therapy. The exact mechanism by which dexamethasone treats AMS is unknown, but may be related to its antiinflammatory effect or by controlling nausea. Keep in mind that high-altitude pulmonary or cerebral edema may rebound once dexamethasone is stopped.

Acetazolamide (a) is the preferred agent for most cases of AMS. However, the patient has an anaphylactic sulfonamide allergy, making acetazolamide contraindicated. Therefore, dexamethasone is indicated for in this case. Acetazolamide is indicated as prophylaxis in patients with a history of altitude illness. It works as a diuretic to decrease the resorption of bicarbonate in the kidneys by inhibiting carbonic anhydrase, resulting in metabolic acidosis and stimulates hyperventilation. This compensatory mechanism is turned off when the pH is close to the physiologic range of 7.4. It is this hyperventilation that counters the altitude-induced hypoxemia thereby relieving symptoms. Nifedipine (c) works by decreasing pulmonary artery pressure in high-altitude pulmonary edema, as does the diuretic effect of furosemide (d). However, furosemide does not provide the beneficial increase in RR. Morphine (e) is thought to reduce pulmonary blood flow and decrease hydrostatic forces in pulmonary edema.

449. The answer is b. This patient sustained a **direct lightning injury** as evidenced by the typical **fern-like pattern** exhibited (known as a Lichtenberg figure). Associated injuries include fractures (from muscle contraction), cardiovascular collapse, burns, blunt abdominal injuries, and neurologic damage. **Tympanic membrane ruptures** are a common associated injury and is believed to be caused by the rapid expansion of surrounding air generating a pressure gradient similar to an explosion. Therefore, it is important to check for blood in the ear canals of these patients. It is important to quickly assess the ABCs of these patients and establish an airway. Immobilization of the cervical spine is often indicated, as well as close ECG monitoring. Patients should be admitted for observation after obtaining a complete blood count (CBC), creatinine kinase, troponin, basic metabolic panel, and appropriate radiographs of injured areas. Although 50 to 100 people die of lightning strikes each year in the United States, most injuries sustained are not lethal. Triage of multiple victims of a single lightning strike is reversed and patients who are pulseless or apneic should be managed first. Respiratory arrest may outlast cardiac arrest as the diaphragm is stunned. This fact may necessitate rescue breathing for a short period of time in the patient with a pulse to give appropriate time for the diaphragm to recover.

Orthostatic vital signs (a) more commonly is seen in vasovagal mediated syncope rather than lightning strikes. Hemoptysis (c) could suggest PE as a potential cause of syncope and is less suggestive of a lightning strike. A systolic murmur (d), especially in the elderly population, could represent critical aortic stenosis. This patient is young with no medical problems, which would decrease the probability that the syncope was secondary to valvular disease. Patients who are struck by lightning often have blunt injuries from being thrown by the blast effect from the current (a tertiary blast injury). Any patient who presents to the ED with paralysis should have cervical spine precautions in place, regardless of whether or not they have cervical spine tenderness (e). Keraunoparalysis is a transient paralysis of both lower extremities due to a lightening injury that will self-resolve over hours and is not due to any spinal cord injury. Initially, such distinction may be difficult to discern so necessary spinal cord precautions should be initiated.

450. The answer is c. Fire ants have proven to be a real threat to humans. Ninety-five percent of clinical cases result from the *Solenopsis invicta* species, a member of the Hymenoptera, which was imported from South America in the 1930s. This ant is found in many of the southern United States given that it cannot survive long winters and is slowly replacing the less dangerous species native to North America. They are small, copper to dark brown in color. Their venom is 95% alkaloid, which is unlike other members of the Hymenoptera Order that they belong to. The venom inhibits Na^+/K^+ ATPase and affects aerobic cellular respiration. It can induce coagulopathy and also has cardiotoxic properties. They are named due to the burning sensation caused by their stings. The sting usually produces a pustule within 24 hours which lasts 1 to 2 weeks. Local **burning, erythema, and pruritus** are common. Anaphylaxis is thought to occur in 0.6% to 6% of cases, resulting in systemic symptoms, including nausea, vomiting, dizziness, respiratory distress, and potential cardiovascular compromise. Therefore, **assessment of this patient's airway, breathing, and circulation is imperative**. Continuous monitoring is indicated to detect hemodynamic instability.

Local wound care **(b)** may be performed after the patient is deemed stable. IV fluids **(d)** should be given if the patient is hemodynamically unstable, but is not the most appropriate next step. Tetanus prophylaxis **(a)** may be administered after the initial assessment and stabilization. Antihistamines **(e)** may be given as indicated; however, they should not be the first step.

451. The answer is d. In all critically ill patients, it is important to remove clothing (especially if wet), obtain a core temperature, and initiate continuous monitoring, including an ECG after performing the primary survey of the patient (ABCs). **Osborne (J) waves** are indicative of a junctional rhythm (the heart is responding to a pacemaker within the AV node or Bundle of His), as seen in this patient, and are consistent with hypothermia. Prolongation of any interval, bradycardia, asystole, atrial fibrillation/ flutter, and ventricular tachycardias may also be seen. The clinician must initiate **advanced cardiac life support** and **rewarm** the patient once a rectal temperature has confirmed **hypothermia** and they are found pulseless and apneic. It is important to remember that severely hypothermic patients who appear dead have a good chance of a normal neurologic outcome with continued resuscitation and rewarming. Remember that **a patient is not dead until he/she is warm and dead!** Those at extremes of age, users of sedative hypnotics, homeless individuals, those with chronic illness, altered mental status, or sepsis are at most risk for hypothermia. Rewarming should begin by removing any wet clothing and placing warm blankets over the patient. Then active rewarming should begin with mechanical warming blankets, warm IV fluids, gastric lavage, bladder lavage, peritoneal warming, and lastly cardiopulmonary bypass (ECMO).

Defibrillation (**a**) and cardiac pacing (**b**) are not currently indicated in this patient as the patient does not have a shockable rhythm (PEA) and is unlikely to respond to pacing as this is not an electrical problem. You should NOT declare the patient deceased (**c**) until they continue to be unresponsive despite elevating core body temperature more than 36°C. Cardiopulmonary bypass (**e**) is a last resort when other methods of warming have failed.

452. The answer is a. There are only **two venomous lizards; the Gila Monster,** which is native to the southwestern United States, and the **bearded lizard** in Mexico. These animals are usually not aggressive, despite the Gila monster's name, and bites are usually a result of direct handling as in this case. Both the Gila monster and the Mexican-bearded lizard are easily identified by their thick bodies and beaded scales (with either a white and black or pink and black configuration), but are rare in the wild. Envenomation occurs via the glands along the lower jaw. The venom is introduced into the victim through grooved teeth that the animal uses to continuously chew after it has bitten down. These **teeth may become embedded in the victim,** distributing more venom, and should be removed on arrival. Initially, symptoms involve pain, erythema, and swelling at the bite site. There is not typically associated skin necrosis. Systemic symptoms can develop later, including nausea, vomiting, diaphoresis, tachycardia, and hypotension. Angioedema has been documented with both species in some cases.

Antivenin (**b**) is not available as these bites are rarely fatal. Broad-spectrum antibiotics (**d**) and tetanus prophylaxis (**c**) should be administered at a later interval. Applying a suction device (**e**) is never warranted in envenomation injury. The patient should be observed for at least 6 hours for systemic effects.

453. The answer is b. The patient should receive **full rabies prophylaxis** against the rabies virus. The Centers for Disease Control and Prevention (CDC) recommends postexposure prophylaxis when a bat is found indoors in the same room with a person. **This immunization is indicated even if**

the person is unaware that a bite or direct contact occurred and rabies cannot be ruled out by testing the bat. Full prophylaxis in the United States includes passive immunization with human rabies immune globulin and active immunization with human diploid cell vaccine. Immunoglobulin is administered in and around a bite wound if visualized and IM at a different site. Human diploid cell vaccine is administered at a distant site from the immunoglobulin, usually in the deltoid, to avoid cross reactivity. Human diploid cell vaccine is subsequently administered on days 3, 7, and 14 for a total of four doses. The immunoglobulin does not need to be repeated and may inhibit antibody production if multiple doses are given.

The patient should not be sent home without treatment (**a**). Ciprofloxacin (**c**) has no role in this patient or in rabies treatment. Admission (**d**) is not warranted as the incubation period for rabies ranges from 30 to 90 days with some reporting up to 7 years. The patient should receive immunoprophylaxis and be sent home. Administering the vaccine alone without immunoglobulin (e) is not recommended as the patient should receive both active and passive immunoprophylaxis unless they already received it in the past.

454. The answer is a. Contact dermatitis from plants including **poison ivy** is the most common cause of plant-induced occupational injury in the United States. Poison ivy is from the plant genus *Toxicodendron* that also includes the poison oak and poison sumac. They all contain an oil (urushiol) that is the causative agent of the hypersensitivity reaction and rash. Patients usually require prior exposure to develop the hypersensitivity, but some people can develop a reaction after a single encounter which is typically delayed for up to 3 weeks. Upon re-exposure to urushiol to someone who is already sensitized, the symptoms develop within 12 to 48 hours. The mildest form manifests as a **vesicular, erythematous, pruritic, and mildly painful rash** in a **linear distribution**. Moderate to severe cases include diffuse areas of erythema and edema with bullae formation and more severe pain. The rash may appear to be spreading; however, this is usually a delayed reaction rather than extension of disease. The best treatment is prevention with the use of long-sleeved clothing and gloves. Treatment is based on severity. In all cases, decontamination should be performed by washing all potentially contaminated clothing and skin. There are many cleansing products available, but soap and water are equally effective. Treatment for mild reactions is symptomatic with oatmeal baths and oral antihistamines. If the **exposure is severe** or involves the genitals or face, then the use of **oral**

systemic steroids is recommended in conjunction with symptomatic relief as previously discussed. This treatment includes prednisone 1 mg/kg/day (maximum 60 mg) tapered over 21 days to prevent disease rebound. Treatment with an oatmeal bath (b) is a good option for mild disease. However, since the rash covers his hands and is very painful, systemic steroids should be given. Aspiration of the bullae (c) is not necessary and may cause more discomfort as well as increase the risk of superinfection. With a clear etiology and no respiratory symptoms, discharge with pain control and oral systemic steroids is appropriate; therefore, the patient does not require admission for additional testing (d). Epinephrine (e) has no role in treatment of contact dermatitis and should only be used in cases of anaphylaxis.

455. The answer is a. This patient has **bilateral Bell's palsy**, which is a known complication of **Lyme disease**. Lyme disease is the most common vector-borne illness in the western world. The causative agent is a tick-born infection called *Borrelia burgdorferi*, which is transmitted by the Ixodes tick. It is endemic in multiple locations worldwide, but, in the United States, is most commonly seen in the Northeast, upper Midwest, and northern California. The clinical course follows a variable pattern ranging from early (weeks to months) to late postexposure manifestations (months to years). Rash and systemic symptoms present first, typically within 1 to 2 weeks of exposure. The rash, *erythema migrans*, appears as a "bull's eye" pattern with annular erythema, a clear inner annulus, and central erythema. Often systemic flu-like symptoms are also seen, including fatigue and lethargy. A disseminated infection can present over the course of weeks or months after onset of the rash and may even be the first manifestation of the illness. It can affect multiple body systems including CNS, cardiovascular, and musculoskeletal. Neurological complications include meningitis, **bilateral Bell's palsy**, and other cranial neuropathies. Cardiac presentations include variable AV block, including third-degree (complete) AV block. Musculoskeletal symptoms include monoarticular large joint arthritis (most commonly the knees), which spontaneously resolves then affects another large joint. Late disease is characterized by arthritic and neurologic symptoms. The arthritis (which is more common) presents with joint effusions and joint pain. It is more indolent and can last multiple months to years. The neurological symptoms can involve a chronic encephalopathy or painful radiculoneuritis. Diagnosis is complicated and includes a two-tier system of ELISA (enzyme-linked immunosorbent assay) followed by a

Western blot. Alternatively, a system of two sequential ELISA tests has also been accepted by the CDC. Further information can be found at the CDC website (https://www.cdc.gov/mmwr/volumes/68/wr/mm6832a4.htm?s_cid=mm6832a4_w). Treatment is similarly complicated and includes prevention as the first step. Prevention is important to decrease disease incidence, including wearing light color clothing and the use of 30% DEET applied to the skin. If the tick is attached, removal is performed with a pair of sharp pointed tweezers. Antibiotic treatment depends on the body system involvement, the symptom severity, the patient's age, and pregnancy status. If the rash is present along with a consistent history, early treatment with doxycycline is recommended without serological testing. Exceptions to doxycycline therapy include pregnancy or age younger than 8 years. In these cases, a beta-lactam, such as amoxicillin, should be prescribed. Early treatment decreases the likelihood of secondary and tertiary sequelae. For late infection, further guidelines are available online on the CDC website.

Snake bites (**b**) present with sharp localized pain at the site of inoculation and do not present with Bell palsy. Muscular dystrophy (**c**) presents with generalized muscle weakness and not Bell palsy. Poison sumac (**d**) presents as a contact dermatitis. A history of atherosclerosis (**e**) increases the probability of having a stroke. However, Bell palsy is not indicative of a stroke.

456. The answer is c. Rocky Mountain Spotted Fever (RMSF) is caused by the bacterium *Rickettsia rickettsii*, which spread most commonly by the American dog tick. It has a high prevalence between April and September, and is most commonly reported in the southeast and south-central states. However, it has been reported throughout the contiguous US states. Signs and symptoms typically begin in 3 to 12 days following exposure and can fatal within days. Initial symptoms typically begin acutely and include a fever, headache, myalgias, and gastrointestinal (GI) symptoms. It may later progress to altered mental status, encephalopathy, coma, pulmonary edema, acute respiratory distress syndrome (ARDS), cardiovascular collapse failure, coagulopathy, DIC, and soft tissue necrosis. The rash of RMSF is a disseminated vasculitic rash that starts **on the wrists, hands, ankles, and feet and spreads centripetally**. It occurs in 90% of affected individuals, but may not be present when the patient presents with the early symptoms. It begins as a blanking pink or red macules and progresses to dark red to black petechiae. Early diagnosis and treatment are crucial to decreasing morbidity and mortality. Therefore, if **suspicion is high, prophylactic treatment** is indicated. Serology is the best confirmatory test but often has high-false negatives early in the disease.

Other laboratory findings that support the diagnosis include **thrombocytopenia, hyponatremia**, and elevated liver function tests (LFTs). Treatment should be initiated in patients who live in endemic areas and develop constitutional symptoms. Before the discovery of effective antibiotics, mortality from RMSF was as high as 80%. However, now it is less than 1%. **Doxycycline** is the drug of choice for **both adults and pediatric patients**. The short course duration for doxycycline does not typically result in staining of pediatric dentition but parents should still be alerted to this possibility.

There are multiple abnormal laboratory findings with RMSF including CSF, skin biopsy, and serology. CSF findings **(a)** can yield an elevated or normal protein level, as well as pleocytosis of lymphocytes and polymorphonuclears (PMNs); however, this is neither a sensitive nor a specific finding; therefore, lumbar puncture is not necessary to initiate therapy. Skin biopsy **(b)** with indirect fluorescent antibody is both sensitive and specific and can detect the disease early. However, this is time consuming and impractical for routine use. Serology (d) often has early high-false negative results. Nasopharyngeal swabs **(e)** can be used to diagnose infections, such as influenza or COVID-19.

457. The answer is a. DEET repellant sprayed on exposed skin and clothing can provide protection from initial tick bites and attachment. This can be safely applied to the skin of children over 2 months, if the repellant concentration is below 30%. In adults, higher concentrations can be used, but effectiveness plateaus at 50%. It can be safely used in pregnancy. A single application provides between 1.5 to 6 hours of protection, with higher concentrations effective for longer periods of time.

Tiki torches **(b)** have been marketed as a mosquito deterrent, not a tick repellent, and have not been shown to be effective. Washing of fruits and vegetables can decrease the risk of contracting infectious gastroenteritis **(c)** but does not decrease the likelihood of contracting RMSF. There is currently not a vaccination for RMSF **(d)**. Living on the west coast of the United States **(e)** decreases the probability of acquiring the disease, but does not eliminate the risk of exposure.

458. The answer is c. If the initial hospital assessment, including history, oxygen saturation, and chest X-ray, are entirely normal and the patient remains asymptomatic without clinical deterioration **at 4 to 6 hours (some pediatric literature suggests 8 hours)**, then the patient can be discharged home. Drowning is defined as a primary respiratory impairment from submersion or immersion in a liquid medium. It is a leading cause of accidental death in the United States, especially in young children. Approximately 80% of drowning victims are male and alcohol is commonly involved. The terms *wet* and *dry drowning* refer to whether or not aspiration of liquid into the lungs has occurred. Dry drowning occurs secondary to laryngospasm and thus minimal water is aspirated into the lungs. However, these terms have largely been abandoned per the latest guidelines. Injury to the lung with a liquid-medium results in a ventilation/perfusion mismatch and a decreased oxygen-diffusing capacity. This mismatch can present as cough, rales, shortness of breath, and wheezing. Cardiac dysrhythmia is also common secondary to acidosis or hypoxia. While the **majority of symptoms** from an immersion or submersion injury will present within the first 4 hours postinjury, **an observation period of 4 to 8 hours is recommended to ensure that those with delayed presentations are not missed**. Depending on the duration of hypoxia, many patients are left with residual neurological sequelae. Treatment is aggressive and quick initiation of ventilation and oxygenation with a high suspicion for concomitant CNS damage secondary to trauma. In cases of cold-water drowning, CPR is continued until the core body temperature is heated to at least 36°C; then resuscitation can be terminated if there is no spontaneous return of circulation. This is similar to the management of other cold-related illnesses.

For a patient who was originally symptomatic, at least 4 hours are needed to ensure the patient is stable for discharge, though some data suggests a longer period of up to 8 hours, particularly in the pediatric population. Immediate discharge or within 2 hours is a dangerous decision (**a and b**). Antibiotics have no role in the initial management of drowning and should only be used if clear evidence of a bacterial pneumonia develops in the coming days. Salt and fresh water (**d and e**) are not independent risk factors. Historically, it was believed that the different mediums of salt water versus freshwater would cause either fluid overload with a dilutional effect (freshwater) or massive pulmonary edema and hypertonic serum (salt water). However, in patients who survive drowning, the aspiration is not enough to cause these changes. There are exceptions to this rule, however, such as the Dead Sea, which is extremely hypertonic and can lead to severe electrolyte disturbances.

459. **The answer is b. Stingray stings** are a commonly encountered marine envenomation. Stingrays are nonaggressive scavengers and bottom-feeders that "attack" as a defensive reaction to being stepped on. These animals are found in both fresh and salt water in tropical or subtropical climates and live partially submerged in shallow water. Stingrays range in size from a few inches to multiple feet in size, are flat, diamond or kite-shaped and have a tail containing a venomous spine. The sting from a stingray can present with a puncture wound or jagged laceration, depending on how the spine hits the skin. Complications include deep and complex lacerations, secondary bacterial infection, and osteomyelitis. Death is a rare complication that occurs secondary to the toxin, secondary infection, or because of direct penetrating trauma (ie, cardiac puncture). The envenomation causes **immediate localized pain, edema, and bleeding.** The pain will peak in 30 to 90 minutes and can last up to 48 hours. Systemic manifestations include nausea, vomiting, diarrhea, diaphoresis, vertigo, lightheadedness, muscle cramps, hypotension, or arrhythmias. Treatment is best approached on multiple fronts. **Immediate irrigation with nonheated tap water or saline is best** followed by **hot water immersion** between 43°C and 45°C for 30 to 90 minutes, with careful attention not to cause burns. This decreases the pain via disruption of the thermolabile components of the venom, but does not decrease the skin necrosis. Next, **debridement and removal of the pieces of sting** are recommended unless the entire spine is embedded in the patient (especially in the chest, abdomen, or neck). This needs to be treated as a penetrating object and left as is and not removed until arrival at a hospital. Once at a medical facility, pain control can be augmented with local anesthetics or narcotics. Radiographs should be performed to assess for retained foreign bodies, followed by sterile debridement, and antibiotic prophylaxis.

Vinegar (a) and seawater immersion are helpful for marine envenomation with nematocysts (eg, jellyfish). They are not effective in stingray stings. Elevation and application of cold compresses (c) is an effective treatment of musculoskeletal sprains and strains. It has no role in stingray envenomation. Urination (d) has no role in marine envenomation. Some areas of Australia use a half-cut onion placed over the wound (e), which has anecdotally provided pain relief but has not been proven. However, hot water immersion is still the best first treatment.

460. The answer is d. Lightning strike multicasualty incidents should be approached with a **"reverse triage" system** that is at odds with the more standard "SMART" triage algorithm. Patients that are found pulseless and apneic are generally given a "black tag" in standard situations and typically do not receive immediate attention as their injuries make them extremely unlikely to survive. However, in cases of lightning strike, these victims are instead treated first as they have a higher survival rate than the general population. This is because the lightning strike itself acts like a **large-voltage defibrillation**, stopping the heart briefly following a massive depolarization that will often recover spontaneously. The strike can also temporarily **paralyze the respiratory center** within the medulla which causes cessation of spontaneous respiration. In some cases, this stunning of the respiratory system can continue despite return of spontaneous cardiac activity. If the patient's airway/breathing is not managed immediately, the patient will likely go on to have a second arrest due to prolonged hypoxia.

The ambulatory patient with hearing loss **(a)** does not require immediate attention and would normally receive a "green tag" per normal triage practices. This patient may have suffered rupture of his tympanic membranes, but does not require immediate transport. The patient with the arm deformity **(b)** would typically receive a "yellow tag" indicating potentially severe injuries, but do not require immediate attention. She most likely suffered a broken arm from being thrown by the lightning strike, which is similar to a tertiary blast injury in cases of explosions. The pregnant patient with abdominal pain **(c)** would also receive a "yellow tag," but is not the immediate priority. There is little data on pregnancy and lightning strikes, but what is available does suggest increased to the fetus and mother. The unconscious patient with tachypnea **(e)** would be given a "red tag" and thus normally require the most immediate attention in standard mass-casualty incidents. This patient is in impending risk of decompensation and death, if he does not receive care soon. He should be the first priority once the pulseless and apneic patient's airway is secured.

461. The answer is b. This patient ingested **Jimson weed** as evidenced by his symptoms and the plant shown in the figure. Jimsonweed ingestion causes symptoms consistent with the **anticholinergic toxidrome** such as tachycardia, hyperthermia, mydriasis, urinary retention, and altered mental status.

Unlike intoxication with sympathomimetic substances (d), the skin is flushed and dry. Ingestion of foxglove (a) typically presents with GI symptoms followed by cardiac dysrhythmia. Ingestion of water hemlock (c) is characterized by bradycardia, hypotension, respiratory distress, and seizure activity that can be difficult to control with standard anticonvulsant therapy. Finally, ingestion of monkshood (e) results in a toxidrome that is the opposite of ingestion with jimson weed including salivation, lacrimation, nausea, vomiting, diarrhea, and cardiac dysrhythmias.

Recommended Readings

Auerbach P. *Wilderness Medicine*. 7th ed. Philadelphia, PA: Elsevier, 2016.

Ingebretsen R. *Advanced Wilderness Life Support*. University of Utah School of Medicine. Adventure Med LLC, 2011.

Wilderness Medical Society Clinical Practice Guidelines. Wilderness & Environmental Medicine. 2019. Available at: https://www.wemjournal .org/issue/S1080-6032(19)X0006-X. Accessed May 1, 2020.

Lyme Disease. Center for Disease Control and Prevention. Available at: https://www.cdc.gov/lyme/index.html. Updated December 16, 2019. Accessed May 1, 2020.

Marx J, Hockerberger R, Walls R, et al. Part IV: Environment and Toxicology. In: *Rosen's Emergency Medicine. Concepts and Clinical Practice*. 8th ed. Philadelphia PA: Elsevier Saunders, 2013.

Eye Pain and Visual Change

Daniel Rutz, MD

Questions

The following scenario applies to questions 462 to 464.

A 65-year-old woman with a history of hypertension, hyperlipidemia, presents to the emergency department (ED) complaining of blurry vision in the left eye, pain in her left eye, and a new rash to her left forehead. One week ago, she was diagnosed with left-sided parotitis by her primary care physician (PCP) and started on antibiotics. On physical examination, you notice a patch of grouped vesicles on an erythematous base located in a dermatomal distribution on her forehead that does not cross midline. There are also a few vesicles located at the tip of her nose. Her visual acuity is 20/20 OD (OD = right eye) and 20/70 OS (OS = left eye), her cornea is cloudy, and her left pupil is mid-dilated with poor reactivity to light. There is no afferent pupillary defect (APD) in either eye. Intraocular pressure (IOP) is noted to be 14 OD and 39 OS. Fluorescein stain of the left eye is normal. Funduscopic exam shows normal appearing optic disc and periphery in the left eye.

462. What is the likely causative organism?

a. Adenovirus
b. *Pseudomonas aeruginosa*
c. Varicella zoster virus (VZV)
d. Herpes simplex virus (HSV)
e. *Chlamydia trachomatis*

463. What ophthalmologic complication(s) of this disease has this patient likely developed?

a. Iridocyclitis and trabeculitis
b. Acute retinal necrosis
c. Keratitis
d. Central retinal vein occlusion
e. Optic neuritis

464. What treatment(s) is/are indicated for this patient's IOP?

a. Acyclovir and erythromycin
b. Preservative free artificial tears
c. Proparacaine and prednisolone acetate
d. Shielding the eye
e. Dorzolamide, brimonidine, and timolol

465. A 31-year-old nurse asks you to evaluate a lesion on her left eye. She denies fever, change in vision, eye pain, or discharge. A picture of her eye is shown in the following figure. Which of the following is the most likely diagnosis?

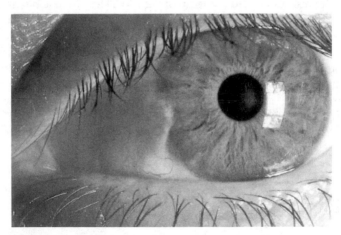

(Reproduced, with permission, from Knoop KJ, Stack LB, Storrow AB. Atlas of Emergency Medicine. New York, NY: McGraw Hill; 2002:43.)

a. Hordeolum
b. Chalazion
c. Dacryocystitis
d. Pinguecula
e. Pterygium

466. A 72-year-old man presents with right eye pain for 1 day. The patient has a history of diabetes, hypertension, and "some type of eye problem." He does not recall the name of his ophthalmic medication. However, he does remember that the eye drop bottle has a yellow cap. Which class of ophthalmic medication is the patient taking?

a. Antibiotic
b. β-Blocker
c. Mydriatic and cycloplegic agent
d. Miotic
e. Anesthetic

467. A 35-year-old woman presents with right eye redness for 3 days. She denies pain and notes watery discharge from the eye. She has been coughing and has felt congested for the past 5 days. On examination, the patient's blood pressure (BP) is 110/70 mm Hg, heart rate (HR) is 72 beats/minute, respiratory rate (RR) is 14 breaths/minute, and temperature is 98.4°F. Her visual acuity is 20/20 bilaterally. On inspection, the right conjunctiva is erythematous with minimal chemosis and clear discharge. The slit-lamp, fluorescein stain, and funduscopic examinations are otherwise unremarkable. The patient has a nontender, preauricular lymph node, and mildly enlarged tonsils without exudates. What is the most likely diagnosis?

a. Gonococcal conjunctivitis
b. Bacterial conjunctivitis
c. Viral conjunctivitis
d. Allergic conjunctivitis
e. Pseudomonal conjunctivitis

468. A 24-year-old woman presents to the ED at 4 am with severe left eye pain that woke her up from sleep. She wears soft contact lenses and does not routinely take them out to sleep. She is in severe pain and wearing sunglasses in the examination room. You give her a drop of proparacaine to treat her pain prior to your examination. On examination, her visual acuity is at baseline and she has no APD. There is some perilimbic conjunctival erythema. On fluorescein examination, a linear area on the left side of the cornea is highlighted when cobalt blue light is applied. No underlying white infiltrate is visualized. No white cells or flare are visualized in the anterior chamber. What is the most appropriate treatment for this condition?

a. Immediate ophthalmology consultation
b. Tobramycin ophthalmic ointment
c. Erythromycin ophthalmic ointment
d. Eye patch
e. Proparacaine ophthalmic drops

469. A 45-year-old woman presents with right eye pain and redness for 1 day. She has photophobia and watery discharge from the eye. She does not wear glasses or contact lenses and has no prior eye problems. On examination, the patient's visual acuity is 20/20 in the left eye and 20/70 in the right eye. She has conjunctival injection around the cornea and clear watery discharge. On slit-lamp examination, the lids, lashes, and anterior chamber are normal. When fluorescein is applied, the following image is seen. The remainder of the head examination is normal and no cutaneous lesions are noted. Which of the following is the most appropriate treatment for this patient?

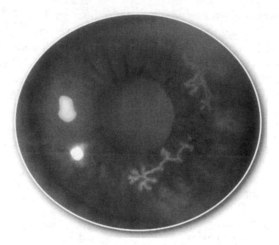

(Reproduced with permission from Adam J. Rosh, MD, and Rosh Review.)

a. Admission for intravenous (IV) antibiotics
b. Admission for IV antiviral agents
c. Discharge home on topical steroids
d. Discharge home on topical antiviral medication
e. Immediate ophthalmology consultation

470. A 21-year-old man presents to the ED with a red eye. The patient complains of rhinorrhea and a nonproductive cough for 3 days. He denies eye pain or discharge. He has no associated ecchymosis, bony tenderness of the orbit, or pain on extraocular eye movements. His vision is 20/20, extraocular movements are intact, and IOP is 12 mm Hg. A picture of his eye is shown in the following figure. What is the most appropriate next step?

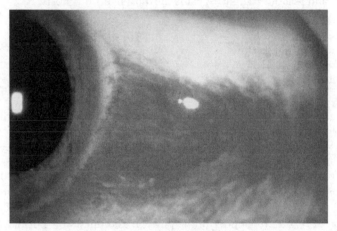

(Reproduced, with permission, from Riordan-Eva P, Asbury T, Whitcher JP. Vaughan & Asbury's General Ophthalmology. New York, NY: McGraw Hill; 2004:124.)

a. Emergent ophthalmology consultation
b. Administer topical 1% atropine
c. Elevate the head of the patient's bed
d. Administer ophthalmic timolol
e. Provide reassurance

471. A 28-year-old mechanic with no past medical history presents to the ED after a small amount of battery acid was splashed in his right eye. He is complaining of extreme pain and tearing from his eye. Which of the following is the most appropriate next step in management?

a. Call for ophthalmology consultation
b. Check visual acuity
c. Check the pH of the tears
d. Irrigation with normal saline
e. Application of erythromycin ointment

472. A 45-year-old man presents to the ED with intense bilateral eye pain, tearing, and foreign body sensation. He denies any trauma, past medical history, or contact lens use. He works as a pipe-fitter and uses a welder regularly. His physical examination is significant for bilateral decreased visual acuity and injected conjunctiva. Fluorescein staining reveals diffuse punctuate corneal lesions with a discrete inferior border. His pupils are equal, round, and reactive to light. What is the most likely diagnosis?

a. Corneal abrasion
b. Traumatic iritis
c. Ultraviolet (UV) keratitis
d. Corneal foreign body
e. Bacterial conjunctivitis

473. A 12-year-old girl presents to the ED for left eye pain and swelling for 2 days. The patient has had cough, congestion, and rhinorrhea for the last week. On examination, BP is 110/70 mm Hg, HR is 115 beats/minute, RR is 12 breaths/minute, and temperature is 101.8°F. On eye examination, there is purplish-red swelling of both upper and lower eyelids with injection of the conjunctiva. Pupils are equal and reactive to light. She has restricted lateral gaze of the left eye. Visual acuity is 20/70 in the left eye and 20/25 in the right eye. The remainder of the physical examination is normal. What is the most appropriate next step in management?

a. Administer oral diphenhydramine
b. Administer oral amoxicillin/clavulanate
c. Administer IV vancomycin and cefotaxime
d. Perform computed tomographic (CT) scan of orbits and sinuses
e. Administer artificial tears

474. A 62-year-old woman with a history of hypertension presents with right-sided blurry vision. She reports unilateral headache, typically more noticeable at night, progressively worsening over the past week. This is associated with episodes of transient blurry vision in her right eye. She also notes jaw pain while eating, especially toward the end of meals. She has taken acetaminophen with mild relief. She endorses tactile fever and malaise. Her vital signs are a temperature of 98.5°F, BP of 167/87 mm Hg, HR of 84 beats/minute, RR of 14 breaths/minute, and pulse oximetry of 98%. Eye exam is notable for visual acuity 20/60 OD and 20/25 OS. She has an APD in her right eye and tenderness to palpation over her right temple.

Remainder of physical exam is unremarkable. What is the treatment of this patient's condition?

a. Topical cycloplegics
b. IV Corticosteroids
c. IOP lowering medications
d. Temporal artery resection
e. BP control

475. A 22-year-old man presents to the ED for left eye pain. He was in an altercation the previous day and was punched in the left eye. On examination, his left eye is ecchymotic and the eyelids are swollen shut. He has tenderness over the infraorbital rim but no step-offs. You use an eyelid speculum to examine his eye. His pupils are equal and reactive to light. His visual acuity is normal. On testing extraocular movements, you find he is unable to look upward with his left eye. He also complains of diplopia when looking upward. Funduscopic examination is normal. What is the most likely diagnosis?

a. Orbital blowout fracture
b. Ruptured globe
c. Retinal detachment
d. Cranial nerve III palsy
e. Traumatic retrobulbar hematoma

476. You are examining a patient's eyes. On inspection, the pupils are 3 mm and equal bilaterally. You shine a flashlight into the right pupil and both pupils constrict to 1 mm. You then shine the flashlight into the left pupil and both pupils slightly dilate. What is this condition called?

a. Anisocoria
b. Argyll Robertson pupil
c. APD
d. Horner syndrome
e. Normal pupillary reaction

477. A 65-year-old man with a history of diabetes, hypertension, coronary artery disease, and atrial fibrillation presents with loss of vision in his left eye since he awoke 6 hours ago. The patient denies fever, eye pain, or discharge. On physical examination of the left eye, vision is limited to counting fingers. His pupil is 3 mm and reactive. Extraocular movements are intact. Slit-lamp examination is also normal. The dilated funduscopic examination is shown in the following figure. Which of the following is the most likely diagnosis?

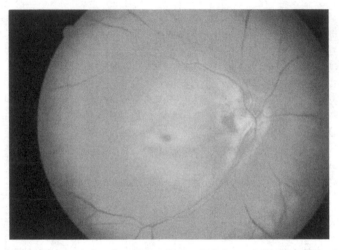

(Reproduced, with permission, from Knoop KJ, Stack LB, Storrow AB. Atlas of Emergency Medicine. New York, NY: McGraw Hill; 2002:82.)

a. Retinal detachment
b. Central retinal artery occlusion (CRAO)
c. Central retinal vein occlusion
d. Vitreous hemorrhage
e. Acute angle-closure glaucoma

478. A 24-year-old man presents complaining of right eye pain. He was punched in the face 2 days ago. Examination reveals a sluggish right pupil with decreased visual acuity and consensual photophobia. His extraocular movements are intact and he denies bony tenderness around the orbit. Which of the following is the most likely diagnosis?

a. Corneal abrasion
b. Retinal detachment
c. Hyphema
d. Traumatic iritis
e. Orbital blowout fracture

479. A 33-year-old woman presents complaining of left eye redness. She notes 3 days of focal redness, mild irritation, and watery discharge in her left eye. She denies trauma, fever, blurry vision, double vision, pain with eye movements, and foreign body sensation. Visual acuity, pupil exam, extraocular movements, visual fields, and IOP are normal. Fluorescein exam is normal. Direct inspection of the affected eye is pictured below. What is the likely diagnosis?

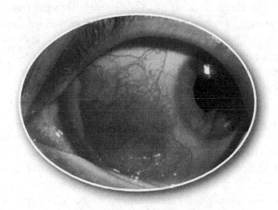

(Reproduced with permission from Adam J. Rosh, MD, and Rosh Review.)

a. Bacterial conjunctivitis
b. Endophthalmitis
c. Keratitis
d. Scleritis
e. Nodular episcleritis

480. A 43-year-old man presents with a painful red eye. He was drilling through metal pipes at his house and states a piece of metal flew into his unprotected right eye. He endorses pain, blurry vision, redness in his eye, and excessive tearing. While viewing the cornea under cobalt blue light after administration of fluorescein, a stream of bright green is noted. What is the next most appropriate treatment?

a. Check IOP
b. Shield the eye and consult ophthalmology
c. CT scan of the orbit
d. Discharge home with cycloplegic and antibiotic eye drops
e. Primary repair of the injury

Eye Pain and Visual Change

Answers

462. The answer is c. At a minimum, the patient has **herpes zoster (shingles)** and may potentially have **herpes zoster ophthalmicus,** an infection caused by the **VZV.** The shingles in this case involves the **ophthalmic division** (V1) of the **trigeminal nerve.** Shingles is diagnosed clinically by visualizing a patch of grouped vesicles on an erythematous base located in a dermatomal distribution. Patients may complain of a prodrome of headache, fever, malaise, unilateral pain, hypesthesia of the affected eye or forehead that can precede the appearance of the rash. Ipsilateral parotitis can be seen with VZV infections.

Adenovirus (**a**) is the most common cause of viral conjunctivitis. *P. aeruginosa* (**b**) is associated with contact lens use, corneal abrasion, and corneal ulceration. HSV (**d**) can cause keratitis and severe ocular infections, but the clinical scenario described is more consistent with VZV. *C. trachomatis* (**e**) can cause conjunctivitis in neonates and sexually active adults. None of these agents are the cause of shingles.

463. The answer is a. The patient likely has **iridocyclitis and trabeculitis. Ocular complications** occur in approximately 50% of the cases involving the ophthalmic division of the trigeminal nerve. The patient in this vignette has elevated IOP due to decreased aqueous humor outflow from her inflamed iris and trabecular network. This produces a clinical syndrome similar to acute angle-closure glaucoma with a blurry vision and a poorly reactive mid-dilated pupil. IOP should be obtained on patients with suspected Zoster ophthalmicus.

Other ocular sequelae include acute retinal necrosis (**b**), keratitis (**c**), conjunctivitis, uveitis, and episcleritis. Keratitis is diagnosed based on signs of anterior chamber inflammation as well as pseudodendrites on fluorescein examination under cobalt blue light. VZV is the leading cause of acute retinal necrosis, characterized by vitritis, necrotizing retinitis, occlusive retinal vasculitis, and eventual retinal detachment. The patient's exam does not support a diagnosis of CRVO (**d**) or optic neuritis (**e**).

464. The answer is e. **Dorzolamide, brimonidine, and timolol** are topical agents given to emergently lower IOP. Timolol is a β-blocker and dorzolamide is a carbonic anhydrase inhibitor that together **decrease aqueous humor production**. Brimonidine is an α-agonist that will **increase trabecular outflow**. These agents can be given repeatedly as needed to lower IOP.

Systemic acyclovir and topical erythromycin ointment **(a)** will likely be used for this patient's VZV, but they do not lower IOP. Preservative free artificial tears **(b)** provide symptomatic relief of dry or irritated eye, but do not have an effect on IOP. Proparacaine and topical prednisolone **(c)** are used in the treatment of traumatic iritis under the guidance of an ophthalmologist. Eye shielding **(d)** is used as a temporizing measure for cases of open globe injuries.

465. The answer is e. This patient has a **pterygium**, a triangular growth of tissue from the bulbar conjunctiva that can encroach on the periphery of the cornea. It is more common on the nasal side of the cornea and may affect one or both eyes. Pterygium is associated with exposure to **wind, dust, and sunlight**. Most cases are asymptomatic and can be followed by an ophthalmologist. In symptomatic cases, surgical excision may be indicated.

A hordeolum **(a)** or stye is an acute infection and abscess of the glands within the eyelids. Chalazions **(b)** are granulomatous inflammations of meibomian glands in the eyelids. In contrast to the erythematous, edematous, and painful hordeolum, a chalazion is usually hard and nontender. Dacryocystitis **(c)** is an inflammation of the lacrimal sac that is characterized by pain, swelling, and erythema of the lacrimal sac on the extreme nasal aspect of the lower lid. Pressure on the lacrimal sac in a patient with dacryocystitis may express pus. Pinguecula **(d)** is a yellow-whitish, fatty lesion of the bulbar conjunctiva that may be on either side of the eye, but does not encroach on the cornea. It is more commonly seen on the nasal side. In contrast to pterygium, a pinguecula does not encroach on the cornea.

466. The answer is b. Ophthalmic medications are **color-coded**. While this question may seem esoteric, it can be clinically useful to know the colors of eye medications. In this case, knowing that **yellow** caps are β-**blockers** suggests that this patient may be currently treated for glaucoma. Medication color knowledge can also help you rapidly locate a specific medication from a large group of eye medications.

Antibiotics **(a)** are usually tan. Mydriatics and cycloplegics **(c)** are red. Miotics **(d)** are green and anesthetics **(e)** are white. Mydriatics and cycloplegics are medications that cause ciliary muscle paralysis and pupil dilation. Miotics are medications that cause pupillary constriction.

467. The answer is c. This patient has classic **viral conjunctivitis** associated with a viral upper respiratory infection. Patients with viral conjunctivitis typically have **conjunctival infection** and **watery discharge**. **Preauricular lymphadenopathy** is also associated with viral etiology. There is no specific antiviral agent for treatment. Supportive measures include warm or cool compresses and ophthalmic antihistamine/α-adrenergic combination medications—naphazoline/pheniramine for example.

Patients with bacterial conjunctivitis **(b)** have thick mucopurulent discharge and often wake up with matted eyelids. These patients are treated with broad-spectrum topical antibiotics. Bacterial and viral conjunctivitis do not always present classically and can be difficult to distinguish between clinically. Therefore, physicians will often treat conjunctivitis patients with antibiotic eye drops until they can be reexamined by an ophthalmologist. Patients who wear contact lenses are at risk for pseudomonal conjunctivitis and keratitis **(e)**. They should be treated with an antibiotic that covers *Pseudomonas*, such as a fluoroquinolone or aminoglycoside. It is very important to always consider gonococcal conjunctivitis **(a)** in sexually active individuals, because this infection can cause permanent visual loss if not rapidly identified and treated. Patients with gonococcal conjunctivitis have a severe conjunctivitis with copious mucopurulent drainage and erythematous conjunctiva. Inpatient IV antibiotics should be started while waiting results of an ocular Gram stain and culture. Allergic conjunctivitis **(d)** presents with watery discharge and eye redness, but itching is the most prominent symptom. Cyclical exacerbations associated with allergen exposure may be a clue to the diagnosis of allergic conjunctivitis.

468. The answer is b. This patient has a **corneal abrasion** from prolonged contact lens use. The abrasion is best visualized after fluorescein staining and cobalt blue illumination of the cornea. **Contact lens wearers** with abrasions are at high risk for **pseudomonal** infection and should be treated with an **antipseudomonal agent**, such as tobramycin. It is critical to distinguish an abrasion from a corneal ulcer. Ulcers are deeper infections of the cornea that develop from corneal epithelial defects (ie, abrasions). Contact lens wearers are also at high risk for corneal ulcers. The hallmark of a corneal ulcer is a shaggy, white infiltrate within the corneal epithelial defect.

Uncomplicated corneal abrasions (in noncontact lenses wearers) may be treated with erythromycin ointment (c). Immediate ophthalmology consultation (a) is necessary for treatment of corneal ulcers, however not corneal abrasion. Some ophthalmologists will see the patient in the ED to perform corneal Gram stain and culture, while other ophthalmologists will examine the patient in 12 hours in the office setting. Eye patches (d) are controversial but should not be given to patients at risk for fungal infections or pseudomonal infections as they are at risk for rapid corneal melting and perforation. Topical anesthetic agents, such as proparacaine (e), may be helpful to facilitate the examination in the ED but should be dispensed with caution as repeated use of these agents may cause corneal injury and vision loss.

469. The answer is d. This patient has **HSV keratitis.** The hallmark of this disease is the branching or **dendritic ulcer.** Patients may also present without corneal involvement but will have typical herpetic skin lesions in the eyelids and conjunctiva. Patients should be treated with topical antivirals, such as acyclovir 3% ophthalmic ointment, and topical antibiotics to prevent secondary bacterial infection. Oral antivirals and topical antivirals are both effective treatment options. If utilizing the former, oral acyclovir 400 mg five times daily or oral valacyclovir 500 three times daily are effective, dosed until 1 week after lesions heal. The choice between oral and topical antivirals is based on patient preference and consultation with ophthalmology.

IV antibiotics (a) are not indicated for herpes simplex keratitis. Corticosteroids (c) must be avoided as they may enhance viral replication and worsen infection. Patients should follow-up with ophthalmology in 1 to 2 days. If there is evidence for herpes zoster ophthalmicus, an infection due to reactivation of the herpes zoster virus involving the trigeminal nerve with ocular involvement, ophthalmology should be consulted immediately (e) and the patient should be admitted for IV antiviral therapy (b).

470. The answer is e. This patient has a **subconjunctival hemorrhage** caused by conjunctival vessel rupture from coughing. This common ED complaint can result spontaneously or from Valsalva-induced pressure spikes (such as coughing, vomiting, or bearing down), trauma, and hypertension. Patients can be **reassured** that subconjunctival hemorrhages **spontaneously resolve** in 1 to 2 weeks.

Subconjunctival hemorrhage is sometimes confused with hyphema or blood in the anterior chamber. A hyphema can be traumatic from a ruptured iris vessel or spontaneous, usually associated with sickle cell disease. Bleeding within the anterior chamber can cause elevated IOP and must be treated aggressively with β-blockers (d) and mannitol. Carbonic anhydrase inhibitors (Diamox) should be avoided in sickle cell patients as these medications lower anterior chamber pH, ultimately enhancing red blood cell (RBC) sickling and increasing IOP. Pupillary activity stretches the iris vessels and exacerbates bleeding with hyphema; therefore, mydriatic agents, such as atropine (b) are used to keep the pupil dilated. The head of the bed can be elevated (c) to minimize elevations of IOP. Many ophthalmologists will admit all patients with hyphemas. This is because 30% of hyphemas rebleed in 3 to 5 days, resulting in dangerously high elevations in IOP necessitating surgical therapy. Some ophthalmologists will follow patients with hyphemas occupying less than one-third of the anterior chamber, on an outpatient basis. However, ophthalmology should be urgently consulted while the patient is in the ED and individual decisions can be discussed (a).

471. **The answer is d.** Chemical injuries to the eye must be **immediately irrigated** with a minimum of 1 to 2 L of normal saline as soon as they arrive in the ED. Topical anesthesia and the use of a Morgan lens (a special device to provide large volume irrigation to the eye) can help facilitate this procedure.

Irreversible eye damage can occur if irrigation is held for physical examination and visual acuity testing (b). Checking the pH of the tears (c) helps determine the effectiveness of irrigation, but should be checked after irrigation has begun. When the ocular pH returns to 7.5 to 8.0, irrigation can be stopped and a complete eye examination should be performed. Remember to check visual acuity and pay special attention to corneal clouding or corneal epithelial defects. Patients with epithelial defects or corneal clouding should receive an ophthalmic antibiotic (e). Patients without corneal or anterior chamber involvement only need erythromycin ointment. The ophthalmologist (a) should be notified, after initial stabilization, of all patients with chemical injury to the eye and follow-up should be arranged within 12 to 24 hours.

472. **The answer is c.** This patient has **UV keratitis**, also known as **welder's flash** or photokeratitis, which is a radiation burn on the cornea from exposure to a **UV-ray-containing light source**. The pathophysiology is desquamation of the corneal epithelium due to inflammation from

UV exposure, thus exposing corneal nerve endings. UV keratitis can result from unprotected exposure to the welder's arc, sun, snow, artificial sun lamps, and tanning booths. Patients usually present 6 to 12-hours postexposure complaining of eye pain, blepharospasm, tearing, photophobia, and foreign body sensation. Physical examination reveals an injected eye with decreased visual acuity. Corneal examination reveals **punctuate lesions** that are clearly demarcated by a protective covering, such as the inferior conjunctiva. Treatment consists of oral analgesics and lubricant antibiotic ointments. Cycloplegics and topical analgesic agents are not currently recommended for outpatient care. Treatment is guided to assist in the quick, natural healing capacity of the cornea, in which the patient should feel better in a couple of days. Follow-up examination with eye exam in 1 to 2 days should be arranged.

A superimposed corneal abrasion (**a**) is possible however does not manifest as bilateral punctate lesions. Traumatic iritis (**b**) usually occurs following blunt trauma and manifests with consensual photophobia and eye pain. Physical examination reveals ciliary flush, cells, and flare in the anterior chamber, and a sluggish pupil. A corneal foreign body (**d**) usually follows a traumatic injury in which the patient can recall something getting into the eye. Corneal foreign bodies can be visualized under slit lamp examination and may present with an associated abrasion or ulceration. The history and physical examination are not consistent with bacterial conjunctivitis (**e**), which manifests as thick purulent discharge, conjunctival inflammation, and irritation.

473. The answer is c. This patient has **orbital cellulitis,** an infection deep to the orbital septum. The patient had a recent upper respiratory infection and probable sinusitis, which likely resulted in orbital extension of the infection. *Staphylococcus aureus* and *Haemophilus influenzae* are common etiologies, and mucormycosis must be considered in diabetics and immunocompromised patients. Distinctive clinical findings of orbital cellulitis include eye pain, fever, **impaired eye mobility,** decreased visual acuity, and proptosis. Patients should be treated with IV **vancomycin plus a third-generation cephalosporin,** such as ceftriaxone or cefotaxime. If intracranial spread of infection is a concern, anaerobic coverage with IV metronidazole is warranted as well. In this case, the diagnosis is clear from the history and physical examination and treatment should be started promptly. Orbital cellulitis must be differentiated from preseptal cellulitis and allergic reactions. Preseptal cellulitis is a superficial infection that does not penetrate the orbital septum. Patients present with swollen, red eyelids, but no visual, pupillary or eye mobility changes.

Orbital and sinus CT scans (**d**) may be performed after antibiotics are started to rule out an abscess. CT scans are also useful when the diagnosis of orbital cellulitis is in consideration but not clinically clear. Patients older than 5 years with preseptal cellulitis may be treated with amoxicillin/clavulanate orally (**b**) and close follow-up with their regular doctor. Children younger than 5 years are at risk for systemic bacteremia and should be admitted for IV antibiotics. Patients with allergic reactions have swelling and erythema of the eyelids but no fever or tenderness to palpation. These patients may be treated with artificial tears (**e**) and antihistamines, such as diphenhydramine (**a**).

474. The answer is b. The patient has **giant cell arteritis (GCA)**, a vasculitis of medium-sized arteries that can affect vision and **lead to irreversible vision loss**. GCA typically affects **women** more than men, with the highest incidence in individuals **50 to 70 years of age**. Symptoms suggestive of GCA include headache over the eye or scalp, low-grade fever, ocular pain, jaw claudication, and decreased vision. Exam findings may include tenderness to palpation over the temporal region of the scalp and a prominent, beady temporal artery. Eye findings may include decreased visual acuity, APD, and, in late stages, a pale and edematous optic disc due to involvement of the ophthalmic artery. Fifty percent of patients with GCA have concomitant polymyalgia rheumatica, so a history of myalgia may be contributory. Erythrocyte sedimentation rate (ESR) is typically elevated, and diagnosis is confirmed via temporal artery biopsy. Treatment is **high-dose IV corticosteroids,** and it should be initiated promptly prior to biopsy to avoid vision loss.

Cycloplegics (**a**) are administered as part of treatment of uveitis and to facilitate funduscopic examination of the eye. IOP lowering medications (**c**) are used for the treatment of glaucoma. While temporal artery biopsy is undertaken to confirm the diagnosis of GCA, resection would not be appropriate treatment in this case (**d**). BP control (**e**) is appropriate long-term care for this patient; however, it is not the most appropriate next step.

475. The answer is a. This patient has an **orbital blowout fracture** of the inferior wall causing **entrapment of the inferior rectus muscle** and **restricted eye movement** resulting in **diplopia**. A CT scan with thin cuts through the orbits can confirm the diagnosis. Patients with this injury are generally started on oral antibiotics because of the risk of infection associated with sinus wall fractures and they may follow-up with the institution's appropriate surgical service in 3 to 10 days. These injuries are associated with other eye problems and a careful eye examination must be performed to rule out corneal abrasion, laceration, foreign body, as well as hyphema, iritis, retinal detachment, and lens dislocation.

The patient has no evidence of a retinal detachment (c), given his normal visual acuity and funduscopic examination. However, even with a normal examination in the ED, patients with orbital blowout fractures should be referred to an ophthalmologist for a repeat examination to rule out traumatic retinal detachment. Globe rupture (b) is more common with penetrating trauma and clues to this diagnosis are shallow anterior chamber, hyphema, irregular pupil, and significant decrease in vision. If a ruptured globe is suspected, a hard eye shield should be applied and ophthalmology should be consulted emergently. Do not check IOP in patients with suspected globe ruptured as this can worsen the injury. Cranial nerve III palsy (d) presents with problems with medial upward, and downward gaze, as well as ptosis. This patient only has difficulty with upward gaze suggesting that cranial nerve III is intact. Traumatic retrobulbar hemorrhage (e) causes anterior displacement of the globe and septum secondary to bleeding into the orbit. Because the globe has limited capacity for expansion, continued bleeding puts pressure on ocular structures and resultant proptosis. Optic nerve compression can result in permanent vision loss. Patients with a traumatic history and clinical signs suggestive of retrobulbar hemorrhage require emergency orbital decompression via lateral canthotomy and cantholysis.

476. The answer is c. This patient has an **APD**, also known as a **Marcus Gunn pupil**. In patients with an APD, light shined into the affected pupil causes a small dilation with no constriction. An APD is the result of a lesion in the anterior visual pathway of the retina, optic nerve, or optic chiasm preventing reception of the light in the affected eye. Neither pupil constricts since constriction is centrally mediated in the midbrain. APDs are sensitive for disease but not specific. The differential diagnosis for an APD includes central retinal artery or vein occlusion, optic neuritis and other optic nerve disorders, tumor, glaucoma, and lesions in the optic chiasm or tract.

Anisocoria (a) is unequal pupil size. Under normal room lighting, normal pupils may be 1 to 2 mm different in size. An Argyll Robertson pupil (b) constricts during accommodation (as expected) but does not constrict in response to light. This is usually seen in both eyes and is associated with neurosyphilis. Horner syndrome (**d**) is decreased sympathetic innervation of the eye from interruption of the sympathetic chain at any point from the brainstem to the sympathetic plexus around the carotid artery. Clinically, patients with Horner syndrome have ptosis, miosis, and anhidrosis. Normal pupillary response (**e**) to light is pupil constriction followed by a small amount of dilation.

477. The answer is b. On funduscopic examination, the patient has a **cherry-red macula** with a **pale retina** and less pronounced arteries. This is diagnostic of **CRAO**. The differential diagnosis for acute painless loss of vision includes retinal detachment, central retinal artery and vein occlusions, vitreous hemorrhage, and transient ischemic attack/cerebrovascular accident (CVA). An ophthalmologist should be called immediately when entertaining these diagnoses because a thorough funduscopic examination and prompt treatment is essential. Occlusion of the central retinal blood supply is commonly caused by emboli, thrombi, vasculitis, or trauma. Treatment aims to dislodge the clot from the main artery to one of its branches and includes digital massage, vasodilation, and lowering IOP.

Acute angle-closure glaucoma (**e**) usually causes painful loss of vision. Central retinal vein occlusion (**c**) presents similarly to retinal artery occlusion but is caused by thrombosis of the central retinal vein from stasis, edema, and hemorrhage. Funduscopic examination shows diffuse retinal hemorrhages and optic disc edema, also called the "blood and thunder" fundus. Treatment involves aspirin and prompt ophthalmology referral. Retinal detachment (**a**) occurs when vitreous fluid accumulates behind a retinal tear displacing the retina. On funduscopy, the retina will be hanging in the vitreous. Clinically, retinal detachment may be heralded by blurry vision or floaters followed by painless vision loss. Vitreous hemorrhage (**d**) is bleeding within the posterior chamber. On funduscopic examination, these patients have blood obstructing the view of the fundus. There are many causes of vitreous hemorrhage, including diabetic retinopathy, retinal detachment, hypertension, trauma, and age-related macular degeneration.

478. The answer is d. The patient has acute **traumatic iritis**, which usually occurs **within 3 days** of experiencing blunt trauma to the eye. Symptoms include pain, decreased visual acuity, photophobia, floaters, and tearing. Physical examination reveals perilimbic conjunctival injection, decreased visual acuity, and a sluggish pupil. The two hallmark findings are **consensual photophobia** and "**cell and flare**" on slit limp examination. Treatment is aimed at the prevention of synechiae formation and includes topical cycloplegics and steroids. Treatment should be initiated in conjunction with ophthalmology.

Corneal abrasions **(a)** are accompanied by pain, photophobia, and tearing. The diagnosis is confirmed by visualizing an epithelial defect on fluorescein staining. Hyphemas **(c)** generally present earlier (soon after the traumatic event) than traumatic iritis. They cause similar symptoms; however, RBCs will be visualized in the anterior chamber. Retinal detachments **(b)** can occur following blunt eye trauma and manifest with non-painful visual field defects, floaters, and flashes of light. Orbital blowout fracture **(e)** is classically a fracture of the inferior orbital wall manifesting with orbital contusion, soft tissue swelling, bony tenderness, infraorbital paresthesia, and potentially **entrapment of the inferior rectus muscle** with **restricted eye movements** and diplopia.

479. The answer is e. The picture shows **nodular episcleritis**, a benign inflammatory condition of the episclera characterized by the presence of namesake episcleral nodules. This is a **self-limited condition** often seen in young women. Origin is typically idiopathic, although it is associated with some underlying autoimmune syndromes such as Crohn's disease and rheumatoid arthritis. On examination, patients will have focal areas of redness and dilated, prominent episcleral vessels, with or without nodular inflammation. Visual acuity is unaffected and there is usually no pain with extraocular eye movements. Treatment is topical lubricants and oral nonsteroidal anti-inflammatory drugs (NSAIDs), and the condition usually resolves in 2 to 3 weeks.

Whereas the inflammation with episcleritis is focal, bacterial conjunctivitis **(a)** has diffuse redness and no accompanying nodules. Endophthalmitis **(b)** is inflammation of deep structures of the eye, presenting as diffuse redness as well as visual acuity loss, headache, discharge, and photophobia. Keratitis **(c)** is inflammation of the cornea, and would be expected to have an abnormal fluorescein examination as well as more diffuse redness. Compared to the benign episcleritis, scleritis **(d)** typically presents with scleral edema, ocular pain radiating to the face, painful extraocular eye movements, and photophobia. Application of topical phenylephrine eye drops causes constriction of episcleral blood vessels. There will be decreased injection and redness in episcleritis but not scleritis. Scleritis is an ophthalmologic emergency and should be promptly referred if suspected.

480. The answer is b. The vignette describes a **positive Seidel sign**, whereby a **full-thickness corneal injury** due to penetrating metallic foreign body is causing leakage of aqueous humor from the anterior chamber. This is a type of open globe injury, and **the eye should be shielded immediately and ophthalmology consulted for evaluation.**

Further manipulation of the eye, such as measuring IOP **(a)** may exacerbate injury. CT scan of the orbit **(c)** may be undertaken to further characterize injury or locate a metallic foreign body, but this should not delay ophthalmologic evaluation. Discharge on cycloplegics and antibiotics **(d)** or primary repair **(e)** is not standard of care for open globe injuries.

Recommended Readings

Banno F, Riccelli T, Banno M. Simultaneous parotitis and ipsilateral herpes zoster ophthalmicus: coincidence?. *BMJ Case Rep.* 2019;12(3):e228897.

Birinyi F, Mauger TF, Hendershot AJ. Ophthalmic conditions. In: Knoop KJ, Stack LB, Storrow AB, et al, eds. *The Atlas of Emergency Medicine.* 4th ed. McGraw-Hill.

Effron D, Forcier BC, Wyszynski RE. Funduscopic findings. In: Knoop KJ, Stack LB, Storrow AB, et al, eds. *The Atlas of Emergency Medicine.* 4th ed. McGraw-Hill.

Guluma K. Chapter 18. Diplopia. In: Marx JA, Hockberger RS, Walls RM, et al, eds. *Rosen's Emergency Medicine: Concepts and Clinical Practice.* 9th ed. Philadelphia, PA: Saunders, 2017.

Sainz de la Maza M, Jabbur NS, Foster CS. Severity of scleritis and episcleritis. *Ophthalmology.* 1994;101(2):389-396.

Sharma R, Brunette DD. Chapter 61. Ophthalmology. In: Marx JA, Hockberger RS, Walls RM, et al, eds. *Rosen's Emergency Medicine: Concepts and Clinical Practice.* 9th ed. Philadelphia, PA: Saunders, 2017.

Walker RA, Adhikari S. Eye Emergencies. In: Tintinalli JE, Ma O, Yealy DM, et al, eds. *Tintinalli's Emergency Medicine: A Comprehensive Study Guide.* 9th ed. McGraw-Hill.

Weaver CS, Knoop KJ. Ophthalmic trauma. In: Knoop KJ, Stack LB, Storrow AB, et al, eds. *The Atlas of Emergency Medicine.* 4th ed. McGraw-Hill.

Prehospital, Disaster, and Administration

Michael Mancera, MD, FAEMS

Questions

The following scenario applies to questions 481 to 483.

During an emergency medical services (EMS) ride along, your team receives a call for multiple injured patients after an explosion at a city building. When you arrive at the scene, there is an incident commander (IC) who instructs you that there are dozens of injured casualties and delegates you to help triage the wounded according to the simple triage and rapid treatment (START) system. You are directed to a secure area where the fire department EMS has brought dozens of injured office workers. You approach a patient who has several abrasions on his torso, face, and extremities. He has no spontaneous respirations. You perform a chin lift and note chest wall movement and audible spontaneous respirations.

481. What color triage tag would you assign this patient?
a. Green
b. Yellow
c. Red
d. Blue
e. Black

482. As responders arrive and begin clearing rubble and debris, significantly more injured patients are found. Additional fire and EMS units are requested. According to the National Incident Management System (NIMS), when an event such as this involves multiple jurisdictions from a variety of backgrounds, which of the following is the most appropriate type of command structure?

a. Area command
b. Regional command
c. Team command
d. Unified command
e. Variable command

483. What is the key defining characteristic of a disaster?

a. Location of the incident
b. Number of patients injured
c. Types of injuries involved
d. Use of chemical, biological, or radiological agents
e. Mismatch between available and required resources

484. While working in the emergency department (ED), you receive a medical control radio call from EMS regarding a 38-year-old woman who developed acute severe respiratory distress while eating a peanut-based dish at a local restaurant. She has erythematous wheals all over her body and has diffuse wheezes on auscultation. Her blood pressure is (BP) 92/55 mm Hg, heart rate (HR) is 115 beats/minute, respiratory rate (RR) is 28 breaths/minute, and oxygen saturation is 98% on room air. EMS informs you that they are a basic unit. What are the most appropriate initial orders for the EMS unit given their level of training?

a. Administer supplemental oxygen and proceed to the ED as quickly and safely as possible
b. Establish intravenous (IV) access and administer IV epinephrine and a normal saline bolus
c. Establish IV access and administer a normal saline bolus
d. Administer intramuscular (IM) epinephrine
e. Perform orotracheal intubation for impending respiratory failure

485. A married couple is hiking a mountain in a large national park, when one partner slips and falls down a steep hill. He hits his chest wall on a tree trunk, and a branch impales his left flank. He also hears a "pop" from his left knee and cannot move his lower leg. He is conscious and tells his partner to go for help because he cannot move and is having difficulty breathing. His partner hikes back to the park ranger's headquarters for assistance. The ranger calls report over the radio requesting assistance in transporting the patient to your ED, which is located approximately 50 miles away. There is a service road adjacent to the hiking trail and it is a clear, sunny day. What is the most appropriate transfer modality to send to the scene?

a. Send an EMS van via the service road to extricate the patient and transfer him to the ED
b. Send the park ranger in his mountain terrain–equipped vehicle to extricate the patient and bring him back to his headquarters where EMS personnel will be waiting for transfer
c. Send a rotary-wing helicopter and have the park ranger mobilize ground transport to the scene for assistance if necessary
d. Send an EMS pickup chassis with an integrated modular patient care compartment as the patient may need advanced monitoring during transfer
e. Send a fixed-wing EMS aircraft and mobilize the park ranger's mountain terrain–equipped vehicle to extricate the patient and transport him to the aircraft

The following scenario applies to questions 486 to 488.

A railroad freight car is overturned while traveling through a suburban area and hundreds of gallons of chemical waste are spilled at the scene. Several railroad crew members were heavily exposed to the chemicals and are reported to be in critical condition. Some have already died from the exposure. The IC sets up a hot-zone perimeter and has designated decontamination zones. You receive a call from a hazardous material (HAZMAT) paramedic unit with a patient in distress who they believe will not survive long.

486. Under which of the following circumstances is it acceptable to immediately transport the patient directly from the hot zone without going through decontamination?

a. If it is reasonably certain that the patient will not survive long enough for the decontamination process
b. If the toxic chemical is identified and the EMS personnel have adequate equipment to reasonably ensure their safety
c. If the IC orders EMS to bypass the decontamination zone due to the patient's impending deterioration
d. If the resources at the incident site are overwhelmed by the number of contaminated people and decontamination cannot be performed rapidly
e. It is never acceptable to bypass the decontamination process after a toxic exposure, especially if the toxin is unknown

487. After successfully passing through the decontamination zone tents, several patients are brought to your ED for medical evaluation and treatment. They are complaining of intense abdominal cramps, vomiting, blurry vision, and sweating after being exposed to the chemicals spilled during the train derailment. What toxidrome do their symptoms most closely resemble?

a. Antimuscarinic
b. Cholinergic
c. Opiate
d. Sedative hypnotic
e. Sympathomimetic

488. You correctly diagnose organophosphate poisoning and quickly get in touch with local medical control. You request mobilization of the county's supply of Mark-1 auto-injector kits because your hospital has a very limited supply. What do these auto-injectors contain?

a. Atropine and pralidoxime
b. Benadryl and physostigmine
c. Clonidine and ondansetron
d. Diazepam and rivastigmine
e. Naloxone and flumazenil

The following scenario applies to questions 489 to 491.

An Emergency Medical Dispatcher receives a 9-1-1 call from a frantic family member who found their 67-year-old mother lying on the ground unresponsive at their home residence. They report that she has a pulse in both wrists, however does not appear to be breathing. After verifying the caller's pertinent demographic information and dispatching the appropriate EMS unit to the scene, the Emergency Medical Dispatcher stays on the line with the caller in order to provide additional pre-arrival instructions.

489. Which of the following is an appropriate pre-arrival instruction that the Emergency Medical Dispatcher is qualified to give to the caller?

a. Administer the patient's home BP medication
b. Establish cervical spine precautions
c. Initiate cardiopulmonary resuscitation (CPR)
d. Open and clear the patient's airway
e. Reposition the patient in an upright seated position

490. EMS arrives on scene in a timely fashion, secures the patient, and begins transporting her to the hospital. En route to the ED, the patient losses pulses and shows ventricular fibrillation on the monitor. On arrival, EMS tells you that she has been pulseless for 10 minutes. You immediately continue resuscitative efforts via advanced cardiac life support (ACLS) guidelines. After several administrations of ACLS medications and several rounds of CPR, you are contemplating terminating the code due to medical futility. Which of the following factors would lead you to continue your resuscitative efforts?

a. The arrest was witnessed by a bystander or EMS who immediately began CPR
b. Before the cardiac arrest, the patient was compliant with taking her cardiac medications
c. The patient has an automated implantable cardioverter-defibrillator (AICD)
d. The patient has previously survived an out-of-hospital cardiorespiratory arrest
e. The patient's initial out-of-hospital rhythm was asystole

491. What is the single most important predictor of survival in adult out-of-hospital cardiac arrest?

a. Bystander aspirin administration
b. Early defibrillation
c. Endotracheal (ET) intubation
d. Epinephrine administration
e. Rapid transportation to the ED

492. A patient is brought in by EMS after sustaining injuries from a motor vehicle accident. Law enforcement arrives with the patient and informs you that the patient is under arrest. Your patient's vital signs are stable. You send basic blood work, including blood alcohol level, a chest radiograph, and a urinalysis. The blood alcohol level comes back above the legal limit for operating a motor vehicle. The rest of the workup is unremarkable. The police officer requests a copy of the patient's medical record. What is the proper response to his request?

a. Because the patient is in police custody, he does not have the same right to privacy as nonincarcerated citizens; hence, you are obliged to give the officer his records
b. Refusal to give the officer the records is considered obstruction of justice and you can be found criminally liable if you do not comply with his request
c. Unless the patient consents, you are obligated to refuse the officer's request for a copy of the medical records as this violates the patient's rights to privacy under the Health Insurance Portability and Accountability Act (HIPAA)
d. As a licensed physician, you are allowed to use your best judgment in a case-by-case basis regarding the release of medical records of incarcerated patients to law enforcement officers as long as you document your rationale in the medical record
e. You may release all pertinent medical information, but can withhold certain data from your workup that may incriminate the patient in order to protect their rights in a subsequent trial

493. A 67-year-old man is brought to the ED by EMS with a chief complaint of chest pain. He is found to be short of breath and diaphoretic. He reports that he vomited 1 hour ago and subsequently feels better. He describes substernal chest pressure that started while doing yard work. He has a history of coronary artery disease and hypertension. He has regularly scheduled appointments with a cardiologist at a neighboring hospital. He requested to be taken to that hospital, but EMS refused and brought him to your ED because it was only 5 minutes away. The patient is angry and requests a transfer to his cardiologist's hospital, which is 20 minutes away. What is the best course of action?

a. You must politely refuse his request and work the patient up for acute coronary syndrome and admit him to your hospital if indicated
b. Contact the neighboring hospital; if the patient's cardiologist accepts the patient, authorize an ambulance transfer for continuity of care
c. Transfer the patient only if he has stable vital signs and his cardiologist is on-call at the neighboring hospital
d. Transfer the patient immediately and inform EMS that they should have respected the patient's wishes in the prehospital setting
e. Perform the appropriate medical screening examination (MSE), in this case at least an electrocardiogram (ECG) and basic laboratory tests including a troponin, before considering a transfer

494. EMS responds to a call for a suicide attempt. The patient is a 58-year-old man who was recently diagnosed with pancreatic cancer and, according to the family, has been extremely depressed. The patient tried to hang himself in his room in a suicide attempt and when family found him gasping for air, they cut him down. He has a weak and thready pulse, sonorous respirations with stridor, and poor air entry. He also has crepitus over the soft tissue of his neck and he appears pale. The family informs EMS that he recently signed a Do Not Resuscitate (DNR) and they have the proper documentation. EMS calls in for your advice on how to proceed. Which of the following is the most appropriate response?

a. The patient has a DNR order; therefore, EMS must abide by his advance directive and take no intervention
b. Advise EMS bring the patient to the ED as quickly as possible and while providing only supportive care
c. Secure the patient's airway, but inform EMS that they cannot proceed with CPR if the patient loses his pulse
d. Secure the patient's airway and provide full supportive care, disregarding the patient's DNR directive due to the suicide attempt
e. Tell EMS to stand by and contact your hospitals medical ethics board for counsel

The following scenario applies to questions 495 and 496.

EMS is responding to a call at a local high school football game. One of the high school football players is unresponsive to verbal stimuli after a helmet-to-helmet collision with another player. His BP is 100/65 mm Hg, HR is 60 beats/minute, and RR is 12 breaths/minute. There is a small crack at the top of the helmet, but it is otherwise intact and strapped tightly to the patient's head.

495. EMS calls medical control to request permission to remove his helmet in order to assess for head trauma. What is the most appropriate prehospital management of this patient?

a. Do not attempt to remove the helmet, maintain cervical spine precautions, and transfer the patient on a backboard to the hospital
b. While maintaining cervical spine precautions, carefully remove the helmet and assess for head injury
c. Check the patient's pupils and if there is asymmetry, remove the helmet with cervical spine precautions
d. Wait at the scene for a physician to arrive with an electric saw for removal of the helmet and further on-scene assessment
e. Do not remove the helmet but assess the cervical spine for step-off or any signs of obvious injury before transfer

496. The patient's overall condition is noted to deteriorate. His BP is 100/60 mm Hg, HR is 60 beats/minute, RR is 6 breaths/minute, and oxygen saturation is 89% on room air. The patient is also noted to have a closed right wrist deformity, with distal pulses intact. Which of the following should be performed first by the paramedic level EMS providers prior to transport?

a. Airway control
b. Disrobing and complete exposure
c. Large bore IV access for volume resuscitation
d. Parenteral analgesic administration
e. Stabilization and splinting of fractures

The following scenario applies to questions 497 to 499.

An EMS physician medical director is called to the scene of a motor vehicle accident to assist EMS providers with field care of an injured patient. The patient is a 41-year-old man who was the driver of a small sedan that struck a tree at a high rate of speed. He was wearing a seatbelt and airbags did deploy. The patient is unresponsive with unstable vitals. The patient is entrapped in the vehicle, with his right lower extremity pinned underneath the vehicle's dashboard. EMS crews and firefighters on-scene have been unable to extricate the patient and called the EMS physician medical director to the scene for further on-scene medical care.

497. Which of the following is a qualification of the medical oversight physician for an EMS agency?

a. Prior experience practicing as a prehospital provider
b. A medical license
c. EMS subspecialty board certification
d. Certification from the National Highway Traffic Safety Administration (NHTSA)
e. Passing the State paramedic level entry exam

498. Which of the following best describes direct medical oversight by a physician EMS medical director?

a. Quality Assurance review process
b. Credentialing of EMS providers
c. Providing real-time treatment orders via radio to an EMS provider
d. Protocol development
e. Setting education standards for EMS providers

499. The extrication process is successful. The patient has a large laceration with pulsatile bleeding from his right lower extremity. Which of the following is most appropriate next step?

a. Apply direct pressure
b. Tourniquet application
c. Emergent field limb amputation
d. Establish large bore IV access
e. Administer tranexamic acid (TXA)

Prehospital, Disaster, and Administration

Answers

481. The answer is c. In mass-casualty incidents, one of the most vital components of triage is to assign the **appropriate acuity level of injury** in an easy to implement, standardized, and efficient manner. The most widely used triage system is the START system that focuses on assessing three parameters. These are as follows:

1. Respirations
2. Perfusion
3. Mental status

Patients are assessed based on these three parameters and then assigned a colored triage tag corresponding to one of the following triage categories:

Immediate: immediate care and transfer necessary
Delayed: delayed transfer and care until all "reds" are cleared
Minor: "walking wounded" and lowest priority to transfer
Deceased: dead at the scene from nonsurvivable injuries

Patients who are wounded but are able to walk on scene are given a green tag (**a**) signifying a low priority and are attended to or transferred last. Next, patients are assessed for ability to breathe. If they are not breathing, the airway is positioned. If breathing resumes, they are labeled "red" (**c**) as depicted in the previously mentioned example. If no spontaneous breathing resumes, they are labeled "black" (**e**). If they are breathing spontaneously and have an RR greater than 30 breaths/minute, they are assigned a red tag (**c**). In patients with a spontaneous RR below 30 breaths/minute, next their perfusion is assessed by checking a radial pulse and capillary refill. If there is no radial pulse or if the capillary refill is greater than 2 seconds, they are assigned a red tag (**c**). For those with a radial pulse or capillary refill under 2 seconds, the next step is a brief mental status examination in which they are asked to follow simple commands (eg, squeeze the examiner's hand). If they cannot do this, they are given a red tag (**c**). However, if they can follow simple commands, they are given a yellow tag (**b**). There is no blue tag (**d**) in the START system. The following image is an example of a START Triage tag, sometimes used by EMS services to designate a patient's triage category.

Simple Triage and Rapid Treatment (START)

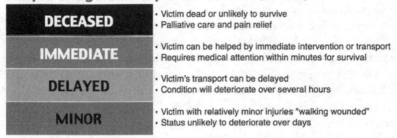

DECEASED	• Victim dead or unlikely to survive • Palliative care and pain relief
IMMEDIATE	• Victim can be helped by immediate intervention or transport • Requires medical attention within minutes for survival
DELAYED	• Victim's transport can be delayed • Condition will deteriorate over several hours
MINOR	• Victim with relatively minor injuries "walking wounded" • Status unlikely to deteriorate over days

482. The answer is d. After the events of September 11th 2001, the United States government and Department of Homeland Security made a concerted effort to better organize and coordinate disaster response, especially when multiple agencies and jurisdictions are responding to an incident. The result was the creation of the **NIMS**, which emphasizes a standardized framework approach to incident commands by focusing on **common terminology, structured multijurisdictional cooperation, and unified command**. NIMS is now overseen by the Federal Emergency Management Agency (FEMA). Within the NIMS incident, command structure responders report to one and only one supervisor to minimize confusion. There are several key command staff positions (safety officer, public information officer, and liaison officer) headed by an IC. The general staff also includes operations, planning, finance, administration, and logistics sections.

There are several different command structure options depending on incident specific factors. The most common is a single IC structure in which there is one IC overseeing the event. **Unified command is used when there are multiple agencies or jurisdictions responding to a single incident.** It involves two or more individuals sharing the authority of the IC position and acting as a single entity. Area command (**a**) is used in the setting of multiple incidents that are all interrelated but spread over a relatively large area. In this situation, each location will have an IC, who then reports to an area command, which assists with coordination among the separate ICs.

Regional, team, and variable command (**b, c, and e**) are not formal terms used in the NIMS system.

483. The answer is e. Disasters can be natural or man-made events. They affect local areas, however can expand beyond that to regional, state, or national levels depending on the underlying incident. A disaster is defined by a **mismatch between available and required resources,** when the available resources are exceeded by the need for additional resources. Resource management is critical during a disaster for all levels of the healthcare system.

Although the location (**a**), number of patients (**b**), types of injuries (**c**), and use of chemical, biological, or radiological agents (**d**) might be important factors in a large-scale incident, these are not defining characteristics of a disaster. EMS agencies play an important role in both disaster preparedness and response. Training exercises for disasters are common for EMS providers, focusing on operational procedures and protocols. These exercises are often coordinated with hospital systems and other public safety agencies.

484. The answer is d. The National Highway Traffic and Safety Administration Act of 1966 set recommendations for first responder and emergency medical technician (EMT) training courses. Because prehospital personnel are covered by state and in some cases local authority, the State Board of Emergency Medical Services is authorized to modify some aspects including recommended course lengths and scope of practice, leading to variances in EMS systems and practices from state to state. There are **four major levels of EMS training and credentialing established within the National EMS Scope of Practice Model. These are as follows:**

1. **First responders** include mandatory training given to firefighters, police officers, and community EMS responders. These are often the first people to arrive on scene. They are trained in CPR, basic life support (BLS), and basic trauma care. Current recommendations are approximately 40 hours of training.
2. **Emergency medical technician basic (EMT-B)** is the lowest EMT level. They can perform BLS, automated external defibrillation (AED), basic assessments, and assist in medication administration. They cannot establish IV access; however, in almost all states they can administer IM medications based on predefined protocols or via a verbal order from an online medical physician. The recommended curriculum is a course length of 110 hours.

3. **Emergency medical technician intermediate (EMT-I)** personnel have completed EMT-B requirements and are trained in procedures such as establishing IV access, ET intubation, and manual defibrillation. Current recommendations are approximately 300 to 400 hours of training.
4. **Emergency medical technician paramedic (EMT-P)** is the most advanced EMT level. They receive all EMT-I training in addition to training to perform advanced airway procedures, needle decompression of the chest, ECG interpretation, external pacing, and advanced drug therapy within predefined standardized protocols. Recommendations for their training curriculum range from 1000 to 1200 hours.

In this case, the patient is having an **anaphylactic reaction** secondary to a peanut allergy. The best initial treatment is IM epinephrine. **EMT-B units** are trained to administer **IM medications**; in some states, they may require an order from the online medical physician before administration. Although the patient requires emergent transport (**a**), an EMT-B unit should be able to provide potentially life-saving care on scene. EMT-I units are trained to establish IV access in order to administer IV fluids (**c**) and medications (**b**), as well as perform ET intubation when indicated (**e**).

485. The answer is c. There are **three modes of transportation** available to most EMS systems: ground transportation, rotary-wing air (helicopter) transportation, or fixed-wing air (small plane) transportation. Ground transportation is used for the vast majority of acutely ill or injured patients. **Air transport is indicated when air transport time would be significantly less than ground transport time. Other indications for air transport** are severe injury in which rapid transport is essential; unstable vital signs; significant trauma in patients younger than 12 years; patients older than 55 years or pregnant; multisystem injuries; ejection from a vehicle; pedestrian struck or motorcyclist struck; death in same passenger compartment; penetrating trauma to the abdomen, pelvis, chest, neck, or head; crush injury to the abdomen, chest, or head; and fall from significant height. This is not an exhaustive list and the specific scenario and clinical assessment must always be factored into every individual case.

Once the decision to use air transportation has been made, the next decision is to employ a rotary-wing or a fixed-wing aircraft. A rotary-wing aircraft has a range of 50 to 150 miles and is indicated in scenarios of entrapped trauma patients with extrication time expected to exceed

20 minutes or locations in a topographically difficult-to-reach area by ground transportation. Keep in mind that rotary-wing air transportation is limited by poor weather and both modes of air transport carry an inherent risk of crashing that must be considered by the physician. A fixed-wing aircraft is indicated for distances longer than 100 miles when rapid transport is essential. This mode of transportation is also limited by weather, lack of runways, and refueling. One must also consider possible altitude problems for the patient such as pneumothorax, ET cuff, and balloon catheters. However, there are no absolute contraindications to fixed-wing air transport.

In this case, even though there is a service road adjacent to the hiking trail, ground transportation (a, b, and d) is not appropriate due to several factors, including prolonged travel time (the nearest hospital is 50 miles away), a topographically difficult-to-reach surface area, and prolonged extrication time. In this scenario, a rotary-winged aircraft (helicopter) would be ideal because it could assist in the extrication process as the hiker fell down a steep hill and cannot move. A fixed-wing aircraft (e) is not the best choice because ground transportation would still be needed and the patient would have to endure a prolonged extrication time. Additionally, the patient has difficulty breathing secondary to blunt chest trauma suggestive of a pneumothorax, which could be significantly worsened by the altitude required by fixed-wing transport.

486. The answer is e. The most important rule of disaster management for chemical agents is **the contaminated patient should never be allowed to enter the ED before being decontaminated**. Each state has a standard operating procedure for mass casualty decontamination. The following are critical steps in the management of chemical mass casualty exposures:

- Recognition of a toxic chemical exposure
- Rapid identification of the agents involved
- Information retrieval on the toxicity and secondary contamination potential of the agent
- Proper protection of self, hospital personnel, already hospitalized patients, and the facility itself from secondary contamination or loss of serviceability to other patients
- Decontamination and triage of victims
- Stabilization and medical treatment of victims
- Protection of the community-at-large from secondary contamination

This question pertains to the decontamination step of a toxic chemical exposure, which is clearly of imminent risk to the surrounding community because some of the crew has already died. Patient decontamination should occur outside the hospital. Hot, warm, and cold zones should be established and cordoned off with brightly colored tape. The **hot zone** is the area of the toxic substance exposure or may be the hospital area where arriving patients with no prior decontamination are held. The **warm zone** is an area where thorough decontamination and further medical stabilization occur. This area should be arranged so that there is no risk of primary contamination, but secondary contamination (transfer of the toxic substance from the victim to personnel or equipment) may occur. Hence, only trained personnel with the proper personal protective equipment (PPE) are allowed in the hot and warm zones. The **cold zone** is the area to which fully decontaminated patients are transferred. The warm and cold zones should be established upwind, uphill, or upstream of the hot zone to minimize extension of the hot zone into other decontamination areas. There is no personnel flow between the different zones. The following figure is a schematic representation of a HAZMAT incident area.

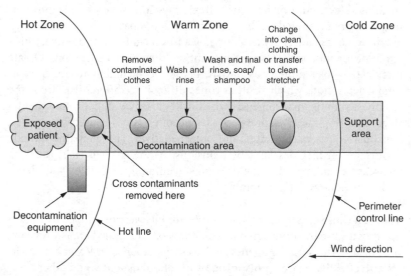

(Reproduced with permission from Shareaf Walid, MD.)

There are no circumstances in which hot and warm zone decontamination can be bypassed, especially in the event of a potentially lethal exposure. Bypassing contamination zones (**a, b, c, and d**) would put the public-at-large, including the ED, which is never acceptable. One salient point to remember is that **clothing should be removed quickly** as this act is thought to accomplish 80% of the decontamination.

487. The answer is b. The patients' symptoms are consistent with a **cholinergic toxidrome**, which can be caused by chemicals (eg, carbamates and organophosphates), chemical weapons that act as nerve agents (eg, tabun, sarin, and VX gas), and several types of mushrooms. The toxidrome can be remembered with the mnemonic **DUMBBELLSS**, which stands for diarrhea, urination, miosis, bradycardia, bronchospasm, emesis, lacrimation, lethargy, salivation, and seizure. Hyperstimulation of cholinergic receptors causes a generalized outpouring of **gastrointestinal (GI) and respiratory secretions**, which is usually the most prominent initial clinical finding. The toxidrome can also be remembered as the **"Killer Bs,"** referring to **bronchorrhea, bronchospasm, bradycardia, and seizure**, which represent the **most common causes of death**.

The antimuscarinic toxidrome **(a)**, also commonly referred to as the anticholinergic toxidrome, will present with hot, flushed and dry skin, mydriasis, fever, and myoclonus, often times in a state of delirium. It is frequently remembered by the phrase "blind as a bat, mad as a hatter, red as a beet, hot as hades, dry as a bone." Causes include antihistamines, antipsychotics, antidepressants as well as antiparkinsonian medications. Opiate intoxication **(c)** manifests as miosis, depressed mental status, and respiratory depression, which is often times difficult to differentiate from the sedative hypnotic toxidrome **(d)** which will present with depressed mental status and respiratory depression as well, often times caused by alcohol, benzodiazepines, barbiturates, and other sedatives. The sympathomimetic toxidrome **(e)** includes anxiety, delusions, paranoia, mydriasis, seizures, tachycardia, and hypertension. It is most commonly associated with drugs such as cocaine and amphetamines.

488. The answer is a. Mark-1 auto-injector kits were developed by the US military for use by servicemen in situations of potential chemical warfare, specifically against **nerve agents** such as sarin, tabun, and VX gas. The kits are also **effective against poisoning by organophosphates** and other similar chemicals that cause inactivation of acetylcholinesterase by irreversibly binding the enzyme and inhibiting it from breaking down acetylcholine. This results in massive amounts of acetylcholine building up in nerve terminals causing hyperstimulation of cholinergic receptors. The Mark-1 kits contain two agents, atropine sulfate and pralidoxime chloride, in a dual-chambered auto-injector that can be self-administered. Atropine acts as a competitive antagonist at the acetylcholine receptor, thereby blocking the effects of the increased acetylcholine in the nerve terminal. Pralidoxime works by binding the organophosphate-inactivated acetylcholinesterase, changing the chemical conformation of the enzyme allowing the organophosphate to be cleaved, resulting in regeneration of functional acetylcholinesterase. Over time, organophosphates and other nerve agents will undergo aging, a process after which the use of pralidoxime is ineffective. For this reason, **prompt administration of the antidotes is critical.** Mark-1 kits are rarely kept in large numbers within hospitals, and for this reason large caches of the kits are kept and managed by many states, as well as the federal government. On the federal level, the Office of Public Health Preparedness manages **CHEMPACK,** a supplemental supply of antidotes suitable for treating large-scale exposures to nerve agents and organophosphate pesticides. Each CHEMPACK is designed to treat a thousand patients, and contains Mark-1 kits, diazepam, and sterile water. Access to these resources should be done in conjunction with local and state officials, as local and state resources should be accessed first in a disaster.

Benadryl (**b**) is an antihistamine that has some anticholinergic properties; however, no role in the treatment of acute cholinergic poisoning. Physostigmine (**b**) and rivastigmine (**d**) are acetylcholinesterase inhibitors and would worsen the cholinergic poisoning. Ondansetron (**c**) is a serotonin antagonist used to control nausea and vomiting, and can be used to aid in symptomatic care but will not treat the underlying cause of poisoning. Clonidine (**c**) is a central α_2-adrenergic agonist which will decrease sympathetic outflow, and is commonly used to treat hypertension as well as opiate withdrawal. Naloxone (**e**) is an opiate reversal agent used in the setting of opiate overdose. Diazepam (**d**) is a benzodiazepine that can be used to treat the seizures associated with cholinergic poisoning, but is not contained within the Mark-1 kit. Flumazenil (**e**) is a gamma aminobutyric acid (GABA) receptor antagonist which can be used to reverse benzodiazepine overdose, although its use is limited by a significant side-effect profile.

489. The answer is d. In the United States, 9-1-1 was adopted as the universal emergency telephone access number in 1973, and since then has been the mainstay of public access to emergency services such as police, fire, and EMS. 9-1-1 Dispatch centers are staffed by specially trained and qualified operators called Emergency Medical Dispatchers who are regulated by the EMS subdivision of the NHTSA, which falls under the oversight of the Department of Transportation (DOT). Emergency Medical Dispatchers are trained to use a chief complaint centered, standardized algorithm to determine the priority and severity of the call, in order to dispatch the appropriate level of EMS unit. After establishing the priority level of the call and dispatching the appropriate unit, the operator can then provide the caller with **simple instructions for potentially life-saving maneuvers** based on the situation.

In the previously mentioned case, the most appropriate action would be to open and clear the patient's airway **(d)** of any potential obstruction. The patient appears to be apneic, and clearing an airway obstruction could be a rapid and lifesaving maneuver. While initiating CPR **(c)** is an instruction that the operator is qualified to give, this patient has a pulse and thus does not require CPR at this time. Many EMS systems have opted to provide compressions-only CPR instructions to bystanders, avoiding the mouth-to-mouth breaths, to simplify telephone instructions and improve bystander compliance. Administering the patient's home medications **(a)** is not a part of the BLS algorithm, and bystanders are generally not advised to give home medications beyond aspirin for cardiac-related complaints. Bystanders are encouraged to leave the patient in the position in which they were found, and to avoid repositioning or moving them in any way **(e)** provided that the scene is safe. However, if CPR is needed, dispatchers will instruct callers to position the patient flat on the floor. While the impetus for encouraging bystanders to leave the patient unmoved is to avoid potential cervical spinal cord injury, there is no recommendation for bystanders to establish or maintain formal cervical spine precautions **(e)**. 9-1-1 dispatch operators are also trained and qualified to give basic instructions regarding hemorrhage control as well as childbirth assistance in the pre-arrival period after appropriate EMS units have been dispatched.

490. The answer is a. In 2010, a metaanalysis of 79 studies spanning 1950-2008 involving 142,740 patients with presumed out-of-hospital cardiac arrest found parameters that **predicted increased survival to hospital discharge**. EMS should be queried about the presence or absence of these factors to help the physician gauge the utility of continuing resuscitative efforts. Survival was found to be more likely among those cardiac arrests that were **witnessed by a bystander** (13.5%-6.4%), **witnessed by EMS** (18.2%-4.9%), **who received bystander CPR** (16.1%-3.9%), were **found**

in ventricular fibrillation/ventricular tachycardia (23.0%-14.8%), **or achieved return of spontaneous circulation** (33.6%-15.5%).

Patients who have a witnessed arrest tend to have EMS arrive quicker and usually have CPR begin sooner. Hence a witnessed arrest, although not the cause of increased survival, correlates with other factors that lead to improved survival. Medication compliance **(b)** is not an independent predictor of out-of-hospital cardiac arrest survival to hospital discharge. Patients who present in cardiorespiratory arrest with AICDs **(c)** are already refractory to cardioversion or defibrillation. Survival of a prior arrest **(d)** has not been shown to favor survival in future arrests. An initial rhythm of asystole **(e)** is actually a poor prognostic indicator for survival.

491. The answer is b. Several studies have demonstrated that **early defibrillation is the single most important predictor of survival** in out-of-hospital cardiac arrest, and thus early bystander AED use should be emphasized and encouraged in the general public. Many organizations, including the American Heart Association, strongly encourage active efforts to decrease time to defibrillation. The most important method of improving the quality and efficacy of resuscitative efforts revolves around public education and awareness in regards to early identification of cardiac arrest, early initiation of CPR, and prompt AED application and use. While aspirin use **(a)** in the setting of cardiac arrest secondary to coronary artery thrombosis could provide important antiplatelet activity, this is not as important as early defibrillation. Control of the airway via ET intubation **(c)** and epinephrine administration **(d)** are important features of full ACLS resuscitation and should be performed by qualified ALCS-certified providers; however, this does not confer the same increase in predicted survival that early defibrillation does. Reduced transport time to a facility capable of managing a cardiac arrest is associated with increased chances of survival; however, AED use should not be delayed for the sake of faster transportation **(e)**.

492. The answer is c. The **HIPAA (1996)** was created to **protect patients' privacy rights** by establishing rules for disclosures of confidential health information. The act was intended to standardize health information transfers, require identification numbers for providers, health plans, and employers, and to protect confidential protected health information (PHI). The inclusion of PHI protection resulted from fears that electronic transfers and ID numbers could be misused. Hence, the law penalizes disclosures of confidential health information that are not authorized in writing by the patient. The secretary of health and human services imposes civil monetary penalties for violation of any HIPAA requirement, up to $25,000 per disclosure. Police officers do not have automatic access to a patient's medical record, even if the patient is in their custody. Only if the police serve you with a subpoena for court-ordered medical records are you obligated to share them without the patient's written consent.

Incarcerated patients (a) are still protected by HIPAA regulations and are entitled to confidentiality of PHI. As a physician, there are no legal ramifications for abiding by HIPAA regulations; in fact, both you and your institution are liable for monetary and civil penalties if HIPAA rules are broken (b). HIPAA privacy regulations are not subject to case-by-case discretionary judgments (d) but rather must be followed with only certain special exceptions, such as psychotherapy notes and disclosures for billing issues, which are outside the physician's scope of practice. Answer choice (e) is incorrect because unauthorized release of medical records violates the HIPAA laws.

493. The answer is e. The **Emergency Medical Treatment and Labor Act (EMTALA)** mandates that **unstable patients cannot be discharged or transferred except for medical necessity**. The purpose of EMTALA was to discourage low-income and high-risk patients from being transferred from one ED to another for financial advantage. Under EMTALA, any patient presenting to an ED has the right to an MSE to determine if an emergency medical condition (EMC) exists without regard to the patient's ability or willingness to pay for services rendered. If an EMC exists, the hospital must stabilize the condition within its capacity. If the hospital cannot stabilize the condition, the staff is further obligated to transfer the patient to a facility capable of providing adequate care. It is important to understand that an MSE is not simply a triage examination, and requires any further indicated workup including consultations if necessary, to determine if an EMC exists. If an EMC is not yet stabilized, a transfer cannot be made unless the transferring physician certifies that the benefits outweigh the risks and the transfer is medically appropriate. Additionally, the transferring hospital must do everything in its capacity to minimize the risk of transfer, and the receiving hospital must have available space and personnel and agree to accept the patient. Any hospital that negligently violates an EMTALA policy can be penalized up to $50,000 per violation and physicians who negligently violate may also have to pay up to $50,000 per violation. Civil money penalties such as EMTALA violations are not covered by malpractice insurance.

In this vignette, the patient has a history of coronary artery disease and presents with shortness of breath, diaphoresis, chest pressure, and vomiting. Given his history, presentation, age, and risk factors, it is clear that the patient is at high risk for a myocardial infarction (MI). Hence, the proper MSE is an ECG and troponin in order to rule out an MI before transfer (**a, b, c, and d**). If the patient is having an MI and the current facility has the capability of providing effective management based on standard-of-care protocols, they are obliged to admit the patient to their facility. If the current facility does not have the capacity to effectively treat the patient (ie, a cardiac catheterization suite), they can transfer the patient if a receiving hospital agrees to accept him and he is deemed stable for transfer.

494. The answer is d. The DNR order was created to allow individuals to provide an advance directive to EMTs regarding their desire for or against resuscitative treatment. This vignette evokes a dilemma where the ethical wishes of rescuers to act for the good of their patient (ie, beneficence) contradicts the individual's autonomous wishes expressed in the DNR order. **In the case of a suicide**, especially within the context of the patient's depression at the news of his recent diagnosis of pancreatic cancer, **treatment is necessary**. The patient must be returned to a level of functioning where it is possible to demonstrate that the decision to end life is truly an autonomous decision. In clinically depressed patients, there is legal precedent that judgment is clouded by disease and the respect for patient autonomy is superseded by beneficence or malfeasance. EMTs are usually not in a position to determine if a patient is autonomous; thus, they should treat the patient by stabilizing them and transporting them to a facility where a definitive evaluation can be performed.

Answer choices (**a, b, and c**) place the patient's autonomy before beneficence based on his EMS-DNR order, which is not appropriate considering the patient's reported depression and suicidal gesture. Answer choice (**e**) is incorrect because the situation does not afford the time to seek counsel from a medical ethics board. Additionally, it is appropriate to override autonomy in suicidal cases without contacting a medical ethics board.

495. The answer is a. A properly fitted football helmet with shoulder pads holds the head in a position of neutral spinal alignment; **field removal of these devices is not recommended**. Instead, the helmet and shoulder pads should remain on as the athlete is immobilized and transported on a rigid backboard. Simultaneous removal of the helmet and shoulder pads should be done after clinical assessment and radiographs at the hospital. Radiographs can be repeated after removal of the helmet as clinically indicated.

The proper removal of a football helmet requires four people and should not be attempted out of hospital (**b**). Even with pupil asymmetry, the EMT's best course of action is to expeditiously transport the patient to the ED for definitive care because EMTs are not trained to perform any techniques to relieve impending uncal herniation (**c**). The use of an electric saw is not indicated and unnecessary prehospital delays should be avoided (**d**). Adequate cervical spine assessment is unreliable and potentially dangerous in the prehospital setting and would also unnecessarily delay transport (**e**).

496. The answer is a. Recommended on-site interventions in the setting of traumatic injury are the subject of much debate, as delays in transportation to a facility capable of providing definitive treatment are associated with worse outcomes. This must be balanced with the need to perform lifesaving maneuvers in the field in order to provide some degree of stability prior to transport and improve patient outcomes. **Rapid transportation should be emphasized; however, life-saving interventions by EMS providers should not be delayed.** If there is significant hypoxia, or inability to protect the airway, then qualified providers should establish **airway control prior to transportation**, as hypoxia can lead to worse neurologic outcomes for the head injured patient. Airway should be prioritized for this specific patient given that he has a decreased RR and is now hypoxic. Advanced airway options for the paramedic level provider generally include ET intubation and supraglottic airway devices. The other routinely indicated on-scene intervention is stoppage of frank uncontrolled hemorrhage as hemorrhagic shock can be rapidly fatal, if left unaddressed.

While disrobing the patient (**b**) in order to completely expose any potential injury is key to accurate diagnosis. This should be performed carefully in a warm environment if possible, such as inside the ambulance, as not to induce hypothermia which is strongly recommended to be avoided in trauma patients. Large bore IV access (**c**) should be obtained as a part of Advanced Trauma Life Support (ATLS) protocol; however, it should not delay transportation to definitive care. He is currently not hypotensive and does not require emergent fluid resuscitation. Parenteral analgesia (**d**) is not indicated emergently for this patient; however, this may be later required if the patient remains intubated for transport depending on postsedation protocols. Splinting of fractures (**e**) may be needed for this patient, however should not be prioritized before airway control for this unstable patient.

497. The answer is b. The NHTSA mandates that all ALS level EMS agencies have a physician medical director, and most states require all levels of EMS services to have physician medical direction. State regulations and laws differ regarding specific qualifications of a physician medical director; however, it **universally required that the physician holds a valid medical license.** Many EMS medical directors are Emergency Medicine trained physicians, likely due to the close working relationship EDs traditionally have with area prehospital services; however, this is not a requirement.

In 2013, the first EMS subspecialty board certification **(c)** was administered by the American Board of Emergency Medicine (ABEM) and currently there are a growing number of Accreditation Council of Graduate Medical Education (ACGME) accredited EMS fellowships within the United States that focus on training highly qualified prehospital physicians. Although this is becoming a common pathway for physicians to become EMS medical directors, fellowship training and board certification are not required by regulation by the any governing authority. The NHTSA also does not offer a certification exam for physicians **(e)**. It is also not mandated that medical directors were prior EMS providers **(a)**, or that they pass a state paramedic level entry exam **(d)**. It is critically important for the physician who practices as a medical director to become familiar with their State's regulations and qualification requirements.

498. The answer is c. Physician medical directors provide oversight and leadership for EMS agencies. The medical director has many responsibilities; however, their oversight duties are commonly described as either **direct or indirect** medical oversight nature. **Direct medical** oversight consists of **real-time participation in clinical care of patients in the prehospital setting.** This most often occurs when a physician provides **real-time treatment orders via radio** to an EMS crew. This could also involve a medical director physician providing clinical care to a patient on-scene in the prehospital setting. Although physician on-scene care is less common in the United States as opposed to some other countries, it is gaining popularity in some EMS systems and some systems have established ground physician response programs staffed by physicians to assist their EMS system.

Indirect medical oversight consists of many responsibilities that do not involve real-time clinical patient care. These often include administrative duties, such as Quality Assurance review **(a)**, credentialing EMS providers **(b)**, developing EMS protocols **(d)**, and setting education standards for

EMS providers (e). These types of medical oversight duties are instrumental to EMS systems.

499. The answer is a. The case describes **life-threatening hemorrhage** from a large laceration. The pulsatile description is highly suspicious for arterial involvement. This requires immediate recognition and treatment to prevent exsanguination. The first-treatment modality for massive hemorrhage is **direct pressure to the wound.** In our case, since the wound is on an extremity that is now accessible following extrication, direct pressure should immediately be applied.

Although tourniquet application (b) does have a role in hemorrhage control, and may be required if bleeding continues despite direct pressure, it is not the first-recommended treatment. Studies have demonstrated that tourniquets provide benefit in massive bleeding and are considered safe to use by EMS providers. Similarly, TXA (e) may provide benefit when administered early to patients with massive hemorrhage by preventing the breakdown of clotted blood; however, it is not the first-line treatment. IV access (d) is important for any critically ill patient, but should not be prioritized over life-saving interventions such as hemorrhage control. Emergent field limb amputation (c) would not be considered in this case, as the patient is described to have already been extricated from the vehicle. This type of advanced procedure would generally be performed by a physician experienced in prehospital field care.

Recommended Readings

American College of Emergency Physicians (ACEP). EMS and disaster preparedness. Available at: http://www.acep.org/disaster. Accessed June 1, 2020.

Bass R, Lawner B, Lee D, et al. Medical oversight of EMS systems. In: Cone D, Brice J, Delbridge T, et al, eds. *Emergency Medical Services: Clinical Practice and Systems Oversight.* 2nd vol. 2nd ed. Hoboken, NJ: Wiley, 2015: 71-84.

Bucher J, Zaidi H. A brief history of emergency medical services in the United States. In: Rogers L, Arshad F, Lenz T. *EMS Essentials: A Residents Guide to Prehospital Care.* Dallas, TX: Emergency Medicine Residents' Association, 2016.

Federal Emergency Management Agency (FEMA) Emergency Management Institute. Available at: http://training.fema.gov/emi.aspxFEMA

Incident Command Systems Resource Center. https://www.fema.gov/incident-command-system-resources. Accessed June 1, 2020.

National Association of State EMS Officials. National EMS Scope of Practice Model 2019 (Report No. DOT HS 812-666). Washington, DC: National Highway Traffic Safety Administration.

Sasson C, Rogers AM, Dahl J, et al. Predictors of survival from out-of-hospital cardiac arrest: a systematic review and meta-analysis. *Circ Cardiovasc Qual Outcomes.* 2009;3:63-81.

Thomas S, Brown K, Oliver Z, et al. An evidence-based guideline for the air medical transportation of prehospital trauma patients. *Prehosp Emerg Care.* 2014;18(1 Suppl):35-44.

Walls R, Hockberger, Gausche-Hill M, et al. *Rosen's Emergency Medicine: Concepts and Clinical Practice.* 9th ed. Part VI: Emergency Medicine Services. Philadelphia, PA: Elsevier, 2017.

Wound Care

Megan E. Gussick, MD

Questions

500. A 25-year-old man presents to the emergency department (ED) with a right forearm laceration that he sustained from a piece of glass during a bar fight. He complains of pain at the laceration site, but denies foreign body sensation. On examination, the laceration is superficial and 4 cm in length. The patient demonstrates intact strength and sensation distally. Which of the following statements regarding radiographic imaging of this patient is true?

a. Imaging can be omitted because he does not have foreign body sensation
b. Imaging is not indicated because retained glass does not cause an inflammatory reaction
c. Plain films are the next best step in the management of this patient
d. Computed tomographic (CT) scan is the most commonly used modality to rule out foreign body
e. Plain films cannot rule out bone, teeth, or glass fragments larger than 2 mm in soft tissues

501. A 30-year-old woman presents to the ED with a left hand laceration. She reports cutting herself while attempting to slice a bagel. She has a superficial 2-cm laceration over the left thenar eminence. No deeper structures are involved. What is the best way to clean the wound?

a. Punch holes in a normal saline bag or bottle and irrigate the wound
b. Use a high-pressure syringe and irrigate with water
c. Wound cleaning is unnecessary because the wound was sustained from a clean knife
d. Soak her hand in normal saline for 30 minutes
e. Apply povidone-iodine to the wound

502. A 40-year-old man presents to the ED with a left foot puncture wound from stepping on a rusty nail. His last tetanus vaccine was during childhood and resulted in a severe allergic reaction and a prolonged hospital stay. Which of the following is true regarding tetanus immunization in this patient?

a. Give tetanus toxoid
b. Give tetanus immunoglobulin
c. Give tetanus immunoglobulin and toxoid
d. Give neither tetanus toxoid nor immunoglobulin
e. Give tetanus toxoid and immunoglobulin with diphenhydramine

The following scenario applies to questions 503 and 504.

A 12-year-old girl presents to the ED with a left index finger laceration that she sustained when her friend accidentally closed the car door on her finger. She has a semicircular laceration distal to the distal interphalangeal (DIP) joint on the volar surface of the left second digit. Sensation distal to the laceration is intact. Range of motion at the DIP joint is intact.

503. Which of the following is the best method to provide anesthesia in this patient?

a. Irrigation of the wound with 3 cc of lidocaine
b. Local infiltration through the wound margins with 3 mL of lidocaine
c. Local infiltration through the wound margins with 3 mL of lidocaine with epinephrine
d. A digital block at the base of the proximal phalanx with 3 mL of lidocaine
e. A digital block at the base of the proximal phalanx with 3 mL of lidocaine with epinephrine

504. Which of the following alternative methods of anesthesia would also be appropriate?

a. Injection of 5 mL of 1% lidocaine with epinephrine in the region of the ulnar nerve
b. Injection of 5 mL of 1% lidocaine with epinephrine in the region of the median nerve
c. Injection of 5 mL of 1% lidocaine with epinephrine in the region of the radial nerve
d. Injection of 5 mL of 1% lidocaine with epinephrine in the region of the musculocutaneous nerve
e. Perform moderate sedation with a combination of ketamine and propofol

505. A 27-year-old man presents to the ED after an altercation with the laceration shown in the following figure. There are no dental fractures and his tetanus immunization is up-to-date. What are the most appropriate next steps in management?

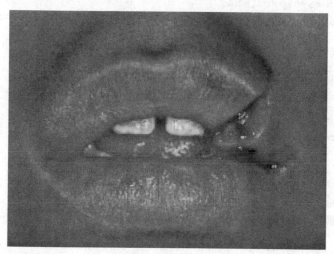

(Reproduced, with permission, from Knoop KJ, Stack LB, Storrow AB. Atlas of Emergency Medicine. New York, NY: McGraw Hill; 2002:162.)

a. Infraorbital nerve block and approximation of the vermilion border
b. Infiltration of local anesthesia into the lip and approximation of the vermilion border
c. Infraorbital nerve block, closure of mucosal defects before the approximation of the vermilion border
d. Infiltration of the lip with local anesthesia, closure of dermis and mucosal defects, and then approximation of the vermilion border
e. Closure with a commercially available tissue adhesive and Steri-Strips to avoid distorting tissue architecture

The following scenario applies to questions 506 and 507.

A 44-year-old woman presents to the ED with a deep puncture wound to her left forearm after she was bitten by her neighbor's dog. The animal is appropriately vaccinated.

506. Which of the following is best initial approach to wound management in this patient?

a. Irrigate the wound thoroughly, reassure the patient that infections following animal bites are rare and thus prophylactic antibiotics are not indicated, and discharge the patient home

b. Irrigate the wound thoroughly, suture it to prevent infection, and discharge the patient home

c. Irrigate the wound thoroughly, begin prophylactic antibiotics, and discharge the patient home with instructions to keep the wound clean and allow it to heal spontaneously

d. Irrigate the wound thoroughly and consult the on-call infectious diseases specialist as dog-bite infections are most commonly secondary to *Pasteurella multocida*

e. Place a dry pressure dressing over the wound, apply topical antibiotics, and discharge the patient home

507. The patient is concerned that she might contract rabies as a result of the dog bite. Which of the following statement is true?

a. Dog bites are the most common source of rabies transmission to humans worldwide

b. Bat bites are the most common source of rabies transmission to humans worldwide

c. Most deaths resulting from rabies occur in the United States

d. Rabies is caused by a gram-positive rod bacterium

e. Human rabies immunoglobulin (HRIG) is an effective treatment for rabies

508. A 23-year-old man presents to the ED complaining of a wound to his left lower extremity. He was pulling branches out of a flooded creek in his backyard, when he punctured his left calf. His legs were in the water when the wound occurred. The puncture wound is 1 cm in diameter, several centimeters deep, and demonstrates surrounding erythema. After irrigating the wound, you discover a splinter within the wound. Which of the following is the most appropriate next step(s)?

a. Obtain radiographs to evaluate for additional foreign bodies

b. Suture the wound using 4-0 nylon suture in a simple interrupted fashion

c. Dress the wound with a sterile bandage and treat with an oral fluoroquinolone

d. Remove the splinter and treat with an oral fluoroquinolone

e. Remove the splinter, suture the wound, and treat with an oral fluoroquinolone

The following scenario applies to questions 509 and 510.

A 21-year-old woman presents to the ED with a superficial 2-cm mid-forehead laceration sustained from a fall. You irrigate and close the wound. She is concerned about her long-term cosmetic outcome and requests detailed wound care instructions.

509. Which of the following statements would be an appropriate wound care instruction to give?

a. Avoid direct sun exposure while the wound is healing
b. The wound should not be washed until sutures are removed
c. Sutures should be removed in 7 to 10 days
d. Appearance of the scar at suture removal will be the final cosmetic outcome
e. Good suturing technique and meticulous wound care guarantee no scar formation

510. While cleaning up after suturing her wound, you inadvertently stick yourself with the dirty needle. You follow the appropriate postexposure procedures and have her blood drawn for hepatitis B and C and HIV testing. When you get home and explain what happened to your spouse, he is concerned that you may contract an infectious disease as a result of the exposure. Which of the following statements is true?

a. Both breast milk and bile contain higher titers of hepatitis B virus (HBV) than blood in persons infected with HBV
b. The most common side effect of HIV postexposure prophylaxis is headache
c. Hepatitis C virus (HCV) is more efficiently transmitted through blood than HBV
d. The average risk of transmission of HIV after a percutaneous exposure to HIV-infected blood is approximately 0.3%
e. Zidovudine therapy for 4 weeks is appropriate postexposure prophylaxis for HIV

511. A 9-year-old girl is brought to the ED by her parents after she sustained a forehead laceration from hitting against a doorknob. The patient is cooperative, but anxious about the upcoming anesthetic injection. She has a 0.5-cm laceration on the mid-forehead with clean edges. Her parents inquire about "skin glue." Which of the following statements is true regarding cyanoacrylate tissue adhesives?

a. Tissue adhesives cannot be applied to mucous membranes and areas with thick hair
b. Tissue adhesives have a higher rate of infection and tissue dehiscence than sutures
c. Tissue adhesives are best suited for forehead lacerations between 5 and 10 cm in length
d. Tissue adhesives are applied inside the wound to pull skin edges together
e. Tissue adhesives must be covered with topical antibiotics and bandages to prevent sloughing

512. A 30-year-old chef presents to the ED with a complete fingertip amputation. Her knife slipped while chopping vegetables. She brought the amputated pulp in a plastic bag. On examination, the patient has a clean, 5 mm in diameter dermal slice on the distal volar tip of the second digit. There is profuse nonpulsatile bleeding. There is no trauma to the DIP joint, proximal interphalangeal (PIP) joint, or the nail. Her most recent tetanus booster was 1 year ago. Which of the following is the most appropriate next step in management?

a. Consult hand surgery for replantation of the pulp in the operating room
b. Irrigate the hand and replant distal tip in the ED as soon as possible
c. Perform a digital block with lidocaine and epinephrine to control bleeding
d. Immediately place the amputated tip on ice to prevent cell death
e. Discharge the patient with a pressure dressing and splint after the wound is irrigated and the bleeding is controlled

513. A 25-year-old graduate student presents to the ED stating that approximately 4 hours ago she burned her left hand after spilling a very small amount of a 5% hydrofluoric (HF) on herself. The patient says the symptoms were initially quite mild, but now the pain is severe. Examination of the affected area reveals a 3-cm area on the dorsal surface of the left hand that is white with surrounding erythema, exquisite tenderness, and edema with multiple small bullae. No other injuries are evident. What is the most initial step in the management of this patient?

a. Perform a wrist block, irrigate the hand with tap water for 10 minutes, place a dry dressing, and discharge home with instructions to follow-up with hand surgery in 1 to 2 days
b. Apply 2.5% calcium gluconate gel to the affected skin
c. Inject 5% calcium gluconate directly into the affected skin
d. Nebulize 2.5% calcium gluconate and have the patient breathe the solution for 30 minutes
e. Update the patient's tetanus and inject 8.4% sodium bicarbonate solution directly into the affected skin

514. A 23-year-old painter is working with a high-pressure paint spray-gun when he inadvertency discharges the spray-gun into his left hand. He had immediate and severe pain and notices a small puncture wound to the left palmar surface of his hand. Upon arrival to the ED, the wound is hemostatic with minimal surrounding erythema, but intense/severe pain reported by the patient. Which of the following is true regarding the presentation and management of high-pressure injection injuries?

a. The degree of damage is often overestimated based on the wound appearance
b. Pain management is best achieved by local infiltration with 1% lidocaine
c. Delayed management leads to better wound healing
d. There is a low risk for compartment syndrome if injury occurs to the hand
e. Early surgery consultation for fasciotomy/debridement should occur

515. A 19-year-old man presents with multiple small lacerations over the dorsum of his right hand. Patient states he is "unsure" of how he sustained the injury and is vague in further questioning. Examination reveals multiple small lacerations (<10 mm) over the third and fourth metacarpophalangeal (MCP) joints with associated swelling and bruising. He has a normal neuro-vascular examination. What is the best management of this injury?

a. Obtain radiographs to identify any foreign body/fractures, clean the wounds with soap and water, leave the wounds open, and place a splint on the hand to promote healing of the wounds over the MCP joints
b. Clean the wounds thoroughly with high-pressure syringe and sterile water, close the wounds with 5.0 nonabsorbable sutures with follow-up for suture removal in 10 to 14 days
c. Clean the wounds thoroughly with high-pressure syringe and sterile water, close the wounds with tissue adhesive
d. Obtain radiographs to identify any foreign body/fractures, clean the wounds thoroughly with high-pressure syringe and sterile water, leave the wounds open, and start patient on amoxicillin-clavulanate
e. Obtain radiographs to identify any foreign body/fractures, clean the wounds thoroughly with high-pressure syringe and sterile water, leave the wounds open, and start patient on doxycycline

516. A mother brings in her 6-month-old baby to the ED because she has been inconsolable and fussy for the past few hours. Mother reports that the infant is otherwise healthy, without recent illness and no history of trauma. After a thorough exam, you find the infant to have swelling and erythema of the left second toe. Which of the following is true regarding this condition?

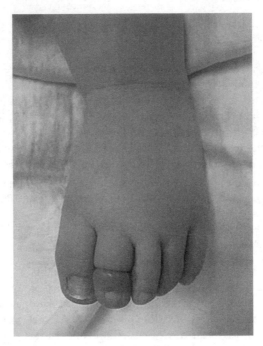

(Reproduced with permission from Adam J. Rosh, MD, and Rosh Review.)

a. This is commonly caused by an infection and should be treated with cephalexin
b. This is commonly caused when the infant's hair becomes wrapped around the digit
c. This commonly requires surgical intervention for successful removal
d. If incision is necessary for removal, it is best to make an incision perpendicular to the hair on the flexor surface of the toe
e. It is safe to trial use of a chemical depilatory agent for removal

The following scenario applies to questions 517 and 518.

A 12-year-old girl is out playing in her backyard when she finds a kitten. She is able to trap the kitten and plans to bring it home as a pet. While carrying the kitten back to her house, the kitten bites her left forearm. The girl drops the kitten and runs home to tell her father who then promptly brings the patient in for evaluation.

517. Evaluation in the ED reveals two small puncture wounds on the left hand over the dorsal surface with no active bleeding, no erythema, and normal neurovascular exam. Which of the following should be avoided in the management of this girl's wound?

a. Thoroughly examine the wound as well as perform a neurovascular exam of the hand
b. Obtain radiographs to identify any foreign bodies including possible teeth
c. Thoroughly clean the wound with high-pressure syringe and sterile water
d. Close the wound with tissue adhesive
e. Provide prophylactic antibiotics

518. Several days later, the patient's father brings the girl back into the ED for fever, swelling, purulent drainage, and erythema extending to the elbow with subsequent streaking to the axilla. What is best course management for this patient on her second ED visit?

a. Broaden patient's oral antibiotics to include methicillin-resistant *Staphylococcus aureus* (MRSA) coverage and have her follow-up in 1 to 3 days
b. Culture the wound and await results to determine need for change in antibiotics
c. Culture the wound, give single dose of IM ceftriaxone, and have her continue the current course of antibiotics until culture results return
d. Culture the wound, start ciprofloxacin, and admit to the hospital for ongoing parenteral antibiotics
e. Culture the wound, start ampicillin/sulbactam, and admit to the hospital for ongoing parenteral antibiotics

519. Which of the following eyelid lacerations can be repaired primarily in the ED without ophthalmology consultation?

a. Laceration involving the medial canthus
b. Laceration involving the upper lid extending into the eyebrow
c. Laceration involving the inner surface of the eyelid
d. Laceration involving the lid margins
e. Laceration involving the tarsal plate

Wound Care

Answers

500. The answer is c. On **plain films**, 80% to 90% of foreign bodies can be seen. **Glass larger than 2 mm** is visible on plain film.

Foreign body sensation **(a)** has a sensitivity of 43% and specificity of 83%. Therefore, lack of a foreign body sensation cannot be used to rule out a foreign body. Retained foreign bodies may lead to a local granulomatous inflammatory response or to local and systemic infection **(b)**. CT is capable of detecting more types of foreign bodies than plain film, but it is not commonly used given the time needed and expense **(d)**. Plain film can usually locate metal, bone, teeth, pencil graphite, gravel, sand, and aluminum **(e)**. Plain film cannot detect wood, thorns, some plastics, and other organic matter.

501. The answer is b. To achieve low bacterial counts through irrigation, a **pressure of 5 to 8 psi is recommended.** This pressure can be generated with an **irrigation syringe** or a **35-mL syringe and a 19-gauge needle.** Water (both sterile or tap) is as equally efficacious as sterile normal saline. The common recommendation for the amount of irrigant to use is **60 to 100 cc per 1-cm wound length.**

Using normal saline bottles or bags with holes **(a)** may not generate adequate pressure. Soaking **(d)** is ineffective in cleansing wounds. Disinfectants **(e)** such as povidone-iodine should not be used on an open wound because they can impair host defenses and promote bacterial growth. Last, irrigation is necessary **(c)** regardless of the method of the sustained injury.

502. The answer is b. Tetanus toxoid is contraindicated in patients who have had a severe allergic reaction, including respiratory distress or cardiovascular collapse. **Tetanus immunoglobulin can be used in these patients.** Local reaction at injection site resulting in redness, pain, and swelling is not considered a contraindication.

The use of tetanus toxoid is contraindicated (**a and c**) even if the patient is given diphenhydramine (**e**). The patient should be given immunoglobulin (**d**), if the injury is high-risk (eg, puncture wound from a rusty nail).

503. The answer is d. Performing a **digital block** with lidocaine at the base of the finger will block the digital nerves allowing for appropriate anesthesia. To perform a digital block, place the patient's hand on a sterile field with the palmar surface flat on a table. Cleanse the appropriate MCP joint and surrounding area and then insert the needle into the dorsal aspect of the web space on either side at a 60 degree angle of insertion toward the palm. Withdraw the plunger slightly to ensure you have not entered the digital artery, and inject approximately 1 mL of anesthetic into the web space slowly withdrawing the needle toward the dorsal aspect of the web space. This is repeated on the opposite side of the affected digit.

Local infiltration and digital block (**c and e**) with lidocaine and epinephrine are incorrect as epinephrine is relatively contraindicated in areas of end-organ circulation (eg, tip of nose, glans penis, scrotum, ears, nose, and fingers). Irrigating a wound with anesthetic (**a**) does not provide adequate anesthesia. Although local infiltration (**b**) will provide adequate anesthesia, it may interfere with good wound approximation and therefore may lead to a poor cosmetic result.

504. The answer is b. The **median** nerve supplies sensation to the volar aspect of the second digit, as well as the radial half of the third and fourth digits, and the ulnar half of the first digit.

The ulnar nerve (**a**) provides sensation to volar aspect of the fifth digit and the ulnar half of the fourth digit. The radial nerve (**c**) supplies the volar radial half of the first digit. On the dorsal surface of the hand, the ulnar nerve supplies the fifth digit and the ulnar half of the fourth digit, the median nerve supplies sensation to the distal aspects of the second and third digit and approximately half of the distal aspect of the fourth digit, and the radial nerve supplies the remaining portions of the dorsal hand. This is shown in the following figure.

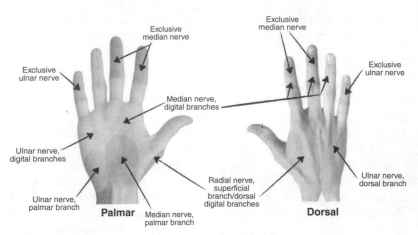

(Reproduced with permission from Adam J. Rosh, MD, and Rosh Review.)

The musculocutaneous nerve **(d)** would be blocked in the area of the axillary portion of the brachial plexus and provides sensation to the forearm and is therefore inappropriate for the wound in question. Moderate conscious sedation **(e)** is inappropriate for a wound of this scope where adequate local or regional anesthesia can be provided.

505. The answer is a. This is a laceration of the face crossing the vermilion border (demarcation of the lip mucosa and facial skin). The goal of repair in this case is **approximation of the vermilion border** with less than 2 mm of displacement because significant displacement is cosmetically unappealing. An **infraorbital nerve block** is required because local anesthesia would distort tissue anatomy, thereby limiting appropriate approximation. The first stitch should focus on approximating the border before closing the other aspects of the wound.

Infiltration with local anesthesia **(b and d)** will distort the tissue anatomy and may make proper alignment unreliable. It should only be used if the patient fails nerve block. Initial alignment of the dermis or mucosal aspects of the laceration **(c and d)** may make approximation of the vermilion border difficult. Tissue adhesive and Steri-Strips **(e)** should not be used to close the lip as it is subject to pulling forces of facial movement. Wound separation in this case could result in a cosmetically unappealing outcome.

506. The answer is c. Puncture wounds, owing to their depth, cannot be cleaned adequately. Often, closure is not necessary in small puncture wounds that, following initial management in the ED, demonstrate adequate healing. However, for large puncture wounds, **delayed primary closure** can improve the cosmetic outcome and decreases the risk of abscess formation and wound infection.

Approximately 5% of dog bites and 40% of cat bites become infected and the risk of infection depends on many host factors (ie, immunity, blood flow in small skin capillaries, etc.) as well as more physician-centered factors such as the ability to cleanse the wound appropriately. Given that this patient suffered a puncture wound that will not be able to be cleaned adequately, discharging the patient without prophylactic antibiotics (**a**) is incorrect. Copious irrigation is crucial in preventing wound infections. Most bite wounds can be repaired with primary closure, however puncture wounds, small lacerations, and hand and foot wounds carry higher risks of infection and therefore are best managed with delayed primary closure and when closed should not be closed "tightly," so that whatever bacterial load has settled into the wound has an portal to exit (**b**). *Pasteurella* is the most common organism in cat bites (**d**) and concern over a possible Pasteurella infection would not be a reason to initiate an emergent consult to an Infectious Disease specialist in the ED. The most commonly used antibiotic for dog and cat bites is amoxicillin/clavulanate (**e**). Clindamycin with a fluoroquinolone can be used for dog bites in penicillin-allergic patients. Doxycycline can be used for cat bites in penicillin-allergic patients. Topical antibiotics are not an appropriate prophylactic antibiotic choice in a patient with a puncture wound suffered from an animal bite.

507. The answer is a. Worldwide, **dog bites** are far and away the most common vector of rabies transmission to humans.

Rabies is an infection caused by a number of Lyssaviruses (**d**) and when contracted by humans, is uniformly fatal. The incubation period between acquisition of the virus and the manifestation of clinical symptoms is anywhere between 2 and 12 weeks. In the United States, bats are the most common vector of transmission to humans (**b**). The United States has approximately one to two deaths (**c**) from rabies each year, and most of the deaths worldwide occur in Asia. There is no known treatment for rabies (**e**); however, HRIG, if given immediately following a potential exposure, can decrease the risk of developing the disease. The Centers for Disease Control and Prevention (CDC) recommends receiving one dose of HRIG immediately following the exposure, with as much of this dose as possible given around the affected area and rabies vaccine, followed by three additional doses of rabies vaccine over a 14-day period.

508. The answer is d. Foreign bodies with potential to cause an infection and inflammatory response **require immediate removal** (eg, thorns, splinters, spines, teeth, and soil-covered objects). These materials may cause intense and excessive inflammatory responses. If the ED physician cannot remove the foreign body, the appropriate specialist should be consulted. After the splinter is removed, the patient should be treated with an outpatient fluoroquinolone. Wounds with stagnant freshwater exposure are at high risk of infection with gram-positive bacteria, *Pseudomonas*, and *Aeromonas* species, and require empiric antibiotic coverage.

Because organic materials are radiolucent, radiographs will not assist in locating organic foreign bodies (**a**). Thorough direct visual inspection is necessary to locate and remove all organic foreign bodies. Treatment with antibiotics (**c**) is necessary, but less important than the removal of the foreign body. Closing a puncture wound, especially with a retained foreign body, will lead to an inflammatory response and likely infection. Closing this patient's wound would not be appropriate management (**b and e**).

509. The answer is a. Direct sun exposure during healing can lead to permanent hyperpigmentation. Therefore, patients should be advised to **avoid direct sun exposure** and use sunblock for up to 12 months after the injury.

Patients should be instructed to wash the wound with gentle soap and water (**b**), as early as 8 hours after sutures are placed. Although the wound should be kept dry, instructing against washing is inappropriate. Healing wounds should be patted dry to avoid dehiscence from forceful wiping. The patient should be informed that all lacerations scar (**e**). Good repair and wound care will improve the appearance of the scar but will not inhibit scar formation. Wounds that heal by delayed closure have the poorest cosmetic outcome. Good wound edge approximation, use of appropriate suture material, and early suture removal all lead to better cosmetic outcomes. The early appearance of the scar is not reflective of the long-term outcome (**d**). Facial sutures should be removed in 3 to 5 days. Leaving sutures in for 7 to 10 days leads to a poorer cosmetic outcome (**c**).

510. The answer is d. The rate of contracting HIV after percutaneous exposure to infected blood is **0.3%,** and the rate of contracting HIV from mucus membrane exposure to infected blood is **0.09%.**

Blood is by far the most efficient transmission medium for HBV (**a**). HCV is not transmitted efficiently through blood, with an average rate of seroconversion in persons exposed to infected blood of 1.8% (compared to a 20% to 30% seroconversion rate in exposure to hepatitis B-infected blood) **(c)**. In persons exposed to HIV-infected blood who go on antiretroviral prophylactic therapy, gastrointestinal side effects **(b)** are by far the most common adverse effects of these drugs. Monotherapy with zidovudine **(e)** is never appropriate postexposure prophylaxis. There are multiple regimens, but the most basic of which is a two-drug regimen involving a nucleoside analogue and a protease inhibitor.

511. The answer is a. **Tissue adhesives** close wounds by forming an adhesive layer that brings the edges of the laceration together. They **cannot be used on mucosal membranes and areas with thick hair**. For optimal results, it should be applied in three to four layers in a dry, bloodless field.

Tissue adhesive rate of infection and dehiscence are comparable to sutures when used appropriately **(b)**. They are best suited for small (<5 cm), clean, straight wounds in low-tensile areas **(c)**. It is applied as a layer on the intact epithelium while holding close approximation of the wound edges. It cannot be used inside the wound because it leads to an intense inflammatory reaction **(d)**. After application, the wound must be left open to air. Applying topical antibiotics and bandages would cause prolonged exposure to moisture leading to weakening of the adhesive layer **(e)**. Patients should be instructed not to pick at the edges of the layer and allow it to slough off naturally in 5 to 10 days.

512. The answer is e. This patient has a less than 10-mm dermal slice that is generally managed with **bleeding control, nonadherent dressings, and a finger splint to prevent reinjury and decrease pain**. Dressing changes have to be performed every 24 to 48 hours. Fingertip amputation greater than 10 mm, exposure of the bone, or involvement of the nail may require a hand surgeon consultation. However, this patient's dermal slice is 5 mm and does not involve the phalanx or nail; therefore, it can be managed conservatively. Pressure dressing is typically sufficient to control bleeding in dermal tip amputations. If hemostasis is not achieved with direct pressure, commercial hemostatic agents can be used.

The management of fingertip amputations is controversial. For amputations involving a significant amount of the distal digit, various techniques, such as partial-thickness skin grafts and full-thickness skin grafts, exist. Most of these are performed in the operating room by a hand surgeon. However, replantation of a less than 10-mm dermal tip is not indicated **(a, b, and d)**. Despite replantation, the amputated tip is most likely to necrose and slough off. Using the amputated piece as a natural dressing is unnecessary given the small size of the wound. Digital blocks (c) are helpful for pain relief while the patient irrigates the distal tip. Epinephrine is not recommended for use on the digits. The most appropriate way to achieve hemostasis is with direct pressure.

513. The answer is b. The most appropriate initial step is to **apply 2.5% calcium gluconate gel to the wound.** HF acid burns can superficially appear very benign, and often the more dilute the solution is, the greater the risk for toxicity because the recognition of symptoms is often delayed. Tissue damage from HF acid burns is caused by both corrosive burns from the hydrogen ions themselves, and also chemical burns from tissue penetration of the fluoride ions. After penetrating, the fluoride ions form insoluble salts with calcium and magnesium and also form soluble salts with other cations that then dissociate rapidly leading to further release of fluoride ions and more tissue destruction. Systemic toxicity occurs when the body's stores of calcium and magnesium become depleted leading to enzymatic dysfunction and subsequently cellular death. The majority of deaths result from fatal cardiac arrhythmias.

While injecting 5% calcium gluconate (c) into the wound may ultimately prove to be the definitive treatment for this patient, this is not the next step. Calcium gluconate acts to bind the fluoride ions at the side of injury. Nebulized calcium gluconate (d) would not allow for the drug to have any impact on the injury. While analgesia and local wound care are important (a), this does not actually treat the HF acid exposure. Although HF acid is classified as a weak acid, injecting sodium bicarbonate (e) is not an appropriate or effective treatment for this injury.

514. The answer is e. High-pressure injection injuries commonly occur in the foot and hand, especially nondominant hand, and occurs typically with paint or oil. **These are high-risk injuries with significant complications.** Although the initial appearance of the wound is innocuous, there is significant risk for damage to the deeper fascial layers. **Hand surgery consultation should occur early as debridement and fasciotomy are recommended to occur within 6 hours to prevent the need for amputation.** Patients and providers can underestimate the underlying damage based on the appearance (a). Patient's will typically present with severe pain despite minimal visible injury. Pain control is best achieved with **parenteral analgesics.** Injection of local anesthetics is contraindicated as this may further worsen the tissue injury and reduce perfusion secondary to increased pressure (**b**). Compartment syndrome is a significant risk for high-pressure injection injuries. This occurs because of the increased pressure in the tissues secondary to the injection of air/liquid itself, but also occurs because of the edema that develops over the next few hours (**d**). If evaluation is delayed, these injuries can lead to amputation in up to 30% of cases (**c**).

515. The correct answer is d. This young male is presenting with an injury/wound suspicious for a **closed-fist injury and secondary human bite**. Any wound over the surface of the third and fourth MCP or PIP of the dominant hand should be considered a closed-fist injury and treated as such. The abrasions/lacerations are sustained when the closed fist strikes the face and/or teeth of the victim. These lead to crushing or tearing of the overlying skin and a potential for inoculation of the tissue with normal human oral flora including most commonly *Eikenella*, staphylococci, and streptococci. Because of this inoculation, these injuries are frequently complicated by infection including cellulitis, lymphangitis, tenosynovitis, abscess, septic arthritis, as well as osteoarthritis. **Amoxicillin-clavulanate** is the first-line antibiotic for prophylactic treatment of such injuries (**e**). Wounds should be thoroughly cleaned with high-pressure syringe and sterile water to help reduce the risk of infection (**a**). Radiographs are also recommended to evaluate for foreign body and underlying fracture (**b, c**). Typically, these wounds are left open to heal by secondary intention as long as the wounds are small and not gaping. Should the wound necessitate closure, sutures should be placed sparingly with 5.0 nonabsorbable sutures with removal in 10 to 14 days (**b**). Tissue adhesive should never be used for suspected human or animal bites as this can trap any potential bacteria and increase the risk of infection/abscess (**c**). Although a splint may be placed if the sutures cross over joint lines to help promote healing, it is not indicated for all closed-fist injuries if no fracture is identified on X-ray (**a**).

516. The correct answer is e. The picture shows a classic finding of a **hair tourniquet**.

Irritability is commonly the chief complaint for hair tourniquets and thorough evaluation to identify a hair tourniquet should occur for any infant brought in for the evaluation of irritability. Hair tourniquets most commonly occur to the digits or penis and are most commonly caused by the mother's hair (**b**). Infection is not the cause of the abnormal findings on exam in this case nor is it a common complication of a hair tourniquet and prophylactic antibiotics are not indicated unless there are secondary findings of infection (**a**). A trial of a chemical depilatory agent may be used on nonmucosal surfaces to dissolve the hair (**e**). If this is unsuccessful or there are other contraindications to use of a chemical depilatory agent, the **hair tourniquet may be released by making an incision perpendicular to the hair on the extensor surface of the digit** (**d**). Surgical consultation may be necessary if there is evidence of ischemia or necrosis, however, most hair tourniquets can be managed by primary care or emergency physicians (**b**).

517. The correct answer is d. The patient has sustained two small puncture wounds secondary to a cat/kitten. Careful examination of the wound should be done through flexion/extension to determine presence of foreign body and/or damage to underlying structures including neurovascular bundles (**a**). Radiographs are recommended for any mammalian bite to identify any potential foreign body or bony involvement (**b**). Mammalian bites are at high risk for infection and these wounds should be cleansed thoroughly and left open with healing by secondary intention (**c**). Tissue adhesive should never be used to close puncture wounds, especially those caused by a bite (**d**). Sutures may be utilized if the laceration is larger/gaping or involves the face but should be placed loosely and with nonabsorbable sutures. **Prophylactic antibiotics are recommended for all mammalian bites including dogs and cats** (**e**).

518. The correct answer is e. The patient has developed a significant infection secondary to the cat bite despite prophylactic antibiotics. On examination, patient has evidence of cellulitis and lymphangitis. Continuing or broadening oral antibiotics is inadequate treatment given the development of infection on appropriate antibiotics and findings of both cellulitis and lymphangitis (**a, b**). Although ceftriaxone may be a good antibiotic choice for cellulitis, it does not provide adequate coverage in this case (**c**). This patient requires hospital admission for ongoing parenteral antibiotics. The appropriate choice of antibiotic would be ampicillin/sulbactam or clindamycin plus ciprofloxacin to cover *P. multocida*, the major pathogen found in cat bites (**d**).

519. The correct answer is b. Eyelid lacerations carry an increased risk of secondary complications due to injuries of underling or surrounding structures. Thorough exam should be performed to assess for ocular foreign bodies, evidence of globe rupture and injury to the lacrimal system, supra-orbital nerve, and infraorbital nerve. **Uncomplicated lid lacerations** can be closed with nonabsorbable 6-0 sutures with removal in 3 to 5 days. Tissue adhesive should be avoided near the eye.

Laceration involving the medial canthus is at greatest risk of injury to the lacrimal system, which can lead to chronic tearing if not recognized (**a**). Other eyelid lacerations that carry risk of secondary injury to surrounding structures include those that involve the lid margin, inner surface of the eyelid, as well as the tarsal plate (**c, d, and e**). These lacerations are indications for emergent consultation with an ophthalmologist for repair.

Recommended Readings

Knoop KJ, Stack LB, Storrow AB. Chapter 18, Wounds and soft tissue injuries. *Atlas of Emergency Medicine*. 4th ed. New York, NY: McGraw-Hill, 2010.

Simon BC, Hern HG. Chapter 52. Wound management principles. In: Marx JA, Hockberger RS, Walls RM, et al, eds. *Rosen's Emergency Medicine: Concepts and Clinical Practice*. 9th ed. Philadelphia, PA: Saunders, 2018.

Thomas SH, Goodloe JM. Chapter 53. Foreign bodies. In: Marx JA, Hockberger RS, Walls RM, et al, eds. *Rosen's Emergency Medicine: Concepts and Clinical Practice*. 9th ed. Philadelphia, PA: Saunders, 2018.

Tintinalli JE, Cline JE, Yealy DM, et al, eds. Section 6. Wound Management. *Tintinalli's Emergency Medicine Manual*. 9th ed. New York: McGraw-Hill Medical, 2019.

U.S. Public Health Service. Updated U.S. Public Health Service guidelines for the management of occupational exposure to HBC, HCV, and HIV and recommendations for post-exposure prophylaxis. *MMWR Recomm Rep*. 2001;50:1-52.

Endocrine Emergencies

Daniel Rutz, MD

Questions

520. A 30-year-old man with type 1 diabetes mellitus (DM) presents to the emergency department (ED). His blood pressure (BP) is 100/70 mm Hg and heart rate (HR) is 140 beats/minute. His blood glucose is 750 mg/dL, potassium level is 2.9 mEq/L, bicarbonate is 5 mEq/L, and arterial pH is 7.1. His urine is positive for ketones. Which of the following is the best initial therapy for this patient?

a. Administer a 2 L normal saline (NS) bolus and 20 units of subcutaneous (SQ) insulin
b. Administer 2 ampules of intravenous (IV) sodium bicarbonate and 10 units of IV insulin
c. Administer a 2 L NS bolus and 40 mEq IV potassium chloride
d. Administer a 2 L NS bolus followed by an insulin drip at 0.1 units/kg/hour
e. Administer 5 mg IV metoprolol and 2L NS bolus

The following scenario applies to questions 521 and 522.

A 39-year-old woman is brought to the ED by her family. She has had diarrhea for the previous 4 days. On the day of presentation, she started "acting crazy" with mood swings and confusion. The family states that she usually takes a medication for a "problem with her neck." Her BP is 130/45 mm Hg, HR is 140 beats/minute, respiratory rate (RR) is 22 breaths/minute, and temperature is 101.5°F. An electrocardiogram (ECG) reveals atrial fibrillation with a normal QRS complex.

521. What laboratory abnormalities would you expect in this patient?

a. Elevated parathyroid hormone and serum calcium
b. Elevated luteinizing hormone (LH) and follicle-stimlating hormone (FSH), low gonadotropin-releasing hormone (GnRH)
c. Low thyroid-stimulating hormone (TSH) and elevated FT4
d. Low adrenocorticotropic hormone ACTH and morning cortisol
e. Elevated TSH and low FT4

522. Which of the following medications inhibits thyroid hormone synthesis and blocks peripheral conversion of T_4 to T_3?

a. Hydrocortisone
b. Oral iodine
c. Propranolol
d. Methimazole
e. Propylthiouracil (PTU)

523. A 65-year-old woman is brought to the ED by her family. She has been weak, lethargic, and "saying crazy things" over the last 2 days. Her family also states that her medical history is significant only for "thyroid disease." Her BP is 120/90 mm Hg, HR is 51 beats/minute, RR is 12 breaths/minute, and temperature is 94°F rectally. On examination, the patient is overweight, her skin is dry, and you notice periorbital nonpitting edema. On neurologic examination, the patient does not respond to stimulation. What is the most appropriate initial treatment?

a. Hydrocortisone
b. T4 and T3
c. PTU
d. Warming blankets
e. Atropine

524. A 74-year-old woman with a history of DM is brought to the ED by emergency medical service (EMS) with altered mental status. Her home health aide states that the patient ran out of her medications 4 days ago. Her BP is 130/85 mm Hg, HR is 110 beats/minute, RR is 18 breaths/minute, and temperature is 99.8°F. On examination, she cannot follow commands but responds to stimuli. Laboratory results reveal white blood cell (WBC) count of 14,000/L, hematocrit 49%, platelets 325/L, sodium 128 mEq/L, potassium 3.0 mEq/L, chloride 95 mEq/L, bicarbonate 22 mEq/L, blood urea nitrogen (BUN) 40 mg/dL, creatinine 1.8 mg/dL, and glucose 1000 mg/dL. Urinalysis shows 3+ glucose, 1+ protein, and no blood or ketones. After addressing the ABCs, which of the following is the most appropriate next step in management?

a. Administer a 2 to 3 L bolus of NS, followed by IV insulin
b. Administer a 2 to 3 L bolus of NS, followed by IV insulin and IV phenytoin
c. Administer 10 units of IV insulin, followed by 2 L of NS
d. Order a computed tomographic (CT) scan of the brain
e. Arrange for emergent hemodialysis

525. A 75-year-old woman is brought to the ED by EMS after she had a witnessed seizure on the street. A bystander reports that the patient fell to the ground, had tonic-clonic activity, and was drooling. Her BP is 162/85 mm Hg, HR is 95 beats/minute, RR is 16 breaths/minute, and temperature is 99.4°F. On examination, the patient is unresponsive and has a bleeding superficial scalp laceration. Which of the following electrolyte disturbances is *least likely* to cause a seizure?

a. Hypoglycemia
b. Hyperglycemia
c. Hyponatremia
d. Hypernatremia
e. Hypokalemia

The following scenario applies to questions 526 to 528.

A 53-year-old woman is brought to the ED by her husband. He states that his wife has been feeling very weak over the last 2 days, is nauseated, and vomited at least three times. She was taking a medication for her joint pain, but ran out of her pills last week. Her vital signs are a BP of 90/50 mm Hg, HR of 87 beats/minute, RR of 16 breaths/minute, and temperature of 98.1°F. You place her on the monitor, begin IV fluids, and send her blood to the laboratory. Thirty minutes later, the metabolic panel results are back and reveal the following:

Na^+	126 mEq/L
K^+	5 mEq/L
Cl^-	99 mEq/L
HCO_3	21 mEq/L
BUN	24 mg/dL
Creatinine	1.6 mg/dL
Glucose	69 mg/dL
Ca^+	11 mEq/L

526. What is the most likely diagnosis?

a. Myxedema coma
b. Thyroid storm
c. Hyperaldosteronism
d. Adrenal insufficiency
e. Diabetic ketoacidosis

527. What are the most appropriate laboratory studies to confirm suspected diagnosis?

a. β-Hydroxybutyrate
b. TSH
c. ACTH and morning cortisol level
d. Adrenal autoantibodies
e. Aldosterone, potassium, and renin

528. Which of the following is the most appropriate definitive therapy?

a. Insulin drip
b. Levothyroxine
c. Norepinephrine
d. Hydrocortisone
e. Dextrose

The following scenario applies to questions 529 and 530.

A 45-year-old man with newly diagnosed type 2 DM treated with glipizide is brought into the ED following a seizure. He is not responding to verbal commands. His airway is patent, with bilateral breath sounds and normal symmetrical pulses. His BP is 90/60 mm Hg, HR is 110 beats/minute, and RR is 26 breaths/minute. His fingerstick glucose is 30 mg/dL.

529. Which of the following is the most appropriate next step in management?

a. Administer lorazepam
b. Intubate for airway protection
c. Administer 1 to 3 ampules of 50% dextrose in water
d. Administer 2 L bolus of NS
e. Order stat CT head without contrast

530. After stabilizing the patient, what additional pharmacological agent should be considered?

a. Somatostatin
b. Octreotide
c. Broad-spectrum antibiotics
d. Glucagon
e. 25% dextrose in water

The following scenario applies to questions 531 and 532.

A 4-year-old boy is brought in by his mother with abdominal pain, irritability, polyuria, and polydipsia. Labs obtained in the ED are consistent with severe diabetic ketoacidosis (DKA), and appropriate treatment is initiated. Approximately 6 hours into his emergency room (ER) stay, the patient develops headache, vomiting, incontinence, and depressed mental status.

531. What is this patient's likely diagnosis?

a. Hyperosmolar hyperglycemic state (HHS)
b. Intraparenchymal hemorrhage
c. Hyperglycemic seizure
d. Cerebral edema
e. Migraine headache

532. What is most appropriate treatment for this patient's condition?

a. Mannitol 1 g/kg intravenously over 15 minutes
b. Insulin infusion 0.1 units/kg/hour
c. Trendelenburg position and continue current care
d. Neurosurgery consultation
e. Increase intravenous fluid (IVF) resuscitation rate to 2 × maintenance

533. A 32-year-old woman presents with a complaint of poor cesarean section wound healing and failure of lactation. The patient had an unremarkable pregnancy and delivered a full-term neonate 2 weeks ago. Her delivery was complicated by maternal hemorrhage and severe hypotension. Her BP is 120/80 mm Hg, HR is 70 beats/minute, RR is 14 breaths/minute, and temperature is 36.6°C. What is the most likely diagnosis?

a. Endometritis
b. Hypothyroidism
c. Toxic shock syndrome
d. Improper lactation technique
e. Sheehan's syndrome

Endocrine Emergencies

Answers

520. The answer is c. While the mainstay of treatment for DKA is aggressive IV fluid resuscitation and IV insulin therapy, this patient's **serum potassium level** is **markedly low**. He requires fluid resuscitation and potassium correction. If the initial serum potassium is below 3.3 mEq/L, **IV KCl** should be given **prior** to administration of insulin. Failure to correct hypokalemia prior to insulin administration could cause respiratory muscle weakness, cardiac arrhythmias, or even cardiac arrest due to intracellular movement of potassium. Once the serum potassium is between 3.3 and 5.3 mEq/L, insulin infusion at 0.1 units/kg/hour is indicated along with IV KCl (20-30 mEq) is added to each liter of IV replacement fluid and continued until the serum potassium concentration has increased to the normal range of 4 to 5 mEq/L.

In DKA, the average adult has a water deficit of 5 to 10 L. After the first 2 L of fluid, **(d)** regular insulin is administered at a rate of 0.1 units/kg/hour. Insulin must be administered for ketosis and acidosis to resolve. There is no consensus on need for an insulin bolus prior to starting an infusion. Such a bolus may negatively affect the already total body deficit of potassium and in recent years has fallen out of favor in the initial treatment of DKA. Intramuscular and SQ insulin administration **(a)** is avoided in DKA as absorption may be erratic secondary to volume depletion and poor perfusion. Currently, no study shows a benefit of using bicarbonate in DKA **(b)**. Bicarbonate administration can cause worsening hypokalemia, paradoxical central nervous system (CNS) acidosis, impaired oxyhemoglobin dissociation, hypertonicity, and sodium overload. Metoprolol **(e)**, a β-blocker, is not indicated in DKA. The tachycardia in DKA is secondary to volume depletion and acidosis. Correcting the underlying cause will treat the tachycardia.

521. The answer is c. This patient is experiencing **thyroid storm**, and would be expected to have **low TSH** and **elevated FT4**. **Thyroid storm** is a **medical emergency** that will lead to death if not treated in time. The manifestations of thyroid storm include **temperature greater than 100°F, tachycardia out of proportion to fever, widened pulse pressure, CNS dysfunction** (eg, confusion, agitation), **cardiovascular dysfunction**

(eg, high-output congestive heart failure, atrial fibrillation), and **gastrointestinal (GI) dysfunction** (eg, diarrhea, abdominal pain). Thyroid storm is a **clinical diagnosis** because no confirmatory tests are immediately available. The most important factor in reducing mortality is blocking peripheral adrenergic hyperactivity with **propranolol**, a β-blocker. **PTU** is used to inhibit new hormone synthesis in the thyroid and has a small effect on inhibiting peripheral conversion of T_4 to T_3. **Iodine** is administered to block hormone release from the thyroid but should be given 1 hour after PTU to prevent organification of the iodine.

Elevated parathyroid hormone and serum calcium would be expected in symptomatic **hyperparathyroidism (a)**, which causes symptoms of hypercalcemia including abdominal pain, emesis, lethargy, confusion, and hallucinations. Elevated LH and FSH and low GnRH **(b)** would be expected in a menstruating female on a monthly basis during normal cycles. Low ACTH and morning cortisol **(d)** are the hallmarks of central adrenal insufficiency. Elevated TSH and low FT4 **(e)** are seen in **hypothyroid** states, the opposite of this patient's condition.

522. The answer is e. PTU is the only medication able to **inhibit thyroid hormone production, as well as block peripheral conversion of T_4 to T_3,** the active and much more potent form of the hormone. Because of this property, PTU is the treatment of choice in thyroid storm.

Hydrocortisone **(a)** is a very potent inhibitor of peripheral conversion of T_4 to T_3, much more so than PTU, but it does not inhibit thyroid hormone synthesis. Oral iodine **(b)** does not inhibit new thyroid hormone synthesis. Propranolol **(c)** is a mainstay of therapy because it blocks adrenergic hyperactivity, but its effect on peripheral T_4 to T_3 conversion is minimal. Methimazole **(d)** targets inhibition of new thyroid hormone synthesis as shown in the table.

	Inhibition of thyroid hormone synthesis	Prevention of preformed thyroid hormone release	Blockade of peripheral T_4 to T_3 conversion
PTU, propylthiouracil	+		+
Methimazole	+		
Propranolol			+
Iodine (after PTU)		+	
Hydrocortisone		+	+

523. The answer is b. Myxedema coma is a syndrome that represents **extreme hypothyroidism**. It is a **life-threatening** condition that has a mortality of up to 50%. Signs and symptoms of hypothyroidism are usually present including dry skin, delayed deep tendon reflexes (prolongation of the relaxation phase), coarse hair, and generalized nonpitting edema. Myxedema coma, however, is better characterized by **profound lethargy or coma** and **hypothermia**. Hypothermia is present in approximately 80% of patients. In addition, patients may present with respiratory depression and sinus bradycardia. Initial treatment involves stabilization of ABCs and the **prompt administration of IV T4 (200-400 μg) and IV T3 (5-20 μg)**. There are no clinical trials comparing efficacy of different hormone treatment regimens, so there is some controversy over the ideal methodology of dosing.

Hydrocortisone **(a)** may be indicated for concomitant adrenal insufficiency, if present. PTU **(c)** is administered for hyperthyroidism—this patient is hypothyroid. Warming blankets **(d)** are adjuncts to treatment, but not the first line for the patient's underlying pathology. Atropine **(e)** may temporarily increase the patient's HR, but her hypothyroid state is driving the bradycardia, so it would recur without administration of thyroid hormone.

524. The answer is a. HHS is a syndrome representing marked **hyperglycemia** (serum glucose > 600 mg/dL), **hyperosmolarity** (plasma osmolarity > 320 mOsm/L), considerable **dehydration** (9 L deficit in a 70-kg patient), and **decreased mental functioning** that may progress to coma. HHS may be the initial presentation of previously unrecognized diabetes in an adult with **type 2 DM**. Elderly diabetics are at greater risk for this illness. Osmotic diuresis is even more pronounced than in DKA. Rapid correction of hyperosmolar state may lead to cerebral edema. Acidosis and ketosis are usually absent or minimal unlike in patients with DKA. **The mainstay of treatment is fluid resuscitation, followed by insulin administration, electrolyte repletion, and identification of the underlying precipitant**.

Phenytoin **(b)** is contraindicated for seizures in HHS because it is often ineffective and may impair endogenous insulin release. Fluid resuscitation is the mainstay of treatment and should always be administered before insulin **(c)**. Although the patient may ultimately receive a CT scan **(d)**, fluid resuscitation is priority because of the profound dehydration in these patients. If a patient has functioning kidneys, then hemodialysis is not necessary **(e)**. However, if the patient has end-stage renal disease, then hemodialysis may be necessary to treat over hydration.

525. The answer is e. **Hypokalemia** can cause **muscle weakness** and characteristic **ECG changes** (flattened T waves and U waves). Hypokalemia is not associated with seizures or altered mental status.

A glucose level can be rapidly obtained from a fingerstick point-of-care glucose check. Hypoglycemia (**a**) is a known reversible cause of seizures and is corrected with administration of dextrose. Significant hyperglycemia (**b**) occurs in DKA (glucose usually is 200-800 mg/dL) or nonketotic hyperosmolar crisis (glucose usually is > 800 mg/dL) and is treated with IV fluids and insulin. Hypo- and hypernatremia (**c and d**) are known causes of seizures.

526. The answer is d. **Adrenal cortical insufficiency** is an uncommon, potentially life-threatening condition that, if recognized early, is readily treatable. The most common cause of adrenal insufficiency is hypothalamic-pituitary-adrenal axis suppression from **long-term exogenous glucocorticoid administration**. This patient abruptly stopped her high-dose steroids prescribed for her chronic knee pain. The clinical presentation of adrenal insufficiency is vague but typically includes **weakness, fatigue, nausea, vomiting, hypotension**, and **hypoglycemia**. Electrolyte abnormalities are common. **Hyponatremia** and **hyperkalemia** are present in more than two-thirds of cases. Management includes supportive care with administration of glucocorticoids and electrolyte correction.

Myxedema coma (**a**) is a syndrome of extreme hypothyroidism, whereas thyroid storm (**b**) is extreme hyperthyroidism. Hyperaldosteronism (**c**) is characterized by hypertension and hypokalemia. DKA (**e**) typically presents with elevated glucose, an anion-gap metabolic acidosis, and ketone production.

527. The answer is c. If adrenal insufficiency is suspected, initial workup includes **ACTH and morning cortisol levels**. The combination of the two levels helps differentiate primary from secondary adrenal insufficiency. Significantly increased plasma value of ACTH in response to low cortisol levels is diagnostic of primary adrenal insufficiency. Cortisol level must be measured in the morning due to diurnal variations and pulsatile production of cortisol throughout the day.

Adrenal autoantibodies (**d**) levels are diagnostic of autoimmune adrenal insufficiency, but useful only after initial diagnosis of adrenal insufficiency is made. β-Hydroxybutyrate (**a**) is used in diagnosis of DKA. TSH (**b**) is used in diagnosis of thyroid disorders. Aldosterone, potassium, and renin (**e**) are used to diagnose primary hyperaldosteronism.

528. The answer is d. High-dose IV hydrocortisone is the treatment of choice in adrenal insufficiency and should be initiated early. Additionally, **IV hydration with dextrose** must be provided to treat associated hypotension and hypoglycemia as soon as possible.

Insulin drip **(a)** is used in treatment of DKA. Levothyroxine **(b)** is a long-term therapy for hypothyroidism. Norepinephrine **(c)** may be used in treatment of adrenal insufficiency in a patient who does not respond to hydration and hydrocortisone therapy, but only after failure to respond to initial appropriate treatment. Dextrose **(e)** is indicated in an acute hypoglycemic episode. It can be added to IV NS in treatment of adrenal insufficiency with significant hypoglycemia.

529. The answer is c. The patient presented with **hypoglycemic seizure**. The initial management step in any patient presenting with altered mental status is **a point-of-care glucose**. Severe hypoglycemia is defined as blood glucose less than 40 to 50 mg/dL and impaired cognitive function. Hypoglycemia is a common problem in DM. Symptoms include tachycardia, diaphoresis, tremor, confusion, seizure, and even coma. Hypoglycemic episodes may be precipitated by decreased PO intake, increased energy expenditure, or increased insulin dose. The initial step in management is **glucose replacement** using 50% dextrose in water (D50W) ampules (which contain 25 mg of dextrose in 50 mL ampule). Patients may require more than 1 ampule as 1 ampule of D50W will unpredictably augment blood glucose in a range from less than 40 mg/dL to greater than 350 mg/dL. Once the patient's mentation is back to baseline, the patient should be provided food as the calories provided to the patient by a meal will exceed those provided in 1 ampule of IV dextrose.

Lorazepam **(a)** is not indicated as an initial management step as it does not address the etiology of seizure secondary to hypoglycemia. The patient's airway is patent and intubation **(b)** is not needed. NS bolus **(d)** may be considered in patients with signs of dehydration as supportive therapy. CT head without contrast **(e)** may be ordered if there is a suspicion for intracranial pathology and not hypoglycemia leading to patient's seizures.

530. The answer is b. Hypoglycemic episodes secondary to **sulfonylurea** medications (ie, glipizide) require special attention and warrant at least **24-hour observation**. Sulfonylurea hyperglycemic agents cause **prolonged, severe hypoglycemia with recurrent episodes**. Newly diagnosed patients treated with these agents are at increased risk for hypoglycemic episodes.

In addition to initial glucose replacement, patients will often require treatment with octreotide to inhibit further insulin release. **Octreotide** is a synthetic somatostatin analog with a half-life of approximately 90 minutes.

Somatostatin hormone (**a**) has a half-life of 2 minutes and would not be recommended. Antibiotics (**c**) would play a role only if an underlying infectious process is identified. Glucagon (**d**), which opposes actions of insulin and increases concentration of blood glucose, may be considered if patient has no IV access; however, its onset of action is can take 10 to 15 minutes. D25W or 25% dextrose in water (**e**) is recommended for use in children younger than 8 years as an initial glucose replacement therapy.

531. The answer is d. This patient has likely developed **cerebral edema**, a feared complication of pediatric DKA that carries a mortality rate of 20% to 25%. Risk factors include severe acidosis at initial presentation, young age (<5 years old), elevated BUN at presentation, and severe hypocapnia. Symptoms include **headache, vomiting, irritability, fluctuating, or depressed mental status**. Prompt recognition and treatment is indicated to avoid morbidity and mortality.

HHS (**a**) is seen in adult type 2 diabetic patients and involves hyperglycemia, elevated serum osmolality, and normal pH. IPH (**b**) is possible based on this patient's presentation, but is not the most likely diagnosis. Hyperglycemic seizure (**c**) typically presents as generalized tonic clonic convulsion in the setting of hyperglycemia. A migraine headache (**e**) would be a consideration in a patient with a known history of migraines, but in this setting with depressed mental status and emesis, is a less likely diagnosis.

532. The answer is a. Following a diagnosis of cerebral edema, efforts to **reduce intracranial pressure (ICP)** should be undertaken rapidly to avoid cerebral herniation and death. This includes **elevating the head of the bed** to 30 degrees and administration of **IV mannitol**. Furthermore, IV fluid infusion should be decreased by 30%. Avoid hypotension to maintain cerebral perfusion.

Insulin infusion (**b**) is the correct treatment for DKA and should continue for this patient, but will not affect his cerebral edema. Trendelenburg position (**c**), which lowers the head of the bed, would increase ICP in this patient. Neurosurgery evaluation (**d**) should be sought, but after starting treatment to lower ICP. IVF infusion rates should be decreased, not increased (**e**) after symptoms of cerebral edema are recognized.

533. The answer is e. **Sheehan's syndrome** is a rare **acute dysfunction of hypothalamic-pituitary axis**, which may be seen after obstetric hemorrhage and maternal hypotension during delivery. The anterior pituitary gland is especially susceptible to ischemia secondary to maternal hypotension resulting in most commonly prolactin and growth hormone deficiencies. Clinically, it is manifested by **failure of lactation, failure of wound healing, and generalized weakness**. Normally, levels of prolactin steadily rise during pregnancy in response to sleep, meals, and increase in thyrotropin-releasing hormone (TRH) produced by hypothalamus. IV TRH may be administered and prolactin can be measured before and 30 minutes after TRH administration in order to diagnose Sheehan's syndrome. Normally, levels of prolactin rise at least threefold following administration of TRH. Failure of prolactin to rise in response to TRH infusion is diagnostic of Sheehan's syndrome.

Endometritis (**a**) and toxic shock syndrome (**c**) would present with signs of systemic illness. Hypothyroidism (**b**) complicates 0.5% of all pregnancies and is most commonly seen with a preexisting Hashimoto's disease. However, isolated decreased thyroid hormone production would not explain all of the presenting symptoms in this patient. Improper lactation technique (**d**) may present with failure of lactation, but would not cause generalized weakness or impaired wound healing.

Recommended Readings

Cydulka RK, Maloney GE. Chapter 118. Diabetes mellitus and disorders of glucose homeostasis. In: Marx JA, Hockberger RS, Walls RM, et al, eds. *Rosen's Emergency Medicine: Concepts and Clinical Practice*. 9th ed. Philadelphia, PA: Saunders, 2017.

Edlow AG, Norwitz ER. Endocrine diseases of pregnancy. *Yen and Jaffe's Reproductive Endocrinology Physiology, Pathophysiology, and Clinical Management*. 7th ed. Philadelphia, PA: Elsevier/Saunders, 2014.

Graffeo CS. Hyperosmolar hyperglycemic state. In: Tintinalli JE, Ma O, Yealy DM, et al, eds. *Tintinalli's Emergency Medicine: A Comprehensive Study Guide*. 9th ed. Newyork, NY. McGraw-Hill, 2019.

Idrose A. Hyperthyroidism and thyroid storm. In: Tintinalli JE, Ma O, Yealy DM, et al, eds. *Tintinalli's Emergency Medicine: A Comprehensive Study Guide*. 9th ed. Newyork, NY. McGraw-Hill, 2019.

Jalili M, Niroomand M. Type 2 diabetes mellitus. In: Tintinalli JE, Ma O, Yealy DM, et al, eds. *Tintinalli's Emergency Medicine: A Comprehensive Study Guide*. 9th ed. Newyork, NY. McGraw-Hill, 2019.

Nyce A, Byrne R, Lubkin CL, et al. Diabetic ketoacidosis. In: Tintinalli JE, Ma O, Yealy DM, et al, eds. *Tintinalli's Emergency Medicine: A Comprehensive Study Guide*. 9th ed. Newyork, NY. McGraw-Hill, 2019.

Sharma AN, Levy DL. Chapter 120. Thyroid and adrenal disorders. In: Marx JA, Hockberger RS, Walls RM, et al, eds. *Rosen's Emergency Medicine: Concepts and Clinical Practice*. 9th ed. Philadelphia, PA: Saunders, 2017.

Sperling M. Diabetes mellitus. *Pediatric Endocrinology*. 4th ed. Philadelphia, PA: Elsevier, 2014.

Psychosocial Disorders

Daniel Rutz, MD

Questions

534. A 31-year-old woman presents to the emergency department (ED) 20 minutes after the sudden onset of chest pain, palpitations, and shortness of breath. She also reports numbness of her mouth, fingers, and toes. She also feels like she has a lump in her throat. Her medical history includes multiple visits to the ED over a period of 6 months with a similar presentation. Her only medication is an oral contraceptive. She occasionally drinks a glass of wine after a busy day of work or when she feels stressed. She tells you that her mom takes medication for anxiety. Her blood pressure (BP) is 125/75 mm Hg, heart rate (HR) is 88 beats/minute, and oxygen saturation is 99% on room air. An electrocardiogram (ECG) shows a sinus rhythm. Her symptoms resolve while in the ED. Which of the following is the most likely diagnosis?

a. Paroxysmal atrial tachycardia
b. Hyperthyroidism
c. Major depressive disorder
d. Panic disorder
e. Posttraumatic stress disorder

535. A 23-year-old woman is brought to the ED for vision loss in her left eye that began shortly after waking up in the morning. She states that she is very depressed after losing her job in the wake of the COVID-19 pandemic. She just got off the phone with her employer prior the vision loss and presented to the ED. Your physical examination is unremarkable. An evaluation by the ophthalmologist is also normal. A computed tomographic (CT) scan of her head is normal. Which of the following is the most likely diagnosis?

a. Somatization disorder
b. Conversion disorder
c. Hypochondriasis
d. Retinal detachment
e. Anxiety disorder

536. Which of the following individuals requires inpatient psychiatric hospitalization?

a. A 25-year-old man with a history of schizophrenia on medication presenting with auditory hallucinations that is cooperative with staff and endorses no homicidal or suicidal ideation
b. A 35-year-old woman who purposefully ingested two sleeping pills after an argument with her boyfriend
c. A 39-year-old man with no previous psychiatric history presents with pressured speech, no sleep for 4 days, is mowing crop circles in his neighbor's yard to communicate with aliens, and states he feels "fantastic"
d. A 22-year-old woman who is having intense hunger after edible tetrahydrocannabinol (THC) brownies
e. A 43-year-old homeless man presented with agitation and alcohol intoxication

537. A 35-year-old woman is eating dinner at a restaurant. Approximately 1 hour after finishing the main course of lamb, red wine, and a fine selection of cheeses, the patient experiences a severe occipital headache, diaphoresis, mydriasis, neck stiffness, and palpitations. Which of the following medications is this patient most likely taking?

a. Paroxetine
b. Alprazolam
c. Phenelzine
d. Citalopram
e. Amitriptyline

538. A 30-year old man presents to the ED with paranoid delusions and agitation. He was combative with emergency medical services (EMS) and shouting loudly that the government is trying to silence him. He is given Haldol 5 mg intravenous (IV) for agitation. While you are examining him, you notice spasms of the patient's neck and face muscles. His airway is patent. Vital signs are within normal limits. What is the cause of the patient's symptoms?

a. Bell's palsy
b. Neuroleptic malignant syndrome
c. Akathisia
d. Dystonic reaction
e. Conversion disorder

539. A 42-year-old man with a history of schizophrenia is brought into the ED by a friend who states that he has not taken his medication for over 2 weeks and is now behaving bizarrely. His BP is 130/70 mm Hg, HR is 89 beats/minute, respiratory rate (RR) is 15 breaths/minute, and oxygen saturation is 99% on room air. On examination, he appears agitated and is shouting, "the aliens are about to get me." He is cooperative enough that you decide to use pharmacologic sedation. Which of the following is the most appropriate choice for sedating this patient?

a. Haloperidol and diphenhydramine
b. Etomidate and succinylcholine
c. Chlorpromazine
d. Ketamine
e. Clozapine

540. A 48-year-old man is brought to the ED by family members who state that the patient has remained homebound for weeks, sleeping for many hours, and appears disheveled. The patient states that he is "fine" and denies any medical symptoms. Initial vitals include a BP of 118/55 mm Hg, HR of 77 beats/minute, RR of 12 breaths/minute, and oxygen saturation of 97% on room air. The patient is afebrile with an unremarkable physical examination. He denies chest discomfort, difficulty breathing, constipation, cold intolerance, weakness, weight changes, or pain. The patient reports that he has had difficulty concentrating, a decreased appetite, and excessive sleeping patterns. The family reports that this has happened before, but that his symptoms self-resolved and were not nearly as severe. Which of the following is the most likely etiology of this patient's symptoms?

a. Hypothyroidism
b. Major depressive episode
c. Diabetes mellitus
d. Subdural hematoma
e. Cushing syndrome

541. A 58-year-old man is brought to the ED by a concerned neighbor. The patient is known to be an alcoholic, consuming 1 pint of vodka daily and little else in terms of nutritional support. The neighbor has not seen the patient outside his house in the past week and the patient's refrigerator was found open and empty. The patient appears intoxicated, thin, and frail. His vital signs are notable for temperature, 98.4°F, BP 105/68 mm Hg, HR 112 beats/minute, RR 14 breaths/minute, and pulse oximetry 94% on room air. Fingerstick glucose is within normal limits. On examination, the patient is oriented to person only. His gait is unsteady, and his eye movements appear abnormal. On closer inspection, he has a bilateral cranial nerve VI palsy. What is appropriate initial treatment for this patient's condition?

a. Normal saline bolus 30 cc/kg IV
b. Magnesium sulfate 2 g IV
c. Multivitamin tab PO
d. Thiamine 500 mg IV
e. Fomepizole 15 mg/kg IV

542. A 23-year-old woman is brought to the ED by police officials who found her standing in the middle of a busy intersection screaming at passing cars. Upon arrival, you see a disheveled woman who is yelling, "You can't get away with this! I'm the Queen of England!" She does not allow the triage nurse to obtain her vitals. She is a young woman of normal habitus without any signs of trauma. Her speech is pressured. She is easily distracted by the commotion of the ED, answers your questions, but then continues to describe grandiose ideas about her social status. What is the most likely etiology of her symptoms?

a. Hypothyroid disorder
b. Manic episode
c. Benzodiazepine overdose
d. Anticonvulsant overdose
e. Barbiturate overdose

543. A mother brings her 7-year-old daughter to the ED stating that child has been weak and not eating for the last 3 days. She has also noted her daughter's urine to be reddish in color and her stools to be smaller in caliber. She brings in urine and stool specimens. Her daughter has been hospitalized multiple times for similar reasons. The mother is a nurse. The child is without distress and sitting quietly. Her mucus membranes are moist, chest is clear to auscultation, abdomen is benign, and her neurologic examination is nonfocal. A urinalysis performed fails to show any blood, myoglobin, or ketones. Stool studies are normal. Which of the following should be included in the differential diagnosis of this child?

a. Malingering
b. Factitious disorder
c. Delusion disorder
d. Medical child abuse (MCA)
e. Conversion disorder

544. An 18-year-old man presents to the ED after telling a school counselor that he wanted to harm himself. His physical examination is unremarkable without any signs of trauma. He reports occasional excessive alcohol use. His parents recently separated and he has been living with either parent on a rotating schedule. Overall, he feels supported by family and friends; however, he continues to feel hopeless despite this. Which of the following factors is most likely to increase his risk of an actual suicidal attempt?

a. Male sex
b. Age
c. Hopelessness
d. Alcohol use
e. Parent separation

545. A thin 16-year-old girl is brought in the ED after collapsing at home. Her initial vitals include a BP of 80/55 mm Hg, HR of 110 beats/minute, RR of 18 breaths/minute, and oxygen saturation of 98% on room air. Upon physical examination, you note a cachectic female in mild distress. Her chest is clear to auscultation. Her abdomen is sunken-in, soft, and non-tender. Upon inspecting her extremities, you notice small areas of erythema over the dorsum of her right hand distally. Which of the following etiologies must be considered in this patient?

a. Bulimia
b. Gastroenteritis
c. Malingering
d. Factitious disorder
e. Suicidal ideation

546. A 55-year-old woman presents to the ED after a reported syncopal event. Her initial vitals include a BP of 125/60 mm Hg, HR of 105 beats/minute, RR of 16 breaths/minute, and oxygen saturation of 98% on room air. Her ECG is shown in the figure. Which of the following substances is associated with the below ECG findings?

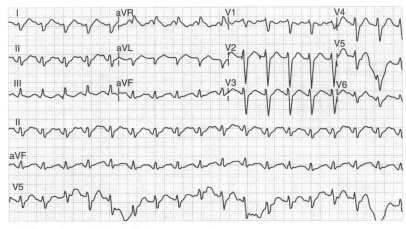

(Reproduced with permission from Adam J. Rosh, MD, and Rosh Review.)

a. Benzodiazepine
b. Ethanol
c. Tricyclic antidepressant (TCA)
d. Insulin
e. Valproic acid

547. A 48-year-old woman presents to the ED complaining of leg pain. She dramatically describes how she injured herself while salsa dancing. She is wearing a sequin cocktail dress, asks to be evaluated by a male doctor, and makes a point to undress in front of the physician. She flirts with him and asks if he is single. Which of the following personality disorders does the patient most likely have?

a. Antisocial
b. Paranoid
c. Narcissistic
d. Histrionic
e. Borderline

548. You are working in the ED when the police bring in a 22-year-old woman who was involved in a fight with her boyfriend. As you enter the room, you overhear her giving the registration clerk a false identity. She is disruptive, rude, shouting profanities, and refuses to give you any information. The patient is well-known to the ED staff as she has frequent visits. She often smokes cigarettes in the bathroom, has urinated on the floor, and been known to steal other patients' belongings. Which of the following personality disorders best fits with this patient's behavior?

a. Antisocial
b. Paranoid
c. Narcissistic
d. Histrionic
e. Schizoid

Psychosocial Disorders

Answers

534. The answer is d. A person with **panic attacks** will often present to multiple EDs and be discharged after a workup is normal. A panic attack is a discrete period of intense fear or discomfort in which four or more of the following symptoms develop acutely and peak within 10 minutes: accelerated HR, palpitations, pounding heart, diaphoresis, trembling or shaking, sensation of shortness of breath or a choking feeling, chest pain, nausea, dizziness, lightheadedness, paresthesia, fear of dying, chills, or hot flushes.

Paroxysmal atrial tachycardia (**a**) is a conduction defect of the heart characterized by random episodes of tachycardia. This disorder is seen on an ECG and her ECG is normal. Hyperthyroidism (**b**) can mimic a panic attack, but there is usually greater autonomic hyperactivity. In addition, thyroid hormone levels are increased. There are no symptoms of depression (**c**) described in the patient's presentation. Nonetheless, panic attacks can occur with major depressive disorder. The diagnosis of posttraumatic stress disorder (**e**) cannot be made with the patient's history.

535. The answer is b. Conversion disorder is diagnosed based on the following criteria:

- One or more symptoms of altered voluntary motor or sensory function
- Clinical findings provide evidence of incompatibility between the symptom and recognized neurological or medical conditions
- The symptom or deficit is not better explained by another medical or mental disorder
- The symptom or deficit causes clinically significant distress or impairment in social, occupational, or other important areas of functioning or warrants medical evaluation

Conversion disorders generally involve neurologic or orthopedic manifestations. The disorder usually presents as a **single symptom** with a **sudden onset** related to a **severe stress**. In this case, the stress is the loss of the patient's job that occurred just prior to presentation. Classic symptoms of conversion disorder include paralysis, aphonia, seizures, coordination disturbances, blindness, tunnel vision, and numbness. The diagnosis cannot be made until **all possible organic etiologies are ruled out**. Treatment involves identifying the stressor and addressing the issue.

Somatization disorder (**a**) involves patients with many complaints with no organic cause. Hypochondriasis (**c**) involves the preoccupation of serious illness despite appropriate medical evaluation and reassurance. Retinal detachment (**d**) can cause unilateral vision loss and generally presents with progressively worsening vision loss with patients complaining of "floaters." This patient's eye examination is normal. Anxiety disorders (**e**) involve excessive fear and apprehension that dominates the psychological life of a person.

536. The answer is c. This patient presents with a **first manic episode**. The core symptom of mania is an **abnormally elevated, irritable, or labile mood**. Classic mania is marked by an unusually good, euphoric, or high mood, which may be accompanied by disinhibition, disregard for social boundaries, expansiveness, and a relentless pursuit of stimulation and social activities. It is necessary to **admit** these patients in order to prevent behavior that is impulsive and dangerous. A full manic syndrome is one of the most striking and distinctive conditions in clinical practice. The main disturbance in mood is one of elation or irritability.

Auditory hallucinations are expected in the setting of schizophrenia, and this patient is not a threat to him or others and can be treated as an outpatient (**a**). This is a suicidal gesture (**b**) and the patient should be evaluated by a psychiatrist after appropriate medical clearance for possible sequelae of the ingestion. She may be able to be managed as an outpatient if reliable family and social support systems are in place and appropriate psychiatric follow-up is arranged. This patient (**d**) is experiencing the expected effect of THC ingestion and can be safely discharged once symptoms resolve. This man (**e**) can be examined for signs of trauma or another medical emergency, then observed for sobriety, reassessed, and likely discharged.

537. The answer is c. Phenelzine is a **monoamine oxidase inhibitor** (**MAOI**) that is used in the treatment of depression. Patients who take this medication should avoid eating or drinking foods that contain **tyramine** (similar structure to amphetamine) such as aged cheese, wine, certain fish, meats, and sauerkraut. The combination of an MAOI and tyramine can lead to a **sympathomimetic reaction** called a **tyramine reaction**. It occurs within 15 to 90 minutes of ingestion of tyramine. The hallmark symptoms include headache, hypertension, diaphoresis, mydriasis, neck stiffness, pallor, neuromuscular excitation, palpitations, and chest pain. Most symptoms gradually resolve over 6 hours; however, deaths have been reported secondary to intracranial hemorrhage and myocardial infarction. Patients who take an MAOI should be instructed to avoid all tyramine-containing foods. Treatment is supportive, including benzodiazepines for agitation, rigidity, and tachycardia. Avoid β-blockers for hypertension.

All of the other answer choices do not cause a tyramine reaction—it is limited only to MAOIs. Paroxetine and citalopram (**a and d**) are serotonin reuptake inhibitors (SSRIs). Alprazolam (**b**) is a benzodiazepine. Amitriptyline (**e**) is a TCA.

538. The answer is d. Dopamine receptor blockade by antipsychotic medications (eg, Haldol) can produce an **acute dystonic reaction** characterized by **involuntary movements and spasms of the neck, face, back, and extremities**. It typically occurs within the first few hours to days of treatment. This occurs in up to 25% of patients treated with Haldol. Rarely, laryngeal dystonia can occur which requires emergent airway intervention. Treatment is administration of **diphenhydramine**, which acts via anticholinergic pathways to abate the symptoms.

Bell's palsy (**a**) presents as cranial nerve VII motor deficit, typically after viral infection, causing unilateral facial muscle weakness. Neuroleptic malignant syndrome (**b**) is a rare, life-threatening disease state that typically occurs after 2 weeks of initiation of antipsychotics. Features include fever, muscle rigidity, altered mental status, tremor, and autonomic instability. Akathisia (**c**) is another extrapyramidal symptom of antipsychotic use and presents as motor restlessness and a compelling urge to move. Conversion disorder (**e**) is neurologic symptoms as a manifestation of underlying psychiatric condition or stressor. While feasible in this scenario, the more likely presentation is acute dystonic reaction.

539. The answer is a. Rapid tranquilization is a method of pharmacologic management of acute agitation or psychosis using high-potency neuroleptics and anticholinergic medication. A suitable regimen used is the combination of **haloperidol** and **diphenhydramine**. There is a synergistic effect between the two medications. Benzodiazepines are an option for blunting extrapyramidal side effects of antipsychotic medications, but there is an association between benzodiazepine use and mortality in schizophrenic patients, so their use should be with caution.

Etomidate and succinylcholine (**b**) are used for rapid sequence intubation, which is not indicated in this patient. Chlorpromazine (**c**) is a low-potency antipsychotic that may cause significant hypotension and is rarely used in the ED setting. Ketamine (**d**) is a dissociative agent that is not typically used in psychotic patients. Clozapine (**e**) is an atypical antipsychotic that is used in schizophrenics when other neuroleptics are ineffective. It is not an agent of choice for acute sedation or psychosis.

540. The answer is b. A **major depressive episode** is characterized by two or more of the following symptoms over a 2-week period: loss of interest in usual activities, depressed or irritable mood, changes in weight or appetite, insomnia or hypersomnia, psychomotor agitation or retardation, loss of energy, difficulty concentrating, recurrent thoughts of death, and suicidal ideation. This patient has three of these symptoms, including excessive sleeping patterns, difficulty concentrating, and a decreased appetite. The danger is that the patient's feelings may be so intensely painful that suicide may be seen as the only way to cope. Some patients may also complain of generalized physical pain, without any clear medical diagnosis able to be made. The cardinal symptom of depression is a **sad or dysphoric mood**.

Hypothyroidism (**a**) and Cushing syndrome (**e**) may also be a medical cause in patients who appear to be depressed. A simple thyroid-stimulating hormone and cortisol level may be drawn to differentiate a medical etiology for these symptoms. Hypothyroidism also presents as generalized sluggishness, difficulty concentrating, constipation, cold intolerance, hair loss of the distal one-third of both eyebrows, dysphagia, and myalgias. A finger-stick glucose should also be performed to evaluate for diabetes mellitus (**c**), which may present as sluggishness, paresthesias, and general malaise. It is also important to keep in mind traumatic causes to this patient's symptoms, given that he lives alone without witnesses to report a fall that may result in a subdural hematoma (**d**). Intracerebral bleeding may present with sluggishness, especially with the relatively slow bleeding from the bridging veins associated with a subdural hemorrhage.

541. The answer is d. The patient requires **thiamine repletion** as he is suffering from symptoms of **Wernicke's encephalopathy**. This occurs in alcoholics and severely malnourished patients and should be on the differential diagnosis for long-term alcoholics presenting with altered mental status. Thiamine (Vitamin B_1) plays a role in energy production pathways, and its depletion causes altered brain metabolism. The classic triad is **altered**

mental status, ataxia, and oculomotor dysfunction. When suspected, Wernicke's encephalopathy should be treated with **high-dose IV thiamine.**

Normal saline (**a**), magnesium (**b**), and multivitamins (**c**) are also indicated for the treatment of a chronically undernourished patient, but this patient's primary issue is thiamine deficiency. Fomepizole (**e**) is the treatment for ethylene glycol or methanol ingestion, which can be seen in chronic alcoholics. Suspect toxic alcohol poisoning in patients presented with intoxication and elevated osmolar gap.

542. The answer is b. This is a typical **manic episode** whose cardinal features are an elevated mood, grandiosity, flight of ideas, distractibility, and psychomotor agitation. Other medical conditions, such as hyperthyroidism, antidepressant, or stimulant abuse, may cause similar symptoms and must be ruled out with laboratory testing. Certain frontal lobe release syndromes that impair executive functioning must also be investigated as a cause of this patient's symptoms. These patients are usually combative, display impaired judgment and impulsivity, and may need to be chemically or physically restrained.

Hypothyroid disorder (**a**), benzodiazepines (**c**), anticonvulsants (**d**), and barbiturates (**e**) may all cause depressive symptoms; however, these do not produce symptoms of mania.

543. The answer is d. MCA, known in the past as **Munchausen syndrome by proxy** or **pediatric condition falsification** is a form of child abuse in which a parent or caregiver cause or fabricates illness in a child. In this example, the mother is placing tincture in the child's urine to mimic blood. The estimated annual incidence is 0.4 to 1.2 children per 100,000 under 16. Over 95% of perpetrators are female, mostly mothers or primary caretakers. MCA presents across a spectrum, and can range from parents seeking or demanding unnecessary care to the child receiving medical treatment that is potentially life-threatening. These children may display incidental characteristics that cannot be linked to the presenting complaints. Affected children often have learning difficulties or clinical depression caused by many hospitalizations. Consultation with a multidisciplinary child abuse team and child abuse specialist is warranted in situations where the physician suspects MCA.

Malingering (**a**) is frequently found in connection with antisocial personality disorder. These patients are often vague about prior hospitalizations or treatments. Patients prefer to counterfeit mental illness given the difficulty in objectively verifying or disproving the etiology of the patient's reported symptoms. Amnesia, paranoia, depression, and suicidal ideation are commonly seen. The idea of an external gain motivates these individuals to fabricate medical symptoms. Conversely, factitious disorders **(b)** are characterized by symptoms or signs that are intentionally produced or feigned by the patient in the absence of external incentives. Delusional disorder **(d)** is characterized by presence of fixed delusions over a period of time (≥ 1 month or greater) in the absence of causative medical condition. Conversion disorder **(e)** is a rare disorder that is characterized by the abrupt, dramatic onset of a single symptom. It typically presents as some nonpainful neurologic disorder for which there are no objective data.

544. The answer is c. Risk factors for suicide include feelings of **hopelessness** or worthlessness, prior suicide attempt in the past, being single, having a formed plan, and access to firearms.

Lower risk factors include male sex **(a)**, age younger than 19 years or older than 45 years **(b)**, excessive alcohol or drug use **(d)**, separation, divorce or widowed status **(e)**, and no social supports. Other risk factors include.

- Poor coping capacity
- History of aggressive behavior directed at others
- Substance abuse
- History of diagnosed psychiatric disorder
- Chronic pain

545. The answer is a. The physical examination in this patient reveals hand abrasions, indicative of **self-purging**. Her general appearance suggests either inadequate food intake or excessive calorie burning. **Bulimics** generally consume an adequate amount of food, albeit low calorie and then purge their intake with the goal of weight loss. Other eating disorders, such as anorexia nervosa, can take the form of starvation, diuretic or laxative use, or excessive exercise. These patients generally suffer from a false visualization of their body, believing that their physical form weighs more than what it does in reality. Social pressures, history of abuse or violence, and other eating disorders may factor into this patient's presentation.

Gastroenteritis **(b)** is unlikely given the lack of history or symptoms. Suicidal ideation **(e)** should be examined in all patients, as their actions may represent a form of occult or hidden self-harm. This patient does not exhibit signs of malingering **(c)** or factitious disorder **(d)**.

546. The answer is c. TCAs are responsible for more drug-related deaths than any other prescription medication. This ECG shows QRS interval prolongation, a common finding with this medication. The mechanism of toxicity is multifold and includes blocking the reuptake of dopamine, serotonin, and norepinephrine. It also binds to the γ-aminobutyric acid (GABA) receptor, thereby lowering seizure threshold. **Sodium channel blockade** produces the widened QRS interval. There are also anticholinergic and antihistamine effects. Sodium bicarbonate is a first-line intervention for dysrhythmias, acting as an alkalizing binder for the acidic TCA. This treatment has been shown to improve conduction and contractility with the goal of preserving a narrow QRS complex.

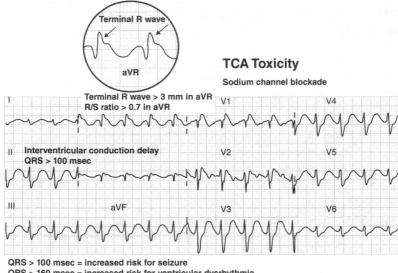

(Reproduced with permission from Adam J. Rosh, MD, and Rosh Review.)

Benzodiazepines (**a**), ethanol (**b**), insulin (**d**), and valproic acid (**e**) have not been shown to exhibit any ECG abnormalities.

547. The answer is d. Individuals with **histrionic** personality disorder display a pervasive pattern of excessive emotionality and attention seeking. They may use physical appearance to draw attention to themselves, show self-dramatization or exaggerated expressions of emotion, and interact with others in an inappropriately sexually seductive manner.

Individuals with antisocial personalities **(a)** have a blatant disregard for and violation of the rights of others; they often violate social norms, exhibit pathological lying, and have a lack of remorse for their actions. Paranoid personality disorder **(b)** manifests as pervasive distrust and suspiciousness of others such that their motives are interpreted as malevolent. Narcissistic **(c)** individuals exhibit grandiosity, a need for attention and admiration, superficial interpersonal relationships, and a lack of empathy. Borderline personality disorder **(e)** is characterized by unstable interpersonal relationships, impulsivity, and disturbances in self-image.

548. The answer is a. Individuals with **antisocial** personality disorder have a blatant disregard for the rights of others; are **aggressive**, irritable, and impulsive; **violate social norms;** and have a **lack of remorse** for their actions. They often **lie and manipulate** situations and frequently give **false identities**.

Paranoid personality disorder **(b)** manifests as mistrust, hypervigilance, and hypersensitivity. Narcissistic **(c)** individuals have a distorted sense of self-importance. People with histrionic personality disorder **(d)** are excessively emotional, demonstrate attention-seeking behavior, and want to be the center of attention. They are often flirtatious, overly dramatic, and may be sexually seductive. Schizoid **(e)** individuals are socially withdrawn, lead a solitary lifestyle, and tend to be emotionally cold and apathetic.

Recommended Readings

American Psychiatric Association. *Diagnostic and Statistical Manual of Mental Disorders.* 5th ed. (DSM-5). Arlington, VA: American Psychiatric Association, 2013.

Colbourne M, Clarke M. Child abuse and neglect. In: Tintinalli JE, Ma O, Yealy DM, et al, eds. *Tintinalli's Emergency Medicine: A Comprehensive Study Guide.* 9th ed. Newyork, NY. McGraw-Hill, 2019.

Colucciello SA. Chapter 105. Suicide. In: Marx JA, Hockberger RS, Walls RM, et al, eds. *Rosen's Emergency Medicine: Concepts and Clinical Practice.* 9th ed. Philadelphia, PA: Saunders, 2017.

DeSelm TM. Mood and anxiety disorders. In: Tintinalli JE, Ma O, Yealy DM, et al, eds. *Tintinalli's Emergency Medicine: A Comprehensive Study Guide.* 9th ed. Newyork, NY. McGraw-Hill, 2020.

Flaherty EG, Macmillan HL, Committee on Child Abuse and Neglect. Caregiver-fabricated illness in a child: a manifestation of child maltreatment. *Pediatrics.* 2013;132(3):590-597.

Hockberger RS, Richards JR. Chapter 100. Thought disorders. In: Marx JA, Hockberger RS, Walls RM, et al, eds. *Rosen's Emergency Medicine: Concepts and Clinical Practice.* 9th ed. Philadelphia, PA: Saunders, 2017.

Ikomi J, O'Malley SS. Alcohol use disorders. In: Ebert MH, Leckman JF, Petrakis IL, eds. *Current Diagnosis & Treatment: Psychiatry.* 3rd ed. Newyork, NY. McGraw-Hill, 2019.

McPheeters R, Tobias JL. Chapter 102. Anxiety disorders. In: Marx JA, Hockberger RS, Walls RM, et al, eds. *Rosen's Emergency Medicine: Concepts and Clinical Practice.* 9th ed. Philadelphia, PA: Saunders, 2017.

Winter AO. Chapter 103. Somatoform disorders. In: Marx JA, Hockberger RS, Walls RM, et al, eds. *Rosen's Emergency Medicine: Concepts and Clinical Practice,* 9th ed. Philadelphia, PA: Saunders, 2017.

Wilson M. Acute agitation. In: Tintinalli JE, Ma O, Yealy DM, et al, eds. *Tintinalli's Emergency Medicine: A Comprehensive Study Guide.* 9th ed. Newyork, NY. McGraw-Hill, 2019.

Young JL, DA Rund. Chapter 101. Mood disorders. In: Marx JA, Hockberger RS, Walls RM, et al, eds. *Rosen's Emergency Medicine: Concepts and Clinical Practice,* 9th ed. Philadelphia, PA: Saunders, 2017.

Emerging Infectious Diseases

Daniel Rutz, MD

Questions

The following scenario applies to questions 549 and 550.

A 33-year-old woman presents to the emergency department (ED) with 8 days of subjective fever, headache, sore throat, and malaise. She states that acetaminophen and ibuprofen have failed to help her symptoms. She recently returned from a 2-year volunteer trip with the Peace Corps in West Africa. She endorses taking her mefloquine weekly. Vitals signs are blood pressure (BP) 115/75 mm Hg, heart rate (HR) 110 beats/minute, respiratory rate (RR) 18 breaths/minute, temperature 101.2°F, and pulse oximetry 98% on room air. She has bilateral conjunctival injection as well as a truncal maculopapular rash.

549. Which of the following tests is most likely to be *abnormal* in this patient?

a. Chest X-ray (CXR)
b. Computed tomography (CT) scan of the chest for pulmonary embolism (PE)
c. Complete blood count (CBC), liver function tests (LFTs), and prothrombin time (PT)
d. Peripheral blood smears
e. Purified protein derivative (PPD) skin test

550. What type of isolation does this patient require?

a. Airborne
b. Contact
c. Droplet
d. Contact and droplet
e. Contact and airborne

The following scenario applies to questions 551 to 553.

A 54-year-old man with a history of hypertension and coronary artery disease presents to the ED with 5 days of intermittent fever associated with dry cough, dyspnea, and myalgias. His wife, with whom he lives, is reporting similar symptoms. Vital signs are notable for temperature 38.4°C, BP 154/87 mm Hg, HR 114 beats/minute, RR 26 breaths/minute, and pulse oximetry 86% on RA. Exam is notable for respiratory distress with accessory muscle use and bilateral inspiratory rales. You suspect COVID-19.

551. What would you expect to see on this patient's CXR?
a. Apical cavitary lesions
b. Single lobar consolidation
c. Bilateral pleural effusions
d. Pneumothorax
e. Bilateral interstitial infiltrates

552. What laboratory finding is most consistent with a diagnosis of COVID-19?
a. Thrombocytosis
b. Hyperkalemia
c. Normal C-reactive protein (CRP)
d. Lymphopenia
e. Macrocytosis

553. You are preparing to perform endotracheal intubation on this patient. In addition to appropriate hand hygiene, which of the following is the most appropriate personal protective equipment (PPE)?
a. Gloves
b. Gloves and gown
c. Gloves, gown, and surgical mask
d. Gloves, gown, N95 mask, and eye shield
e. Gloves and level A [Biosafety level 4 (BSL4)] suit

The following scenario applies to questions 554 to 556.

A 50-year-old man with a history of congestive heart failure and tobacco use presents to the ED with fever, cough, and dyspnea that started 4 days ago. He started feeling ill soon after returning from a religious pilgrimage to Mecca 7 days ago. His vitals include BP 85/60 mm Hg, HR 120 beats/minute, RR 26 breaths/minute, temperature 103°F, and pulse oximetry 92%

on room air. He is toxic appearing, in respiratory distress, and has mild abdominal tenderness to palpation.

554. Which of the following pathogens is responsible for this patient's presentation?
a. H5N1 avian flu
b. Middle East respiratory syndrome coronavirus (MERS-CoV)
c. Human immunodeficiency virus
d. Plasmodium falciparum
e. Severe acute respiratory syndrome coronavirus 2 (SARS-CoV-2)

555. What is the most likely complication to result from this patient's illness?
a. Acute respiratory distress syndrome (ARDS)
b. PE
c. Myocardial infarction
d. Pneumothorax
e. Peripheral edema

556. Which of the following is the most appropriate management and disposition plan for this patient?
a. Discharge home on acetaminophen with instructions for oral hydration
b. Discharge home on oral antibiotics with close primary care follow-up
c. Admit him for 24-hour observation and intravenous fluid therapy
d. Admit to the telemetry floor on intravenous nitroglycerin and furosemide drips
e. Admit to the intensive care unit for careful monitoring for respiratory decompensation

557. An otherwise healthy 45-year-old man is brought from a local jail to the ED with respiratory distress. There is a known cluster of COVID-19 cases at the jail among both inmates and guards. The patient's vitals include temperature 38.1°C, BP 149/78 mm Hg, HR 110 beats/minute, RR 24 breaths/minute, and pulse oximetry 89% on 4 L by nasal cannula (NC). He is awake, alert, and following commands. Rapid polymerase chain reaction (PCR) testing for COVID-19 is positive. Which of the following is the best initial step to manage the patient's hypoxia?
a. Increase flow rate via NC to 8 L
b. 100% fraction of inspired oxygen (Fio_2) via nonrebreather (NRB)
c. Rapid sequence intubation
d. Continuous positive airway pressure (CPAP)
e. Bilevel positive airway pressure (BiPAP)

558. An otherwise healthy 36-year-old woman presents to the ED for evaluation of fever, joint pain, and rash that began yesterday. She returned from a cruise in the Caribbean 2 days ago. She denies cough, vomiting, or diarrhea. On physical examination, she appears generally well. Vital signs include BP 112/68 mm Hg, HR 104 beats/minute, RR 18 breaths/minute, temperature 101°F and pulse oximetry 99%. Her conjunctivae are injected bilaterally. You note several bites on her ankles and legs, which she reports are from mosquitoes and a maculopapular rash on her torso. What is the most likely diagnosis?

a. Lyme disease
b. Zika virus
c. COVID-19
d. Ebola virus disease (EVD)
e. Anaplasmosis

Emerging Infectious Diseases

Answers

549. The answer is c. This patient is presenting with signs and symptoms concerning for infection with **EVD**. EVD symptoms are initially nonspecific and include fever, arthralgia, conjunctivitis, vomiting, and diarrhea. She should be evaluated for abnormal CBC, LFTs, and coagulation profile. Early in the disease course, laboratory testing will show **leukopenia, lymphocytopenia, mild thrombocytopenia** (50,000-100,000 platelets), and **transaminitis** [aspartate transaminase (AST) > alanine transaminase (ALT) and in the 1000 IU/L range]. Later in the disease course, there will be leukocytosis with a left shift on the differential (increased neutrophil count) and signs of disseminated intravascular coagulation (**DIC**) [prolonged PT/PTT (partial thromboplastin time) and elevated fibrin degradation products].

CXR **(a)** would be nonspecific and indicated in patients in which tuberculosis (TB) would be suspected. Travel history alone increases the risk for PE **(b)**; however, other signs and symptoms of Epstein-Barr virus (EBV) infection make this less likely. While patients returning from Malaria endemic areas are susceptible, the lack of cyclical fever, presence of rash, and adherence to prophylaxis makes this less likely. In the absence of prophylaxis, peripheral blood smears **(d)** would be useful. Thick smears allow for detection of the intracellular parasites while thin smears allow for speciation. The patient's presentation is not consistent with TB infection and therefore a PPD skin test **(e)** is not indicated.

550. The answer is e. EVD spreads through **direct contact** (mucous membranes, breaks in skin, and needles) with **blood or body fluids** of patients infected with EVD disease. Given the high pathogenicity (fatality rate) and virulence of the disease (ease of spread), **high-level contact precautions are recommended alongside airborne precautions** when there is a chance of generating aerosols. The CDC recommends **full-body coverage** (including eye protection) by PPE and the use of either **N95 masks or personal air purifying respirators (PAPRs)** for protection from aerosols.

Health care workers who are potentially at risk for exposure to EBV should be trained and observed on the donning and doffing of PPE as this is a high-risk activity.

Airborne isolation alone (a), contact isolation alone (b), droplet isolation (c), and contact and droplet isolation (d) are not adequate for preventing the spread of EBV.

551.   The answer is e. The classic CXR findings for COVID-19 are **bilateral interstitial infiltrates**. CT scans of the chest may show patchy ground glass opacities in the lung periphery.

The patient lacks risk factors (homelessness, incarceration, high-risk exposure, hemoptysis, night sweats, or weight loss) for TB infection, which most commonly presents with apical cavitary lesions on CXR (a). While the patient could have community-acquired pneumonia (CAP) manifested as a single lobar consolidation (b), COVID-19 does not typically present this way radiographically, nor does it typically cause pleural effusions (c). The patient's presentation is not consistent with pneumothorax (d).

552.   The answer is d. In early case series of COVID-19 patients, **lymphopenia** is commonly seen. A cutoff of less than 1500 b/L increases sensitivity of diagnosis. A normal overall WBC count or leukocytosis may be present, along with thrombocytopenia, not thrombocytosis (a). Other lab findings consistent with COVID-19 include elevated PT/INR (international normalized ratio), elevated D-dimer, elevated fibrinogen, elevated ferritin, and elevated inflammatory markers, in particular CRP.

Hyperkalemia, normal CRP, and macrocytosis are not associated with acute COVID-19 infection (**answers b, c, and e**).

553.   The answer is d. The most common mechanism that **SARS-CoV-2** spreads is via **respiratory droplets** and via **aerosols in close proximity**. Rapid sequence intubation (RSI) is a high-risk procedure for aerosol generation. Therefore, current National Institutes of Health (NIH) guidelines recommend using **fit-tested respirators (N95 respirators)** or **powered air-purifying respirators** rather than surgical masks, in addition to **gloves, gown, and eye protection** such as a face shield or safety goggles. In addition, the most experienced operator should perform the intubation, and it should be done via video laryngoscopy, if possible.

Gloves (a) are appropriate for all patient encounters. Gloves and gown (b) are not adequate PPE for encounters with this patient. Gloves, gown, and surgical mask (**c**) are not correct, as there is no eye protection in this answer choice. Gloves and BSL4 suit (**e**) is indicated for dangerous/exotic agents which post high individual risk of aerosol-transmitted laboratory infections that are frequently fatal and for which there are no vaccines or treatments.

554. The answer is b. The MERS-CoV causes a respiratory viral syndrome with predominant symptoms of **cough, fever, and shortness of breath,** infecting patients who live in the Middle East or have traveled to this region. The biggest risk factor for contracting MERS-CoV is **travel to the Arabian Peninsula**. MERS-CoV is endemic to countries in the Arabian Peninsula including Jordan, Kuwait, Lebanon, Oman, Qatar, Saudi Arabia, the United Arab Emirates, and Yemen. More than 85% of the reported cases occur in Saudi Arabia. It is thought that **camels** in the Arabian Peninsula are the primary vector for transmission of MERS-CoV.

H5N1 Avian flu (**a**) is a subtype of influenza A that causes symptoms of fever, cough, conjunctivitis, and muscle aches. Human immunodeficiency virus (**c**) can present with similar symptoms but is not limited to transmission from the Middle East. Plasmodium falciparum (**d**) is a parasitic protozoan that is transmitted by mosquitoes in endemic regions. It causes malaria with the primary symptom of recurrent, cyclic fever. SARS-CoV-2 (**e**) is the virus responsible for the COVID-19 pandemic.

555. The answer is a. **ARDS** is a severe and common complication of MERS-CoV. ARDS is a life-threatening condition characterized by widespread inflammation in the lungs secondary to cytokine release, affecting the alveoli leading to impaired gas exchange. ARDS has a high mortality between 20% and 50%. The mortality rate with ARDS varies widely based on disease severity, a person's age, and the presence of other medical conditions. Patients with **preexisting comorbidities** such as diabetes, cancer, and chronic lung, heart, or kidney disease are more likely to develop complications.

PE, myocardial infarction, and pneumothorax (**b, c, and d**) are not reported to be directly associated with or complications of MERS-CoV. Peripheral edema (**e**) may result from this patient's congestive heart failure but is not likely to be caused by MERS.

556. The answer is e. This patient is toxic-appearing with abnormal vital signs including high fever, tachycardia, hypotension, tachypnea, and hypoxia. Given his presentation, this patient warrants **admission to the**

intensive care unit for close monitoring. MERS-CoV infection is thought to be transmitted via **respiratory droplets** and **close contact with infected animals**. Therefore, patients suspected of having MERS-CoV should be placed in both **contact and droplet isolation**.

The patient requires admission and discharging him home **(a and b)** would be inappropriate. Observation status **(c)** is not appropriate for such an ill patient who exhibits respiratory distress and may require intubation. Admission to the telemetry floor on intravenous nitroglycerin and furose-mide drips **(d)** would be appropriate management for acute decompensated heart failure, but that is not the underlying issue in this patient.

557. The answer is d. The patient is hypoxic and tachypneic on oxygen via NC, therefore an intervention is indicated. In patients with COVID-19, hypoxia seems to be driven by lung injury and atelectasis, both of which can be remedied with **CPAP**. Compared to other forms of noninvasive ventila-tion, CPAP provides the highest mean airway pressure and thus effective recruitment of atelectatic lung. However, it requires a cooperative patient and the use of a **viral filter on a closed circuit** in order to decrease aerosol-ization of viral particles.

Increasing the NC flow rate **(a)** or placing the patient on an NRB **(b)** may improve oxygenation, but not work of breathing and provides little positive pressure for lung recruitment. RSI **(c)** is indicated if the patient fails noninvasive ventilation or does not have the mental status to support CPAP. BiPAP **(e)** will recruit less collapsed lung owing to decreased man airway pressure, and, theoretically could cause lung damage from encour-aging large tidal volumes from inspiratory pressure support. Other options for oxygenation in this patient could include awake proning and high-flow NC.

558. The answer is b. This patient most likely has **Zika virus**. Zika virus is spread to humans primarily via infected Aedes mosquito bites. Cases of perinatal, sexual, and transfusion transmission have been reported. The most common symptoms include **fever, maculopapular rash, conjunctivi-tis, arthralgia, myalgia, and headache**. Zika virus has been associated with **microcephaly** and other birth defects, therefore pregnant women should be extremely cautious to avoid potential exposure. Cases of Zika virus have been reported in many countries worldwide, including the United States and Caribbean. Many individuals are asymptomatic and the majority recover following a self-limited viral illness.

While both Lyme disease **(a)** and anaplasmosis **(e)** are acute febrile illnesses; however, these are tick-borne illness; not mosquito borne. COVID-19 **(c)** is also an acute viral illness caused by SARS-CoV-2 and can present in a variety of ways; most commonly with fever and respiratory symptoms (eg, cough, rhinorrhea, pharyngitis). SARS-CoV-2 is spread by respiratory droplets, not mosquitoes. EVD **(d)** symptoms are initially nonspecific and include fever, arthralgia, conjunctivitis, vomiting, and diarrhea. Patients are acutely ill and can ultimately develop DIC and hemorrhage. This patient is generally well and did not travel to an EVD endemic region.

Recommended Readings

Centers for Disease Control. Pandemic Influenza. Resources for clinical providers. Available at: https://www.cdc.gov/flu/pandemic-resources/index.htm. Accessed on June 17, 2020.

Centers for Disease Control. Zika Virus. Resources for clinical providers. Available at: https://www.cdc.gov/zika/hc-providers/index.html. Accessed on June 26, 2020.

Centers for Disease Control and Prevention. Ebola virus disease (EVD) information for Clinicians in US Healthcare Settings. Available at: https://www.cdc.gov/vhf/ebola/clinicians/index.html. Accessed on June 17, 2020.

Centers for Disease Control and Prevention. Guidance on Personal Protective Equipment (PPE) To Be Used By Healthcare Workers during Management of Patients with Confirmed Ebola or Persons under Investigation (PUIs) for Ebola who are Clinically Unstable or Have Bleeding, Vomiting, or Diarrhea in U.S. Hospitals, Including Procedures for Donning and Doffing PPE. Available at: https://www.cdc.gov/vhf/ebola/healthcare-us/ppe/guidance.html. Accessed on June 17, 2020.

Internet Book of Critical Care. COVID-19. Available at: https://covid19treatmentguidelines.nih.gov/critical-care/. Accessed on May 24, 2020.

National Institutes of Health. Care of Critically Ill patients with COVID-19. Available at: https://covid19treatmentguidelines.nih.gov/critical-care/. Accessed on May 26, 2020.

Professionalism, Ethics, and Communication

Jonah Gunalda, MD

Questions

559. A 41-year-old woman presents to the emergency department (ED) for evaluation of fever and headache. She initially went to her primary care physician's office for evaluation. A rapid influenza test and strep screen were negative. She says she was instructed to come to the ED to rule out meningitis. She denies neck stiffness, photophobia, pain with extraocular movements, or focal neurologic complaints. Her vital signs on arrival to the ED are temperature 100.1°F, blood pressure (BP) 118/80 mm Hg, heart rate (HR) 98 beats/minute, respiratory rate (RR) 12 breaths/minute, and oxygen saturation 100% on room air. Her neurologic exam is normal, including her alertness and awareness, and she has no petechial rash or meningismus. You are unable to contact the referring provider and there is no documentation of the patient's encounter with her primary care physician. Which of the following is the best approach regarding lumbar puncture in this patient?

a. Consult neurology for lumbar puncture as she likely has atypical meningitis
b. Do not perform the lumbar puncture because she is no longer febrile
c. Explain the benefits, risks, and alternatives of the procedure and utilized shared decision-making with the patient
d. Perform lumbar puncture because her primary care doctor recommended it
e. Perform lumbar puncture because the patient had a fever and headache

560. A physician colleague of yours arrives to work and smells of alcohol. Her speech is slurred and she is making repeated errors in ordering medications and diagnostic studies for patients. You are concerned about the safety of patients. Who of the following should be notified first about this physician's behavior?

a. The hospital administrator
b. The hospital ethics committee
c. The patients
d. The physician
e. The police

561. A 23-year-old transgender man presents to the ED for abdominal pain. Which of the following options is the most appropriate way to begin this patient encounter?

a. Elicit a detailed sexual history
b. Inquire how the patient wishes to be addressed
c. Inquire why the patient wishes to be transgender
d. Perform a through urogenital examination
e. Determine the human immunodeficiency virus (HIV) status of the patient

562. A 51-year-old man presents to the ED for altered mental status and intoxication. He was found outside a liquor store and brought in by emergency medical services. He is shouting at medical personnel and is demanding to speak to the doctor. He is threatening to kill everyone and their families if he does not see a doctor. He is not physically aggressive and remains in bed. Which of the following should the physician do upon entering the room?

a. Place physical restraints on the patient and place an involuntary hold
b. Tell the patient he will not be evaluated until he lowers his voice
c. Restrain the patient with intramuscular antipsychotic medication
d. Introduce himself or herself and his or her role
e. Turn the lights off and remove any stimulating distractions

563. A 45-year-old man with a history of HIV infection presents to the ED for chest pain. He is accompanied by a man who appears near his age. The patient appears well upon general inspection and has normal vital signs. Which of the following is the most appropriate introduction by the physician?

a. Does your friend mind stepping outside while we talk?
b. Have you been taking your HIV medications?
c. Is this your husband or boyfriend with you?
d. Tell me about your abdominal pain.
e. Who is this you have with you today?

564. A 55-year-old man with a history of hypertension and diabetes presents with shortness of breath and a rash that began while he was at dinner. He has a known allergy to peanuts. His vital signs on arrival are temperature 98.7°F, BP 89/45 mm Hg, HR 124 beats/minute, RR 28 breaths/minute, and oxygen saturation 88% on room air. He is given epinephrine 1 mg intramuscularly for anaphylaxis instead of the recommended 0.3 to 0.5 mg. His symptoms resolve and he is monitored for 4 hours without return of symptoms. Which of the following should be disclosed to the patient?

a. He was given an inappropriate dose of medication
b. He was given the wrong medication for his condition
c. Because his symptoms improved, nothing needs to be disclosed
d. Because he was given the correct medication, nothing needs to be disclosed
e. Because he improved after epinephrine, he should receive a higher dose in future anaphylaxis events

565. A 23-year-old woman presents for the ED for right leg pain. She denies recent trauma or hospitalization, hemoptysis, cancer, estrogen use, or asymmetric leg swelling. Her vital signs are temperature 98.6°F, BP 135/85 mm Hg, HR 76 beats/minute, RR 12 beats/minute, and oxygen saturation 100% on room air. Her breath sounds are clear and she has a normal lower extremity examination. Which of the following is the most appropriate management strategy at this time?

a. Admit under observation status for lower extremity Doppler examinations
b. Admit under observation status for chest computed tomography angiography (CTA)
c. Explain the low likelihood of a deep venous thrombosis (DVT) and discharge
d. Reassure the patient does not have a DVT
e. Obtain serial D-dimer levels

566. A 39-year-old man is transferred to the ED from an outside facility for fever and altered mental status because the patient needed a higher level of care. According to emergency medical services, the patient had laboratory tests, urine studies, blood cultures, a chest X-ray, and lumbar puncture performed at the sending facility. It is unknown if the patient received antibiotics or intravenous fluids at the other facility. The patient was not sent with any paperwork or imaging studies from the sending facility. His vital signs on arrival are temperature 102.4°F, BP 90/54 mm Hg, HR 118 beats/minute, RR 24 breaths/minute, and oxygen saturation 93% on 2 L/minute by nasal cannula. Which of the following is the next best step in management?

a. Administer empiric antibiotics and admit the patient for sepsis
b. Administer empiric antibiotics and call the sending facility for supplemental history and documentation
c. Arrange transportation back to the sending facility where his diagnostic workup began
d. Repeat laboratory tests, blood cultures, urine studies, and chest X-ray
e. Repeat laboratory tests, blood cultures, urine studies, and chest X-ray and administer antibiotics

567. You have evaluated a 39-year-old woman in the ED for acute coronary syndrome and have consulted cardiology to admit the patient. The patient has a history of chronic pain and substance abuse and has presented to the ED multiple times for various pain-related complaints. While in the ED, she has had multiple chest pain episodes, has become diaphoretic, and her pain improves with nitroglycerin. Serial electrocardiograms (ECGs) demonstrate dynamic ST-T wave changes. The cardiologist evaluates the patient and then tells you she is not admitting her because she feels that the patient is malingering. You have a high index of suspicion for acute coronary syndrome. After insisting on the patient's admission, the cardiologist yells at you and demands you discharge the patient from the ED. Which of the following is the best response to the cardiologist in this situation?

a. I am calling the police
b. I am happy to have a professional conversation about what is best for the patient
c. You should do your job and admit the patient
d. I will discharge the patient
e. You should lower your voice

568. A 39-year-old woman presents to the ED for shortness of breath. She has no significant past medical history and does not smoke cigarettes or use drugs. Her family history is significant for breast cancer in her maternal grandmother and her sister. She denies nipple discharge, overlying skin changes, or a palpable breast mass. She says, "before my grandmother was diagnosed with breast cancer, she complained of breathing problems." She then begins to cry. Which of the following is the best response to the patient at this time?

a. I doubt that your symptoms are caused by cancer
b. Let me examine your breasts
c. We will get a CT scan to rule out cancer
d. What I'm hearing you say is you are concerned that you may also have cancer
e. Your vital signs are normal so you are going to be just fine

Professionalism, Ethics, and Communication

Answers

559. **The answer is c.** **Shared decision-making** with patients means allowing patients who have medical decision-making capacity to play a key role in their care. By explaining the risks, benefits, and alternatives of diagnostic or therapeutic interventions, patients are given autonomy to engage in their health care choices. The patient's **core values and goals** must be communicated, understood, and adhered to when shared decision-making is implemented. Oftentimes, shared decision-making leads to less resource utilization (eg, less testing, fewer consultations) and improved patient experience. When an invasive procedure is being considered (such as a lumbar puncture) and the likelihood that such a procedure will change the outcome of the patient's care, shared decision-making can be a decision tool to aid providers in delivering the best **patient-centered care**.

Answer choice (**a**) is incorrect because the patient does not have clinical findings that strongly suggest meningitis and neurology does not need to be consulted. Answer choice (**b**) is incorrect because the reason for not performing lumbar puncture is not because the patient has defervesced, but because it does not seem to be clinically indicated since the likelihood of her having meningitis based on clinical assessment is low (at least low enough to engage the patient in a shared decision to forego the procedure). Answer choice (**d**) is incorrect because providers should not blindly perform invasive procedures at the request of other providers without supporting clinical evidence. There is no documentation of the patient's earlier encounter to support her claim that her physician wanted her to have a lumbar puncture, and you are unable to clarify this yourself with the referring provider. The best action is to utilize logical clinical judgment and shared decision-making with the available information present. Answer choice (**e**) is incorrect because headache and fever are nonspecific symptoms that can be caused by a range of medical conditions, not just meningitis. These symptoms alone are not enough to justify performing a lumbar puncture.

560. The answer is d. Health care providers have a duty to protect patients from impaired physicians when the impaired are unable or unwilling to seek help for themselves. Impairment is the inability of a provider to safely and effectively care outpatient care duties. Signs of impairment include failure to meet job responsibilities (eg, arriving late to work), forgetfulness during tasks, or evidence of substance use. The American College of Emergency Physicians (ACEP) Code of Ethics states, "Emergency physicians shall deal fairly and honestly with colleagues and take appropriate action to protect patients from health care providers who are impaired or incompetent." Handling an impaired colleague should begin in a stepwise fashion. When a colleague notices **impairment** of skill or judgment, he or she should approach **the physician** about their concerns first.

If the physician fails to respond to this direct approach or patient safety or wellbeing is at risk, reporting to the other answer options **(a)**, **(b)**, **(c)**, and **(e)** may need to be utilized.

561. The answer is b. Patients who identify as lesbian, gay, bisexual, transgender, or queer/questioning (LGBTQ) should be asked **how they wish to be addressed**, including which gender pronouns they prefer. Ideally, this should be done at the beginning of the patient encounter during the initial introduction. Providers should not make assumptions about gender identity, sexual orientation, sexual preferences, or sexual history. It is best to use an unbiased and inquisitive approach to gathering such history.

Eliciting a detailed sexual history **(a)** or performing a thorough urogenital examination **(d)** may or may not be indicated in LGBTQ patients depending on their reason for seeking ED care. Inquiring why the patient wishes to be transgender **(c)** is usually irrelevant to medical care and may be offensive to patience. Determining the HIV status of an LGBTQ patient **(e)** may or may not be indicated, and may be presumptuous (ie, not all patients who identify as LGBTQ are at risk for contracting HIV infection).

562. The answer is d. The patient encounter begins by **introducing oneself and explaining his or her role** in the care of the patient. This allows patients to designate who is in charge of their care and what roles each person plays in their ED visit. Patients who are aggressive or combative may require pharmaceutical or physical restraints prior to evaluation. This is to provide safety for the medical staff, the patient, and other patients and visitors. Once the physician introduces himself or herself and explains his or her role, it is often best (especially in this case) to lay some "ground rules" of the ED, including voice volume, behavior, language, and gestures that will and will not be tolerated or accepted without appropriate intervention. The patient's safety and medical care must always be considered when handling an acutely agitated patient.

Placing physical restraints on the patient and placing an involuntary hold (a) or restraining the patient with intramuscular antipsychotic medication (c) should not occur before the physician has had a chance to introduce himself or herself and try to de-escalate the situation. If the patient becomes physically aggressive or combative, these interventions take precedence before attempting to engage in interpersonal communication. Telling the patient that he will not be evaluated before he lowers his voice (b) will likely make the patient more agitated because he is receiving instructions from someone who has not introduced himself or herself or explained their role as the overseeing physician of the patient. Turning the lights off and removing any stimulating distractions (e) is a passive and indirect way of handling an acutely agitated patient and does not seek to address their needs or medical reason for being in the ED. A history and physical examination are still warranted as safely possible in an agitated patient.

563. The answer is e. Patients in the ED are frequently accompanied by guests or visitors. These may be children, parents, friends, spouses, coaches, clergy, or have some other relationship or acquaintance with the patient. It is in the best interest of the physician to **ask the relationship of the accompanying person or persons to the patient** rather than assume or attempt to guess the relationship. This has several obvious pitfalls. But it is also important to identify this relationship early in the encounter because the next question should be, "Do you mind if your guest is present while we talk about your medical care, or would you like them to step out?" Patients should be given autonomy to share protected health information with their provider in the absence of guests should the patient choose. In this case, the patient's history of HIV may or may not be known to his accompanying guest. It is a violation of doctor-patient confidentiality to discuss the patient's medical history without consent from the patient. Always seek to acknowledge everyone in the room and ask the patient whether or not he or she wants to be interviewed or examined in private.

Answer choice (a) assumes that the accompanying guest is the patient's friend, when it could be a family member or other acquaintance. Answer choice (b) is grossly inappropriate because it reveals private health information to someone who is not the patient without the patient's consent. While answer choice (c) is an attempt to seek understanding of the role of the patient's guest, it is presumptive that he is a same-sex partner of the patient because the patient has HIV. Answer choice (d) does not acknowledge the patient's guest and assumes the patient wants to discuss his medical care in the presence of his guest.

564. The answer is a. The patient was **given an inappropriate dose of medication**. The recommended dose of intramuscular epinephrine for anaphylaxis in an adult patient is 0.3 to 0.5 mg. This patient received 1 mg IM, which is at least twice the recommended dose. The patient's clinical condition improved, and he was monitored without any recurrent anaphylaxis. One might be tempted to assume that because the patient did not suffer any harm that nothing needs to be disclosed to the patient. However, an error was made, and **although it did not lead to harm or a bad clinical outcome (a nonharmful event), it still should be disclosed to the patient**. Other types of clinical errors include near misses, harmful events, and death. The Code of Ethics of the American Medical Association states that physicians should always deal honestly and openly with patients. Recommendations for disclosing medical errors include timely disclosure (ie, not waiting for the patient to find out later than an error occurred), communicate clearly without ambiguity or misleading, explain potential outcomes as a result of the error, elicit questions from the patient or family, and offer a sincere apology to the patient.

Answer choice (b) is incorrect; he was given the correct medication for his condition, but an incorrect dose. Answer choices (c) and (d) are incorrect because the error should be disclosed to the patient. Answer choice (e) is incorrect because this deviates from medical guidelines suggesting recommended dosage of therapy.

565. The answer is c. Based on the patient's history, risk factors, and physical examination, there appears to be no evidence to suggest a DVT or pulmonary embolism. Risk factors for DVT include active cancer, three or more days of recent immobility, major surgery within the last 12 weeks, asymmetric calf swelling, the presence of superficial collateral veins in the legs, an entirely swollen leg, localized tenderness along the deep venous system, pitting edema in the symptomatic leg, paralysis or paresis of the leg, recent plaster immobilization of the leg, or a previously documented DVT. The pretest probability of a DVT in this patient is low. Therefore, **no further clinical workup is indicated.** The most appropriate step at this time would be to **explain the low likelihood of a DVT and discharge** the patient.

Admitting the patient under observation status for lower extremity Doppler examinations **(a)** or chest CTA **(b)** or obtaining serial D-dimer levels **(e)** are not clinically indicated due to the low pretest probability of the patient having a DVT. Reassuring the patient that she does not have a DVT **(e)** seems tempting, but history and physical examination alone are not 100% accurate at fully ruling out DVT, only lowering the clinical suspicion or likelihood that a DVT is present.

566. The answer is b. Patients are often transferred for higher level of care or specialty evaluation. Transferring a patient is a complex and coordinated effort between the sending and receiving facilities. Ideally, the patient's medical documentation and study results are made available to the receiving facility for review upon patient arrival or shortly thereafter. This aids in continuity of care, reduces redundancy of testing, reduces cost, increases ED workflow and throughput, and improves patient satisfaction. However, in the event that a patient arrives without any documentation from the sending facility, the accepting physician has an **obligation to care for the patient regardless of the available information**. Additionally, **attempts should be made to contact the sending facility to request records and documentation** to prevent unnecessary testing and reduce medical errors from occurring. Therefore, given the limited information available to the treating physician, the patient requires treatment of sepsis including **empiric antibiotics while the physician attempts to call the sending facility for supplemental history and documentation.**

Answer choice **(a)** is incorrect insomuch as it neglects the important task of contacting the sending facility to gather information about care provided to the patient (eg, fluid resuscitation, antibiotics, blood cultures obtained, imaging studies) prior to transfer. Answer choice **(c)** is incorrect because it is inappropriate to send a critically ill patient (or any patient for that matter) from a higher level of care to a lower level of care. Additionally, this sort of patient "dumping" or "shuffling" is fraught with litigation potential under the Emergency Medical Treatment and Labor Act (EMTLA), which dictates that patients must be stable prior to discharge or transfer to another facility. Answer choice **(d)** and **(e)** are incorrect because this patient requires treatment for sepsis, including empiric antibiotic administration, and the sending facility should be contacted to gain additional information about the patient's care.

567. The answer is b. Physicians are expected to uphold professionalism values and standards at all times. This is true in our interactions with patients, family members, ancillary staff, consultants, and hospital administrators. Our first and ultimate responsibility is to the patient. The ACEP Code of Ethics states that patient welfare is the primary professional responsibility of the emergency physician and that providers should strive to protect the pest interest of their patients. Emergency physicians have an especially challenging task of advocating for patients when health care resources are limited. The most appropriate response to this consultant is to **suggest engaging in a professional conversation regarding what is best for the patient**. This illustrates an interpersonal tactic of de-escalating a heated situation by redirecting the focus on the patient. This upholds the ethical principle of beneficence, which states to do good by the patient as much as one is able.

Threatening to call the police (**a**) is rarely a helpful strategy in handling interprofessional conflict. Additionally, it is not a patient-centered approach to problem solving. Answer option (**c**) is condescending and is unlikely to change the consultant's mind about admitting the patient after she has already refused. Discharging the patient (**d**) is not the right choice given the strong clinical concern for acute coronary syndrome. A consulting physician refusing to care for a patient does not justify discontinuing to care for the patient and advocating for their clinical needs. Comments such as answer choice (**e**) are often taken defensively and is unlikely to de-escalate the situation.

568. The answer is d. Fear is a frequent concern of patients presenting to the ED. Fear of death, injury, disability, a life-limiting diagnosis, or not having an explanation for one's symptoms are all frequently experienced by patients. However, these fears are not always articulated by patients or drawn from them by the physician. Patients may communicate with their actions or other nonverbal cues that an underlying fear or concern lies beneath their presenting complaint that is registered at triage. Emergency physicians ought to have enough interpersonal awareness to identify these cues and seek to understand any underlying fears or concerns the patient may have. In this case, the patient seems quite anxious and afraid that her symptoms may be related to an underlying cancer diagnosis because her family member who did have cancer experienced these symptoms. By **voicing to the patient what you understand them to be saying** is a helpful tool to gain clarity and avoid missing important indicators of suffering. Therefore, the best response is, "What I'm hearing you say is you are concerned that you may also have cancer." This allows the patient the opportunity to confirm the physician's inference or correct him or her. Whether or not the physician's interpretation of the patient's behavior is true is less important than the act of acknowledging the patient's concerns and seeking to gain understanding.

Answer choice (a) is dismissive of the patient's concerns and offers no empathy or compassion. Although a breast exam (b) may be indicated to further evaluate the patient's concerns, conveying concern for and understanding of the patient is an opportunity that should occur before the patient is examined. Ordering diagnostic studies such as CT scans (c) may or may not be indicated in this case based on the overall suspicion of malignancy. This is determined after careful history taking and physical examination. Answer choice (e), while attempting to provide reassurance to the patient, still dismisses her concerns about having cancer. Additionally, abnormal vital signs do not equal absence of disease.

Recommended Readings

American Medical Association. Physician responsibilities to impaired colleagues: Code of medical ethics opinion 9.3.2. Available at: https://www.ama-assn.org/delivering-care/ethics/physician-responsibilities-impaired-colleagues. Accessed June 1, 2020.

Candilis PJ, Kim DT, Sulmasy LS. Physician impairment and rehabilitation: reintegration into medical practice while ensuring patient safety: A position paper from the American College of Physicians. *Ann Intern Med.* 2019;170:871-879.

Chamberlain CJ, Koniaris LG, Wu AW, et al. Disclosure of "nonharmful" medical errors and other events. *Arch Surg.* 2012;147(3):282-286.

Code of ethics for emergency physicians. American College of Emergency Physicians Policy Statement. 2017.

Gustin AN Jr. Shared decision making. *Anesthesiol Clin.* 2019;37(3):573-580.

Iserson KV, Heine CE. Chapter e10. Bioethics. In: Walls RM, Hockberger RS, Gausche-Hill M, eds. *Rosen's Emergency Medicine: Concepts and Clinical Practice*, 9th ed. Philadelphia, PA: Elsevier, 2018.

Kaplan JA, Weichenthal L. Chapter e13. Wellness, stress, and the impaired physician. In: Walls RM, Hockberger RS, Gausche-Hill M, eds. *Rosen's Emergency Medicine: Concepts and Clinical Practice*, 9th ed. Philadelphia, PA: Elsevier, 2018.

Rubin R. AIDET in the medical practice: More important than ever. Studor Group. Available at: https://www.studergroup.com/resources/articles-and-industry-updates/insights/november-2014/aidet-in-the-medical-practice-more-important-than. Accessed June 1, 2020.

Shorey JM, Spollen JJ. Approach to the patient. Post TW, ed. UpToDate. Waltham, MA: UpToDate Inc.

Welch SJ. Twenty years of patient satisfaction research applied to the emergency department: a quality review. *Am J Med Qual.* 2010;25:64-72.

Welch SJ. AIDET: A popular way of improving patients' care experience. *ACEPNow.* 2015.

Index